ALTERNATIVE TOXICOLOGICAL METHODS

ALTERNATIVE TOXICOLOGICAL METHODS

Edited by
Harry Salem
Sidney A. Katz

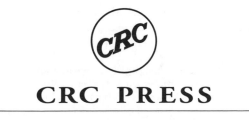

CRC PRESS

Boca Raton London New York Washington, D.C.

Library of Congress Cataloging-in-Publication Data

Alternative toxicological methods / edited by Sidney A. Katz, Harry Salem.
    p. cm.
Includes bibliographical references and index.
ISBN 0-8493-1528-X (alk. paper)
    1. Alternative toxicity testing. I. Katz, Sidney A., 1935- II. Salem, Harry, 1929-

RA1199.4.A46 A45 2003
    619--dc21
                                                   2002041396

Visit the CRC Press Web site at www.crcpress.com

Dedication

*This book is dedicated to all scientific investigators
who are committed to the principles of the three Rs
plus the fourth R, which signifies responsibility,
without compromising human and animal health and welfare,
as well as to our families who encompass compassion
and gentleness in their lives: to Flo, Jerry, Amy,
Joel, Marshall, and Abby Rose, and to Sheila, Craig,
Ji, Kevin, Hana, Jeff, Wendy, Sydney, and Daniel,
who continue to encourage and inspire
us to follow our dreams.*

Preface

Alternative Toxicological Methods brings together the recent and relevant contributions of over 125 scientists from government, industry, and academia in North American, the U.K., and Western Europe for meeting the needs for developing and validating replacement, reduction, and refinement alternatives to animal testing. These internationally recognized scientists present what has been accomplished thus far in developing acceptable alternatives to traditional animal toxicological assessment as well as providing potentially new initiatives. This is done in 44 chapters focusing on seven themes.

The first theme focuses on the validation and regulatory acceptance of alternatives in both the United States and the European Union. In addition, this section deals with the history of humane treatment of animals, humane endpoints, and pain and distress management in animal research and testing.

This is followed by themes on the development of predictive methods based on the mechanisms of eye irritation at the ocular surface, dermal toxicity testing and molecular biomarkers, and transgenics for assessing neurotoxicity. Subsequent themes include a case study in the use of alternatives to study the mechanisms of sulfur mustard action, the role of transgenics and toxicokinetics in the development of alternative toxicity tests. The final theme is recent innovations in alternatives. These include the use of archival data in *in silico* techniques and the next generation biochips.

Our interest in alternatives and the three Rs plus one (responsibility) goes back two decades to the early 1980s. This interest was recognized by the invitation to participate in the Interagency Regulatory Alternatives Group (IRAG) even though we were not employed by a government regulatory agency. This *ad hoc* group was formed by Doctor Sidney Green, who at the time was with the Food and Drug Administration (FDA), and also included representatives from the Environmental Protection Agency (EPA) and the Consumer Product Safety Commission. This group ultimately evolved into the *ad hoc* Interagency Coordinating Committee for the Validation of Alternative Methods (ICCVAM) established by Bill Stokes of the National Institute of Environmental Health Sciences (NIEHS) and Dick Hill of the EPA in 1993. This committee resulted from a mandate in the National Institutes of Health (NIH) Revitalization Act of 1993 (public law 103-43 Section 1301) in which Congress instructed the NIH to research replacement, reduction, and refinement alternatives and to establish the criteria for validation of regulatory acceptance, as well as to recommend a process for scientifically validated alternatives to be accepted for regulatory use. ICCVAM became established as a committee in 1997 and was made official in the year 2000. One of us has served as the official Department of Defense (DoD) representative since 1993 and continues to serve on the committee.

At the same time in 1993, the National Defense Authorization Act (H.R. 10 2-257; 102nd Congress, second session) directed the Secretary of Defense to establish aggressive and targeted programs to replace, reduce, and refine the current use of animals in the DoD.

Even prior to this, in 1990, we sponsored our first biennial Alternative Conference titled DoD Initiatives in Alternatives to Animal Testing. This was followed until 2000 by biennial conferences cosponsored by the NIEHS, the FDA, the EPA, the Consumer Product Safety Commission (CPSC), the Army (Soldier and Biological Chemical Command, Medical Research Institute of Chemical Defense, Center for Health Promotion and Preventive Medicine), the Air Force, the Navy, and the Association of Government Toxicologists, National Capital Area Chapter of the Society of Toxicology, Sigma Xi, and other agencies and industrial firms.

The scientists who have contributed chapters to this book include those who are well known in the alternative field and have presented and published in various alternative forums, as well as those whose methodologies are consistent with the three Rs and are applicable to the alternative field, but who have routinely presented and published in other scientific disciplines.

Thus, this book frames a broader pool of work relevant to alternatives and involves a wide array of additional contributing scientists. In addition, *Alternative Toxicological Methods* includes succinct, concise presentations on the state-of-the-art material, such as updates from ICCVAM and the European Centre for the Validation of Alternative Methods (ECVAM) on the validation and regulatory acceptance, the application of genomics and proteomics to toxicological sciences, the cutting edge of research on engineered tissue equivalents for screening ocular injury, and the utility of gene array technology in skin biology, endocrine disruptor screening, and recent innovations in alternatives.

We thank all of the contributors to this book as well as all scientists who promote the three Rs and embrace the fourth R, responsibility. We also thank Doctor Max Klein of Booze Allen and Hamilton for his help, as well as Stephen Zollo and Erika Dery of CRC Press for their guidance and efforts in making this book possible.

Harry Salem
U.S. Army Edgewood Chemical Biological Center

Sidney A. Katz
Rutgers University

The Editors

Harry Salem is chief scientist at the U.S. Army Edgewood Chemical Biological Center. He has been a visiting professor at Drexel University, Rutgers University, Temple University, and the University of Pennsylvania, and he has held a variety of positions in the pharmaceutical industry and in commercial toxicology laboratories. He is the editor-in-chief of the *Journal of Applied Toxicology*. During 2001, he was the Society of Toxicology's Congressional Fellow.

Sidney A. Katz is professor of chemistry at Rutgers University. He has been a visiting professor in Canada, England, Germany, Hungary, and Yugoslavia, and he was employed as a chemist by E.I. du Pont de Nemours and by R.M. Hollingshead. His research activity is in the area of environmental bioanalytical chemistry. Until July 2002, he was a New Jersey state commissioner for hazardous waste facilities siting.

Contributors

Kashif Ali
Applied Pharmacology Branch
Pharmacology Division
U.S. Army Medical Research Institute
  of Chemical Defense
Aberdeen Proving Ground, Maryland

Douglas P. Avery
Applied Pharmacology Branch
Pharmacology Division
U.S. Army Medical Research Institute
  of Chemical Defense
Aberdeen Proving Ground, Maryland

Seyoum Ayehunie
MatTek Corporation
Ashland, Massachusetts

Michael C. Babin
U.S. Army Medical Research Institute
  of Chemical Defense
Aberdeen Proving Ground, Maryland

Michael Balls
FRAME
Nottingham, U.K.

Steven I. Baskin
Pharmacology Division
U.S. Army Medical Research Institute
  of Chemical Defense
Aberdeen Proving Ground, Maryland

Martin Béliveau
University of Montreal
Research Group in Human Toxicology
Faculty of Medicine
Montreal, Quebec, Canada

Kristen L. Bellavance
MatTek Corporation
Ashland, Massachusetts

Hilma R. Benjamin
Applied Pharmacology Branch
Pharmacology Division
U.S. Army Medical Research Institute
  of Chemical Defense
Aberdeen Proving Ground, Maryland

Roger W. Beuerman
Louisiana State University School
  of Medicine
Department of Ophthalmology
Lions Eye Research Laboratories
Laboratory for Molecular Biology of
  the Ocular Surface
LSU Eye Center
New Orleans, Louisiana

Bas Blaauboer
Division of Toxicology
Institute for Risk Assessment Sciences
Division of Toxicology
Utrecht University
Utrecht, The Netherlands

Bridget A. Breyfogle
MatTek Corporation
Ashland, Massachusetts

Robert L. Bronaugh
Skin Absorption and Metabolism
  Section
U.S. Food and Drug Administration
Laurel, Maryland

Clarence A. Broomfield
Pharmacology Division
U.S. Army Medical Research Institute
  of Chemical Defense
Aberdeen Proving Ground, Maryland

Christof Buehler
Paul Scherrer Institut
Villingen, Switzerland

Maria Bykhovskaia
Department of Biological Sciences
Lehigh University
Bethlehem, Pennsylvania

Jean Lud Cadet
Molecular Neuropsychiatry Section
National Institutes of Health
Baltimore, Maryland

Robert P. Casillas
Medical Research
 and Evaluation Facility
Battelle Memorial Institute
Columbus, Ohio

Phillip L. Casterton
Alticor Corporation
Ada, Michigan

Daniel R. Cerven
MB Research Laboratories
Spinnerstown, Pennsylvania

Wiley A. Chambers
Division of Anti-Inflammatory,
 Analgesic, and Ophthalmologic
 Drug Products
U.S. Food and Drug Administration
Rockville, Maryland

Stephen Chevalier
Molecular and Cellular Toxicology
 Department
Pfizer Global Research and
 Development
Amboise, France

James H. Clark
Applied PharmacologyBranch
Pharmacology Division
U.S. Army Medical Research Institute
 of Chemical Defense
Aberdeen Proving Ground, Maryland

Offie E. Clark III
Cellular Pharmacology Team
Pharmacology Division
U.S. Army Medical Research Institute
 of Chemical Defense
Aberdeen Proving Ground, Maryland

Kathleen M. Conlee
The Humane Society of the United
 States
Washington, D.C.

Charlene M. Corun
Drug Assessment Division
U.S. Army Medical Research Institute
 of Chemical Defense
Aberdeen Proving Ground, Maryland

Fred M. Cowan
Cellular Pharmacology Team
Pharmacology Division
U.S. Army Medical Research Institute
 of Chemical Defense
Aberdeen Proving Ground, Maryland

Charisse Davenport
Cellular Pharmacology Team
Pharmacology Division
U.S. Army Medical Research Institute
 of Chemical Defense
Aberdeen Proving Ground, Maryland

George L. DeGeorge
MB Research Laboratories
Spinnerstown, Pennsylvania

Maura E. DeJoseph
Cellular Pharmacology Team
Pharmacology Division
U.S. Army Medical Research Institute
 of Chemical Defense
Aberdeen Proving Ground, Maryland

Michael Dellarco
U.S. Environmental Protection Agency
Washington, D.C.

Bart DeWever
SkinEthic Laboratories
Nice, France

Francine Dolins
Department of Psychology
Polytechnic University
Brooklyn, New York

Chen-Yuan Dong
National Taiwan University
Taiwan, Republic of China

Lori Donley
York, Pennsylvania

Henry F. Edelhauser
Department of Ophthalmology
Emory University School
  of Medicine
Atlanta, Georgia

Mohyee E. Eldefrawi
Department of Pharmacology
  and Experimental Therapeutics
University of Maryland School
  of Medicine
Baltimore, Maryland

Julia H. Fentem
Unilever Colworth
Sharnbrook, Bedfordshire, U.K.

Melissa M. Fitzgerald
DermTech International
San Diego, California

George C. Fonger
Division of Specialized
  Information Services
Toxicology and Environmental Health
  Information Program
National Library of Medicine
Bethesda, Maryland

Anna Forsby
The Arrhenius Laboratories
  for Natural Sciences
Department of Neurochemistry
  and Neurotoxicology
Stockholm University
Stockholm, Sweden

Maximo Gacula, Jr.
Gacula Associates
Scottsdale, Arizona
and
Arizona State University
Tempe, Arizona

Boris L. Gelmont
Department of Electrical Engineering
University of Virginia
Charlottesville, Virginia

T.R. Globus
Department of computer Engineering
University of Virginia
Charlottesville, Virginia

Sidney Green
Department of Pharmacology
Howard University College of Medicine
Washington, D.C.

May Griffith
University of Ottawa Eye Institute
Ottawa, Ontario, Canada

Clark L. Gross
Cellular Pharmacology Team
Pharmacology Division
U.S. Army Medical Research Institute
  of Chemical Defense
Aberdeen Proving Ground, Maryland

Juanita J. Guzman
Drug Assessment Division
U.S. Army Medical Research Institute
  of Chemical Defense
Aberdeen Proving Ground, Maryland

Thomas D. Hancewicz
Unilever Research, Inc.
Edgewater, New Jersey

Patrick J. Hayden
MatTek Corporation
Ashland, Massachusetts

Jerry Heindel
National Institute of Environmental
  Health Sciences
Division of Extramural Research
  and Training
Research Triangle Park, North Carolina

J. Hesler
University of Virginia
Charlottesville, Virginia

Lily Hsu
Department of Mechanical Engineering
Massachusetts Institute of Technology
North Cambridge, Massachusetts

Stacey B. Humphrey
DermTech International
San Diego, California

G. Robert Jackson
MatTek Corporation
Ashland, Massachusetts

Abigail C. Jacobs
Center for Drug Evaluation
  and Research
U.S. Food and Drug Administration
Rockville, Maryland

Nirmala Jayakumar
DermTech International
San Diego, California

J. O. Jensen
U.S. Army Edgewood Chemical
  Biological Center
Aberdeen Proving Ground, Maryland

Akbar S. Kahn
Molecular Engineering Team
Research and Technology Directorate
Edgewood Chemical Biological Center
U.S. Army Soldier Biological
  Chemical Command
Aberdeen Proving Ground, Maryland

Peter D. Kaplan
Unilever Research Inc.
Edgewater, New Jersey

Sidney A. Katz
Rutgers University at Camden
Camden, New Jersey

Susan A. Kelly
Drug Assessment Division
U.S. Army Medical Research Institute
  of Chemical Defense
Aberdeen Proving Ground, Maryland

Maha Khalil
Department of Pharmacology
  and Experimental Therapeutics
University of Maryland School
  of Medicine
Baltimore, Maryland

Akbar S. Khan
Molecular Engineering Team
Research and Technology Directorate
Edgewood Chemical Biological Center
Aberdeen Proving Ground, Maryland

Ki-Hean Kim
Department of Mechanical Engineering
Massachusetts Institute
  of Technology
North Cambridge, Massachusetts

Ian Kimber
Syngenta Central
  Toxicology Laboratory
Macclesfield, Cheshire, U.K.

Robyn C. Kiser
Medical Research
  and Evaluation Facility
Battelle Memorial Institute
Columbus, Ohio

Mitchell Klausner
MatTek Corporation
Ashland, Massachusetts

Harvey J. Kliman
Department of Obstetrics and
  Gynecology
Yale University School of Medicine
New Haven, Connecticut

James Knoben
Division of Specialized Information
  Services
Toxicology and Environmental Health
  Information Program
National Library of Medicine
Bethesda, Maryland

Benjamin C. Kramer
U.S. Army Center for Health Promotion
  and Preventive Medicine
Aberdeen Proving Ground, Maryland

Kannan Krishnan
University of Montreal
Research Group in Human Toxicology
Faculty of Medicine
Montreal, Quebec, Canada

Joseph Kubilus
MatTek Corporation
Ashland, Massachusetts

Sarah Kupfer-Lamore
MatTek Corporation
Ashland, Massachusetts

Thomas J. Last
MatTek Corporation
Ashland, Massachusetts

Glen J. Leach
U.S. Army Center for Health Promotion
  and Preventive Medicine
Aberdeen Proving Ground, Maryland

Claire F. Levine
Applied Pharmacology Branch
Pharmacology Division
U.S. Army Medical Research Institute
  of Chemical Defense
Aberdeen Proving Ground, Maryland

W.R. Loerop
U.S. Army Edgewood Chemical
  Biological Center
Aberdeen Proving Ground, Maryland

Janna S. Madren-Whalley
U.S. Army SBCCOM
Aberdeen Proving Ground, Maryland

Millard M. Mershon
Biomedical Modeling
  and Analysis Program
Science Applications International
  Corporation
Joppa, Maryland

Vera B. Morhenn
DermTech International
San Diego, California

Janet Moser
U.S. Army Medical Research Institute
  of Chemical Defense
Aberdeen Proving Ground, Maryland

Martin Nau
Walter Reed Army Institute of Research
Rockville, Maryland

Adrienne M. Navarro
Veterinary Resources Program
Office of Research Services
National Institutes of Health
Bethesda, Maryland

Eric W. Nealley
U.S. Army Medical Research Institute
  of Chemical Defense
Aberdeen Proving Ground, Maryland

Marian R. Nelson
Drug Assessment Division
U.S. Army Medical Research Institute
  of Chemical Defense
Aberdeen Proving Ground, Maryland

D.H. Nguyen
Department of Ophthalmology
Lions Eye Research Laboratories
Laboratory for Molecular Biology
  of the Ocular Surface
LSU Eye Center
New Orleans, Louisiana

Kevin P. O'Connell
Molecular Engineering Team
Research and Technology Directorate
Edgewood Chemical Biological Center
U.S. Army Soldier Biological
  Chemical Command
Aberdeen Proving Ground, Maryland

Melissa M. Osborn
MatTek Corporation
Ashland, Massachusetts

James D. Paauw
Calvin College
Grand Rapids, Michigan

William D. Pennie
Department of Drug Safety Evaluation
Pfizer Global Research
  and Development
Groton, Connecticut

Peter L. Platteborez
Virology Division
U.S. Army Medical Research Institute
  of Infectious Diseases
Frederick, Maryland

Stephanie Publicker
Division of Specialized
  Information Services
Toxicology and Environmental Health
  Information Program
National Library of Medicine
Bethesda, Maryland

Martin Reim
Eye Clinic
Faculty of Medicine
Technical University Aachen
Aachen, Germany

Lawrence A. Rheins
DermTech International
San Diego, California

Martin Rosdy
SkinEthic Laboratories
Nice, France

Laurie E. Roszell
U.S. Army Center for Health Promotion
  and Preventive Medicine
Aberdeen Proving Ground, Maryland

Andrew N. Rowan
The Humane Society
  of the United States
Washington, D.C.

Joyce E. Royland
National Health
  and Environmental Effects
U.S. Environmental Protection Agency
Research Triangle Park, North Carolina

Denise M. Sailstad
NHEERL, Experimental
  Toxicology Division
U.S. Environmental Protection Agency
Research Triangle Park, North Carolina

Harry Salem
U.S. Army SBCCOM
Edgewood Chemical Biological Center
Aberdeen Proving Ground, Maryland

A.C. Samuels
U.S. Army Edgewood Chemical
  Biological Center
Aberdeen Proving Ground, Maryland

John J. Schlager
Operational Toxicology Branch
AFRL/HEST
Wright-Patterson Air Force Base, Ohio

Jennifer W. Sekowski
Molecular Engineering Team
Research and Technology Directorate
Edgewood Chemical Biological Center
U.S. Army Soldier Biological Chemical
  Command
Aberdeen Proving Ground, Maryland

Frank D. Sistare
Center for Drug Evaluation and
  Research
U.S. Food and Drug Administration
Laurel, Maryland

James E. Sistrunk
Pharmacology Division
Vanderbilt University
Nashville, Tennessee

William J. Slikker, Jr.
National Center for Toxicology
  Research
U.S. Food and Drug Administration
Jefferson, Arkansas

William J. Smith
Cellular Pharmacology Team
Pharmacology Division
U.S. Army Medical Research Institute
  of Chemical Defense
Aberdeen Proving Ground, Maryland

Peter T.C. So
Department of Mechanical Engineering
Massachusetts Institute of Technology
North Cambridge, Massachusetts

Thomas J. Sobotka
Center for Food Safety and Applied
  Nutrition
U.S. Food and Drug Administration
Laurel, Maryland

Martin L. Stephens
The Humane Society of the United
  States
Washington, D.C.

William S. Stokes
National Toxicology Program
  Interagency Center for the Evaluation
  of Alternative Toxicological Methods
National Institute of Environmental
  Health Sciences
Research Triangle Park, North Carolina

Erik Suuronen
University of Ottawa Eye Institute
Ottawa, Ontario, Canada

Bethany S. Toliver
U.S. Army Medical Research Institute
  of Chemical Defense
Aberdeen Proving Ground, Maryland

John L. Ubels
Calvin College
Grand Rapids, Michigan

Maryanne Vahey
Walter Reed Army Institute of Research
Rockville, Maryland

James J. Valdes
Molecular Engineering Team
Research and Technology Directorate
Edgewood Chemical Biological Center
Aberdeen Proving Ground, Maryland

Sherry L. Ward
U.S. Army Medical Research
& Material Command
Congressionally Directed Medical
Research Programs
Ft. Detrick, Maryland

Robert J. Werrlein
U.S. Army Medical Research Institute
of Chemical Defense
Aberdeen Proving Ground, Maryland

Philip Wexler
Division of Specialized Information
Services
Toxicology and Environmental Health
Information Program
National Library of Medicine
Bethesda, Maryland

William White
U.S. Army Edgewood Chemical
Biological Center
Aberdeen Proving Ground, Maryland

Georgette Whiting
Division of Specialized Information
Services
Toxicology and Environmental Health
Information Program
National Library of Medicine
Bethesda, Maryland

Neil L. Wilcox
Gillette Medical Evaluation
Laboratories
The Gillette Company
Gaithersburg, Maryland

D.L. Woolard
Army Research Office
Research Triangle Park, North Carolina

Roman B. Worobec
Medical Sciences and Biotechnology
Team
Library of Congress
Washington, D.C.

Ke-Ping Xu
Department of Cellular Biology and
Anatomy
Medical College of Georgia
Augusta, Georgia

Fu-Shin Yu
Department of Cellular Biology and
Anatomy
Medical College of Georgia
Augusta, Georgia

Errol Zeiger
National Institute of Environmental
Health Sciences
and
Errol Zeiger Consulting
Chapel Hill, North Carolina

Robert P. Zendzian
U.S. Environmental Protection Agency
Washington, D.C.

Csaba K. Zoltani
U.S. Army Research Laboratory
Computational and Information
Sciences Directorate
Aberdeen Proving Ground, Maryland

Contents

Progress in the Validation and Regulatory Acceptance of Alternatives

NEIL L. WILCOX

Part I begins with the historical developments in the humane care and use of research animals and presents an update on the current status of validation and regulatory acceptance on alternatives to animal testing. Two government organizations, the Interagency Coordinating Committee for the Validation of Alternative Methods (ICCVAM) and the European Center for the Validation of Alternative Methods (ECVAM), reviewed new toxicological testing methods to determine their validity and promote regulatory acceptance. Each organization has successfully validated new methods that have also received regulatory acceptance by the U.S. Federal Government and the European Union, respectively. Associated with the emergence of these organizations are several issues that need to be addressed. How many new methods will realistically be proposed for formal review, and will the ICCVAM and the ECVAM have the resources to meet high expectations? What are these organizations doing to identify and prioritize new testing methods to meet regulatory needs? What steps are being taken to harmonize the acceptance of methods that have been validated by both organizations?

Although the operations of these two organizations are inherently different, their foundations are similar. That is, as a result of international workshops conducted by both the ICCVAM and the ECVAM, there is fundamental agreement related to the criteria that need to be met for a test method to be considered valid. Clearly, the process for data review is different between the two groups, but the scientific standards upon which the methods are reviewed are consistently high. It is imperative that the U.S. and the European Union bilaterally accept methods validated by the ICCVAM and the ECVAM through mutual recognition.

Dr. Bill Stokes and Dr. Julia Fentem, representing the ICCVAM and the ECVAM, respectively, provide updates on the current status of their programs, in Chapters 3 and 4. Of similar international interest are the recent activities to assess integrated *in vitro* approaches to acute toxicity testing and the validation and regulatory acceptance of alternative methods to replace the conventional LD_{50} test. To this end, Drs. Anna Forsby and Bas Blaauboer, Stockholm University, provide

Chapter 5, "Integrated *In Vitro* Approaches for Assessing Systemic Toxicity." In addition, Dr. Errol Zeiger, National Institute of Environmental Health Sciences (NIEHS), provides Chapter 6, a summary of the Organization for Economic Cooperation and Development document on the recognition, assessment, and use of clinical signs as humane endpoints for experimental animals used in safety evaluation. This part is completed by Dr. Martin Stephens and his colleagues from the Humane Society of the United States with Chapter 7, "Pain and Distress Management in Animal Research and Testing."

The collective expertise of the authors in this part represents some of the best innovative and progressive thinking in the world.

CHAPTER 1

Historical Developments in the Humane Care and Use of Research Animals: The First 4000 Years

Harry Salem and Sidney A. Katz

CONTENTS

BIBLICAL ORIGINS

Concerns for the humane treatment of animals have biblical origins. According to Genesis 1:29, humankind was given "every seed-bearing plant that is upon the earth, and every tree that has seed-bearing fruit" for food. Permission to eat meat wasn't given until after the Flood. Even then, the slaughter of an animal was made an act that demanded thought, care, and responsibility. In Leviticus 20:25 and 22:8, the Children of Israel were given laws on which animals could be eaten and on how these animals must be slaughtered.

Included in the Jewish dietary laws is the separation of meat and milk. The prohibition on mixing animal flesh and dairy products is attributed to the verse "You shall not boil a kid in its mother's milk." This verse shows a special sensitivity and respect toward the animal slaughtered for food by not adding insult to injury by mixing its flesh with its mother's milk. The importance of this sensitivity is

Table 1.1   Chronology for the Enactment of Animal Welfare Legislation

Year	State	Year	State	Year	State
1828	New York	1864	Idaho	1880	Ohio
1835	Massachusetts	1864	Oregon	1881	North Carolina
1838	Connneticut	1867	New Jersey	1881	South Carolina
1938	Wisconsin	1868	California	1883	Alabama
1842	New Hampshire	1868	West Virginia	1883	Maine
1845	Missouri	1869	Illinois	1884	Hawaii
1848	Virginia	1871	District of Columbia	1887	New Mexico
1851	Iowa	1871	Michigan	1887	South Dakota
1851	Minnesota	1871	Montana	1889	Florida
1852	Kentucky	1872	Colorado	1890	Maryland
1854	Vermont	1873	Delaware	1891	North Dakota
1856	Texas	1873	Indiana	1893	Oklahoma
1857	Rhode Island	1873	Nebraska	1895	Wyoming
1858	Tennessee	1875	Georgia	1898	Utah
1859	Kansas	1879	Arkansas	1913	Alaska
1859	Washington	1879	Louisiana	1913	Arizona
1860	Pennsylvania	1880	Mississippi	1921	Virgin Islands
1861	Nevada				

reflected in the verse's repetition twice in Exodus, 23:19 and 24:26, and again in Deuteronomy 14:21.

Biblical expressions of animal welfare are found in the Ten Commandments (Exodus 20:8–10).

> Remember the Sabbath day, to keep it holy. Six days shall you labor, and do all your work; but the seventh day is a Sabbath unto the Lord, your God; in it you shall not do any manner of work, you, nor your son, nor your daughter, nor your man-servant, nor your maid-servant, nor your **cattle**, nor the stranger that is within your gates.

COLONIAL AMERICA

The Puritan's "Body of Liberties" brought animal welfare to Colonial America in 1641. The chronology for the enactment of subsequent animal welfare legislation in the United States is tabulated above (Animal Welfare Institute, 1990) (see Table 1.1).

Animals have been used for laboratory experiments for more than two centuries. Their increased use in the 19th century brought numerous challenges alleging the use of animals in research cruel, inhumane, unethical, medically unpredictive, unnecessary, and even misleading.

VICTORIAN ENGLAND

During the first half of the 19th century, Marshall Hall, a British physician, proposed five principles for eliminating unnecessary and repetitive procedures and for minimizing suffering in animal experimentation. Although he earned his living as a medical practitioner, he was active in research. His most important contributions were in the area of circulatory physiology. Hall felt compelled to defend his experiments with animals, which were coming under increased scrutiny and criticism from the antivivisectionist movement. He argued "The whole science of medicine and surgery, indeed, is dependent upon physiology. To exclude physiological investigation, would be to erect an utter barrier to the practice of our art." In his *A Critical and Experimental Essay on the Circulation of the Blood*, he proposed five principles for experimental physiology (Fye, 1997):

1. We should never have recourse to experiment, in cases in which observations can afford us the information required.
2. No experiments should be performed without a distinct and definite objective.
3. We should not needlessly repeat experiments which have been performed by physiologists of reputation.
4. Experiments should be performed with the least possible infliction of suffering.
5. Every physiological experiment should be performed under such circumstances as will secure a due observation and attestation of its results, and to obviate, as much as possible, the necessity for its repetition.

He also recommended the use of phylogenetically lower, less sentient animals.

In 1876, the Cruelty to Animals Act was passed in the House of Commons. Under the act, no experiment calculated to cause pain could be performed on a vertebrate animal:

1. By a person unlicensed either by the Secretary of State or, when necessary in a criminal case, by a judge,
2. Or to acquire manual skill
3. Or as a public exhibition
4. Or without a view to the advancement of new discovery of physiological knowledge or of knowledge which will be useful for saving or prolonging life or alleviating pain
5. Or without complete anesthesia of the animal during the whole of the experiment
6. Or without the animal being killed before recovery from the anesthetic, if it is in pain or seriously injured
7. Or as an illustration of lectures in medical schools, hospitals, colleges or elsewhere
8. Or on a dog or cat
9. Or on a horse, ass or mule

The first three provisions of the act are binding; the last six can be dispensed with by means of certificates. Conviction of unlawful experiments is subject to fines and up to three months imprisonment.

Toward the end of the 19th century, the American Humane Association increased pressures for laws prohibiting the repetition of painful experiments for the purpose of teaching or demonstrating already known or accepted facts. Legislation was proposed in the U.S. Congress to restrict vivisection in the District of Columbia by way of a system of regulation and periodic inspection of laboratories. The bill was defeated on the floor of the Senate largely through the testimonies offered by members of the medical community including William Henry Welch, Dean of the

Johns Hopkins Medical School. The legislation was reintroduced in 1900 as Senate Bill 34 and was once again defeated.

RUSSELL AND BURCH

Animal activism waned after World War I, remained at a low level until the early 1950s, and then increased again. It was at this time that William Russell and Rex Burch undertook a systematic study of laboratory techniques and their ethical aspects. In 1956, they prepared a general report, which led to the publication of the *Principles of Humane Experimental Techniques* (Russell and Burch, 1959). At the end of this book, they conclude

In the course of this book, many problems have been raised and many fields reviewed. It is proper to close with the comment that research in this whole subject has barely started as a systematic discipline. The key branches of fundamental science for the whole enterprise are those of animal behavior and psychosomatics, though many others, such as statistical methods and black box theory, must be pressed into service. In this book, we have sought only to limn the barest outlines; it will remain for others to fill the interior. We hope the book may stimulate some experimentalists to devote special attention to the subject, and many others to work in full awareness of its existence and possibilities. Above all, we hope it will serve to present to those beginning work a unified image of some of the most important aspects of their studies. If it does any of these things, this book will have amply served its purpose.

THE THREE Rs

The book has indeed served its purpose. Their three Rs (replacement, reduction, and refinement) have become fundamental guidelines for conducting basic and applied research, implementing quality control and quality assurance procedures, and performing clinical and environmental assessments. Federal regulations subsequently endorsed the principles of the three Rs. Some of the relevant legislation include:

Animal Welfare Act of 1966, public law (PL) 89-544
Animal Welfare Act of 1970, PL 91-579
Animal Welfare Act of 1976, PL 94-279
Food Security Act of 1985, PL 99-198
Food, Agriculture, Conservation and Trade Act of 1990, PL 101-624

Of at least equal importance are the ongoing efforts to promote the principles of the three Rs on a worldwide basis. These are described in the subsequent chapters of this section.

REFERENCES

Animal Welfare Institute (1990) *Animals and Their Legal Rights: A Survey of American Laws from 1641 to 1990,* Animal Welfare Institute, Washington, D.C., p. 4.

Fye, W.B. (1997) Profiles in cardiology: Marshall Hall, *Clin. Cardiol.,* 20(10), 904–905.

Russell, W.M.S. and Burch, R.L. (1959) *The Principles of Humane Experimental Techniques,* Methuen, London.

CHAPTER 2

A History of Interagency Approaches to Alternatives and Establishment of the Interagency Regulatory Alternatives Group

Sidney Green

CONTENTS

INTRODUCTION

This history will describe activity, particularly in the initial stages, associated with the Food and Drug Administration (FDA). This focus is a consequence of the attention animal rights activists have given to the Draize eye test, used to test personal care products, which fall under the jurisdiction of the FDA. This attention led to the recognition early on of the need for interagency approaches to developments relative to the eye test in particular and alternatives in general.

It may surprise some to learn that the first test method in toxicology to draw attention of the animal rights activists was not the Draize test. The LD_{50} became the focus of FDA efforts in 1984. In that year an FDA-wide steering committee on animal welfare issues was organized. Each bureau (foods, drugs, medical devices, etc.) was represented on this committee and was requested to provide a list of procedures or tests that require use of animals and that were requested of regulated industry either routinely or occasionally. The number of animals used per dosage or per test was also requested. Responders were asked "whether there was an implied requirement for LD_{50} data" and "whether all individuals associated with regulatory, research activities of their division/office were aware that the LD_{50} test was not required by the FDA." If there were any documents, guidelines, recommendations, etc., suggesting a requirement for the classical LD_{50}, copies were to be provided. This activity culminated in a policy statement being issued in the Federal Register in 1988 clarifying the FDA's position relative to this test.

Prior to the 1988 policy statement, more and more attention was directed to the Draize eye test on the part of animal rights activists and, consequently, FDA personnel. Industry had also begun to devote resources to the development of alternatives to the eye test. FDA representatives indicated in meetings and symposia that the agency was willing to hold discussions with those developing alternative tests and that the government wanted to be consulted and become an integral part of the developments. Industry recognized that the development of an alternative was only one facet of eventual acceptance and that such an alternative had to meet certain federal requirements. Thus it would be beneficial to learn of those requirements early in the process of development. Investigators were encouraged to meet with FDA personnel to discuss their plans.

Several cosmetic companies met with FDA personnel. These discussions resulted in an understanding between FDA personnel and industry that, in general, the procedures under development could be used as screens but could not replace the Draize test. It was also understood that the methods were product-specific and may not be useful for cosmetics in general. After several such meetings, FDA personnel realized that it would be useful to expand discussions to include other regulatory and government organizations. This would allow the agencies to comment jointly and provide feedback to industry on an approach or a specific test. This would also require regulatory agencies to broaden their view of the application of a test and perhaps forge a common approach to its further development. Additionally, it would provide industry a better understanding of the philosophies and positions of the agencies without having to organize separate meetings with each (Green, 1994).

ESTABLISHMENT OF IRAG

After much discussion within the Center for Food Safety and Applied Nutrition, which had responsibility for cosmetics, and before contacting other federal entities, clearance and opinions regarding such an approach were obtained from the Commissioner of the FDA and other centers, respectively. Comments from all centers were supportive of the effort. Responses were received from the Center for Drug Evaluation and Research, the Center for Biologic Evaluation and Research, The National Center for Toxicological Research, the Center for Veterinary Medicine, and the Center for Devices and Radiologic Health. After concurrence within the FDA was reached, the Environmental Protection Agency (EPA) and the Consumer Product Safety Commission (CPSC) were contacted. At the first meeting of agency representatives in 1988 it was decided to name the organization the Interagency Regulatory Alternatives Group (IRAG). Richard Hill, M.D. of the Environmental Protection

Agency agreed to serve as chairman. Charter members of the group were Sidney Green of the FDA, Richard Hill of the EPA, and Kailash Gupta of the CPSC. Other federal organizations were invited to join. Those agencies were the Department of Transportation represented by George Cushmac, the U.S. Army represented by Harry Salem, the National Institute of Environmental Health Sciences represented by William Stokes, and the Occupational Safety and Health Administration represented by Surender Ahir. Neil Wilcox of the Center for Veterinary Medicine of the FDA was also invited to become a member given the fact that the center had the major responsibility for alternatives within the FDA.

The purpose of the group was to provide a forum for the discussion of alternatives to whole animal toxicological test methods. The *ad hoc* group was to identify issues of common interest to the scientific community in both the private and public sectors; participate in the collection and exchange of information; assist in setting priorities for the evaluation of *in vivo* and *in vitro* methods development, validation, and acceptance; analyze information and make recommendations consistent with good science; and function as a liaison with international regulatory bodies, industry, academia, and public interest groups to facilitate initiatives that lead to international harmonization (Bradlaw and Wilcox, 1997).

IRAG WORKSHOPS

The first workshop was held in September of 1988 in Arlington, VA, and focused on the Draize test. The state of alternatives was discussed in the context of that time frame, 1988. This workshop represented an initial effort intended to set the stage for additional planning and focus. Representative of the presentations at this meeting was a discussion of "regulatory considerations for alternatives to the Draize eye test" (Green, 1989).

The second workshop was titled "Workshop on Updating Eye Irritation Test Methods: Proposals for Regulatory Consensus" and was held on September 26–27, 1991 in Washington, D.C. The original intent was to discuss *in vitro* and *in vivo* test methods. It became clear that specific *in vitro* methods were not at a stage of development to be considered at that time. Thus a second workshop was planned for the *in vitro* methods. The purpose of the first workshop was to identify different testing and evaluation practices, develop proposals for change that minimized differences in those methods, and determine areas of consensus in the scientific community. Thus the emphasis was, by default, on reduction and refinement procedures.

At this workshop seven papers were presented: "Criteria for *In Vitro* Alternatives for the Eye Irritation Test" by Sidney Green, "Screening Procedures for Eye Irritation" by Pamela Hurley, "Use of Ophthalmic Topical Anesthetics" by Van Seabaugh, "The Use of Low-Volume Dosing in the Eye Irritation Test" by Lark Lambert, "Number of Animals for Sequential Testing" by Janet Springer, "Scoring for Eye Irritation Tests" by Wiley Chambers, and "An Eye Irritation Test Protocol and an Evaluation and Classification System" by Kailash Gupta. The workshop concluded that "with respect to reduction and refinement, the strongest consensus was related to use of the two-stage testing in which only one or two animals were studied initially and the nature and consistency of the findings dictated further testing, the low volume test provoked the sharpest debate and participant consensus was not evident, much information is lost when the number of grades or classes of irritants is reduced, thus elimination of a 'corrosive class' would require more discussion, international practices and conventions prevented a consensus regarding the definition of a positive test, either as number of animals responding or as the mean score, and the use of total acidity or alkalinity as a substitute for pH required further study." The entire proceedings of the workshop were published in one volume of *Food and Chemical Toxicology,* Volume 31, 1993, and the reader is referred to that publication for a full discussion of the workshop.

The third workshop was held in November 1993 in Washington, D.C. and was titled "Workshop on Eye Irritation Testing: Practical Applications of Non-Whole Animal Alternatives." The goal of the workshop was to set a course for the scientific approval and acceptance of non–whole animal alternatives to the Draize eye test. A retrospective review of then existing *in vitro* and *in vivo* data by expert working groups was conducted with the intent to examine the status of a practical application of *in vitro* alternatives used to predict eye irritation (Bradlaw and Wilcox, 1997). It was concluded that "data was insufficient to support the total replacement of *in vivo* ocular irritancy testing with *in vitro* methods, alternative methods to the *in vivo* Draize were being used extensively by industry as screens, based on then current practice some models may have the potential to reduce the need for new animal testing provided they are validated and conducted under well defined conditions." It was also concluded that "basic research needed to be encouraged to identify mechanistic endpoints for human ocular injury, test batteries identified to test novel substances, a third party take the lead to identify promising methods and to facilitate validation and international harmonization of method development, validation and acceptance be given high priority." The entire proceedings of the workshop were published in one volume of *Food and Chemical Toxicology,* Volume 35, 1997, and the reader is referred to this publication for a full discussion of the workshop.

EVOLUTION OF ICCVAM

The federal employees participating in various IRAG activities, such as meetings, organizing symposia, and participating in expert workgroups, all had other primary responsibilities. Support of these individuals was crucial to the success of the group. Since its inception there had been no formal budget to support the group's activities. As competition for scarce resources materialized, it became increasingly more difficult for this cohort to devote the time and effort needed to continue the work of the group and to seek agency and other funding sources.

The establishment of the Interagency Coordinating Committee for the Validation of Alternative Methods (ICCVAM) in 1997 was viewed as a complement to the work of the IRAG. Its mission was to develop and validate new test methods and to establish criteria and processes for the validation and regulatory acceptance of toxicological testing methods. Although never formally stated, I believe the IRAG viewed itself as concentrating on what were considered major regulatory alternative issues such as eye and skin testing. There had not been much thought given to other toxicological methods. The ICCVAM's mandate was broader. The ICCVAM is now, as then, composed of representatives from 15 federal regulatory and research agencies that generate, use, or provide information from toxicity test methods for risk assessment purposes (NIEHS, 1997). Almost all members of the IRAG served on the ICCVAM. As the ICCVAM, supported by resources from the National Institute of Environmental Health Sciences, began to assemble its program, it became apparent that much of the work contemplated by the IRAG could be accomplished under the ICCVAM. There certainly seemed to be no reason for the existence of two groups within the federal government having such closely related activities. Thus the activity of the IRAG was gradually diminished and, after some time, the ICCVAM was accepted as the group within the federal government having responsibility for coordinating activities related to animal alternatives.

I think it is fair to state that the work of the IRAG was the stimulus for the establishment of the ICCVAM and that much of the work of the ICCVAM, at least initially, benefited tremendously from the experience of those who organized and executed the programs of IRAG.

REFERENCES

Bradlaw, J.A. and Wilcox, N.L. (1997) Workshop on eye irritation testing: practical applications of non-whole animal alternatives, *Food Chem. Toxicol.,* 35, 1–11.

Green, S. (1989) Regulatory considerations for alternatives to the Draize eye test, *J. Toxicol. Cutaneous Ocular Toxicol.,* 8(1), 59–68.

Green, S. (1994) Progress of various US regulatory agencies in reviewing alternative test methods, *J. Toxicol. Cutaneous Ocular Toxicol.,* 13(4) 339–343.

National Institute of Environmental Health Sciences) (1997) Validation and Regulatory Acceptance of Toxicological Test Methods: A Report of the *ad hoc* Interagency Coordinating Committee on the Validation of Alternative Methods, NIH publication 97-3981, NIEHS, Research Triangle Park, NC.

CHAPTER 3

The Interagency Coordinating Committee on the Validation of Alternative Methods (ICCVAM): Recent Progress in the Evaluation of Alternative Toxicity Testing Methods

William S. Stokes

CONTENTS

INTRODUCTION

Toxicological test methods are used to assess the safety or potential adverse health effects of chemicals and products. In recent years, there has been growing interest in development of new test methods that provide more accurate assessments of toxicity and that can be used to evaluate new toxicity endpoints of interest. New methods are also sought that provide improved efficiency in terms of time and expense and that will replace, reduce, and refine animal use (Stokes, 1997; Stokes and Marafante 1998; Hill and Stokes, 1999). However, before a new method is used to generate information for regulatory purposes, it must be found to be valid and acceptable for its proposed use (NIEHS, 1997). Demonstrating validity requires scientific evidence of the method's accuracy and reproducibility. Acceptance requires a determination that the method will fulfill a specific regulatory need.

Increasing societal concerns about animal welfare and difficulties in achieving regulatory acceptance of alternative test methods contributed to new laws that led to establishment of the Interagency Coordinating Committee on the Validation of Alternative Methods (ICCVAM) (U.S. Code, 1993; Purchase et al., 1998; U.S. Code, 2000; Stokes and Hill, 2001). An *ad hoc* ICCVAM established criteria for test method validation and acceptance and a process for federal agencies to coordinate the review of proposed test methods that are of interest to other federal agencies (Table 3.1). A standing ICCVAM established in 1997 to evaluate new and alternative test methods became a permanent committee in 2000 (U.S. Code, 2000). This chapter will provide an overview of the ICCVAM test method evaluation process and describe alternative test methods that have been evaluated by the ICCVAM.

BACKGROUND AND HISTORY OF THE ICCVAM

The National Institutes of Health (NIH) Revitalization Act of 1993 (Public Law 103-43) directed the National Institute of Environmental Health Sciences (NIEHS) to establish criteria for the validation and regulatory acceptance of alternative testing methods and to develop a process by which scientifically valid alternative methods could become accepted for regulatory use (U.S. Code, 1993). The law also directed NIEHS to develop and validate alternative toxicological testing methods that could reduce or eliminate the use of animals in acute and chronic toxicity testing. The director of the NIEHS established an *ad hoc* ICCVAM to develop a report on validation and regulatory acceptance criteria and a process for achieving regulatory acceptance of alternative methods. The *ad hoc* ICCVAM was comprised of representatives from the 15 agencies that are now represented on the ICCVAM (Table

3.2) (ICCVAM, 1997). In developing its report, the committee sought broad input and participation from interested stakeholders including industry, academia, animal welfare organizations, and the international community. The *ad hoc* ICCVAM

Table 3.1 Member Agencies

Interagency Coordinating Committee on the Validation of Alternative Methods (ICCVAM)
Consumer Product Safety Commission
Department of Defense
Department of Energy
Department of Health and Human Services
    Agency for Toxic Substances and Disease Registry
    Food and Drug Administration
    National Institute for Occupational Safety and Health
    National Institutes of Health, Office of the Director
    National Cancer Institute
    National Institute of Environmental Health Sciences
    National Library of Medicine
Department of the Interior
Department of Labor
    Occupational Safety and Health Administration
Department of Transportation
    Research and Special Programs Administration
Department of Agriculture
Environmental Protection Agency

Table 3.2 Test Method Validation and Acceptance Criteria[a]

Validation Criteria

Clear statement of proposed use
Biological basis/relationship to effect of interest provided
Formal detailed protocol
Reliability assessed
Relevance assessed
Limitations described
All data available for review
Data quality: Ideally good laboratory practices (GLPs)
Independent scientific peer review

Acceptance Criteria

Fits into the regulatory testing structure
Adequately predicts the toxic endpoint of interest
Generates data useful for risk assessment
Adequate data available for specified uses
Robust and transferable
Time and cost effective
Adequate animal welfare consideration (3 Rs)

[a] These are shortened versions of the adopted criteria. For the full text see: National Institute of Environmental Health Sciences (NIEHS), *Validation and Regulatory Acceptance of Toxicological Test Methods: A Report of the ad hoc Interagency Coordinating Committee on the Validation of Alternative Methods (ICCVAM),* NIH publication 97-3981, Research Triangle Park, NC, 1997.

published its final report, *Validation and Regulatory Acceptance of Toxicological Test Methods,* in 1997 (ICCVAM 1997). The report describes validation and acceptance criteria and processes for new and revised test methods (Table 3.2). The principles embodied in these criteria are based on good science and the need to ensure that the use of new test methods will provide for equivalent or better protection of human health and the environment than previous testing methods or strategies.

Establishment of the ICCVAM

A standing ICCVAM was established in 1997 to implement a process by which new test methods of interest to federal agencies could be evaluated (ICCVAM, 1997; Stokes and Hill, 2001). This committee, which replaced the *ad hoc* ICCVAM, evaluates test methods of multiagency interest and provides recommendations regarding their usefulness to appropriate agencies. The ICCVAM also coordinates cross-agency issues on the development, validation, acceptance, and national/international harmonization of toxicological test methods. The ICCVAM serves as a way for test developers to communicate with applicable agencies during test method development and validation. Federal agencies designate representatives to serve on the committee. These representatives function as agency points of contact and help identify technical experts from their agencies to serve on specific test method workgroups.

ICCVAM Authorization Act of 2000

The ICCVAM was designated as a permanent committee with the enactment of the ICCVAM Authorization Act of 2000, Public Law 106-545 (U.S. Code, 2000). The law was enacted "to establish, wherever feasible, guidelines, recommendations, and regulations that promote the regulatory acceptance of new or revised scientifically valid toxicological tests that protect human and animal health and the environment while reducing, refining, or replacing animal tests and ensuring human safety and product effectiveness." The Act established the ICCVAM as a permanent interagency committee composed of the heads or their designees from the 15 federal agencies that originally agreed to participate on the *ad hoc* ICCVAM (Table 3.1). The Act mandates specific purposes and duties of the ICCVAM (Tables 3.3 and 3.4). The ICCVAM also continues to coordinate interagency issues on test method development, validation, regulatory acceptance, and national and international harmonization (ICCVAM, 2001a).

Table 3.3 The Purposes of the ICCVAM[a]

Increase the efficiency and effectiveness of federal agency test method review
Eliminate unnecessary duplicative efforts and share experiences between federal regulatory agencies
Optimize use of scientific expertise outside the federal government
Ensure that new and revised test methods are validated to meet the needs of federal agencies
Reduce, refine, or replace the use of animals in testing where feasible

[a] ICCVAM Authorization Act (U.S. Code, 2000).

Table 3.4   The Duties of the ICCVAM[a]

Consider petitions from the public for review and evaluation of new and revised test methods
for which there is evidence of scientific validity

Coordinate the technical review and evaluation of new and revised test methods of
interagency interest

Submit ICCVAM test recommendations to each appropriate federal agency

Facilitate and provide guidance on validation criteria and processes

Facilitate:

  Interagency and international harmonization of test protocols that encourage the reduction,
  refinement, and replacement of animal test methods

  Acceptance of scientifically valid test methods and awareness of accepted methods

Make ICCVAM final test recommendations and agency responses available to the public

Prepare reports on the progress of this act and make these available to the public

[a] ICCVAM Authorization Act (U.S. Code, 2000).

THE NATIONAL TOXICOLOGY PROGRAM INTERAGENCY CENTER FOR THE EVALUATION OF ALTERNATIVE TOXICOLOGICAL METHODS (NICEATM)

A National Toxicology Program Interagency Center for the Evaluation of Alternative Toxicological Methods (NICEATM) was established by NIEHS in 1997 to provide operational support for the ICCVAM and its activities (ICCVAM, 1997, 2001a; Stokes and Hill, 2001). NICEATM is a part of the Environmental Toxicology Program, Division of Intramural Research, NIEHS, with offices in Research Triangle Park, North Carolina. The components of NICEATM are a center office, the ICCVAM, peer-review and expert panels, and a scientific advisory committee. The NICEATM office provides committee management and operational support for the ICCVAM, ICCVAM working groups, peer-review and expert panels, and the scientific advisory committee.

NICEATM collaborates with the ICCVAM to carry out scientific peer review and interagency consideration of new test methods of multiagency interest. The center also performs other functions necessary to ensure compliance with provisions of the ICCVAM Authorization Act of 2000 (U.S. Code, 2000). The public health goal of the NICEATM and the ICCVAM is to promote the scientific validation and regulatory acceptance of new toxicity testing methods that are more predictive of human health and ecological effects than currently available methods. Methods are emphasized that provide for improved toxicity characterization, savings in time and costs, and refinement, reduction, and replacement of animal use whenever feasible.

The ICCVAM Scientific Advisory Committee

In order for the ICCVAM and the NICEATM to obtain constructive advice from knowledgeable scientists outside of government, an Advisory Committee on Alternative Toxicological Methods (ACATM) was established in 1997 (NIEHS, 1998). The advisory committee was composed of professionals from academia, industry, animal welfare groups, and other organizations. The committee provided advice on the activities and priorities of NICEATM and ICCVAM and on ways to foster partnership activities and interactions among interested parties. To comply with provisions of the ICCVAM Authorization Act of 2000, the ACATM was rechartered in 2002 as an NIH advisory committee and renamed the Scientific Advisory Committee on Alternative Toxicological Methods (SACATM) (NIEHS, 2002).

As directed by the Act, the SACATM provides advice to the ICCVAM and the NICEATM on ICCVAM activities (U.S. Code, 2000). Like the ACATM, the SACATM operates in accordance with provisions of the Federal Advisory Committee Act (U.S. Code, 1972). Accordingly, meetings are open to the public and there is an opportunity for the public to comment at meetings. Meetings and tentative agenda are announced to the public in advance in the *Federal Register* and other notices. Representation on the SACATM is specified by law and the SACATM charter (U.S. Code, 2000; NIEHS, 2002). The charter calls for 15 voting members of the SACATM, and the act specifies that ICCVAM agency representatives serve as *ex officio* nonvoting members.

THE ICCVAM TEST METHOD EVALUATION PROCESS

Test Method Validation

A major function of the ICCVAM is to evaluate the validation status of proposed new, revised, and alternative test methods and to provide test recommendations to federal agencies. Validation is defined as the process by which the reliability and relevance of a test method are established for a specific purpose (ICCVAM, 1997). Reliability is a measure of the extent to which a test can be performed reproducibly within and among laboratories over time, while relevance is the extent to which a test method will correctly predict or measure the biological effect of interest (ICCVAM, 1997). Adequate validation is considered a prerequisite for regulatory acceptance consideration. A test method typically evolves through a process involving research, development, prevalidation, and validation before gaining acceptance as an approved test method (ICCVAM, 1997). Test methods for which there are completed validation studies can be submitted to the ICCVAM for consideration.

Test Method Submissions

Following completion of appropriate validation studies, the sponsor submits all available information and supporting documentation for a test method to ICCVAM in accordance with the ICCVAM submission guidelines (Figure 3.1) (ICCVAM, 1999a). The extent to which each of the established validation and acceptance criteria have been addressed must be described in the submission (ICCVAM, 1997). Submissions must contain sufficient information for (1) an independent scientific peer-review panel to assess the validation status of the proposed test method and (2) for agencies to assess the acceptability of the proposed test method for providing useful information for hazard or risk assessment. Submissions should include all relevant

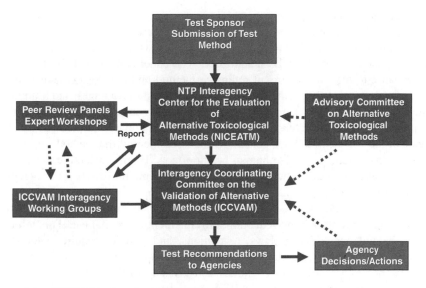

Figure 3.1 ICCVAM test method evaluation process.

data, detailed protocols, statistical analyses, publications, and other information as described in the submission guidelines.

ICCVAM Interagency Working Groups

Once a decision is made to review a test method and resources are available, an ICCVAM Interagency Working Group is organized to collaborate with NICEATM to carry out the technical evaluation of the test method (Figure 3.1) (ICCVAM, 1997; Stokes and Hill 2001). Working groups are composed of government scientists recommended by ICCVAM agencies. The working group assesses the submission and may request additional information or analyses deemed necessary to make decisions about the method. The group recommends expert scientists to serve on the peer-review panel and prepares questions that should be addressed by the panel. Working group members provide information to the panel about current agency test requirements and test methods used or approved by their agency. Members attend peer-review meetings to provide additional information as necessary. Following the peer-review meeting, the working group develops draft test method recommendations for consideration by the ICCVAM.

Independent Scientific Peer-Review Panels

When adequate information is available for a test method and it has been accepted for ICCVAM evaluation, an independent scientific peer-review panel is usually convened. The panel is charged with developing a scientific consensus on the validation status of the proposed test method, including its usefulness for generating information for specific human health and/or ecological risk assessment purposes (Figure 3.1). The panel consists of experts from around the world who are knowledgeable in the field and who do not have a conflict of interest with the outcome of the evaluation. In assessing the validation status of a method, peer-review panels are asked to consider all available information and to evaluate the extent to which the ICCVAM validation and acceptance criteria have been addressed. The panel compares the test method's performance to that of the current reference method and develops conclusions and recommendations regarding the test method's usefulness, advantages, and limitations. Where available and appropriate, the panel considers information available about human toxicity for the reference chemicals used to evaluate the predictive performance of the test method. Such data allow for assessment of the method's usefulness in predicting potential adverse human health effects. From a scientific perspective, the panel addresses how and when the new test method might partially or fully replace existing methods or approaches.

Peer-review panels are also asked to evaluate the extent to which the test method provides for the replacement, reduction, or refinement of animal use. This information is helpful because U.S. laws, regulations, and policies require scientists to consider scientifically valid alternative methods and approaches prior to their use of animals for research or testing (Stokes and Jensen, 1995; Stokes, 1997). These requirements are prescribed by the 1985 Amendment to the Animal Welfare Act (U.S. Code, 1985a) implemented as regulations in 1989 (U.S. Department of Agriculture, 1989), and the Health Research Extension Act of 1985 (U.S. Code, 1985b), which was implemented by the Public Health Service Policy on the Humane Care and Use of Laboratory Animals in 1986 (Public Health Service, 1986).

In order to ensure that all interested stakeholders have the opportunity to provide comments on proposed test methods, test method submissions are made available to the public prior to peer-review meetings. Public comments and published and unpublished information are requested and provided to the peer-review panel for consideration. Peer-review panel meetings are conducted in public session, and opportunities for public comment are provided during the meeting. The peer-review panel prepares a report of their evaluation, conclusions, and recommendations, which is published and made available to the public.

Expert Panels and Workshops

ICCVAM may be asked to review the current validation status of test methods where adequate validation studies are not available. In these situations, expert workshops or expert panel meetings are convened (ICCVAM, 2001a). These workshops and meetings may:

- Evaluate the interim validation status of methods
- Evaluate proposed validation studies
- Develop recommendations for research, development, and validation studies needed to further characterize or improve the usefulness of test methods
- Evaluate the adequacy of current methods for assessing specific toxicities
- Identify testing areas in need of new or improved methods

Federal agencies and other funding sources can then use this information to establish priorities for appropriate research, development, and validation efforts.

ICCVAM Test Recommendations

Following a peer-review meeting, the ICCVAM reviews the meeting report and public comments and develops recommendations regarding potential usefulness, limitations, and applicability of the test method to federal testing requirements. The test method submission, peer-review panel report, public comments, and ICCVAM test method recommendations are compiled in an ICCVAM test method evaluation report, which is published and made available to the public. All reports are publicly available at no charge on the ICCVAM/NICEATM web site in a readily download-able format (http://iccvam.niehs.nih.gov).

REGULATORY AGENCY CONSIDERATION OF ICCVAM RECOMMENDATIONS

ICCVAM test recommendations and test method evaluation reports are forwarded to federal agencies for their consideration through the Secretary of Health and Human Services or his/her designee (U.S. Code, 2000). In accordance with Public Law 106-545, agencies must review the ICCVAM test recommendations and notify the ICCVAM within 180 days of their findings (U.S. Code, 2000). Each federal agency makes a decision regarding the applicability and acceptability of the test method, based on their specific statutory mandates, and determines when and how they can be used to meet agency testing requirements. If the test method is accepted, appropriate action is taken by an agency, such as the revision or issuance of regulations, guidelines, or guidance documents. The ICCVAM is required to make both its recommendations and federal agency responses available to the public (U.S. Code, 2000).

ICCVAM TEST METHOD EVALUATIONS

The Local Lymph Node Assay

The first test method evaluated by the ICCVAM was the murine local lymph node assay (LLNA), a new alternative method for assessing the allergic contact dermatitis potential of chemicals (ICCVAM, 1999b; Sailstad et al., 2001; Dean et al., 2001; Haneke et al., 2001). The LLNA is a mechanism-based test method that provides dose-response information, uses fewer animals, and eliminates pain and distress compared to the standard testing method for which it can be substituted (Dean et al., 2001). A scientific peer-review panel concluded that the LLNA is a valid substitute to the currently accepted test methods that use guinea pigs (ICCVAM, 1999b; Dean et al., 2001). The panel also concluded that the LLNA provides for the refinement and reduction of animal use. The ICCVAM forwarded test recommendations to agencies for their consideration, and the LLNA was subsequently accepted by the U.S. Environmental Protection Agency (EPA), Food and Drug Administration (FDA), and Occupational Safety and Health Administration (OSHA) (Sailstad et al., 2001). A new internationally harmonized test guideline (test guideline

429) for the LLNA has been adopted by the Organization for Economic Cooperation and Development (OECD, 2002).

ICCVAM organized a training workshop on the LLNA in January 2001, in collaboration with the International Life Sciences Institute (ILSI) and other federal agencies. The purpose of the workshop was to train regulatory scientists and industry toxicologists on how to correctly perform the LLNA and interpret data in accordance with regulatory testing requirements. Such training is expected to facilitate effective use of the LLNA.

Skin Corrosivity

Corrositex® (In Vitro International, Inc., Irvine, California) is an *in vitro* method for assessing the dermal corrosivity potential of chemicals. The method was submitted to ICCVAM for evaluation and subsequently underwent review by an independent scientific peer-review panel in January 1999 (ICCVAM, 1999c). The panel concluded that Corrositex® could be used to assess the corrosivity potential of certain chemical classes for specific regulatory testing purposes such as for transportation hazard classification (ICCVAM, 1999c). The panel also concluded that the method was useful for screening the corrosivity potential of some chemical classes in a stepwise tiered testing approach such as that endorsed by the OECD (ICCVAM, 1999c; ICCVAM, 2002). When used in this manner, the method provides for the refinement, reduction, and partial replacement of animal use.

The European Center for the Validation of Alternative Methods (ECVAM) conducted validation studies on three other *in vitro* test methods for assessing skin corrosivity: EpiDerm ™ (MatTek, Ashland, MA), Episkin™ (Episkin SNC, Lyon, France), and the rat skin transcutaneous electrical resistance (TER) assay (Barratt et al., 1998; Fentem et al., 1998; Liebsch et al., 2000). EpiDerm ™ and Episkin™ use a three-dimensional tissue culture model of human skin comprised of a reconstructed epidermis and a functional stratum corneum composed of human keratinocytes. The rat skin TER assay measures the extent to which a chemical alters the transcutaneous electrical resistance of a skin disc during a defined exposure period. These methods have been accepted by the European Commission (EC, 2000). Evaluation by ICCVAM using an expedited review process was completed in 2002 (ICCVAM, 2002).

Frog Embryo Teratogenesis Assay in *Xenopus* (FETAX)

ICCVAM and NICEATM convened an expert panel meeting in May 2000, to evaluate the frog embryo teratogenesis assay—*Xenopus* (FETAX), a screening method proposed for evaluating the developmental toxicity potential of chemicals. The panel of expert scientists developed a consensus on the current validation status of FETAX and developed recommendations on current and potential uses of FETAX. Although the panel concluded that FETAX was not adequately validated for regulatory testing applications, the panel recommended ways that the FETAX protocol might be further optimized to improve reproducibility and performance. The panel also recommended additional research and test method development that might improve the accuracy of FETAX for predicting developmental toxicity to humans and environmental species (ICCVAM, 2000). Minutes of the meeting are on the ICCVAM/NICEATM web site at http://iccvam.niehs.nih.gov.

Up-and-Down Procedure for Acute Oral Toxicity

ICCVAM and NICEATM completed evaluation of a revised up-and-down procedure (UDP) for determining the acute oral toxicity of chemicals in 2001 (ICCVAM, 2001b). Revision of the UDP was prompted by the OECD's proposed deletion of the conventional acute oral toxicity test guideline (ICCVAM, 2001b). The EPA revised the UDP so that it could provide equivalent hazard identification and dose-response information as the conventional test guideline (OECD, 1987; EPA, 1999). The independent peer-review panel concluded that the UDP could replace the conventional acute oral toxicity test to estimate an LD_{50} for hazard classification and labeling purposes. However, the UDP does not provide dose-response and slope information, so other testing would be necessary if this information was required.

The UDP significantly reduces the number of animals necessary for determining acute toxicity, using an average of seven to nine animals compared to the 25 or more used in the conventional test method (ICCVAM, 2001b). The procedure involves sequential testing in single animals, with the dose adjusted up or down based on the outcome of the previously dosed animal. The UDP limit test uses only three to five animals and can be used to evaluate relatively nontoxic substances that have a LD_{50} of more 5,000 mg/kg (or 2,000 mg/kg, depending on the regulatory requirement). A software program is available to (1) facilitate calculation of doses, (2) determine when testing is completed, and (3) calculate an estimated LD_{50} and confidence interval (ICCVAM, 2001b). The revised UDP was subsequently adopted by the OECD as an internationally harmonized test guideline (OECD, 2001a).

Following evaluation of the UDP, the ICCVAM, in partnership with the U.S. EPA and the International Life Sciences Institute (ILSI), organized a training workshop on acute toxicity testing methods in February 2002. The workshop provided practical information and case studies to facilitate understanding and the implementation of the UDP and two other *in vivo* alternative methods, the acute toxic class procedure and the fixed dose procedure (OECD, 2001b,c). The workshop also discussed how to use *in vitro* methods to estimate starting doses for animal studies (Spielmann, 1999; ICCVAM, 2001b) and the application of humane endpoints to acute toxicity studies (OECD, 2000).

In Vitro Methods for Assessing Acute Systemic Toxicity

ICCVAM and NICEATM organized an international workshop on *in vitro* methods for assessing acute systemic toxicity in October 2000 (NIEHS, 2000; ICCVAM, 2001a). The workshop experts developed recommendations on the extent that current *in vitro* test methods might be used to evaluate acute systemic toxicity potential of chemicals. The experts also recommended research, development, and validation efforts needed to further improve the usefulness of *in vitro* methods for acute toxicity. Four breakout groups addressed each of the following topics:

- *In vitro* screening methods for assessing acute toxicity
- *In vitro* methods for toxicokinetic determinations
- *In vitro* methods for predicting organ-specific toxicity
- Chemical data sets for validation of *in vitro* acute toxicity test methods

The final workshop report and a guidance document on using *in vitro* data to estimate *in vivo* starting doses for acute toxicity were developed and published in September 2001 (ICCVAM, 2001c,d). The report concludes that although *in vitro* methods cannot currently replace animals for acute toxicity testing, they can be used to screen chemicals for their relative toxicity. The guidance document provides standardized protocols for two *in vitro* cytotoxicity methods that can be used to estimate the starting doses for *in vivo* acute toxicity studies (ICCVAM, 2001b). Preliminary data suggest that use of the *in vitro* methods can reduce the number of animals required in the UDP procedure by up to 30%–40%.

SUMMARY

The ICCVAM provides an efficient process for the interagency evaluation of new, revised, and alternative methods of multiagency interest. The ICCVAM and the NICEATM have now evaluated several test methods that reduce, refine, and partially replace animal use for regulatory testing. Continued development, validation, and adoption of improved testing methods can be expected to support enhanced protection of public health and the environment. Adoption of scientifically valid alternative methods will also benefit animal welfare by the reduction, replacement, and more humane use of laboratory animals.

ACKNOWLEDGMENTS

The author acknowledges Debbie McCarley for her expert editorial assistance in preparing this manuscript, and the contributions and support of Dr. Richard N. Hill, U.S. EPA, who served as co-chair of the ICCVAM from its inception in 1994 until 2002.

REFERENCES

Balls, M., Blaauboer, B.J., Fentem, J.H., Bruner, L., Combes, R.D., Ekwall, B., Fielder, R.J., Guillouzo, A., Lewis, R.W., Lovell, D.P., Reinhardt, C.A., Repetto, G., Sladowski, D., Spielmann, H., and Zucco, F. (1995) Practical aspects of the validation of toxicity test procedures. The report and recommendations of ECVAM Workshop 5. *Alt. Lab. Anim.*, 23, 129–147.
Barratt, M.D., Brantom, P.G., Fentem, J.H., Gerner, I., Walker, A.P., and Worth, A.P. (1998) The ECVAM international validation study on *in vitro* tests for skin corrosivity. Selection and distribution of test chemicals. *Toxicol. In Vitro,* 12, 471–482.

Dean, J., Twerdok, L., Tice, R., Sailstad, D., Hattan, D., and Stokes, W. (2001) Evaluation of the murine local lymph node assay (LLNA) II: conclusions and recommendations of an independent scientific peer review panel, *Regul. Toxicol. Pharmacol.*, 34(3), 274–286.

EC (European Commission) (2000) EU Commission Directive 2000/33/EC of 25 April 2000 (Official Journal of the European Communities), Skin Corrosion, Rat Skin TER and Human Skin Model Assay, *Off. J. Eur. Communities*, June 8.

EPA (Environmental Protection Agency) (1999) Health Effects Test Guidelines OPPTS 870.1100 Acute Oral Toxicity, Washington, D.C., Office of Pesticides, Prevention, and Toxic Substances, url: http://www.epa.gov/OPPTS Harmonized/870 Health Effects Test Guidelines/Series/870-1100.pdf.

Fentem, J.H., Archer, G.E.B., Balls, M., Botham, P.A., Curren, R.D., Earl, L.K., Esdaile, D.J., Holzhutter, H.G., and Liebsch, M. (1998) The ECVAM international validation study on *in vitro* tests for skin corrosivity. II. Results and evaluation by the management team, *Toxicol. In Vitro*, 12, 483–524.

Haneke, K., Tice, R., Carson, B., Margolin, B., and Stokes, W.S. (2001) Evaluation of the murine local lymph node assay (LLNA). III. Data analyses completed by the national toxicology program (NTP) interagency center for the evaluation of alternative toxicological methods, *Regul. Toxicol. Pharmacol.*, 34(3), 287–291.

Hill, R. and Stokes, W.S. (1999) Validation and regulatory acceptance of alternatives, *Cambridge Quart. Healthcare Ethics*, 8, 74–80.

ICCVAM (Interagency Coordinating Committee on the Validation of Alternative Methods) (1997) Validation and regulatory acceptance of toxicological test methods: a report of the ad hoc interagency coordinating committee on the validation of alternative methods, NIH publication 97-3981, Research Triangle Park, NC, ICCVAM, url: http://ntp-server.niehs.nih.gov/htdocs/ICCVAM/iccvam.html.

ICCVAM (Interagency Coordinating Committee on the Validation of Alternative Methods) (1999a) Evaluation of the validation status of toxicological methods: general guidelines for submissions to ICCVAM, NIH publication 99-4496, National Institute of Environmental Health Sciences, Research Triangle Park, NC, ICCVAM, url: http://iccvam.niehs.nih.gov/docs/guidelines/subguide.htm.

ICCVAM (Interagency Coordinating Committee on the Validation of Alternative Methods) (1999b) The murine local lymph node assay: a test method for assessing the allergic contact dermatitis potential of chemical/compounds, NIH publication 99-4494, Research Triangle Park, NC, ICCVAM, url: http://iccvam.niehs.nih.gov/methods/llnadocs/llnarep.pdf.

ICCVAM (Interagency Coordinating Committee on the Validation of Alternative Methods) (1999c) Corrositex®: an in vitro test method for assessing dermal corrosivity potential of chemicals, NIH Publication 99-4495, Research Triangle Park, NC, ICCVAM, url: http://iccvam.niehs.nih.gov/docs/reports/corprrep.htm.

ICCVAM (Interagency Coordinating Committee on the Validation of Alternative Methods) (2000) Minutes of the expert panel meeting on the frog embryo teratogenesis assay—xenopus (FETAX): a proposed screening method for identifying the developmental toxicity potential of chemicals and environmental samples, Research Triangle Park, NC, ICCVAM, url: http://iccvam.niehs.nih.gov/docs/minutes/fetaxMin.pdf.

ICCVAM (Interagency Coordinating Committee on the Validation of Alternative Methods) (2001a) Annual progress report of the Interagency Coordinating Committee on the Validation of Alternative Methods, NIEHS, Research Triangle Park, NC, ICCVAM, url: http://iccvam.niehs.nih.gov/about/annrpt/annrpt.htm.

ICCVAM (Interagency Coordinating Committee on the Validation of Alternative Methods) (2001b) The revised up-and-down procedure: a test method for determining the acute oral toxicity of chemicals, NIH publication 02-4501, Research Triangle Park, NC, ICCVAM, url: http://iccvam.niehs.nih.gov/methods/udpdocs/udpfin/vol 1.pdf.

ICCVAM (Interagency Coordinating Committee on the Validation of Alternative Methods) (2001c) Report of the international workshop on *in vitro* methods for assessing acute systemic toxicity, results of an international workshop organized by the Interagency Coordinating Committee on the Validation of Alternative Methods (ICCVAM) and the National Toxicology Program (NTP) Interagency Center for the Evaluation of Alternative Toxicological Methods (NICEATM), NIH publication 01-4499, Research Triangle Park, NC, ICCVAM, url: http://iccvam.niehs.nih.gov/methods/invidocs/finalall.pdf.

ICCVAM (Interagency Coordinating Committee on the Validation of Alternative Methods) (2001d) Guidance document on using *in vitro* data to estimate *in vivo* starting doses for acute toxicity, based on recommendations from an international workshop organized by the Interagency Coordinating Committee on the Validation of Alternative Methods and the National Toxicology Program (NTP) Interagency Center for the Evaluation of Alternative Toxicological Methods (NICEATM), NIH publication 01-4500, Research Triangle Park, NC, ICCVAM, url: http:iccvam.niehs.nih.gov/methods/invidocs/guidance/iv guide.pdf.

ICCVAM (Interagency Coordinating Committee on the Validation of Alternative Methods) (2002) ICCVAM Evaluation of EPISKIN™, Epiderm™ (EPI-200), and the Rat Skin Transcutaneous Electrical Resistance (TER) Assay: In Vitro Test Methods for Assessing Dermal Corrosivity Potential of Chemicals, NIH Publ. No. 02-4502, Research Triangle Park, NC, ICCVAM, url: http://iccvam.niehs.nih.gov/methods/epiddocs/cwgfinal/cwgfinal.pdf.

Liebsch, M., Traue, D., Barrabas, C., Spielmann, H., Uphill, P., Wilkins, S., McPherson, J.P., Wiemann, C., Kaufmann, T., Remmele, M., and Holzhutter, H.G. (2000) The ECVAM prevalidation study on the use of EpiDerm™ for skin corrosivity testing, *Alt. Lab. Anim.,* 28, 371–401.

NIEHS (National Institute of Environmental Health Sciences) (1997) Notice of meeting to discuss the procedures and activities of the National Toxicology Program (NTP), Center for the Evaluation of Alternative Toxicological Methods and the Interagency Coordinating Committee on the Validation of Alternative Methods (ICCVAM), 62 FR 55649, url: http://iccvam.niehs.nih.gov/docs/FR/6255649.pdf.

NIEHS (National Institute of Environmental Health Sciences) (1998) Notice of meeting of the Advisory Committee on Alternative Toxicological Methods, 63 FR 40302, url: http:iccvam.niehs.nih.gov/docs/FR/6340303.pdf.

NIEHS (National Institute of Environmental Health Sciences) (2000) Notice of International Workshop on *In Vitro* Methods for assessing acute systemic toxicity, cosponsored by NIEHS, NTP, and the U.S. EPA: request for data and suggested expert scientists, 65 FR 37400, url: http:iccvam.niehs.nih.gov/methods/invidocs/6537400.pdf.

NIEHS (National Institute of Environmental Health Sciences) (2002) Notice of Establishment: Scientific Advisory Committee on Alternative Toxicological Methods, 67 FR 11358, url: http://iccvam.niehs.nih.gov/docs/FR/6711358.pdf.

OECD (Organization for Economic Cooperation and Development) (1987) OECD Test Guideline 401: acute oral toxicity, Paris, France, Organization for Economic Cooperation and Development.

OECD (Organization for Economic Cooperation and Development) (2000) Guidance document on the recognition, assessment, and use of clinical signs as humane endpoints for experimental animals used in safety evaluation, Paris, France, Organization for Economic Cooperation and Development.

OECD (Organization for Economic Cooperation and Development) (2001a) Harmonized integrated classification system for human health and environmental hazards of chemical substances and mixtures, Paris, France, Organization for Economic Cooperation and Development.

OECD (Organization for Economic Cooperation and Development) (2001b) OECD Test Guideline 425: acute oral toxicity-up-and-down procedure, Paris, France, Organization for Economic Cooperation and Development.

OECD (Organization for Economic Cooperation and Development) (2001c) OECD Test Guideline 423: acute oral toxicity-acute toxic class method, Paris, France, Organization for Economic Cooperation and Development.

OECD (Organization for Economic Cooperation and Development) (2001d) OECD Test Guideline 420: acute oral toxicity—fixed dose method, Paris, France, Organization for Economic Cooperation and Development.

OECD (Organization for Economic Cooperation and Development) (2002) OECD Test Guideline 429: sensitization: local lymph node assay, Paris, France, Organization for Economic Cooperation and Development.

Public Health Service (1986) Public health service policy on humane care and use of laboratory animals, U.S. Department of Health and Human Services, Washington, D.C..

Purchase, I.F.H., Botham, P.A., Bruner, L.H., Flint, O.P., Frazier, J.M., and Stokes, W.S. (1998) Scientific and regulatory challenges for the reduction, refinement, and replacement of animals in toxicity testing, *Toxicol. Sci.*, 43, 86–101.

Sailstad, D., Hattan, D., Hill, R., and Stokes, W.S. (2001) Evaluation of the murine local lymph node assay (LLNA). I. The ICCVAM review process, *Regul. Toxicol. Pharmacol.*, 34(3), 258–273.

Spielmann, H., Balls, M., Liebsch, M., and Halle, W. (1999) Determination of the starting dose for acute oral toxicity (LD50) testing in the up-and-down procedure (UDP) from cytotoxicity data, *Alt. Lab. Anim.*, 27, 957–966.

Stokes, W.S. (1997) Animal use alternatives in research and testing: obligation and opportunity, *Lab. Anim.*, 26, 28–32.

Stokes, W.S. and Hill, R. (2001) The role of the interagency coordinating committee on the validation of alternative methods in the evaluation of new toxicological testing methods, in *Progress in the Reduction, Refinement, and Replacement of Animal Experimentation,* Balls, M., van Zeller, A.M., and Halder, M., Eds., Elsevier Science, Amsterdam, pp. 385–394.

Stokes, W.S. and Jensen, D.J. (1995) Guidelines for institutional animal care and use committees: consideration of alternatives. *Contemporary Top. Lab. Anim. Sci.,* 34(3), 51–60.

Stokes, W.S. and Marafante, E. (1998) Alternative testing methodologies: the 13th meeting of the scientific group on methodologies for the safety evaluation of chemicals: introduction and summary, *Environ. Health Perspect.,* 106, 405–412.

U.S. Code (1972) Federal Advisory Committee Act, Public Law 92-463, U.S. Government Printing Office, Washington, D.C.

U.S. Code (1985a) Animal Welfare Act Amendment, Public Law 99-198, U.S. Government Printing Office, Washington, D.C.

U.S. Code (1985b) Health Research Extension Act of 1985, Public Law 99-158, U.S. Government Printing Office, Washington, D.C.

U.S. Code (1993) National Institutes of Health Revitalization Act of 1993, Public Law 103-43, U.S. Government Printing Office, Washington, D.C.

U.S. Code (2000) ICCVAM Authorization Act of 2000, Public Law 106-545, U.S. Government Printing Office, Washington, D.C., url: http://iccvam.niehs.nih.gov/about/PL106545.pdf.

U.S. Department of Agriculture (1989) Animal Welfare, Final Rules: Code of Federal Regulations, Parts 1, 2, and 3, 54 FR 36112.

CHAPTER 4

Validation and Regulatory Acceptance of Alternative Test Methods: Current Situation in the European Union

Julia H. Fentem and Michael Balls

CONTENTS

INTRODUCTION

Considerable progress has been made in recent years in validating *in vitro* alternatives to animal tests. In February 2000, the European Union (EU) Member States approved the first replacement alternative (*in vitro*) methods to be mandated for use for regulatory toxicity testing. *In vitro* tests for skin corrosion (the rat skin transcutaneous electrical resistance [TER] method and tests employing human skin models; Fentem et al., 1998; Liebsch et al., 2000) and phototoxicity (the 3T3 neutral red uptake [NRU] phototoxicity test; Spielmann et al., 1998a,b) had both been shown unequivocally to be reliable and relevant in extensive prevalidation and formal validation studies conducted under the auspices of the European Center for the Validation of Alternative Methods (ECVAM). The EU process and procedures for the validation and regulatory acceptance of alternative test methods are outlined in this chapter, with particular reference to the various stages involved in the prevalidation, validation, and regulatory acceptance of *in vitro* tests for skin corrosion (Botham et al., 1995; ECVAM, 1998b, 2000; Fentem et al., 1998; Liebsch et al., 2000).

VALIDATION AND REGULATORY ACCEPTANCE

It has been agreed, internationally, that validation (i.e., the process by which the reliability and relevance of a procedure are established for a specific purpose) is a prerequisite for the regulatory acceptance of new test methods (Balls et al., 1990, 1995a; Goldberg et al., 1993; Balls and Karcher, 1995; Bruner et al., 1996; OECD, 1996; Fentem and Balls, 1997; ICCVAM, 1997). The validation process has been well documented in various reports (e.g., Balls et al., 1995a; OECD, 1996; ICCVAM, 1997). Typically, it involves conducting an interlaboratory blind trial as a basis for assessing whether a test can be shown to be useful and reliable for a specific purpose according to predefined performance criteria. Validation studies are conducted principally to provide objective information on new tests, to show that they are robust and transferable between laboratories, and to show that the data generated can be relied upon for decision-making purposes (e.g., for the identification and labeling of a potential skin corrosive, severe eye irritant, teratogen, etc.). If a new test is to be endorsed as being scientifically valid, the outcome of the validation study must provide sufficient confidence in the precision and accuracy of the predictions made on the basis of the test results (Fentem, 2000). The successful validation of a new toxicological test method is seen as a route to securing (1) regulatory acceptance of that test (where appropriate), (2) routine use of a new method in-house, and (3) the wider acceptance and uptake of the method by other scientists.

Validation studies, as well as the independent review of data on potential new test methods, are generally conducted under the auspices of sponsors, such as government organizations (e.g., ECVAM, the U.S. Interagency Coordinating Committee on the Validation of Alternative Methods [ICCVAM], the Japanese Ministry of Health and Welfare [MHW]) or industry trade organizations, or as collaborative activities initiated by industrial companies in association with other interested groups (e.g., the validation of the mouse local lymph node assay [LLNA] by Procter and Gamble, Unilever, and Zeneca; Loveless et al., 1996; Basketter et al., 2000).

Several successful validation studies have now been conducted in the EU, most notably those funded by ECVAM on *in vitro* tests for phototoxicity (Spielmann et al., 1998a) and skin corrosion (Fentem et al., 1998), both of which adhered to the theoretical framework and recommendations for undertaking practical validation studies outlined by Balls et al. (1995a). Other examples of completed and ongoing practical prevalidation (Curren et al., 1995; Fentem and Balls, 1997) and validation studies in the EU include those on *in vitro* tests for eye irritation (Balls et al., 1995b; Brantom et al., 1997), skin irritation (Fentem et al., 1999, 2001), embryotoxicity (Scholz et al., 1999), and haematotoxicity (Pessina et al., 2000). In addition, ECVAM has also funded prevalidation and validation studies on alternative methods for the potency and quality control testing of vaccines and other biologicals (Hendriksen, 2000; ECVAM, 2001b).

The ECVAM approach to validation has been described previously (Balls et al., 1995a; Balls and Karcher, 1995; Fentem and Balls, 1997). It covers both (a) the conduct of practical validation studies and critical review of their outcome and (b) the peer review of information and data supporting the validity of any new alternative test that may be submitted directly to ECVAM for its consideration and opinion.

With respect to (a), following the completion of a validation study, the management team (MT) prepares a report for publication in the peer-reviewed scientific literature (e.g., Balls et al., 1995b; Loveless et al., 1996; Brantom et al., 1997; Fentem et al., 1998; Spielmann et al., 1998a). In the case of those methods considered to be scientifically valid by the MT, an independent review/assessment is then undertaken (Balls et al., 1995a; ICCVAM, 1997). In the EU, the process for this independent review initially involves the ECVAM scientific advisory committee (ESAC), which can agree upon a statement endorsing the validity of a new test method (e.g., ECVAM, 1998a, 2000). Other services of the European Commission (EC) and various independent expert committees are then asked to review the outcome of the validation study from the perspective of their specific roles, interests, and legal responsibilities. For example, the scientific validities of the *in vitro* tests for phototoxicity and skin corrosion were subsequently also endorsed by DG Environment (responsible for EU chemicals testing legislation) and DG Enterprise (responsible for cosmetics, medicines, and vaccines testing legislation) of the EC, and by the Scientific Committee on Cosmetic Products and Non-Food Products intended for consumers (SCCNFP; the EC's expert advisory committee on cosmetics), following review of all relevant documentation.

The scientific validity of the LLNA for skin sensitization (NIH, 1999a), as well as of Corrositex® for skin corrosion (NIH, 1999b), has been endorsed by peer-review panels convened in the U.S. by ICCVAM, based on evaluations of data submitted by industry. In accordance with point (b) above, the ESAC has reviewed the submission on the LLNA made to ICCVAM and has endorsed the validity of the LLNA as a reduction and refinement alternative for skin sensitization testing (ECVAM, 2000). In December 2000, the ESAC also reviewed the submission on Corrositex made to ICCVAM and the findings of the ICCVAM peer-review panel (ECVAM, 2001a). Thus, the EU has in place processes for critically reviewing and endorsing the validities of alternative methods evaluated both with and without direct ECVAM involvement.

Following independent endorsement of the validity of a new test method, the next step (if appropriate) may be to draft a new test guideline or to draft a revision to an existing guideline for subsequent consideration by the relevant regulatory authorities. For example, draft guidelines on the *in vitro* tests for phototoxicity and skin corrosion were prepared by the MTs for the respective validation studies and were submitted to the OECD Secretariat in December 1998. Similarly, a draft test guideline on the use of the LLNA for predicting skin sensitization was submitted to the OECD during 1999, following the successful ICCVAM review. As is the case for the independent assessment of the validity of new tests, the process of regulatory acceptance involves various stages of critical review of the new test method and all supporting data. For example, drafts of potential new OECD test guidelines are reviewed by national experts in all of the OECD Member Countries; a similar process is followed in the EU for Annex V Test Methods (Directive 67/548/EEC—Dangerous Substances Directive [DSD]).

To illustrate the process and procedures adhered to in the EU, the main stages involved in the validation and regulatory acceptance of alternative test methods for skin corrosion are described, from an EU perspective, in the following sections. For the purposes of this chapter, skin corrosion has been taken as a suitable case study, but note that the various steps and procedures were basically the same for the validation and regulatory acceptance of the 3T3 NRU phototoxicity test. As a follow up to the successful validation of *in vitro* tests for skin corrosion, a prevalidation study of *in vitro* tests for skin irritation has been funded by ECVAM during 1999–2000; the outcome of this study is also outlined briefly later in this chapter.

SKIN CORROSION

The assessment of acute skin corrosion/irritation potential is included in international regulatory requirements for the testing of chemicals. The standard approach used involves applying the test material to the shaved skin of albino rabbits (OECD, 1992). Testing for skin corrosion in laboratory animals has the potential to cause them considerable discomfort or pain, and it is recognized that the response in the rabbit is not always predictive of that found in humans. For these reasons, in recent years considerable effort has been directed toward the development and evaluation of alternative test methods for predicting chemical-induced acute dermal corrosion and irritation (Botham et al., 1998; Fentem et al., 1998).

Skin corrosivity testing is a relatively simple procedure in biological terms. The endpoint is severe and irreversible tissue destruction, not a subtle biological change, and the application route is topical, with no problems of dilution or distribution. These two factors made the development of non-animal methods for the prediction of skin corrosion easier than for other toxic effects exerted by more subtle, multifactorial, mechanisms. Nevertheless, the successful validation of *in vitro* tests for skin corrosion represents a significant achievement in relation to the replacement of toxicity tests known to cause considerable animal pain due to the nature of the endpoint under evaluation.

A prevalidation study on *in vitro* skin corrosivity testing was conducted during 1993 and 1994 (Botham et al., 1995) as a first step toward defining those alternative tests that could be used within the context of OECD testing guideline 404 (OECD, 1992). Three tests were included in the prevalidation study: (a) the rat skin transcutaneous electrical resistance (TER) assay; (b) Corrositex® (In Vitro International, Irvine, CA); and (c) the Skin²™ ZK1350 corrosivity test (Advanced Tissue Sciences, La Jolla, CA). Fifty coded chemicals [25 corrosives (C), 25 non-corrosives (NC)] were tested. The report on the outcome of the prevalidation study recommended that a formal validation study on alternative methods for skin corrosivity testing should be conducted (Botham et al., 1995).

An international validation study on *in vitro* tests for replacing the *in vivo* rabbit test for skin corrosivity was conducted during 1996 and 1997 under the auspices of ECVAM (Fentem et al., 1998). The main objectives of the study were to (a) identify tests capable of discriminating C from NC for selected types of chemicals and/or all chemicals and (b) determine whether these tests could correctly identify known R35 (UN packing group I) and R34 (UN packing groups II and III) chemicals. The tests evaluated were the rat skin TER assay, Corrositex, the Skin² ZK1350 corrosivity test, and Episkin™ (Episkin, Chaponost, France). Each test was conducted in three independent laboratories. Sixty coded chemicals were tested (Barratt et al., 1998).

Two of the tests evaluated, the TER and Episkin assays, met the criteria agreed upon by the MT concerning acceptable reproducibility and predictive ability (Fentem et al., 1998) so that they could be considered scientifically valid replacements for the rabbit test for distinguishing between C and NC chemicals for all of the chemical types studied [objective (a)]. Episkin was also able to distinguish between known R35/UN packing group 1 and R34/UN packing groups II and III chemicals, for all of the chemical types included in the study, on an acceptable number of occasions [objective (b)] (Fentem et al., 1998). Following formal presentation of the findings of the validation study to the ESAC and its critical review of the data, the scientific validity of the rat skin TER and Episkin tests was endorsed by the ESAC in March 1998, and a signed statement to this effect was issued jointly by ECVAM (DG Joint Research Center) and DG Environment of the EC. This was disseminated widely and was also published in the scientific literature (ECVAM, 1998b).

An ECVAM-funded prevalidation study on the EpiDerm skin corrosivity test was coordinated by ZEBET (German Centre for the Documentation of Alternative Methods) during 1997 and 1998 (Liebsch et al., 2000). Phase III of this study was considered to be a catch-up validation activity for a test protocol that was similar to one that had already been successful in a formal validation study (Balls, 1997). The objective of the study was to determine whether a test protocol developed for another human skin model (i.e., in addition to that for Episkin) could similarly discriminate C from NC for various chemical types.

The test was conducted in three independent laboratories, according to the ECVAM prevalidation scheme (Curren et al., 1995). In phase III, 24 coded chemicals (12 C, 12 NC) were tested; these were independently selected to be representative of the set of 60 chemicals tested in the ECVAM validation study (Barratt et al., 1998; Fentem et al., 1998).

The results obtained were reproducible, both within and between the three laboratories. As had been found with the rat skin TER and Episkin assays, the EpiDerm test proved applicable to testing a diverse group of chemicals (both liquids and solids). The concordances between the skin corrosivity classifications derived from the *in vitro* data and from the *in vivo* data were very good, and the test was able to distinguish between C and NC chemicals for all of the chemical types studied (Liebsch et al., 2000).

Following critical review of the test protocol and all data supporting the validity of the EpiDerm test for skin corrosion, it was endorsed as scientifically valid by the ESAC in March 2000 (ECVAM, 2000); the committee stated that "the EpiDerm human skin model can be used for distinguishing between corrosive and non-corrosive chemicals within the context of the draft EU and OECD test guidelines on skin corrosion." Again, a signed statement to this effect was issued and circulated by the EC, and this was published (ECVAM, 2000).

Furthering the endorsement of the scientific validity of the rat skin TER and Episkin assays by the ESAC, several EC services (DG Environment and DG Enterprise) and the SCCNFP reviewed all relevant documentation and subsequently added their endorsements to the ESAC statements. A draft guideline on the use of the TER and human skin model assays for skin corrosion testing was prepared by the MT of the validation study, which was jointly submitted to the OECD Secretariat in December 1998 by DG Environment (on behalf of the EC) and the U.K. government authorities. A draft Annex V test method on skin corrosion was also prepared in February 1999 for discussion with the EU national coordinators for test methods.

On 4 February 2000, the EU Competent Authorities approved the draft Annex V test method on skin corrosion, which makes the use of validated *in vitro* tests for this endpoint mandatory in the EU Member States. In June 2000, test method "B.40 Skin Corrosion" was incorporated into the DSD via Commission Directive 2000/33/EC of 25 April 2000, the 27th adaptation to technical progress of Council Directive 67/548/EEC (EC, 2000). Meanwhile, the OECD national coordinators submitted their comments on the initial draft test guideline prepared in 1998, and these were discussed at their meeting in 2001. Following an OECD nominated experts meeting in November 2001, OECD test guidelines on the rat skin TER assay (TG 430) and the human skin model assays (TG 431) were finally accepted in May 2002.

Corrositex, one of the *in vitro* methods included in the ECVAM validation study (Fentem et al., 1998), was subsequently evaluated by a peer-review panel convened in the U.S. by ICCVAM (NIH, 1999b). The MT for the ECVAM validation study had concluded that Corrositex may be valid for testing specific classes of chemicals, such as organic bases and inorganic acids. The database reviewed in the ICCVAM evaluation was considerably larger than that generated in the ECVAM prevalidation (Botham et al., 1995) and validation (Fentem et al., 1998) studies, and the peer-review panel was able to be more specific in its conclusions, stating that "in limited testing situations the assay is valid for evaluating the corrosivity potential of acids, acid derivatives, and bases." The peer-review panel concluded that in other testing situations, and for other chemical and product classes, the assay is appropriate as part of a tiered testing strategy (NIH, 1999b).

In April 2000, an ESAC working group reviewed the submission on Corrositex made to ICCVAM and the findings of the peer-review panel, and a statement on Corrositex endorsing the ICCVAM findings was agreed upon at the ESAC meeting in December 2000 (ECVAM, 2001a). The ESAC concluded that "the Corrositex assay is a scientifically validated test, but only for those acids, bases and their derivatives which meet the technical requirements of the assay."

SKIN IRRITATION

A prevalidation study on *in vitro* tests for acute skin irritation was conducted during 1999 and 2000, as a follow up to the successful validation of *in vitro* tests for skin corrosion (Botham et al., 1998; Fentem et al., 1999, 2001). The overall objective of validation in this area, of which the prevalidation study was an initial stage, is to identify tests capable of discriminating irritants (I) from non-irritants (NI), as defined according to EU risk phrases ("R38," no classification) and the harmonized OECD criteria ("irritant," no label). The prevalidation study specifically addressed aspects of protocol refinement (phase I), protocol transfer (phase II), and protocol performance (phase III), in accordance with the prevalidation scheme defined by ECVAM (Curren et al., 1995). The tests evaluated were EpiDerm™ (phases I, II, and III), Episkin™ (phases I, II, and III), Prediskin™ (BIOPREDIC, Rennes, France; phases I and II, and additional protocol refinement), the non-perfused pig ear method (phases I and II, and additional protocol refinement), and the mouse skin integrity function test (SIFT, phases I and II) (Fentem et al., 2001).

Modified, standardized test protocols and well-defined prediction models were available for each of the tests at the end of phase I. The results of phase I (intralaboratory reproducibility) were sufficiently promising for all of the tests to progress to phase II. Protocol transfer between the lead laboratory and laboratory 2 was undertaken for all five tests during phase II, and additional refinements were made to the test protocols. For EpiDerm, Episkin, and the SIFT, the intralaboratory and interlaboratory reproducibilities were acceptable; however, better standardization of certain aspects of the test protocols was needed prior to commencing phase III. Neither Prediskin nor the pig ear test performed sufficiently well in phase II to progress to phase III. The Prediskin protocol was overly sensitive, resulting in the prediction of all the NI chemicals as I. The variability in the pig ear test results was too great, indicating that the test would show limited predictive ability. In additional studies (a repeat of phase I), further modification of the Prediskin protocol and a change in the prediction model considerably improved the ability of the test to distinguish I from NI chemicals. However, attempts to improve the intralaboratory reproducibility of the pig ear test were unsuccessful.

In phase III, an initial assessment of the reproducibility and predictive ability in three independent laboratories per test was undertaken for the EpiDerm and Episkin tests (the SIFT was a late inclusion in the prevalidation study and was subsequently evaluated in a separate phase III study). A set of 20 coded chemicals (10 I, 10 NI) were tested with the final, refined, test protocols. The intralaboratory reproducibility was acceptable for both EpiDerm and Episkin. The interlaboratory reproducibility was considered to be acceptable for Episkin; however, for EpiDerm, analysis of variance (ANOVA) indicated that there was a statistically significant laboratory effect on the overall variability, suggesting that the interlaboratory transferability of the test needed to be improved. The EpiDerm test had an overall accuracy of 58%, with an overprediction rate of 37% and an underprediction rate of 47%. The Episkin test had an overall accuracy of 58%, showing an underprediction rate of 23% and an overprediction rate of 60% (Fentem et al., 2001). The MT concluded that none of the tests evaluated in the prevalidation study were yet ready for inclusion in a formal validation study on in vitro tests for acute skin irritation.

Further studies have been undertaken to improve the test protocols and prediction models for EpiDerm, Episkin, and the SIFT. An ECVAM task force reviewed the status of these tests in November 2002 and concluded that they now meet the criteria for inclusion in a validation study. ECVAM will conduct this study during 2003 and 2004.

DISCUSSION

The procedures for conducting formal practical prevalidation and validation studies adopted by ECVAM have now been shown to be successful in reality, not just in theory (Fentem, 2000). In the EU, *in vitro* tests for skin corrosion and phototoxicity have been shown to be reliable and relevant in prevalidation and formal validation studies and, following independent peer review, they have now been incorporated into the pertinent chemicals testing regulations (Directive 67/548/EEC as amended to technical progress). In addition, the ESAC has endorsed the scientific validity of the mouse LLNA for skin sensitization (ECVAM, 2000) based on critical review of the ICCVAM peer-review documentation and other published studies. Similarly, it has endorsed the findings of the ICCVAM peer-review panel on Corrositex (ECVAM, 2001a).

Thus, the EU now has in place processes for critically reviewing and, where appropriate, endorsing the validities of alternative methods evaluated, both with and without direct ECVAM involvement, anywhere in the world. Once such processes for mutual recognition of validated methods have also been agreed upon within other key countries/regions, it is hoped that we should begin to see more timely and more efficient progress in implementing validated alternative methods into regulatory testing requirements at an international level in addition to that at a national/regional level.

ACKNOWLEDGMENTS

The key involvement of the following individuals in the studies outlined in this paper is acknowledged: Graeme Archer, Philip Botham, David Briggs, Christoph Chesné, Rodger Curren, Lesley Earl, Graham Elliott, David Esdaile, John Harbell, Jon Heylings, Manfred Liebsch, Roland Roguet, Han van de Sandt, Horst Spielmann, and Andrew Worth.

REFERENCES

Balls, M. (1997) Defined structural and performance criteria would facilitate the validation and acceptance of alternative test procedures, *Alt. Lab. Anim.,* 25, 483–484.

Balls, M. and Karcher, W. (1995) The validation of alternative test methods, *Alt. Lab. Anim.,* 23, 884–886.

Balls, M., Blaauboer, B., Brusick, D., Frazier, J., Lamb, D., Pemberton, M., Reinhardt, C., Roberfroid, M., Rosenkranz, H., Schmid, B., Spielmann, H., Stammati, A.-L., and Walum, E. (1990) Report and recommendations of the CAAT/ERGATT workshop on the validation of toxicity test procedures, *Alt. Lab. Anim.,* 18, 339–344.

Balls, M., Blaauboer, B.J., Fentem, J.H., Bruner, L., Combes, R.D., Ekwall, B., Fielder, R.J., Guillouzo, A., Lewis, R.W., Lovell, D., Reinhardt, C.A., Repetto, G., Sladowski, D., Spielmann, H., and Zucco, F. (1995a) Practical aspects of the validation of toxicity test procedures. The report and recommendations of ECVAM workshop 5. *Alt. Lab. Anim.,* 23, 129–147.

Balls, M., Botham, P.A., Bruner, L.H., and Spielmann, H. (1995b) The EC/HO international validation study on alternatives to the Draize eye irritation test, *Toxicol. In Vitro*, 9, 871–929.

Barratt, M.D., Brantom, P.G., Fentem, J.H., Gerner, I., Walker, A.P., and Worth, A.P. (1998) The ECVAM international validation study on *in vitro* tests for skin corrosivity. I. Selection and distribution of the test chemicals, *Toxicol. In Vitro*, 12, 471–482.

Basketter, D., Gerberick, F., and Kimber, I. (2000) Validation in Practice—the Reality for Skin Sensitization, paper presented in Progress in the Reduction, Refinement and Replacement of Animal Experimentation, Proceedings of the Third World Congress on Alternatives and Animal Use in the Life Sciences, Bologna, 1999—*Developments in Animal and Veterinary Sciences*, Vol. 31A, Balls, M., van Zeller, A.M., and Halder, M., Eds., Elsevier, Amsterdam, pp. 395–399.

Botham, P.A., Chamberlain, M., Barratt, M.D., Curren, R.D., Esdaile, D.J., Gardiner, J.R., Gordon, V.C., Hildebrand, B., Lewis, R.W., Liebsch, M., Logemann, P., Osborne, R., Ponec, M., Régnier, J.-F., Steiling, W., Walker, A.P., and Balls, M. (1995) A prevalidation study on *in vitro* skin corrosivity testing. The report and recommendations of ECVAM workshop 6. *Alt. Lab. Anim.*, 23, 219–255.

Botham, P.A., Earl, L.K., Fentem, J.H., Roguet, R., and van de Sandt, J.J.M. (1998) Alternative methods for skin irritation testing: the current status. ECVAM Skin Irritation Task Force report 1, *Alt. Lab. Anim.*, 26, 195–211.

Brantom, P.G. et al. (1997) A summary report of the COLIPA international validation study on alternatives to the Draize rabbit eye irritation test, *Toxicol. in Vitro*, 11, 141–179.

Bruner, L.H., Carr, G.J., Chamberlain, M., and Curren, R.D. (1996) Validation of alternative methods for toxicity testing, *Toxicol. In Vitro*, 10, 479–501.

Curren, R.D., Southee, J.A., Spielmann, H., Liebsch, M., Fentem, J.H., and Balls, M. (1995) The role of prevalidation in the development, validation and acceptance of alternative methods, *Alt. Lab. Anim.*, 23, 211–217.

EC (2000) Annex I to Commission Directive 2000/33/EC adapting to technical progress for the 27th time Council Directive 67/548/EEC on the approximation of laws, regulations and administrative provisions relating to the classification, packaging and labeling of dangerous substances, *Off. J. Eur. Communities*, L136, 91–97.

ECVAM (1998a) ECVAM News and Views, *Alt. Lab. Anim.*, 26, 7–8.

ECVAM (1998b) ECVAM News and Views, *Alt. Lab. Anim.*, 26, 275–280.

ECVAM (2000) ECVAM News and Views, *Alt. Lab. Anim.*, 28, 366–367.

ECVAM (2001a) ECVAM News and Views, *Alt. Lab. Anim.*, 29, 96–97.

ECVAM (2001b) ECVAM News and Views, *Alt. Lab. Anim.*, 29, 93–96.

Fentem, J.H. (2000) Validation in Practice—from Theory to Reality, paper presented in Progress in the Reduction, Refinement and Replacement of Animal Experimentation, Proceedings of the Third World Congress on Alternatives and Animal Use in the Life Sciences, Bologna, 1999—*Developments in Animal and Veterinary Sciences*, Vol. 31A, Balls, M., van Zeller, A.M., and Halder, M., Eds., Elsevier, Amsterdam, 365–373.

Fentem, J.H. and Balls, M. (1997) The ECVAM Approach to Validation, paper presented in Animal Alternatives, Welfare and Ethics, Proceedings of the Second World Congress on Alternatives and Animal Use in the Life Sciences, Utrecht, 1996—*Developments in Animal and Veterinary Sciences*, Vol. 27, van Zutphen, L.F.M. and Balls, M., Eds., Elsevier, Amsterdam, pp. 1083–1089.

Fentem, J.H., Archer, G.E.B., Balls, M., Botham, P.A., Curren, R.D., Earl, L.K., Esdaile, D.J., Holzhütter, H.-G., and Liebsch, M. (1998) The ECVAM international validation study on *in vitro* tests for skin corrosivity. II. Results and evaluation by the Management Team, *Toxicol. In Vitro*, 12, 483–524.

Fentem, J., Botham, P., Earl, L., Roguet, R., and van de Sandt, J. (1999) Prevalidation of *in vitro* tests for acute skin irritation, in *Alternatives to Animal Testing II*, Proc. 2nd Int. Scientific Conf. organised by the European Cosmetic Industry, Brussels, Belgium, Clark, D.G., Lisansky, S.G., and Macmillan, R., Eds., CPL Press, Newbury, pp. 228–231.

Fentem, J.H., Briggs, D., Chesné, C., Elliott, G.R., Harbell, J.W., Heylings, J.R., Portes, P., Roguet, R., van de Sandt, J.J.M., and Botham, P.A. (2001) A prevalidation study on *in vitro* tests for acute skin irritation: results and evaluation by the Management Team, *Toxicol. In Vitro*, 15, 57–93.

Goldberg, A.M., Frazier, J.M., Brusick, D., Dickens, M.S., Flint, O., Gettings, S.D., Hill, R.N., Lipnick, R.L., Renskers, K.J., Bradlaw, J.A., Scala, R.A., Veronesi, B., Green, S., Wilcox, N.L., and Curren, R.D. (1993) Framework for validation and implementation of *in vitro* toxicity tests: report of the Validation and Technology Transfer Committee of the Johns Hopkins Center for Alternatives to Animal Testing, *J. Am. Coll. Toxicol.*, 12, 23–30.

Hendriksen, C.F.M. (2000) Replacement, Reduction and Refinement and Biologicals: about Facts, Fiction and Frustrations, paper presented in Progress in the Reduction, Refinement and Replacement of Animal Experimentation, Proceedings of the Third World Congress on Alternatives and Animal Use in the Life Sciences, Bologna, 1999, *Developments in Animal and Veterinary Sciences*, Vol. 31A, Balls, M., van Zeller, A.M., and Halder, M., Eds., Elsevier, Amsterdam, pp. 51–63.

ICCVAM (1997) Validation and Regulatory Acceptance of Toxicological Test Methods, A Report of the *ad hoc* Interagency Coordinating Committee on the Validation of Alternative Methods, NIEHS, Research Triangle Park, NC.

Liebsch, M., Traue, D., Barrabas, C., Spielmann, H., Uphill, P., Wilkins, S., McPherson, J.P., Wiemann, C., Kaufmann, T., Remmele, M., and Holzhütter, H.-G. (2000) The ECVAM prevalidation study on the use of EpiDerm for skin corrosivity testing, *Alt. Lab. Anim.*, 28, 371–401.

Loveless, S.E., Ladics, G.S., Gerberick, G.F., Ryan, C.A., Basketter, D.A., Scholes, E.W., House, R.V., Hilton, J., Dearman, R.J., and Kimber, I. (1996) Further evaluation of the local lymph node assay in the final phase of an international collaborative trial, *Toxicology*, 108, 141–152.

NIH (1999a) The murine local lymph node assay, the results of an independent peer review evaluation coordinated by the Interagency Coordinating Committee on the Validation of Alternative Methods (ICCVAM) and the National Toxicology Program Center for the Evaluation of Toxicological Methods (NICEATM), NIH publication 99-4494, NIEHS, Research Triangle Park, NC.

NIH (1996b) Corrositex: an *in vitro* test method for assessing dermal corrosivity potential of chemicals, NIH publication 99-4495, NICEATM, Research Triangle Park, NC.

OECD (1992) OECD guideline for the testing of chemicals, 404: Acute Dermal Irritation/Corrosion, OECD, Paris.

OECD (1996) Final report of the OECD workshop on harmonization of validation and acceptance criteria for alternative toxicological test methods, OECD, Paris.

Pessina, A., Albella, B., Bueren, J., Brantom, P., Casati, S., Corrao, G., Gribaldo, L., Parchment, R., Parent-Massin, D., Piccirillo, M., Rio, B., Sacchi, S., Schoeters, G., and van den Heuvel, R. (2000) Method development for a prevalidation study of the *in vitro* GM-CFU assay for predicting myelotoxicity, in Progress in the Reduction, Refinement and Replacement of Animal Experimentation. Proceedings of the Third World Congress on Alternatives and Animal Use in the Life Sciences, Bologna, 29 August – 2 September 1999, *Developments in Animal and Veterinary Sciences, Vol. 31A*, Balls, M., van Zeller, A.M., and Halder, M., Eds., Elsevier, Amsterdam, pp. 679–692.

Scholz, G., Genschow, E., Brown, N., Piersma, A., Brady, M., Clemann, N., Huuskonen, H., Paillard, F., Bremer, S., and Spielmann, H. (1999) First results of a validation study of three *in vitro* embryotoxicity tests, *Alt. Lab. Anim.,* 27, 296.

Spielmann, H., Balls, M., Dupuis, J., Pape, W.J.W., Pechovitch, G., de Silva, O., Holzhütter, H.-G., Clothier, R., Desolle, P., Gerberick, F., Liebsch, M., Lovell, W.W., Maurer, T., Pfannenbecker, U., Potthast, J.M., Csato, M., Sladowski, D., Steiling, W., and Brantom, P. (1998a) EU/COLIPA "*in vitro* phototoxicity" validation study, results of phase II (blind trial). I. The 3T3 NRU phototoxicity test, *Toxicol. In Vitro,* 12, 305–327.

Spielmann, H., Balls, M., Dupuis, J., Pape, W.J.W., de Silva, O., Holzhütter, H.-G., Gerberick, F., Liebsch, M., Lovell, W.W., and Pfannenbecker, U. (1998b) A study on UV filter chemicals from Annex VII of European Union Directive 76/768/EEC, in the *in vitro* 3T3 NRU phototoxicity test, *Alt. Lab. Anim.,* 26, 679–708.

CHAPTER 5

Integrated *In Vitro* Approaches for Assessing Systemic Toxicity

Anna Forsby and Bas Blaauboer

CONTENTS

INTRODUCTION

Classical toxicological risk assessment is based on quantification of acute, subchronic, or chronic toxic doses to animals, which can be expressed as, for example, the dose generating 50% lethality in a population (LD_{50}), lowest observed effect dose (LOED), or no observed effect dose (NOED). A number of safety factors are then used in order to extrapolate these doses to the human situation and to establish safety standards for human exposure. However, the increasing number of chemicals and the public criticism toward the use of animal experimentation have contributed to the development of cell test systems for toxicological risk assessment. The drawbacks of such systems are that results obtained are not easily extrapolated to the intact organism: concentrations are determined (not dose), and generally there is a lack of biotransformation and kinetic considerations. Furthermore, *in vitro* assays have been developed to measure general cytotoxicity, rather than on mechanisms of importance *in vivo*. It is therefore necessary to find a strategy by which cellular toxic concentrations determined *in vitro* can be "converted" to doses that are relevant for risk assessment. One approach is to integrate the *in vitro* data with computer-based biokinetic models.

THE STEPWISE APPROACH FOR INTEGRATED TESTING

To be able to construct a biokinetic model it is necessary to determine relevant parameters on physiological characteristics of an organism and physicochemical characteristics of the compounds. The integrated approach for assessing toxicity can be performed in a stepwise procedure.

1. Model building on the basis of nonanimal data by determination of:
   - Physicochemical properties, e.g., lipophilicity and protein binding, from which blood–tissue partition, air–blood partition can be estimated
   - Parameters in cell culture systems, e.g., biotransformation, passage over cell layers with barrier functions.
2. Validation of the biokinetic model by comparison with known *in vivo* data.
3. If necessary, improve or construct the biokinetic model by using *in vivo* data. This should be done by extrapolation of data from nontoxic doses.
4. Use *in vitro* assays to determine dynamic data for:
   - (Aspecific) cytotoxicity
   - Tissue-specific toxicity
   - Relevant concentrations for functional cellular disorders, e.g., the concentrations giving 20% effect (EC_{20}). These concentrations are then used as response surrogates (target tissue levels) at given doses (i.e., LOEDs).
5. Integrate kinetic and dynamic data to find relevant critical tissue concentration–effect relationships.
6. Predict surrogate doses resulting in *in vivo* effects.
7. Evaluate results by comparing with known *in vivo* data.

THE ECITTS PROJECT

In 1991, the European Research Group for Alternatives in Toxicity Testing (ERGATT) initiated an interlaboratory project in association with the Swedish Board for Laboratory Animals (Centrala Försöksdjursnämnden, CFN). The project was called the ERGATT/CFN Integrated Toxicity Testing Scheme (ECITTS), and its aim was to investigate the possibility of estimating toxic doses from *in vitro* toxicity data, which were integrated with computer-based biokinetic models (Walum et al., 1991). A prevalidation study was constructed on the basis of three fundamental sections of building blocks. First, experimental data for biokinetic models, as well as cytotoxicity and target toxicity data, were determined; second, physiologically based biokinetics, target tissue concentrations, toxicological response, and systemic toxicity were modeled; and, third, the model was validated against *in vivo* kinetics and *in vivo* toxicity parameters (Figure 5.1).

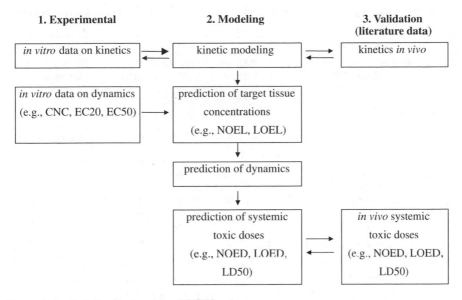

1. Experimental

2. Modeling

3. Validation
(literature data)

| *in vitro* data on kinetics | ⟷ | kinetic modeling | ⟵ | kinetics *in vivo* |

in vitro data on dynamics
(e.g., CNC, EC20, EC50) →

prediction of target tissue
concentrations
(e.g., NOEL, LOEL)

prediction of dynamics

prediction of systemic
toxic doses
(e.g., NOED, LOED,
LD50) →

in vivo systemic
toxic doses
⟵ (e.g., NOED, LOED,
LD50)

Figure 5.1 Building blocks of the ECITTS scheme.

Compounds and Test Battery

Eight well-characterized test compounds, which possess activity in the central or peripheral nervous systems, were selected. These were acrylamide, caffeine, diazepam, n-hexane/2,5-hexanedione, lindane, parathion/paraoxon, phenytoin, and toluene. An *in vitro* test battery with general and neurospecific endpoints was designed in order to cover endpoints for basal cytotoxicity, morphology, physiology, and neurochemistry (Walum et al., 1993; Forsby et al., 1995).

The human neuroblastoma cell line SH-SY5Y has been used extensively as a model for sympathetic ganglion cells (Ross et al., 1980) and was chosen for these studies. The cells can be further differentiated when cultured in serum-free medium with retinoic acid (N2-RA), which induces the cells to develop an extensive network of neurites (Påhlman et al., 1984) (Figure 5.2). Furthermore, the excitability and

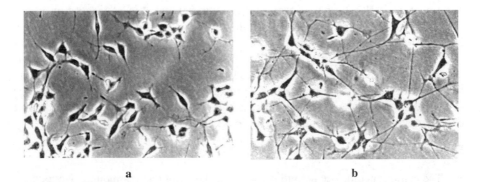

a   b

Figure 5.2 (a) Native and (b) retinoic acid-differentiated SH-SY5Y cells.

Table 5.1   **Endpoints Studied in the** *in Vitro* **Neurotoxicity Test Battery for the ECITTS Project**

Endpoint	Assay	Toxicity level
Cytotoxicity/Inhibition of cell growth	Total cellular protein content	Basal cytotoxicity
Neurite degeneration (ND)	Number of neurites per cell	Morphology
Protein synthesis rate (PSR)	[^{3}H] leucine incorporation in proteins during 2 hr	Physiology
Basal intracellular free Ca^{2+} concentration (basal Ca^{2+})	Fura-2/Ca^{2+}, fluorescence	Physiology
Voltage operated Ca^{2+} channels (VOCC)	High potassium-induced Ca^{2+} flux, fluorescence	Neurochemistry
Phospholipase C-coupled acetylcholine receptor signal transduction (mAChR peak)	Carbachol-activated, immediate transient Ca^{2+} peak, fluorescence	Neurochemistry
Acetylcholine-induced capacitive Ca^{2+} entry (mAChR plateau)	Carbachol-activated, secondary Ca^{2+} plateau, fluorescence	Neurochemistry

receptor functions are enhanced. Hence, the cells were cultured in N2-RA for 72 hr before the 72 hr of exposure with the test compounds. After exposure, the effects on several endpoints were investigated and EC_{20} values were estimated. The endpoints and the assays used for the study are listed in Table 5.1.

Critical neurotoxic concentrations (CNCs) were defined as the EC_{20} value determined in the most sensitive endpoint for each compound. The CNCs were hypothesized to mimic the toxic target tissue concentrations at the lowest observed effect levels (LOELs). The CNCs for each compound were integrated with computer-based biokinetic models for rats, and acute and subchronic LOEDs were estimated. For acrylamide the study was extended by integrating the EC_{20} value reflecting lowest basal cytotoxicity as determined by total cellular protein content (see Table 5.1), in order to estimate the LOED for acute, nonlethal systemic toxicity. It has previously been suggested that slightly cytotoxic concentrations, determined after 24 hr of exposure, are good surrogates for acute toxic blood concentration in man 4 hr after exposure to a dose that gives mild to moderate intoxication (Walum et al., 1990). Time-dependent neurite degeneration was also determined for acrylamide for estimation of subchronic LOEDs after different exposure times (DeJongh et al., 1999). To estimate lindane-induced subchronic LOED for convulsions, which occur at considerably higher doses than the LOED for learning deficiencies (Desi, 1974), additional data (EC_{20}) on increased intracellular free calcium concentration in the cells after 72 hr of exposure were integrated in the model for lindane. Furthermore, in order to study the correlation between basal cytotoxicity data and acute lethal toxicity *in vivo* (LD_{50}) for lindane, EC_{50} from the protein determination was used as the basis for the evaluation. Ekwall and coworkers have shown that EC_{50} values for cytotoxicity, i.e., inhibition of cell growth and/or cell death determined after several cell cycles in unaffected cells, are good surrogates for lethal blood peak concentrations in humans after acute exposure (Ekwall et al., 1998).

Results

The cellular neurotoxic activities for six of the eight test compounds were determined after 72 hr of exposure. The CNCs and the additional EC_{20} and EC_{50} values

Table 5.2   Effects of the Test Compounds, Determined in Differentiated Human Neuroblastoma SH-SY5Y Cells, on *in Vitro* Endpoints as Presented in Table 5.1

Compound	*In vitro* effect	Concentration (µM or µM/hr)
Acrylamide	20% cytotoxicity	920
Acrylamide	CNC; neurite degeneration/time	11
Caffeine	CNC; inhibition of VOCC	10
Diazepam	CNC; inhibition of VOCC	49
Lindane	CNC; inhibition of VOCC	3.4
Lindane	20% increased basal $[Ca^{2+}]_i$	35
Lindane	50% cytotoxicity	150
Parathion/paraoxon	CNC; neurite degeneration/time	0.5
Phenytoin	CNC; inhibition of protein synthesis	87

CNC, critical cellular neurotoxic concentration; VOCC, voltage operated calcium channels.

that were used as LOEL surrogates are given in Table 5.2. Toluene and n-hexane could not be tested in the present battery due to technical obstacles such as volatility and reaction with the plastic used for the cell cultures. Nevertheless, a successful simulation of toluene kinetics was determined (DeJongh and Blaauboer, 1996).

Integration of the *in vitro* data with the biokinetic model showed that there was a very good correlation between estimated and experimental toxic doses for most compounds (Figure 5.3). However, the correlation between estimated and experimental LOED for diazepam differed about 10,000 times. The reason was that the cellular mechanism (GABA$_A$ receptor activation), most probably underlying the experimental *in vivo* effect (time to emerge) after acute LOED exposure (Schulz and Feuer 1986), was not included in our neurotoxicity test battery. However, when literature *in vitro* data on diazepam-activated GABA$_A$ receptor function were integrated with the biokinetic model, an acceptable estimation of LOED (0.09 mg/kg) as compared to experimental LOED (0.01 mg/kg), was obtained (Blaauboer et al., 2000).

CONCLUSIONS AND FUTURE PERSPECTIVES

The prevalidation study showed that it is possible to estimate LOEDs and LD$_{50}$s by integrating *in vitro* derived toxicity data with computer-based biokinetic modeling. However, there are some remarks that have to be considered.

Refinement of the Neurotoxicity Test Battery

The results of diazepam indicated that the *in vivo* endpoints are dependent on relevant *in vitro* endpoints, which describe the molecular mechanisms of the compounds. Thus, the neurotoxicity test battery, which can be designed as a tiered stepwise test strategy, should consist of a fixed part for estimation of a specific systemic toxicity (basal cytotoxicity), physiology (for instance, energy metabolism and basal intracellular Ca^{2+} concentrations), and possibly axonopathy (neurite degeneration). The second part (neurochemistry) should be flexible and individually

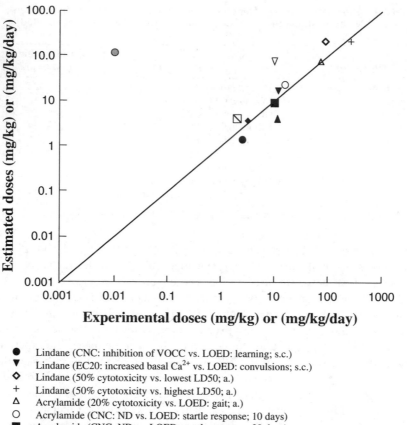

Lindane (CNC: inhibition of VOCC vs. LOED: learning; s.c.)
Lindane (EC20: increased basal Ca^{2+} vs. LOED: convulsions; s.c.)
Lindane (50% cytotoxicity vs. lowest LD50; a.)
Lindane (50% cytotoxicity vs. highest LD50; a.)
Acrylamide (20% cytotoxicity vs. LOED: gait; a.)
Acrylamide (CNC: ND vs. LOED: startle response; 10 days)
Acrylamide (CNC: ND vs. LOED: startle response; 30 days)
Acrylamide (CNC: ND vs. LOED: startle response; 90 days)
Caffeine (CNC: inhibited VOCC vs. LOED: anti-nociception; a.)
Diazepam (CNC: inhibited VOCC vs. LOED: time to emerge; a.)
Phenytoin (CNC: inhibition of PSR vs. operant learning; a.)
Parathion/paraoxon (CNC of paraoxon: ND vs. LOED: tail-pinch response of parathion; a.)

Figure 5.3   Estimated versus experimental doses after (a) acute and/or (s.c.) subchronic
exposure. See Table 5.1 for endpoint definitions. The line represents the identity.

designed for different classes of compounds. The specific endpoints should be chosen
based on knowledge about toxicological mechanisms of related compounds. *In vivo*
data, human data, and knowledge about structure-activity relationships will be useful.

Different Exposure Times

The neurotoxic activities should be determined after various exposure times *in
vitro*. Determination of acrylamide-induced degeneration of neurites over time markedly improved the estimation of neurotoxicity after subchronic exposure (DeJongh
et al., 1999). Furthermore, neurochemical properties may be different after short-
term (minutes) as compared to long-term (days) exposure.

In conclusion, the ECITTS prevalidation study indicated that the strategy of using cellular *in vitro* methods integrated with computer-based biokinetic modeling can be a powerful tool for risk assessment. However, general as well as specific toxicological mechanisms must be considered for the design of test batteries. The results of the project also revealed that it is possible to build computer-based biokinetic models on *in vitro* data for the rat. In extension, computer-based biokinetic models of humans can be constructed when *in vitro* methods for determination of human metabolism, blood–brain barrier, partition coefficients, etc. are available. One general problem of validation is the limited amount of reliable human toxicity data, which makes it difficult to validate alternative tests for a larger set of test compounds. Nevertheless, our studies have shown that alternatives can estimate toxic doses with the same quality as traditional animal tests.

ACKNOWLEDGMENTS

This investigation was financed by grants from the European Center for Validation of Alternative Methods (ECVAM) and the Swedish Board for Laboratory Animals (CFN). We thank all participants in the ECITTS project for valuable contribution to the biokinetic model and scientific discussions.

REFERENCES

Blaauboer, B.J., Forsby, A., Houston, B.J., Beckman, M., Combes, R., and DeJongh, J. (2000) An integrated approach to the prediction of systemic toxicity using computer-based biokinetic models and biological *in vitro* test methods, in *Progress in the Reduction Refinement and Replacement of Animal Experimentation,* Balls, M., van Zeller, A.-M., and Halder, M.E., Eds., Elsevier, Amsterdam.

DeJongh, J. and Blaauboer, B.J. (1996) Simulation of toluene kinetics in the rat by a physiologically based pharmacokinetic model with application of biotranformation parameters derived independently *in vitro* and *in vivo, Fund. Appl. Toxicol.,* 32, 260–268.

DeJongh, J., Nordin-Andersson, M., Ploeger, B.A., and Forsby, A. (1999) Estimation of systemic toxicity of acrylamide by integration of *in vitro* toxicity data with kinetic simulations, *Toxicol. Appl. Pharmacol.,* 158, 261–268.

Desi, I. (1974) Neurotoxicological effect of small quantities of lindane, *Int. Arch. Arbeitsmed.,* 33, 153–162.

Ekwall, B., Barile, F., Castano, A., Clemedson, C., Clothier, R., Dierickx, P., Ekwall, B.A., Ferro, M., Fiskesjö, G., Garza-Ocañas, L., Gómez-Lechón, M.J., Gülden, M., Hall, T., Isomaa, B., Kahru, A., Kerzman, G., Kristen, U., Kunimoto, M., Kärenlampi, S., Lewan, L., Loukianov, A., Ohno, T., Persoone, G., Romert, L., Sawyer, T.W., Shrivastava, R., Segner, H., Stammati, A., Tanaka, N., Valentino, M., Walum, E., and Zucco, F. (1998) MEIC Evaluation of acute systemic toxicity. VI. The prediction of human toxicity by rodent LD50 values and results from 61 *in vitro* methods, *Alt. Lab. Anim.,* 26, 617–658.

Forsby, A., Pilli, F., Bianchi, V., and Walum, E. (1995) Determinations of critical cellular neurotoxic concentrations in human neuroblastoma (SH-SY5Y) cell cultures, *Alt. Lab. Anim.,* 23, 800–811.

Påhlman, S., Ruusala, A.I., Abrahamsson, L., Mattsson, M.E.K., and Esscher, T. (1984) Retinoic acid-induced differentiation of cultured human neuroblastoma cells: a comparison with phorbol ester-induced differentiation, *Cell Differentiation*, 14, 135–144.

Ross, R.A., Hyub Joh, T., Reis, D.J., Spengler, B., and Biedler, J. (1980) Neurotransmitter-synthesizing enzymes in human neuroblastoma cells: relationship to morphological diversity, in *Advances in Neuroblastoma Research*, Evans, A.E., Ed., Raven Press, New York, pp. 151–160.

Schulz, H. and Feuer, L. (1986) Anticonflict properties of the dipeptide Litoralon and of diazepam in rats, *Acta Physiol. Hung.*, 67, 331–338.

Walum, E., Gómez-Lechón, M.J., Hellberg, S., and Ekwall, B. (1990) Presentation of some pertinent data from the recent evaluation of acute, sublethal toxicity for the first 10 MEIC chemicals, *MEIC Newsletter*, 2, 1–4.

Walum, E., Balls, M., Bianchi, V., Blaauboer, B., Bolcsfoldi, G., Guillouzo, A., Moore, G.A., Odland, L., Reinhardt, C., and Spielmann, H. (1991) ECITTS: an integrated approach to the application of *in vitro* test systems to the hazard assassment of chemicals, *Alt. Lab. Anim.*, 20, 406–428.

Walum, E., Nordin, M., Beckman, M., and Odland, L. (1993) Cellular methods for identification of neurotoxic chemicals and estimation of neurotoxicological risk, *Toxicol. In Vitro*, 7, 321–326.

CHAPTER 6

Summary of the OECD's New Guidance Document on the Recognition, Assessment, and Use of Clinical Signs as Humane Endpoints for Experimental Animals Used in Safety Evaluation

Errol Zeiger

CONTENTS

INTRODUCTION

In November 2000, the Organization for Economic Cooperation and Development (OECD) released its new guidance document, "Recognition, Assessment and Use of Clinical Signs as Humane Endpoints for Experimental Animals Used in

Safety Evaluation" (OECD, 2000). This consensus document was developed for use with the OECD's existing and future health effects test guidelines, and as guidance to laboratory researchers, in general. It is also intended to provide international harmonization on the use of humane endpoints in testing and research.

Humane endpoints are defined as the earliest indicators in an animal of severe pain, distress, suffering, or impending death. The guidance document defines these terms and addresses the concept of refinement of animal testing (i.e., the minimizing of pain, distress, and suffering) through the use of humane endpoints. The need for careful design and monitoring of experiments, as well as expert judgment in the application of humane endpoints, is emphasized. The goal of the experimenter should be to use humane endpoints to minimize pain, distress, or suffering to the extent possible without compromising the scientific objectives of the experiment.

The document provides guidance on the humane conduct of specific types of toxicity tests, including acute and long-term tests, and on the recognition of clinical signs. The annexes to the document contain an extensive listing and description of clinical signs that should be considered as indicators of pain or distress or impending death and information on how to determine whether the earliest possible clinical endpoints have been addressed. There also is a one-page annex to the document that is designed to be displayed in animal rooms that addresses the recognition and management of clinical signs.

The following description of the OECD guidance document is not designed to replace or substitute for the document, but to briefly summarize its philosophy and content. As a result, this article quotes extensively from the guidance document.

DEVELOPMENT OF THE GUIDANCE DOCUMENT

Current OECD health effects test guidelines contain a general statement that animals that are moribund or obviously in pain and showing signs of severe and enduring distress should be humanely killed. In 1994, an *ad hoc* working group was formed to develop an OECD guidance document that would provide guidance and criteria for determining when an animal is in a moribund condition, expected to become moribund, or experiencing significant pain and distress, and should therefore be euthanized for humane reasons.

This guidance document applies the principles of the three Rs (replacement, reduction, refinement) to the use of animals in regulatory toxicity tests. It specifically addresses refinement and the principles of humane experimentation that are applicable to all mammalian toxicology studies. It is generally accepted that there are differences among species in many signs of pain or distress. However, variables due to the type of study being performed, the types of materials being tested, and the species and strain of animal involved are not addressed in detail. Although there are a number of similarities between mammals and other vertebrate species, the differences among the different families do not allow them to be easily addressed in a single document. The general principles presented are based on studies with rats and mice but are applicable for all mammalian species used in toxicity testing and experimental studies. The guidance document was not designed to address nonmammalian animal studies.

In addition to providing general guidance on the recognition of humane endpoints, the document also includes four annexes.

Annex 1 presents the list of expert participants who initially drafted this document in November 1998.

Annex 2 provides a list of questions to help determine whether earliest possible humane endpoints have been sought.

Annex 3 provides a list of common conditions and clinical signs, and their descriptions, that may indicate that an animal is experiencing pain or distress. The list is primarily based on observations in rats and mice, but many of the signs also apply to other mammals used in toxicity testing. The indications described in this annex are not sufficient, in themselves, for humane killing. Additional factors have to be considered. It is also recognized that many of these signs are highly objective, and different diagnoses and conclusions may be reached by different investigators.

Annex 4 is designed for display in animal rooms and facilities. It summarizes the clinical signs and conditions of animals requiring action by animal care staff and study directors and provides guidance as to what those actions should be.

This guidance document is intended to be flexible so that it can change with improved knowledge in the future. It is expected that with increasing knowledge and experience, investigators in animal research will be able to identify more specific, early humane endpoints in the form of clinical signs of impending death or severe pain and distress.

DEFINITIONS

A *humane endpoint* is defined as the earliest indicator in an animal experiment of severe pain, severe distress, suffering, or impending death.

The purpose of the application of humane endpoints to toxicology studies is to be able to accurately predict severe pain, severe distress, suffering, or impending death before the animal experiences them. Unfortunately, the science of toxicology is not yet to the point where such accurate predictions can be made prior to the onset of severe pain and distress. However, it is possible to identify pain, distress, or suffering very early after their onset by careful observation and clinical examination of animals being tested. The adverse conditions causing these symptoms should be minimized or eliminated, either by humanely killing the animal or, in long-term studies, by temporary termination, modification, or reduction of exposure. It is recognized, however, that different animal species and animals at different stages of development may respond differently to similar test conditions and exhibit different indications of distress.

Pain is defined as an unpleasant sensory and emotional experience associated with actual or potential tissue damage or described in terms of such damage. Objective signs of pain can include vocalization, evidence of infection, aversion or avoidance by active withdrawal from stimuli, guarding affected body parts, self-mutilation, or reduced food intake.

There are three general categories of pain:

- Acute nociceptive pain: the pain response evoked by a brief noxious stimulus that produces no tissue damage. This form of pain is not regarded as severe.
- Persistent (chronic) inflammatory pain: the pain resulting from tissue damage lasting for the duration of the damage or the ensuing inflammatory process, which may persist after the local damage has healed. This type of pain may be severe or distressing, particularly if it is long lasting or permanent.
- Neuropathic pain: pain as a result of compromised function or abnormal activation of the peripheral or central nervous system. Neuropathic pain is always considered to be severe and distressing pain.

Distress is defined as an aversive state resulting from maladaption or inability to adapt to stressors. Physical or behavioral alterations may be signs of stress. The major stressors associated with distress are situations that may give rise to marked pain, fear, or anxiety. Retreat to the corner of the cage or excessive struggling or vocalizing on dosing are examples of distress in anticipation of an experimental procedure.

Suffering is defined as a negative emotional state that (in humans) is produced by persistent pain and/or distress. If something is known to cause pain or suffering in humans, it is assumed to cause suffering in animals, in the absence of evidence to the contrary.

The guidance document recognizes three levels of response that could be included under the category of *death:*

- Predictable death: the presence of clinical signs indicative of death before the planned end of the experiment.
- Impending death: when a moribund state or death is expected, based on clinical signs, prior to the next planned time of observation.
- Moribund state: when the animal is in state of dying, or will be unable to survive, even if treated.

GUIDING PRINCIPLES

Briefly, the guiding principles with respect to the use of humane endpoints include the following:

- There is strong scientific evidence that pain and distress are present in animals in comparable situations as they occur in humans.
- Severe pain, suffering, and death are to be avoided as test endpoints.
- Studies must be designed to minimize pain, distress, or suffering experienced by the animals, consistent with the scientific objective of the study.
- The earliest possible endpoints that are indicators of distress, severe pain, or impending death that could be used as indications for humanely killing the animals should be determined prior to the animals' reaching a moribund state.

- Studies should be terminated prior to their anticipated termination time if the objectives of the study have been satisfied or if it is obvious that they will not be achieved.
- Studies should build on information about the substance to be tested. This enables better prediction of the likely signs and timing of adverse effects and allows the incorporation of these adverse effects into the protocol and standard operating procedures (SOPs).
- The successful application of humane endpoints is dependent on the involvement of all members of the study team, who should be adequately trained and aware of their individual roles and responsibilities.
- Study directors and the other responsible individuals should be free to exercise professional judgment in the design and conduct of the experiments.
- Conditions under which interventions should be made to alleviate pain and distress by humane killing, as well as the individuals who are adequately trained and authorized to kill the animals, should be clearly defined.
- All aspects of animal studies should be subject to an ethical review process.

All decisions related to the application of humane endpoints should be made by the study director or designated responsible person, after consultation with the team of experts, which includes the principal investigator, the veterinarian, and an experienced animal technician. The study protocol should clearly define the conditions under which it is necessary to immediately and humanely kill an animal. The goal of the experimenter should be to use humane endpoints to minimize pain, distress, or suffering, to the extent possible, without compromising the scientific objectives of the experiment.

INITIAL CONSIDERATIONS IN THE DESIGN OF ANIMAL EXPERIMENTS

In order to meet the intended objectives of the experiment while minimizing pain, distress, and suffering, it is essential to collect as much information as possible about the substance to be tested prior to designing the experiment. Such information can include the following:

- Literature searches for studies using the test substance or related substances
- Physicochemical parameters
- Molecular modeling
- Results from *in vitro* or prior *in vivo* tests
- Statistical determinations to identify the fewest number of animals and doses that can be used without compromising the objectives of the study

This preliminary information can serve many purposes. It can help to define the objectives of the test, determine whether the results would duplicate previous work, select the most appropriate species, determine how best to design the protocol to satisfy the objectives, identify potential clinical signs and estimate the timing and duration of their occurrences, and determine any special training needed by personnel involved in the conduct of the study.

Preliminary range-finding studies are often used to determine the appropriate dose range or limit dose to use in an experiment. The dose-range study should also be used to obtain data that can provide information useful to the identification of early endpoints as indicators of severe pain or distress that could then be used in the decision to either complete the study, to terminate the study before the animals experience severe pain or suffering, or to determine whether analgesia or anesthesia will be needed and can be used. When the study is performed, it should use only the minimum number of animals consistent with the objectives of the study.

RECOGNITION AND ASSESSMENT OF PAIN, DISTRESS, AND SUFFERING AS AN APPROACH TO DETECTING CLINICAL SIGNS AND ABNORMAL CONDITIONS

The principal investigator and the responsible committees (e.g., animal care and use, ethics) have the obligation for assuring that all individuals involved in a study have the necessary expertise and training to be able to assess the animal's physiology, behavior, and appearance and to determine whether they are, or will be, experiencing pain or suffering. In order to recognize clinical signs of pain and distress, the observer must be familiar with the characteristics of the animal species used in a study. This is important because some species may not show obvious physical or behavioral changes even when in severe pain and/or distress. Awareness of clinical signs and conditions and the ability to identify them increases the likelihood of their accurate and timely detection. (See Table 6.1 for some common conditions and clinical signs.)

Careful and regular observation and examination of the animals being tested is essential for the detection of clinical signs and abnormal conditions. The types and frequency of the observations will depend on the type of study being performed, the species, whether any previous effects have been observed, the timing and nature of anticipated toxic effects, and the objectives of the study. Such observations and measurements can also be important indicators of the condition of the animal and can be used to determine whether the condition is irreversible and therefore an indication of impending death. In addition, postmortem examination can be helpful to relate postmortem findings to previous clinical signs. If the animal is experiencing severe pain or distress, the study director must determine whether further information useful for the purposes of the study is likely to be obtained from that animal. If not, then the animal should be humanely killed.

There are a number of effects to be considered in the adequate evaluation of an animal to determine its condition and whether there might be evidence of pain or distress. These include the following:

- Changes in physical appearance, and other clinical signs. A list of commonly observed clinical signs and conditions is provided as Annex 3 to the document. This list is not inclusive. Each study could have its own standard list of clinical signs that might be observed for that particular type of study and that are appropriate for the species used.
- Behavioral changes in response to external stimuli (e.g., excitability, righting reflex), appearance, posture, grooming patterns, and activity levels.

Table 6.1 Common Conditions and Clinical Signs

Abdominal rigidity	Discharge, abnormal	Pinna reflex
Abortion	Dyspnea (difficult breathing)	Prostrate
Agalactia	Epistaxis (nasal bleeding)	Pruritis
Anemia	Excitable	Pupillary
Analgesia	Eyelid closure	constriction/dilation
Anuria	Eyes fixed/sunken	Rales, pulmonary
Apathy	Fractured bone	Rectal prolapse
Ataxia/incoordination	Gasping	Recumbency, prolonged
Bleeding	Grooming—failure to do	Red eye(s)/nose
Blepharospasm	Hunched/stiff posture	Reflexes
Blood in feces or urine	Hyperreflexia	Retention of feces
Blood around nose, eyes	Immobile/inactive	Righting reflex
Boarded abdomen	Jaundice (icterus)	Salivation, excessive or
Body temperature, abnormal	Joints swollen	abnormal
Body weight loss or	Kyphosis	Seizures
emaciation	Lateral position	Self-mutilation
Breathing difficulties	Limping/lameness	Skin bruising/color/crepitus
(Dyspnea)	Locomotory behavior	Spasm
Cachexia	Lordosis	Staggering
Chewing, persistent	Loss of condition, body	Sunken flanks
Chromodachryorrhea	muscle	Suppuration
Circling	Mammary gland	Swellings
Comatose	abnormalities	Tenesmus
Compulsive behavior	Moribund	Tetany
Constipation	Motor excitation	Tremor
Convulsions	Not eating/drinking	Urine retention
Corneal ulceration	Oedema	Vaginal prolapse
Coughing/sneezing	Pale mucous membranes	Vocalization
Cyanosis	Paralysis	Vomiting
Dehydration	Paresis	
Diarrhea	Piloerection	

- Changes in body weight (specifically, weight loss) and related changes in food and water consumption.
- Changes in clinical parameters (e.g., body temperature, heart and respiration rate, clinical chemistry and hematology).

These parameters can serve as indicators of a deteriorating clinical condition of an animal.

MAKING AN INFORMED DECISION TO HUMANELY KILL ANIMALS

Impending death and moribund condition are criteria for humane killing to avoid unnecessary pain or distress that the animal may be experiencing at the present or in the future. Impending death or moribund condition is indicated by various clinical signs and objective measurements. A lesser degree of severity of these signs and measurements may also be useful indicators. The signs and conditions of impending death typically include one or more of the following:

- Prolonged, impaired ambulation preventing the animal from reaching food or water, or prolonged anorexia
- Excessive weight loss or extreme emaciation or severe dehydration

- Significant blood loss
- Evidence to suggest irreversible organ failure
- Prolonged absence of voluntary responses to external stimuli
- Persistent, difficult, labored breathing
- Prolonged inability to remain upright
- Persistent convulsions
- Self-mutilation
- Prolonged diarrhea
- Significant and sustained decrease in body temperature
- Substantial tumors

Animal-care staff must be adequately trained for each type of toxicity study so that they can differentiate between clinical signs indicative of a moribund condition and similar clinical signs that may be transient effects from acute dosing procedures.

SEVERE PAIN AND DISTRESS AS CRITERIA FOR HUMANE KILLING

The following clinical signs may indicate that an animal is experiencing significant pain and distress. Pain and distress should be alleviated with appropriate treatment if it does not interfere with the conduct or the objectives of the study. Consideration should be given to humane killing of the animal if any of the following are present:

- Abnormal vocalization
- Abnormal aggressiveness
- Abnormal posture
- Abnormal reaction to handling
- Abnormal movements or reluctance to move
- Self-induced trauma
- Difficulties in respiration
- Bone fractures, open wounds, significant bleeding, corneal or skin ulceration
- Abnormal external appearance
- Rapid weight loss, emaciation, or severe dehydration
- Any other factor(s) that suggests that the animal may be in pain or distress

A short list of severe signs and conditions that are indicators that the well being of an experimental animal may be compromised is provided in Annex 4 of the document. That annex is designed for use in animal rooms and facilities as a guide to alert the staff to clinical signs that require discussion or action. The decision to humanely kill the animal must be made with appropriate clinical judgment, taking into account the severity of the condition, the amount of pain or distress, the prognosis, and the potential loss of valuable data. Ideally, maximum achievable information should be obtained from every animal used, while limiting pain and distress to an absolute minimum.

Animal tests require a team approach and include those responsible for ethical review. Study directors should work with and coordinate staff to establish the time and frequency of observations, how and when invasive measurements are to be made, and SOPs for identifying, documenting, and reporting of clinical signs. The animal care technician will generally be the first to observe the clinical signs and should bring this information to the attention of the attending veterinarian and the designated responsible person, usually the study director. Experiments should not be allowed to proceed longer than is necessary to achieve the purpose of the study.

GUIDANCE ON THE HUMANE CONDUCT OF SPECIFIC TYPES OF TOXICITY TESTING

This section of the guidance document briefly describes the protocols for a number of short- and long-term toxicology studies and identifies potential areas of pain and distress and approaches to relieving this distress without compromising the purpose of the testing. The assays addressed are acute single dose studies, ocular irritation studies, systemic repeated-dose studies, reproductive toxicity studies, sensitization studies, and chronic toxicity and carcinogenicity studies.

REFERENCE

OECD, Guidance Document 19, Guidance Document on the Recognition, Assessment and Use of Clinical Signs as Humane Endpoints for Experimental Animals Used in Safety Evaluation, Paris, November 2000, url: http://www1.oecd.org/ehs/test/monos.htm.

CHAPTER 7

Pain and Distress Management in Animal Research and Testing: The Humane Society of the United States Pain and Distress Initiative*

Martin L. Stephens, Francine Dolins, Lori Donley, Adrienne M. Navarro, Kathleen M. Conlee, and Andrew N. Rowan

CONTENTS

* This chapter is adapted from Animal Welfare Perspectives on Pain and Distress Management in Research and Testing, *MSMR News,* Spring 1999, Massachusetts Society for Medical Research, North Chelmsford, MA.

INTRODUCTION

The public's perception that animals suffer in biomedical research and testing is a key factor fueling the controversy over animal experimentation. This public concern has brought about laws and regulations that specifically address laboratory animal pain and distress and call for efforts to limit or at least report when animal pain and distress occur. However, the identification and management of pain and distress in research animals are complex issues that have received insufficient attention to date. To address the gaps in our knowledge of pain and distress, and to promote laboratory animal welfare, The Humane Society of the United States (HSUS) has launched an initiative to eliminate significant pain and distress in laboratory animals by the year 2020 by working with Institutional Animal Care and Use Committees (IACUCs) and scientists. While this is an ambitious goal, it is arguably within the ingenuity and skills of those who use and care for laboratory animals and the scope and responsibility of the scientific community. More importantly, while not widely recognized outside the research community, most scientists and laboratory personnel support efforts to minimize pain and distress in laboratory animals.

PUBLIC CONCERN ABOUT PAIN AND DISTRESS IN RESEARCH

Polls and surveys have begun to document the influence of animal suffering on people's views toward animal research. The results of a 2001 poll commissioned by The HSUS indicate that public approval of animal research varies dramatically according to the amount of pain and distress that the animals experience. Sixty-two percent of Americans approve of animal research when little or no pain and distress are experienced, but this approval drops to 21% when the pain and distress are severe. A poll commissioned by the *New Scientist* (Aldous et al., 1999) found that the British public's support for research on mice or monkeys declines 16% to 35% (depending on the species and field of research) when the animals are subjected to pain, illness, or surgery. In another survey, Plous (1996a,b) canvassed professional psychologists and psychology students in the U.S. and found that support for research involving "pain or death" is approximately 40% lower than for studies simply involving confinement (the influence of pain and death were not analyzed separately). Finally, a survey carried out in the U.S. in the mid-1980s (Foundation for Biomedical Research, 1985) asked if participants agreed or disagreed with the statement that "most animals used in research suffer more pain and distress than they should." The respondents supported this statement by a five to one margin. Not surprisingly, when the same survey asked participants whether the government should impose regulations "to reduce or eliminate pain and suffering," 74% of the public and 81% of students said yes.

In the U.S., the IACUC system is specifically charged with reducing the likely pain and distress that animals may experience when used in research. Thus, IACUCs are required by Animal Welfare Act (AWA) regulations to ensure that investigators have searched for alternatives to any research likely to cause animal pain and distress, even if anesthetics and analgesics are used to prevent such outcomes. By contrast, investigators do not have to demonstrate that they have considered alternatives if the research project is placed in the nonpainful/nondistressful category. The implicit message is that inflicting animal pain and distress is of greater public concern than killing the animals (euthanasia). Despite this regulatory emphasis on alleviating pain and distress, the U.S. Department of Agriculture (USDA), which enforces the AWA, provides little explicit guidance on the topic or on the potential impact of specific experimental procedures, such as infecting animals with pathogenic organisms, on pain, distress, or animal well-being generally (see USDA Policy 11, available at http://www.aphis.usda.gov/ac/policy/policy11.pdf).

THE CHALLENGE

The systematic reduction of animal pain and distress in research is a formidable task for several reasons. First, there is much conceptual confusion over such terms as pain, distress, and suffering. Second, animal use in the laboratory is quite varied; refinements developed for any one specific procedure will not necessarily translate to other procedures. Third, animal pain, distress, and suffering are not easy to recognize or measure unambiguously, even in the commonly used laboratory species, and there is considerable opportunity for legitimate disagreement over assessment and treatment (Hellyer et al., 1999). Fourth, there is limited published information about animals' experience of pain, distress, and suffering caused by typical laboratory procedures.

The use of analgesics in laboratory rodents has become generally accepted practice only in the past decade. Before that, animals typically were not given the benefit of the doubt when treating pain or distress. Even infant humans did not routinely receive anesthesia for major surgery 20 years ago (Bouwmeester et al., 1999).

While the subject of laboratory animal pain is now receiving increased attention, animal distress that is not the result of pain (e.g., fear, anxiety, or depression) is still largely overlooked, in our experience. The AWA regulations and policies do not even define "distress." However, in July 2000, the USDA published a *Federal Register* notice stating that the agency is considering defining "distress" and replacing or modifying the current pain and distress classification system. The USDA solicited comments on these issues, which are currently under review within the agency. In its submitted comments, The Humane Society of the United States (HSUS) argued that "distress" is perhaps best defined as an aversive state resulting from an inability to adapt to stressors or from maladaption (OECD, 2000). Stressors can be physiological (e.g., disease), environmental (e.g., restraint), or psychological (e.g., anxiety) (ILAR, 1992). The HSUS further emphasized that a definition should include several operational endpoints and examples of procedures that might cause distress.

Sensitive, practical measures to gauge levels of distress in common laboratory animal species do not presently exist. For the most part, animal-care staff rely on *ad hoc* observations or on relatively insensitive measures such as a weight loss to ascertain whether animals are experiencing pain or distress. If principal investigators, lab personnel, and IACUCs do not currently have the tools to document distress objectively or do not recognize distress caused by disease, toxic agents, or psychological factors, then it is unlikely that they will take meaningful action to alleviate such distress when it occurs. It is therefore essential to promote a discussion on when distress occurs and to achieve some consensus on those procedures that cause either pain or distress.

EXPERIMENTAL PROCEDURES THAT CAUSE PAIN AND DISTRESS IN RESEARCH

The animal pain and distress caused by specific research models and techniques raise serious concerns from both a scientific perspective as well as an animal welfare perspective (Russell and Burch, 1959; Fox, 1986; Flecknell, 1997). The HSUS has compiled a preliminary list of research models/areas and techniques from the perspective of pain and distress (Table 7.1). The research models are divided into two categories depending on whether the resulting distress is pain induced or non-pain induced. There are overlaps between the two categories, of course, yet the distinction serves to draw attention to the relatively neglected issue of distress in research animals. Judging from this preliminary list, an extensive array of models, research areas, and specific techniques induce distress in laboratory animals. Some do so directly, others indirectly by first inducing pain, fear, anxiety, or some other adverse state.

THE HSUS PAIN AND DISTRESS INITIATIVE

Based on data from Canada, Switzerland, and the Netherlands, The HSUS estimates that up to 25% of laboratory animals experience moderate to severe pain and distress as a result of what is done to them. Given the pervasiveness of pain and, especially, distress in animal research and testing and the challenges of eliminating animal suffering in the laboratory, The HSUS believes that a more systematic approach to pain and distress management is warranted. That it why we have launched our Pain and Distress Initiative and adopted as our goal the elimination of all significant pain and distress in animal research. Our initiative has the following four elements:

Outreach to IACUCs

In the past, the animal protection community's campaigns aimed at animal research have typically selected individual scientists or research projects as targets of protests. In the Pain and Distress Initiative, by contrast, the HSUS has invited the collaboration of the scientific community—those who will ultimately develop the techniques and implement the approaches that will make our goal attainable. Specifically, The HSUS has invited IACUCs to join in the initiative. They already have a statutory mandate to minimize pain and distress.

The HSUS began facilitating an exchange of information and policies among IACUCs so that new ideas and initiatives, including "best practices," could be disseminated quickly. Initially, The HSUS sent a series of five letters and attachments to the chairs of all IACUCs nationwide. These mailings were primarily informational

Table 7.1   Models and Areas of Research and Specific Techniques That Cause Distress

Research Models or Areas

Non-Pain-Induced Distress

Aggression	
Anxiety	(e.g., Vogel conflict-drinking model)
Cancer	(tumor burden, cachexia, carcinogenicity testing)
Depression	(e.g., learned helplessness, forced swimming, maternal deprivation)
Diabetes	
Drug addiction and withdrawal	
Environmental stress	(e.g., hot, cold)
Fear	
Immunological research	(e.g., vaccine potency testing)
Infectious disease	
Motion sickness	
Nutrition research	(e.g., nutrient deprivation)
Panic	
Pharmacology (some)	(e.g., tumor necrosis factor, capsaicin research)
Psychopathology	(other than anxiety, depression, fear, etc., mentioned above)
Radiation research	
Stress (psychological)	
Toxicology (induced effects)	
Transgenic research	

Pain-Induced Distress

Arthritis	
Burn research	
Cancer research	(tumor pain)
Chronic pain studies[1]	
Dental studies	
Inflammation studies	
Experimental surgery	(e.g., organ transplantation/rejection)
Muricide	(as a model of aggression, neophobia, etc.)
Orthopedic studies	
Trauma research	

Specific Techniques

Non-Pain-Induced and Pain-Induced Distress

Anesthesia aftereffects	
Antibody production	(polyclonal and monoclonal)
Aversive stimuli	(e.g., electric shock)
Bleeding techniques	(including retro-orbital bleeding)
Complete Freund's Adjuvant	
Control group	(animals denied experimental treatments)
Deprivation	(e.g., water, food, sleep, or social partners/experiences)
Dosing techniques	(e.g., gavage)
Granuloma techniques	
Gut loop studies	

(continued)

Table 7.1 (continued) Models and Areas of Research and Specific Techniques That Cause Distress

Knockout technology
Restraint
Surgery sequelae

[1] Acute pain should not be a problem if the guidelines of the International Association for the Study of Pain (IASP, 1979) are followed.

in nature, alerting IACUC chairs to upcoming meetings and new publications, as well as informing them about the Pain and Distress Initiative. Feedback from IACUC chairs on the first two mailings was minimal, so we included a stamped, self-addressed response card in the third. Though we heard from less than 100 out of the approximately 1,800 IACUCs, over 90% of the respondents indicated that they found the mailings helpful and wanted to continue receiving them, and over 25% took the additional step of joining in the initiative.

The HSUS eventually discontinued sending letters to IACUC chairs and, instead, created a newsletter specifically aimed at IACUCs and others in the field of laboratory animal science. In the fall of 2000, the inaugural issue of the *Pain and Distress Report* was sent to over 2,000 IACUCs and others. This newsletter provides up-to-date information regarding pain and distress in laboratory animals. The *Pain and Distress Report* includes information on policies and perspectives, resources and services, recent publications, summaries of publications found in the technical literature, upcoming conferences, pain and distress statistics, and helpful web sites. All issues of the *Pain and Distress Report* can be found at http://www.hsus.org/ace/11401.

As part of our efforts to raise the profile of pain and distress issues with IACUCs, The HSUS has begun to focus on specific research areas, practices, and techniques (such as infectious disease research) where relatively little attention has been given to animal suffering. Our aim is to seek out new approaches to recognizing, measuring, and alleviating animal distress. In our first such effort, in 1999, we held a workshop focused on toxicology research. A group of international experts addressed topics such as humane endpoints to lethality, noninvasive research techniques, and dose–volume guidelines. Information about this workshop is available at http://www.hsus.org/ace/11447. We were particularly interested in the new technology described by the Xenogen Corporation as a possible refinement and reduction in infectious disease studies. Another workshop was held in August 2002, which addressed issues in immunology research, including polyclonal antibody production, adjuvant use, welfare concerns, and possible alternatives.

Regulatory Aspects

The USDA enforces the Animal Welfare Act, which regulates animal pain and distress, while the National Institutes of Health's Office of Laboratory Animal Welfare (OLAW) enforces Public Health Service (PHS) guidelines on animal research, which include provisions against causing unnecessary animal pain and distress. As part of its responsibilities under the AWA, the USDA issues annual animal welfare enforcement reports that summarize data on the number of animals of regulated species used in research, testing, and education, grouped under column headings that correspond to the USDA's pain and distress categories. Animals used in painful or distressful experiments for which pain- or distress-relieving drugs were withheld are listed under column E. Facilities listing animal use in column E are required to describe these experiments and explain why drugs for pain and distress relief were withheld (see Stephens et al., 1998, for an analysis of these descriptions).

Unfortunately, the USDA's pain and distress classification system is out of date and in need of reform (Orlans, 1990; Stephens, 1994). When the current pain categories (column C = no pain, column D = pain relieved by drugs, and column E = pain without relief) were first introduced nearly 30 years ago, they may have served a useful purpose. However, the categories are ambiguous and incomplete, and they do not adequately address the issue of *levels* of pain and distress (the current categories boil down to a yes/no dichotomy), nor do they specifically address the issue of distress. In addition to these inherent problems with the system, the situation is further complicated by the paucity of USDA guidance to institutions on assigning protocols to categories as well as the lack of USDA oversight of institutional decisions on categorization of actual experiments. However, as previously mentioned, the USDA is currently considering replacing or modifying its pain and distress classification system.

The important issue today is how much pain and distress the animals actually experience given that some pain-relieving drugs may have been administered. A straightforward but informative system would assess the levels of pain and distress as minor, moderate, or severe. The national policies of several countries including Canada, the Netherlands, and Switzerland incorporate such systems (Canada and the Netherlands report between approximately 25% and 48% of animal use in the moderate to severe pain and/or distress categories).

The HSUS supports a proposal to adopt a similar system in the U.S. The proposal (Table 7.2) was developed in the mid-1990s by a working group consisting of representatives of academia, animal protection, and the USDA. It was originally presented to the USDA several years ago and is currently under review as the USDA considers modifications to its current scheme. The proposed new system divides pain and distress into none/minor, moderate, and severe categories (whether or not analgesics or anesthetics are used). It has some continuity with the existing one, with its heavy emphasis on pain relief, but it too has generated some criticism. In a report on "regulatory burden" (see http://grants.nih.gov/grants/policy/regulatory-burden/animalcare.htm), convened under the auspices of the NIH, the authors expressed concern about any additional administrative burden that the proposed reporting scheme would entail. Their endorsement of the current system appears to be based more on its convenience and familiarity than its merits.

In fact, the proposed system has advantages in terms of relief of regulatory burden. Researchers proposing to conduct an experiment that falls in the minor/no-pain-relief-needed category could have the requirement waived for an alternative literature search and full IACUC review. The same exemptions could also be considered for protocols in the minor/pain-relief-needed category (see Table 7.2).

The proposed new system offers a meaningful scheme for tracking a primary issue in laboratory animal welfare and in the public controversy over animal research,

Table 7.2   The USDA's Current Pain and Distress Categories and a Proposed Modification, as Well as Related Features of the Two Systems

A. Current Scheme

USDA Category	Pain and/or Distress	Anesthesia/ Analgesia	Full ACUC Review	Alternative Literature Search
C (63%)[1]	Little or None	No	Yes	No
D (29%)	Yes or No[2]	Yes	Yes	Yes
E (8%)	Yes	No	Yes	Yes

B. Proposed Scheme

Category	Pain and/or Distress	Anesthesia/ Analgesia	Full IACUC Review	Alternative Literature Search
I	Minor or None	No	No	No
II	Minor or None	Yes	Perhaps	Perhaps
III	Moderate	Yes or No	Yes	Yes
IV	Severe	Yes or No	Yes	Yes

[1] Numbers in parentheses are USDA figures for 2000.
[2] Animals listed in USDA category D were given pain- or distress-relieving drugs, but these drugs may not have been sufficient to relieve all pain and distress throughout the experiment.

namely, the levels of pain and distress actually experienced by the animals. As such, it could be used to monitor trends in pain and distress across institutions and over time and provide data for comparisons with countries with similar systems. Also, IACUCs might use the new system to gauge the intensity of their protocol review, with protocols in the severe category being assigned the most intense review.

Until the current USDA pain classification system is revised, The HSUS will seek to develop more consistency in how pain and distress are reported. In its annual reports, the USDA aggregates pain and distress data across all facilities within each state. There is considerable variation across states in the reporting of column E usage (Table 7.3). Many states repeatedly report few or no animals in column E (Table 7.4). It is possible that the numbers in Table 7.4 accurately reflect the way that animals were used. However, our analyses reveal obvious discrepancies between the types of research and publications emerging from institutions in some states, on the one hand, and their lack of reporting of animal use in column E, on the other. The HSUS has done a similar analysis of the top 50 research institutions (based on 1998 NIH funding) in the U.S. and has found that these institutions reported that less than 1% of their animals experienced unrelieved pain and/or distress for the years 1996–1998 (the most recent years for which individual facility reports are available). Given the extent of research conducted at these institutions, The HSUS believes that this percentage represents significant underreporting of pain and distress, and we have since sent a letter to each of those institutions indicating this concern. We will continue to pressure individual institutions in order to bring these issues to the forefront.

If institutions do not report animals experiencing distress in column E, then The HSUS fears that the needs of these animals are being overlooked. If the USDA data

Table 7.3   State to State Variation in Reporting Animal Use in Column E (Unalleviated Pain or Distress) for States Using Greater Than 20,000 Animals

State	Percentage of Animals in Column E	State	Percentage of Animals in Column E
Nationwide	8	Missouri	22
California	4	Nebraska	15
Delaware	15	New Jersey	6
Georgia	2	New York	11
Illinois	3	North Carolina	6
Indiana	18	Ohio	3
Iowa	28	Pennsylvania	8
Kansas	16	Texas	3
Maryland	12	Virginia	0
Massachusetts	1	Washington	20
Michigan	15	Wisconsin	9
Minnesota	3	Federal Agencies	7

Note: USDA data from 2000.

Table 7.4   States That Reported Less Than 1% of Animal Use in Column E between 1995 and 1997

Alaska	(300)	Mississippi	(2,000)	Tennessee	(10,900)
Arizona	(5,000)	Nevada	(3,000)	Utah	(4,600)
Hawaii	(500)	Oklahoma	(4,300)	Vermont	(1,100)
Kentucky	(5,300)	Oregon	(4,700)	Virginia	(19,200)
Louisiana	(16,800)	Rhode Island	(2,100)	West Virginia	(1,700)
Maine	(800)	S. Carolina	(6,100)	Wyoming	(300)

Data from the USDA. Figures in parentheses indicate the average number of animals used across all pain categories.

are to be at all useful, then better reporting guidelines should be developed. The task will not be easy, but this is no excuse for maintaining the current uninformative and inconsistent system.

In addition to our outreach to the USDA, The HSUS will encourage the NIH's OLAW to issue "best practice" guidelines covering specific techniques. The regulatory burden report mentioned above also encourages the agency to do the same. An example of such an initiative is the NIH Office of Protection from Research Risks (now OLAW) letter stating that ascites production causes animal distress and should be used only if *in vitro* production of monoclonal antibodies is unsuccessful (the text of the letter is available at http://grants.nih.gov/grants/olaw/references/dc98–01.htm).

Financial Support for Research on Pain and Distress

One of the problems in advancing our knowledge of how to assess and alleviate animal pain and distress is that there is virtually no funding to support research on this topic. Clearly there are impediments to encouraging agencies to provide funds for projects that deliberately cause animal distress, but it may be possible to piggy-back such assessments onto ongoing (and approved) investigations of other topics. The HSUS plans to urge both private and government entities to fund studies aimed at developing more sensitive and practical measures of animal distress and methods by which such distress can be alleviated. The HSUS has submitted testimony to Congress requesting that $2.5 million of the NIH's 2003 research and development budget be earmarked to identify and eliminate pain and distress in laboratory animals, with the caveat that the research be piggybacked, as previously mentioned.

Development of a Technical Report on Animal Pain and Distress

The HSUS will draft a comprehensive, detailed, and referenced report on the subject, with the help of international experts in veterinary medicine, animal behavior, physiology, neurology, anesthesiology, philosophy, and other fields. The topics covered by the report, which will be published by The HSUS, will include the following:

- Definitions of animal pain, distress, discomfort, anxiety, fear, and suffering
- Biology of pain, distress, and suffering
- Recognition and assessment of animal pain and distress: current and potential approaches
- Alleviation of animal pain and distress
- Housing issues (excluding general care and feeding)
- Pain and distress caused by specific techniques and research endpoints

The HSUS invites collaboration on the Pain and Distress Initiative from all parts of the scientific community, including investigators, animal caretakers, veterinarians, regulatory officials, funding agency representatives, and, especially, IACUCs. For more information, visit The HSUS web site at http://www.hsus.org/ace/15808.

BEST PRACTICES AND POLICIES

Many institutions and animal facilities have developed in-house policies and guidelines for conducting common animal-based procedures, such as blood collec-tion and euthanasia. One of the typical aims of these documents is to minimize any pain or distress caused to the animals. Unfortunately, many of these guidelines are available only in-house and are not disseminated to other institutions and labs through professional publications. This limits the comparison of such guidelines across institutions and the formulation of industry-wide "best practices." The HSUS encourages institutions to make their guidelines available to other institutions so that best practices can evolve more rapidly.

A preliminary review of available guidelines covering specific techniques sug-gests that there is considerable variation in standard practice among institutions. The HSUS has begun summarizing the available information on guidelines for specific techniques and encouraging a discussion of the different practices. We initiated this process with an analysis of policies on monoclonal antibody production gathered

Table 7.5 Selected Elements of Institutional Policies on Monoclonal Antibody Production Available on the World Wide Web

	Penn State	Stanford	U Iowa	U Minnesota
Monitoring subj. with solid tumors	Not specified	3×/week	Not specified	3×/week
Priming	As low as 0.1 ml pristane	Not specified	0.2 ml max pristane	0.5 ml max pristane
Number of taps	Max 3 taps, last terminal	Not specified	2 taps, last after euthanasia	Not specified
Monitoring postinoculation	Daily	3×/week for first week, then daily	Daily	Daily
Replacement fluid after ascites harvest	Not specified	Not specified	1–2 ml of saline subcutaneous	Not specified
Anesthesia during tap	Anesthesia can be used	Anesthesia used for new personnel	Not specified	Not specified

from the World Wide Web (Table 7.5). We assume each of these guidelines is effective in producing antibodies. The question is, which one causes the least pain and distress to the animals, and what can be considered to be best practice? It is clear that more interinstitutional discussion and empirical studies are needed to assist scientists and IACUCs in making a determination on this and other practices. The HSUS has conducted similar analyses for Freund's complete adjuvant, anesthesia and analgesia use, tail clipping, and blood collection techniques.

The HSUS also has begun work on comprehensive critiques of certain techniques that are likely to cause pain and distress in animals, but continue to be used in animal research. For example, we have drafted an extensive review on the use of carbon dioxide for euthanasia and anesthesia (see http://www.hsus.org/ace/11427). The review emphasizes the growing body of evidence that carbon dioxide causes more than momentary pain and distress in animals, at least under some circumstances. Additionally, carbon dioxide clearly causes pain in humans, which is relevant to the policies and regulations pertaining to animal use, such that if a procedure causes pain and/or distress in humans, it should be assumed to do so in animals. The HSUS is currently conducting a similar critique on the use of Avertin as an anesthetic in rodents. We will use such critiques to bring these issues to the attention of the laboratory animal science community and oversight agencies, in the hope that alternatives to these procedures are explored and implemented.

CONCLUSIONS

The public's support for animal use in biomedical research has declined in recent years (Plous, 1998), perhaps reflecting an increasing perception or appreciation that such research involves animal suffering (see above) and that little is being done about this suffering (see Phillips, 1994). Given the public's interest in the humane treatment of animals in laboratories, greater attention should be paid to minimizing pain and distress in research animals. The HSUS Pain and Distress Initiative seeks to encourage that effort.

We are aware that some in the animal research community distrust the HSUS and the rest of the animal protection community and that this attitude will impede progress on forging working relationships on pain and distress issues. We have deliberately developed an initiative (elimination of pain and distress) whose premises are already widely embraced by the scientific community. We therefore hope that any skeptics within the scientific community will at least support the aims of the initiative, if not The HSUS's efforts per se.

For the moment, our limited knowledge of pain and distress in laboratory animals leaves us with far more questions than answers. The need for increased knowledge of these issues is gaining further attention in the scientific community. For example, a recent editorial in *Nature* emphasizes the importance of making the science of animal suffering and cognition a higher priority (Editorial, 2002). Fortunately, there has been an increase in attention to pain and distress issues within science and academia. The result of this increased attention is a steady trickle of experimental data addressing animal distress and well being and an increase in the debate about the conceptual issues. Activities such as these will lead to greater improvements for both animals and science, and therefore should be encouraged.

ACKNOWLEDGMENTS

The authors wish to thank the Kenneth Scott Trust and the Doerenkamp-Zbinden Fund for helping to fund the HSUS Pain and Distress Initiative.

References

Aldous, P., Coghlan, A., and Copley, J. (1999) Let the people speak, *New Scientist*, 22 May.

Bouwmeester, J., van Dijk, M., and Tibboel, D. (1999) Human neonates and pain, in *Humane Endpoints in Animal Experiments for Biomedical Research,* Hendriksen, C.F.M. and Morton, D.B., Eds., Royal Society of Medicine, London, pp. 20–25.

Editorial (2002) Right, wrongs and ignorance, *Nature*, 416, 351.

Flecknell, P.A. (1997) Assessment and alleviation of post-operative pain, *AWIC Newsletter,* 8, 8–14.

Foundation for Biomedical Research (1985) Members of the American public comment on the use of animals in medical research and testing, Foundation for Biomedical Research, Washington, D.C.

Fox, M.W. (1986) *Laboratory Animal Husbandry: Ethology, Welfare and Experimental Variables,* State University of New York, Albany.

Hellyer, P.W., Frederick, C., Lacy, M., Salman, M.D., and Wagner, A.E. (1999) Attitudes of veterinary medical students, house officers, clinical faculty, and staff toward pain management in animals, *J. Am. Vet. Med. Assoc.*, 214(2), 238–244.

IASP (International Association for the Study of Pain) (1979) Report of international association for the study of pain: subcommittee on taxonomy, *Pain*, 6, 249–252.

ILAR (Institute for Laboratory Animal Resources) (1992) Recognition and Alleviation of Pain and Distress in Laboratory Animals, National Academy of Sciences, Washington, D.C.

OECD (Organization for Economic Cooperation and Development) (2000) Guidance Document on the Recognition, Assessment, and Use of Clinical Signs as Humane Endpoints for Experimental Animals Used in Safety Evaluation, OECD Environmental Health and Safety Publications Series on Testing and Assessment 19, OECD, Paris.

Orlans, B. (1990) Animal pain scales and public policy, *Alt. Lab. Anim.,* 18, 41–50.

Phillips, M.T. (1994) Savages, drunks and lab animals: the researcher's perception of pain, *Society and Animals* 1, 61–81.

Plous, S. (1996a) Attitudes toward the use of animals in psychological research and education: results from a national survey of psychologists, *Am. Psychol.,* 51, 1167–1180.

Plous, S. (1996b) Attitudes toward the use of animals in psychological research and education: results from a national survey of psychology majors, *Psychol. Sci.,* 7, 352–358.

Plous, S. (1998) Opinion research on animal experimentation: areas of support and concern, paper presented in the proceedings of Pain Management and Humane Endpoints Workshop, Washington, D.C., url: http://altweb.jhsph.edu/meetings/pain/plous.htm.

Russell, W.M.S. and Burch, R.L. (1959) *The principles of humane experimental technique,* London, Methuen.

Stephens, M.L. (1994) Request for changes in USDA regulations, in *Rabbits and Rodents: Current Research Issues,* S.N. Niemi, J.S. Venable, and H.N. Guttman, Eds., Greenbelt, MD, Scientists Center for Animal Welfare, and Washington, D.C., Working for Animals in Research, Drugs and Surgery, pp. 3–12.

Stephens, M.L., Mendoza, P., Weaver, A., and Hamilton, T. (1998) Unrelieved pain and distress in animals: an analysis of USDA data on experimental procedures, *J. Appl. Anim. Welfare Sci.,* 1(1), 15–26.

PART II

Development of Predictive Methods Based on Mechanisms of Eye Irritation at the Ocular Surface: Meeting Industry and Regulatory Needs

SHERRY L. WARD AND WILEY A. CHAMBERS

The rationale for this section is to provide the reader with an update on the most current developments in alternative methods for the evaluation of eye irritation.

This section is highlighted by the contribution from Dr. Martin Reim on the pathology and clinical features of thermal and chemical eye injuries. Dr. Reim's Chapter 9 provides insight into the basic mechanisms of chemical injury to the human eye and describes useful methods for collecting human clinical data following ocular exposure to noxious materials.

Overviews of the industry and regulatory perspectives related to the development, validation, and application of Draize eye test alternative methods are presented in Chapter 8.

A number of scientists present their research findings in Chapter 10 through 15 on the development of alternative methods that can be used to assess the eye irritation potential of chemical and product formulations. Many alternative methods have been developed. The methods selected for inclusion in this section were those that had been developed to the stage where comparative data to the Draize rabbit eye test, the reference method, were available. These methods can broadly be divided into two groups: cell-based or corneal equivalent models, and corneal organ culture models. The authors were asked to address three key points: the biological relevance of the model, the mechanistic basis for the assay of the endpoint or biomarker, and the performance of the new test method relative to the reference method.

Alternative methods for the Draize rabbit eye test have progressed both scientifically and in predictive capability over the past decade due to the increased sophistication of the biological models and the technology applied. Exploring the performance of these alternatives to the Draize test provides the framework needed to move forward into the new decade, where we expect to have one or more validated non-animal test method(s) for the evaluation of human eye irritants.

CHAPTER 8

Meeting Industry and Regulatory Needs for Alternative Test Methods to the Draize Rabbit Eye Irritation Test

Sherry L. Ward

CONTENTS

INTRODUCTION

Animal-based toxicological test methods evolved earlier in this century in response to a recognized need, by both industry and government regulatory agencies, for providing safe products to ensure consumer safety. As a result of a number of injuries and deaths from consumer products in the 1930s, Congress passed the Federal Food, Drug, and Cosmetic Act of 1938 (21 U.S. Code), which mandated premarket safety testing for certain products.

One component in the risk assessment of many products is the evaluation of its potential to cause eye injury or eye irritation. The Draize rabbit eye irritation test, the standard method for evaluating the ocular irritation potential of a substance, was developed in response to the need for this type of information (Draize et al., 1944; Friedenwald et al., 1944). In this test, a material is instilled into one eye of albino rabbits (different modifications of the test require different numbers of animals) and the ocular response of the animals is monitored, using a standardized scoring system for the cornea, the conjunctiva, and the iris, for up to 21 d.

Animal welfare concerns over the use of animals for all types of testing and research purposes arose in the early 1950s. At that time, Charles Hume, founder of the Universities Federation for Animal Welfare, proposed "a scientific study of humane technique in laboratory animal experiments" (Balls, 1997). This study led to the publication of Russell and Burch (1959), *The Principles of Humane Experimental Technique*, in which the concepts of reduction, refinement, and replacement (the three Rs) regarding the use of animals in experimentation were defined.

The mandate for both industry and government regulatory agency scientists is to ensure the safety of products that are made available for consumer use. Both groups have confidence in using the currently accepted Draize rabbit eye test method for estimating the human eye safety of a product. To maintain this integrity and provide adequate safety information, new test methods developed to replace the Draize test will have to be validated and will have to provide information that is useful in the risk assessment process.

For validation, new toxicological test methods must demonstrate they are reliable, which means repeatable and reproducible, and that they are relevant, which means the method is predictive and has a biological basis for the stated purpose (NIEHS, 1997). To ensure the standardization of these determinations, validation and regulatory acceptance criteria for evaluating new toxicological test methods were developed by three different international organizations in the 1990s: the Organization for Economic Cooperation and Development (OECD) (OECD, 1996), the European Center for the Validation of Alternative Methods (ECVAM) (Balls, et al., 1995), and the Interagency Coordinating Committee on the Validation of Alternative Methods (ICCVAM) (National Institute for Environmental Health Sciences [NIEHS], 1997).

An alternative method that can replace the Draize rabbit eye test has not yet been validated by any of these organizations. This paper provides an overview of industry and U.S. regulatory perspectives related to the validation and regulatory agency acceptance of Draize alternative test methods.

INDUSTRY PERSPECTIVE

The development and use of animal-alternative methods by industry are driven by current scientific, social, economic, and political considerations. Both government agency and industry scientists are encouraging development and use of validated non-animal toxicological test methods, since they have the potential to provide better scientific and mechanistic data and therefore better human risk assessment.

An industry-wide problem has been the lack of available non-whole animal, validated, and regulatory-accepted toxicological test methods for product safety evaluations. The competitiveness of many manufacturers hinges on their ability to develop and market new products. All global companies are faced with potential legislation regarding the sale of animal-tested products. Organizations that have to engage in product safety testing are faced with an unusual type of technological discontinuity

(Utterback, 1994)—the dilemma of needing to adopt animal replacement test methods without having adequate methods available for this purpose. Unfortunately, efforts toward developing appropriate alternative test methods are progressing slowly relative to the strategic needs of industry for the new technology. The dilemma of industry at this time is that validated and regulatory-accepted, animal-alternative test methods are not available.

A major effort of industry scientists for more than a decade has been the development and validation of new alternative tests methods for the replacement of the Draize rabbit eye test. A number of Draize alternative test methods have been developed. Several of these methods, like the bovine corneal opacity and permeability (BCOP) assay (Gautheron et al., 1992) and the chorioallantoic membrane vascularization assay (CAMVA) (Bagley et al., 1994), are used by some industrial and contract toxicology laboratories as components of a testing scheme for in-house product safety evaluations or for product development. If validated, these or other Draize alternative test methods could also be used to generate data to support product-labeling claims and to support risk assessments for regulatory submissions.

During the late 1980s and early 1990s a number of companies established *in vitro* toxicology laboratories dedicated to meeting the company's needs for non-animal toxicity testing. As an example, the Gillette *In Vitro* Testing and Research Laboratory (IVTRL) was established in 1991 as part of the company's response to the need for nonclinical (*in vitro* or alternative) toxicological test methods for product safety evaluations. One of the major objectives of the IVTRL was to develop new *in vitro* test methods, with the goal being their eventual validation and regulatory acceptance. The first goal was the development of nonclinical test methods for the assessment of the human eye irritation potential of chemicals and product formulations. Company scientists developed a new human corneal epithelial cell line, the HCE-T cell line, and used these cells to develop an *in vitro* corneal model, the HCE-T model. The HCE-T model was used to develop several different *in vitro* test methods for the assessment of the eye irritation potential of chemicals and products (Kahn and Walker, 1993; Ward et al., 1996, 1997; Kruszewski et al., 1997; Clothier et al., 2000). One of the methods, the HCE-T TEP assay, has been used to provide data on the eye irritation potential of products to staff toxicologists and has undergone formal interlaboratory prevalidation and validation studies (Ward et al., 2003). This test method and the results of the prevalidation study for the HCE-T TEP assay are the topic of Chapter 15 in this volume.

The validation and regulatory acceptance of the HCE-T TEP test method will provide industry scientists with an alternative to the Draize rabbit eye test. Validation will facilitate the wider acceptance and use of the test method. Validation of the HCE-T TEP assay will confer industry-wide recognition and will demonstrate the goodwill effort of the company in promoting the three Rs. These same principles are true for companies that are supporting the development and validation of other Draize alternative methods such as MatTek's EpiOcular™ test method (Stern et al., 1998; Klausner et al., 1999).

Replacing the Draize rabbit test with a non–animal-based test scheme will promote the competitive advantage of an organization by providing some or all of the following advantages: (1) scientifically superior product safety evaluations—the potential to provide better scientific and mechanistic data, and therefore better human risk assessments; (2) product differentiation—scientifically superior product development and reformulation due to more sensitive and specific measures of relevant biological responses; (3) cost savings—these may be indirect, for example, a reduction in adverse responses due to better product reformulation or increased customer loyalty; (4) maintenance of competitive position in potentially restricted future markets (for example, the European Union countries); and (5) enhanced corporate image and public relations (PR capital).

A number of interindustry cooperative efforts have been conducted to address the issues of alternative methods development and validation. These include activities by industry trade associations and by the International Life Sciences Institute (ILSI) Technical Committee for Alternatives to Animal Research (AAT). The trade associations have supported numerous workshops and validation studies. The many interlaboratory validation studies for alternatives to the Draize eye test that have been supported by industry are too numerous to discuss here, but they have been summarized by Spielmann (1997). In general, the conclusions of these validation studies have been that different methods differ in their ability to predict the *in vivo* Draize results and that none of the alternative methods that were evaluated could be accepted as replacements for the Draize test based on the existing data.

The ILSI AAT brought together industry, academic, and regulatory scientists to address issues that would promote the development and validation of Draize alternative test methods. Their unique activities have included the following: activities to inform the ophthalmology community of industry's needs for nonclinical ocular test methods, meetings with panels of ophthalmology experts to identify mechanisms of human eye irritation that might be modeled by *in vitro* systems, the development of a chemical-induced human eye injury classification scheme, and a pilot study to evaluate the availability and utility of retrospective human chemical-induced eye injury data (ILSI AAT, 1996; Blazka et al., 2003; Nussenblatt et al., 1998). To alleviate the concerns in conducting human testing, the ILSI AAT has worked with a panel of ophthalmology experts to develop a human eye injury classification scheme that can be used to collect data prospectively or retrospectively from accidental human eye exposures to chemicals and products (Blazka et al., 2003). Since the consumer-product industry has recently curtailed much of its former support for alternative methods development, the ILSI AAT has disbanded. Future work in this area is uncertain.

REGULATORY PERSPECTIVE

The accepted method for determining the eye irritation potential of a substance is the Draize rabbit eye irritation test (Draize et al., 1944). A number of regulatory agencies in different countries require Draize test data as a part of their testing guidelines for risk assessment (Williams, 1994; ILSI AAT, 1996). In the original test, nine rabbits were used. The test has been modified to use fewer animals, and various modified versions have been specified by the Federal Hazardous Substances Act (FHSA); the Environmental Protection Agency (EPA) under the Federal Insecticide, Fungicide, and Rodenticide Act (FIFRA) and the Toxic

Substances Control Act (TSCA); and the Organization for Economic Cooperation and Development (OECD). A list of the regulatory guidelines for the various eye irritation test protocols is provided in DiPasquale and Hayes (2001). Wilhelmus (2001) has provided an excellent historical review of ocular toxicology and the development of the Draize test.

Regulatory agencies need data to evaluate the potential for a product to cause acute eye irritation as one of the components in the assessment of its overall risk to human health. The Food and Drug Administration (FDA), the Environmental Protection Agency (EPA), the Consumer Product Safety Commission (CPSC), the Department of Transportation (DOT), the Occupational Safety and Health Administration (OSHA), and other regulatory agencies worldwide accept and/or require Draize eye test data for risk assessment and for labeling purposes.

Among regulatory agencies, the FDA has taken the lead in encouraging the submission of Draize alternative test data. The Center for Food Safety and Applied Nutrition (CFSAN) is the FDA division involved with the safety of cosmetics (the Federal Food, Drug, and Cosmetic Act). Although they do not require premarket approval for cosmetics, the FDA/CFSAN has relied on the Draize eye irritation test "for evaluating the safety of a substance introduced into or around the eye" (FDA, 1998). In their 1992 position paper on animal use, the FDA said they encourage efforts to develop and implement non-whole animal techniques (FDA, 1998). The FDA's Center for Drug Evaluation and Research (CDER) regulates over-the-counter drugs, and they do not use the Draize test and actively discourage its use. The FDA's Center for Biologics Evaluation and Research (CBER) follows CDER's lead in this area.

The EPA Office of Prevention, Pesticides, and Toxic Substances reviews testing procedures to meet the data requirements of the Toxic Substances Control Act (15 U.S. Code 2601) and the Federal Insecticide, Fungicide, and Rodenticide Act (7 U.S. Code 136, *et seq.*). The substances regulated by the EPA are typically more hazardous to human health than those regulated under the Federal Food, Drug, and Cosmetic Act; thus premarket review is required. The guidelines indicate use of the Draize rabbit eye test to evaluate eye corrosion (irreversible tissue damage) and eye irritation (reversible eye injury). The guidelines state that "results from well validated and accepted *in vitro* test systems may serve to identify corrosives or irritants such that the test material need not be tested *in vivo*" (EPA, 1996). However, *in vitro* test systems that are well validated and accepted do not yet exist to meet this criterion.

Prior to regulatory agency acceptance, a new Draize alternative method will have to become a validated method. New toxicological test methods developed in the United States are evaluated and recommended to a peer-review panel for validation by the ICCVAM. The ICCVAM has defined the criteria and processes for the validation and regulatory acceptance of new and revised toxicological test methods. These guidelines are described in the report titled *Validation and Regulatory Acceptance of Toxicological Test Methods* (NIEHS, 1997). Validation has been defined as "the process whereby the reliability and relevance of a procedure are established for a particular purpose" (Balls et al., 1995). Validation is defined by the ICCVAM as "a scientific process designed to characterize the operational characteristics, advantages, and limitations of a test method, and to demonstrate its reliability and relevance" (NIEHS, 1997). The relevance of a test method describes the extent to which a test method will correctly predict or measure the biological effect of interest and describes whether the test is meaningful and useful for a particular purpose (NIEHS, 1997). Reliability is a measure of the degree to which a test can be performed reproducibly, both within and between laboratories (NIEHS, 1997).

Regulatory agency acceptance is the acceptance of a validated test method for regulatory use. Regulatory acceptance criteria have been defined by the ICCVAM, and ICCVAM will provide recommendations regarding a reviewed test method to the appropriate agencies; however, the process for the acceptance of a new test method is left up to the individual agency (NIEHS, 1997). The ICCVAM submission guidelines require that the "intended regulatory use(s) and rationale (e.g., screen, substitute, replacement, or adjunct)" for a new test method be described in the submission document (ICCVAM, 1999). The type(s) of data provided by an alternative test method will become evident during the validation process, and each agency will have to determine whether it will accept an alternative method and what type of data it requires from the method. Alternative test method data could be submitted to agencies in several contexts, including (1) stand alone new test method data (i.e., the new test method has been validated and accepted for that particular purpose); (2) new test method data that is supplemented by additional information (i.e., a tier scheme and/or historical Draize data on similar products) that is submitted as a "preponderance-of-evidence" approach; or (3) new test method data that is submitted as a supplement to Draize test data that will serve to reduce the number of animals.

An issue of special concern to many regulatory agency scientists is the use of Draize rabbit eye data to evaluate the performance of new test methods that are developed to predict the human response to eye irritants (Nussenblatt et al., 1998; Chambers, 2000). The ICCVAM regulatory acceptance criteria related to this issue states that "data generated by the method should adequately measure or predict the endpoint of interest and demonstrate a linkage between either the new test and an existing test, or the new test and effects in the target species" (NIEHS, 1997). The reference method data used to evaluate the performance of new Draize alternative methods has been the Draize rabbit eye irritation test. The continued use of the rabbit as the test species is due in part to the large database of ocular response data that is available for the rabbit; thus toxicologists feel comfortable in the use of the method. However, the Draize test has been cited as a poor test for many reasons, including the species/biological differences, and the large coefficient of variations seen in Draize rabbit data (Beckley, 1965; Beckley et al., 1969; Weil and Scala, 1971; Gershbein and McDonald, 1977; ILSI AAT, 1996). The rabbit ocular response to many types of irritating materials frequently overpredicts the human ocular response (Walker, 1985). One large study that compared ocular responses in the rabbit and the monkey eye, which is considered to be an excellent model for the human eye, concluded that the rabbit eye was a poor predictor of the monkey, and therefore the human, ocular response (Green et al., 1978).

Many scientists support the alternative use of human data for test method development and validation and claim that it should replace the Draize rabbit eye irritation test as the "gold standard" (Nussenblatt et al., 1998; Chambers, 2000; Blazka et al.,

2003). However, sufficient human eye irritation data, in the quantitative form needed for new test method evaluation, does not exist. There is the potential for using retrospective or prospective accidental human eye injury data, but there is also a concern about its probable lack of sufficient information. Some scientists think that human eye testing is adequately regulated under current guidelines, and that additional testing can be conducted to develop the data needed. Chambers (2000) has described a plan for prospectively collecting human eye data for products not expected to cause injury and for collecting accidental exposure information for products that could be expected to result in eye injury. Other scientists are of the opinion that sufficient human eye testing could not be performed to obtain the range of data needed to validate a new method. There are dichotomies in both the scientific and the ethical issues associated with the collection and use of human data that need to be addressed before this type of data will be available.

DISCUSSION AND CONCLUSIONS

The main goal of the symposium entitled "Development of Predictive Methods Based on Mechanisms of Eye Irritation at the Ocular Surface: Meeting Industry/Regulatory Needs" was to present alternative eye irritation test methods that have a demonstrated relevance, and therefore could be considered as candidates for future validation studies. The methods selected for presentation have produced data that have some correlation to the reference method (the Draize rabbit eye test), and have a mechanistic basis for their use as a test method for human eye irritation. At the present time, only two of the test methods, the HCE-T TEP assay and the EpiOcular™ assay, are being considered for submission to the ICCVAM for validation. Both of these methods are discussed in different chapters of these proceedings.

The ICCVAM was only recently established, first as an *ad hoc* committee in 1997, and then as a permanent committee in 2000 by the ICCVAM Authorization Act (Public Law 106-545). At the time of this symposium (November 2000), ICCVAM had already facilitated the validation of two alternative methods, the Corrositex® assay for assessing the dermal corrosivity potential of chemicals and the murine local lymph node assay (LLNA) for assessing the allergic contact dermatitis potential of chemicals, and it had about six additional methods in different stages of evaluation (ICCVAM-NICEATM, 2002). ICCVAM-NICEATM has been making excellent progress toward meeting the needs of industry and regulatory scientists for new validated toxicological test methods.

The ICCVAM validation criteria and processes evolved from the ongoing international efforts of the ECVAM and the OECD and other groups in defining test method validation criteria. However, at this time none of these organizations have validated an alternative method to the Draize rabbit eye test. A number of reasons have been proposed to explain the failure of previous studies to validate an alternative method to the Draize test (Purchase et al., 1998). The early validation studies were conducted before the current concepts of validation criteria were established. In many cases the mechanistic basis of the test methods that were evaluated were not known or were not defined. Previous validation studies were set up to validate a replacement test for the Draize eye test and are considered to be rather rigid in the criteria and processes that were used.

Draize alternative methods have their own unique challenges when it comes to test method validation. Only a few of these issues will be discussed here. Many scientists think that test batteries rather than one test method will be needed to replace the Draize test. The essential components for a replacement scheme for the Draize test are not well defined at this time. One approach is to validate individual tests as screens until they can be assembled into more predictive test batteries. Another approach is to validate individual methods that are expected to be part of a battery with the limitations clearly defined and the method validated for only the specific purpose for which it is defined. This process is compatible with the ICCVAM guidelines. This means that a Draize alternative test could be validated for a limited range of *in vivo* irritation, chemical class, or physical form of the test material. The importance of this concept cannot be overstated. All non-animal methods evaluated thus far as Draize alternatives have had at least one of these limitations.

Another unique challenge for the validation of Draize alternative methods is that the *in vivo* test evaluates the biological response to a material in three different ocular tissues, the cornea, the iris, and the conjunctiva. Many regulatory agencies use a specific part of the Draize test data, frequently the corneal opacity score, in making their risk assessments. Both statistical and empirically derived data support the conclusion that the results from a relevant corneal test method alone should be sufficient to model all of the ocular surface responses. Lovell (1996) analyzed Draize tissue scores using principal component analysis and showed that the Draize scores from the different ocular tissues are statistically related to one another and that little information is missed in using only the total Draize score (MAS or MMAS). Analysis of the data obtained by testing 25 surfactant formulations in the HCE-T TEP assay also support this conclusion (Kruszewski et al., 1997; S. Ward, 2000). The Draize tissue scores for the conjunctival and the iris responses for the 25 materials correlated with the endpoint of the HCE-T TEP assay as well as the corneal score and the Draize maximum average score (MAS).

The ICCVAM validation criteria require that a test method provide data that are useful for risk assessment and not necessarily replace an existing test method (NIEHS, 1997). Under the ICCVAM criteria a test method can be validated as a replacement method, but the criteria also provide for validation of methods that would be part of a tier testing scheme, part of a test battery, or used as an adjunct or screening assay. ICCVAM has established criteria that are flexible, and the validation process establishes test method performance and effective outcome (NIEHS, 1997).

Scientists involved in the validation process of Draize alternative methods must look at the unique challenges to replacing the Draize rabbit eye test, some of which have been discussed in this chapter. The test method developers, the regulatory agency scientists, and other ICCVAM stakeholders need to work together to address these issues for each method that is evaluated. The ICCVAM validation criteria are compatible with this process and must be interpreted with these principles in mind so that both industry and regulatory agencies can obtain the new technologies they need to replace animal testing. This will ensure that better science is used in risk assessments and that industries sustain their competitive edge for the development of safe new products.

REFERENCES

Bagley, D.M., Waters, D., and Kong, B.M. (1994) Development of a 10-day chorioallantoic membrane assay as an alternative to the Draize rabbit eye irritation test, *Fund. Chem. Toxicol.*, 32, 1155–1160.

Balls, M. (1997) The three Rs concept of alternatives to animal experimentation, in *Animal Alternatives, Welfare and Ethics,* van Zutphen, L.F.M. and Balls, M., Eds., Elsevier, Amsterdam, pp. 27–41.

Balls, M., Blaauboer, B.J., Fentem, J.H., Bruner, I., Combes, R.D., Ekwall, B., Fielder, R.J., Guillouzo, A., Lewis, R.W., Lovell, D.P., Reinhardt, C.A., Repetto, G., Sladowski, D., Spielmann, H., and Zucco, F. (1995) Practical aspects of the validation of toxicity test procedures. The report and recommendations of the ECVAM Workshop 5, *Alt. Lab. Anim.*, 23, 129–147.

Beckley, J.H. (1965) Comparative eye testing: man versus animal, *Toxicol. Appl. Pharmacol.*, 7, 93–101.

Beckley, J.H., Russell, T.J., and Rubin, L.F. (1969) Use of the rhesus monkey for predicting human response to eye irritants, *Toxicol. Appl. Pharmacol.*, 15, 1–9.

Blazka, M.E., Casterton, P.L., Dressler, W.E., Edelhauser, H.F., Kruszewski, F.H., McCulley, J.P., Nussenblatt, R.B., Osborne, R., Rothenstein, A., Stitzel, K.A., Thomas, K., and Ward, S.L. (2003) Proposed new classification scheme for chemical injury to the human eye, in preparation.

Chambers, W. (2000) Regulatory perspective—Meeting regulatory agency needs for Draize alternatives, Alternative Toxicological Methods for the New Millennium Program Guide, U.S. Army (DoD), Bethesda, MD, 33.

Clothier, R., Orme, A., Walker, T.L., Ward, S.L., Kruszewski, F.H., DiPasquale, L.C., and Broadhead, C.L. (2000) A comparison of three cytotoxicity assays using the corneal HCE-T model, *Alt. Lab. Anim.*, 28, 293–302.

DiPasquale, L.C. and Hayes, A.W. (2001) Acute toxicity and eye irritancy, in *Principles and Methods of Toxicology*, 4th ed., Hayes, A.W., Ed., Taylor and Francis, Philadelphia, 853–916.

Draize, J.H., Woodard, G., and Calvery, H.O. (1944) Method for the study of irritation and toxicity of substances applied topically to the skin and mucous membranes, *J. Pharmacol. Exp. Ther.*, 82, 377–389.

EPA (Environmental Protection Agency) (1996) Health effects test guidelines, 870.2400 Acute eye irritation, url: www.epa.gov.

FDA (Food and Drug Administration) (1998) Animal use in testing FDA-regulated products, url: http://vm.cfsan.fda.gov.

Friedenwald, J.S., Hughes, W.F., and Herrmann, H. (1944) Acid-base tolerance of the cornea, *Arch. Ophthalmol.* 31, 279–283.

Gautheron, P., Dukic, M., Alix, D., and Sina, J.F. (1992) Bovine corneal opacity and permeability test: an *in vitro* assay of ocular irritancy, *Fundam. Appl. Toxicol.*, 18, 442-449.

Gershbein, L.L. and McDonald, J.E. (1977) Evaluation of the corneal irritancy of test shampoos and detergents in various animal species, *Food Cosmet. Toxicol.*, 15, 131–134.

Green, W.R., Sullivan, J.B., Hehir, R.M., Scharpf, L.G., and Dickinson, A.W. (1978) *A Systematic Comparison of Chemically Induced Eye Injury in the Albino Rabbit and Rhesus Monkey,* The Soap and Detergent Association, New York.

ICCVAM (Interagency Coordinating Committee on the Validation of Alternative Methods) (1999) *Evaluation of the Validation Status of Toxicological Methods: General Guidelines for Submissions to ICCVAM* (NIH Publication 99-4496), url: http://iccvam.niehs.nih.gov/docs/guidelines/subguide.htm.

ICCVAM-NICEATM (2002) Test methods under review, url: http://iccvam.niehs.nih.gov/methods/review.htm.

ILSI AAT (International Life Sciences Institute Technical Committee on Alternatives to Animal Testing) (1996) Replacing the Draize eye irritation test: scientific background and research needs, *J. Toxicol. Cutaneous Ocular Toxicol.*, 15, 211–234.

Kahn, C.R. and Walker, T.L. (1993) Human corneal epithelial cell lines with extended lifespan: transepithelial permeability across membranes formed *in vitro, Invest. Ophthalmol. Vis. Sci.*, 34, 1010.

Klausner, M., Sheasgreen, J., Breyfogle, B., Sennott, H., Liebsch, M., Kubilus, J. (1999) The EpiOcular prediction model: a reproducible *in vitro* means of assessing ocular irritancy potential, *Alt. Lab. Anim.*, 27, 299.

Kruszewski, F.H., Walker, T.L., and DiPasquale, L.C. (1997) Evaluation of a human corneal epithelial cell line as an *in vitro* model for assessing ocular irritation, *Fundam. Appl. Toxicol.*, 36, 130–140.

Lovell, D.P. (1996) Principal component analysis of Draize eye irritation tissue scores from 72 samples of 55 chemicals in the ECETOC data bank, *Toxicol. In Vitro*, 10, 609–618.

NIEHS (National Institute of Environmental Health Sciences) (1997) Validation and regulatory acceptance of toxicological test methods: a report of the *ad hoc* Interagency Coordinating Committee on the Validation of Alternative Methods (NIH publication 97-3981). NIEHS: Research Triangle Park, NC, url: http://ntp-server.niehs.nih.gov/htdocs/ICCVAM/ICCVAM.html or http://iccvam.niehs.nih.gov/docs/guidelines/validate.pdf.

Nussenblatt, R., Bron, A., Chambers, W., McCulley, J., Pericoi, M., Ubels, J., and Edelhauser, H. (1998) Ophthalmologic perspectives on eye irritation testing, *J. Toxicol. Cutaneous Ocular Toxicol.*, 17, 103–109.

OECD (Organization for Economic Cooperation and Development) (1996) Final report of the OECD Workshop on harmonization of validation and acceptance criteria for alternative toxicological test methods (ENV/MC/CHEM/TG(96)9), OECD, Paris.

Purchase, I.F., Botham, P.A., Bruner, L.H., Flint, O.P., Frazier, J.M., and Stokes, W.S. (1998) Workshop overview: scientific and regulatory challenges for the reduction, refinement, and replacement of animals in toxicity testing, *Toxicol. Sci.*, 43, 86–101.

Russell, W.M.S., and Burch, R.L. (1959, reprinted 1992) *The Principles of Humane Experimental Technique*, Universities Federation for Animal Welfare, Herts, U.K.

Spielmann, H. (1997) Ocular irritation, in *In Vitro Methods in Pharmaceutical Research*, Academic Press, New York, 265–287.

Stern, M., Klausner, M., Alvarado, R., Renskers, K., and Dickens, M. (1998) Evaluation of the EpiOcular™ tissue model as an alternative to the Draize eye irritation test, *Toxicol In Vitro*, 12, 455-461.

Utterback, J.M. (1994) *Mastering the Dynamics of Innovation*, Harvard Business School Press: Boston.

Walker, A.P. (1985) A more realistic animal technique for predicting human eye response, *Food Chem. Toxicol.*, 23, 175–178.

Ward, S.L., Walker, T.L., and Dimitrijevich, S.D. (1997) Evaluation of chemically-induced toxicity using an *in vitro* model of human corneal epithelium, *Toxicol. in Vitro*, 11, 121–139.

Ward, S.L. et al. (2000) Pre-Study Plan for the Validation of the HCE-T TEP Assay. Submission to the ICCVAM Ocular Toxicity Working Group (OTWG).

Ward, S.L., Gacula, M., Jr., Cao, C., DiPasquale, L., Edelhauser, H., Kruszewski, F., Valdes, J., Walker, T., and Hayes, A.W. (2003) Prevalidation study results for the human corneal epithelial fluorescein transepithelial permeability assay for eye irritation, the HCE-T TEP assay, *J. Toxicol. Cutaneous Ocular Toxicol.*, submitted.

Weil, C.S. and Scala, R.A. (1971) Study of intra- and inter-laboratory variability in the results of rabbit eye and skin irritation test, *Toxicol. Appl. Pharmacol.*, 19, 276–360.

Wilhelmus, K.R. (2001) The Draize eye test, *Surv. Ophthalmol.*, 45, 493–515.

Williams, P.D. (1994) Alternatives to ocular testing *in vivo:* scientific and regulatory considerations, *Toxicol. Methods*, 4, 24–25.

CHAPTER 9

The Ocular Surface: Barrier Function and Mechanisms of Injury and Repair

Martin Reim

CONTENTS

THE OCULAR SURFACE

The optical quality of the eye is largely dependent on the integrity of the cornea and the overlying tear film. The interaction of the ocular surface fluid with corneal epithelium and stroma has been investigated repeatedly using various methods (Thoft and Friend, 1978; Reim et al., 1997). To understand the pathology of the cornea, the special structure of the epithelium and stroma must be considered. The corneal epithelium shows distinct layers consisting of basal, intermediate, and superficial cells. Zonulae occludents form diffusion barriers preventing diffusion of even rather small molecules and penetration of microorganisms. The epithelial cells are attached to the basement membrane by hemidesmosomes (Rohen, 1977). In addition, special anchoring complexes protrude from the epithelium into the stroma (Gipson et al., 1989). From its anatomical structure, the epithelium consists mainly of cellular material; its extracellular space is very small.

The stroma forms the major part of the cornea. In contrast to the epithelium, about 90% of the stromal volume is made up by the extracellular space. It is filled with the delicate structure of collagens and glycosaminoglycans. Normally, the stroma contains 78% water (Reim, 1992a). The extracellular water of the cornea represents a large volume for solutes such as electrolytes, metabolites like glucose and lactate, and low molecular weight proteins, including cytokines. The cells of the stroma, the keratocytes, form a syncytium, which was perceived more clearly when confocal microscopy was introduced (Thaer and Geyer, 1997).

ELECTROLYTES AND METABOLITES IN CORNEAL STROMA AND EPITHELIUM

Electrolytes, for example sodium (Na^{1+}), potassium (K^{1+}), chloride (Cl^{1-}), calcium (Ca^{2+}), and sulfate (SO_4^{2-}), form important parts of the ionic milieu for living cells (Schrage et al., 1993, 1996). Glucose is known to be a major nutrient metabolite of the corneal tissues (Reim, 1982b). Lactate is the product of the anaerobic energy-producing metabolism (Table 9.1). In the cornea, like in many other tissues, adenosine triphosphate (ATP) and adenosine diphosphate (ADP) are major carriers of cellular energy. Therefore, ATP levels are considered to indicate the vitality of tissues and cells (Reim et al., 1966, 1967; Hennighausen et al., 1972). Since ATP levels

Table 9.1   Stroma of rabbit cornea, mean ± SD,
             hydration = 3.2 ± 0.4

µMol/g H₂O (n = 20)	µMol/g net weight (n = 15)
Na 125 ± 42	Lactate 9.66 ± 1.2
Cl 123 ± 25	Glucose 3.63 ± 0.8
K 24 ± 4	ATP 0.20 ± 0.05
S 105 ± 21	ADP 0.07 ± 0.03
P 12 ± 4	ASC 4.72 ± 1.44

Note: ASC = ascorbate. Levels of some metabolites and electrolytes in the corneal stroma. Adenosine triphosphate (ATP) and adenosine diphosphate (ADP) are strictly intracellular metabolites. Since the corneal stroma contains keratocytes only in about 10% of its volume, their levels are much lower than in the epithelium (see Table 9.2). Lactate is present in the extracellular as well as in the intracellular space and consequently shows levels close to those of the epithelium (Reim et al., 1970, 1978; Fischern, 1996).

Table 9.2   Metabolite levels of rabbit
             corneal epithelium µMol/g wet
             weight, m ± SEM

ATP	3.03 ± 0.10 ($n = 14$)
ADP	0.26 ± 0.02 ($n = 14$)
ATP/ADP	12.23 ± 0.89 ($n = 14$)
AMP	0.93 ± 0.08 ($n = 14$)
Glucose	2.02 ± 0.22 ($n = 14$)
Lactate	9.89 ± 1.02 ($n = 14$)
GSH	3.03 ± 0.43 ($n = 21$)
GSSG	0.28 ± 0.05 ($n = 21$)
ASC	11.55 ± 1.05 ($n = 24$)

GSH = reduced glutathione, GSSG = oxidized
glutathione, ASC = ascorbate.

Note: Levels of some metabolites in the
corneal epithelium, which may be significant to estimate vitality, to indicate
microtrauma, and to show levels of
radical scavengers (Hennighausen et
al., 1972; Reim et al., 1966, 1967,
1970, 1976, 1982).

can be assayed with the bioluminescence method in tissue samples of a few milli-
grams (Salla et al., 1996), even in histological sections, analyses of ATP levels may
be used more widely in clinical and experimental eye research. ATP/ADP ratios
represent the state of cellular energy independent from absolute metabolite levels
(Table 9.2).

Na^{1+}, Cl^{1-}, and SO_4^{2-} are distributed mainly in the extracellular space of the
stroma. The energy dispersive x-ray analysis method (EDXA) was recently adapted
and calibrated to analyze quantitatively elements in corneal samples not larger than
10 µm. This procedure evaluates backscattered x-ray spectra in the scanning electron
microscope. The peaks obtained from the elements contained in the sample irradiated
by the x-ray beam could be quantitatively evaluated when the background scatter
was eliminated by a special peak-background calculation procedure (Schrage et al.,
1993). In addition, a microtrephine was constructed to take corneal biopsies of 160
µm in diameter allowing for a minimal invasive diagnostic examination (Schrage et
al., 1994, 1996). This new technique gave the opportunity, among other experiments,
to investigate concentrations of electrolytes and some other elements in various parts
of the cornea *in situ*.

While glucose remains mainly outside the cells, lactate is found in the intracellular as well as in the extracellular fluid. Both of these metabolites can be assayed
now with more sensitive micro methods (Frantz et al., 1998). Contrary to glucose
and lactate, ATP and ADP are restricted to cells (Table 9.2). In addition, glutathione
occurs mainly intracellularly. It is an important reducing metabolite. Its generation
is closely connected with the energy-producing metabolism (Reim et al., 1978). So
is ascorbic acid. In the cornea, this compound achieved an extraordinary high
concentration (Reim et al., 1978). In the epithelium, the ascorbic acid concentration
was found to be ten times higher than in the aqueous humour and 50 to 100 times
higher than in the blood plasma. It is assumed that in the anterior eye segment,

ascorbic acid serves for scavenging oxygen and hydroxyl radicals, which are generated to a large extent in the light exposed tissues of the eye (Reim and Becker, 1995; Ringvold et al., 1998).

TRAUMA TO OCULAR SURFACE

Trauma, defined as an adverse influence including mechanical, chemical, or physical impact, is considered to be a quantitative process. In this context, quantity is understood as a function of adverse impact and time. Severe trauma, like alkali burns, immediately causes severe damage [Reim et al., 1984]. On the other hand, mild irritation, such as gently touching the surface, rinsing with indifferent fluids, or little alteration of pH, induced only little alteration to the tissue, which disappeared quite soon. Minute lesions of the epithelium may produce tissue responses, which can be detected with various methods of examination, such as confocal microscopy, biochemical analyses of the cornea, or the tear fluid.

Repeated or continuous alteration may become chronic irritation with time. Then, low traumatic stimulus may accumulate and cause more severe damage. An example of chronic subthreshold trauma is contact lens wear or the application of eye drops, which usually contain disinfectants (Morley and McCulloch, 1961; Turss and Schebitz, 1972; Kilp, 1974; Kilp and Heisig, 1975; Thoft and Friend, 1975). Small trauma and disease is easily overcome by defense mechanisms of a healthy organism. However, severe trauma or chronic disease may induce violent and exaggerated responses, such as those following chemical injuries.

The ocular surface fluid is not only composed of tears, but is influenced by various eye drops and rinsing solutions. As long as the corneal epithelium is intact, interaction between cornea and ocular surface fluid is slight and of little importance. However, surface trauma may damage the epithelial barrier and induce interactions between surface fluid and corneal tissues. Erosions or complete defects of the epithelium involve the stroma. By its special anatomical structure and its swelling pressure, the denuded stroma soaks fluid from the surface like a sponge (Dohlman, 1971; Reim, 1972). Clinically, this condition appears with edema. However, as revealed by EDXA and other analyses, corneal edema from surface lesions brings about dramatic changes of the chemical composition of the stroma (Reim et al., 1969, 1972; Schrage et al., 1996).

CHEMICAL AND THERMAL INJURIES TO THE OCULAR SURFACE

Since the prognosis of chemical or thermal injuries of the eyes depends on the severity of the damage, a classification is necessary. In Table 9.3, signs of chemical injuries to the eye were compiled and graded in order to define stages of damage.

In mild burns, stage I, surface epithelia became defective and the conjunctiva was hyperemic (Figure 9.1).

Stage II of eye burn injuries showed chemosis and some ischemia of conjunctiva in addition to epithelial defects and hyperaemia (Figure 9.2). Some parts of the limbal

Table 9.3   Grading of Eye Burns

I	II	III	IV
		Immediate signs	
Erosion	Large erosion	Surface defect	Epithelia destroyed
Hyperemia	Ischemia 1/3	Ischemia >1/2	Deep ischemia >3/4
	Chemosis	Rose chemosis	Dense corneal opacity
		Corneal opacity	Conjunctival necroses
			Sclera porcelain white
			Discoloration and atrophy of iris
			Fibrin exudate
		Later signs	
Regeneration	Recirculation	Persistent erosion	Proliferation
	Regeneration	Ulceration	Large ulcerations
		Vascularization	Melting of cataract
		Scars	Glaucoma
			Scarification

Note: Grading of eye burns according to clinical signs. The upper part lists immediate
damage visible, the lower one later secondary events. The classification of signs
was developed from various authors and by clinical experiences (Hughes, 1946;
Roper-Hall, 1965; Thoft, 1978; Reim and Kuckelkorn, 1995)

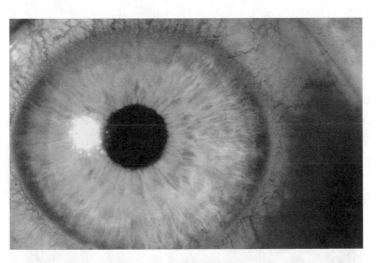

Figure 9.1   Eye with a mild alkali burn stage I (Table 9.3). The corneal epithelium was completely
lost, but the stroma remained undamaged and clear. The conjunctiva showed hype-
remia, but no swelling or ischemia. The damage healed within a few days.

zone might have been included, but deeper tissues remained unaffected. Surrounding
conjunctiva was more or less infiltrated with leukocytes (Reim et al., 1980). However,
surface epithelia regenerated within two or three weeks (Reim et al., 1982).

More severe injuries were seen in stage III burns. All signs listed in Table 9.3
were found. The healing period was extended and complicated by long-standing
epithelial defects, ulceration, scar formation, and permanent corneal turbidities. Most

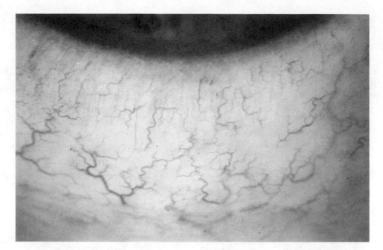

Figure 9.2   Lime burn stage II (Table 9.3). The whole corneal and some conjunctival epithelium
was destroyed. The corneal stroma exhibited little superficial turbidities. The lower
conjunctiva is demonstrated by upgaze. It was swollen (chemosis). Superficially
in the conjunctiva, ischemia is recognized by the interrupted blood columns. With
the lit lamp microscope, bloodstream could not be detected. Underneath the
otherwise pale conjunctiva, intact sclera appeared with a faint rose background.

severe burns exhibited disastrous stage IV damage (Figures 9.3 and 9.4) and late
complications induced by the severe and long-standing secondary inflammation.
Surface epithelia did not heal after years. Secondary corneal scarification, neovascularization, and shrinking of conjunctiva resulted often in blindness.

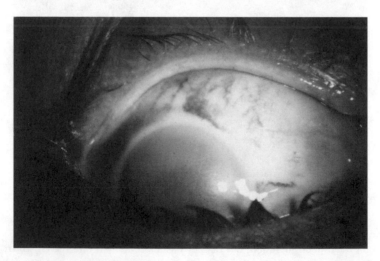

Figure 9.3   Clinical appearance of a severe chemical injury grade IV. The inner margin of the
upper lid showed a white line of necrosis. The conjunctiva appeared flat and white,
also from necrosis, which presumably included visible parts of the sclera. In the
upper left region, some hemorrhages were deposited in necrotic conjunctiva.
Ischemia was evident. The cornea was completely turbid. The outlines of iris and
pupil could be hardly identified.

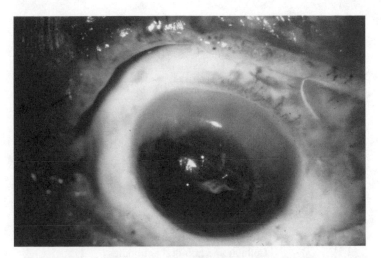

Figure 9.4   Melting of the anterior eye segment, nine days after most severe burn from liquid metal. There were extended necroses of all conjunctival, subconjunctival, and scleral tissues, appearing homogeneously white and slippery. Only in the right upper region, some hemorrhages in necrotic tissues showed red color. The cornea was opaque in the upper marginal parts. The lower and central cornea was melted away and the iris and lens exposed. Since at that time (1977) corneal donor material was not available, the eye was lost and had to be removed. In the melting tissues of the anterior eye segment, high activities of N-acetylglucose aminidase (NAcGA, E.C.3.2.1.50) and cathepsin-D (E.C.3.4.23.5) were found (Reim, 1982a).

PATHOPHYSIOLOGY OF CHEMICAL EYE INJURIES

Ischemia and Necrosis

The damage by chemical injuries is quantitative and depends upon the quantity of corrosive agent, its concentration, and the pressure of a splash hitting the eyes. Surface epithelia are destroyed by chemical agents, which then may penetrate the corneal stroma and the subconjunctival tissues including Tenon's capsule and even sclera. There, keratocytes, conjunctival fibrocytes, and other living cells become necrotic. In addition, blood circulation is disturbed. Consequently, limbus, conjunctiva, and even sclera become ischemic (Figures 9.3 and 9.4; Reim, 1992b). The amount of limbal ischemia marks clinically the extent and the severity of the damage. Penetration of the corrosive agents into the anterior chamber and the ciliary body is marked by discoloration of the iris, ectropium uveae, and lens turbidities (Reim, 1992b; Reim and Kuckelkorn, 1995). Damage to the ciliary body results in hypotonia, and necroses in the trabecular meshwork induce glaucoma.

Inflammatory Response

Mediators of inflammation are released in necrotic cells and in cells bordering on necrosis. Many compounds as shown in Figure 9.5 were assayed in corneal and conjunctival samples from both model experiments and clinical patients

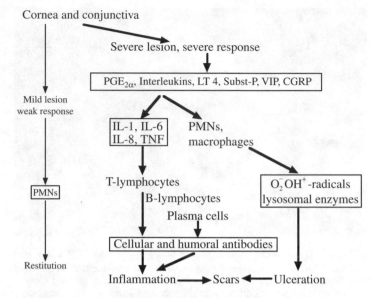

Figure 9.5   Flow diagram of inflammatory cascade following chemical and thermal injuries of
the eye. The inflammatory response is a quantitative process produced by the
affected tissues and the leucocytes involved (Ghattacherjee et al., 1979; Reim et
al., 1980, 1993, 1997; Reim, 1982a; Rochels et al., 1982; Kulkarni and Srinivasan,
1983; Becker et al., 1991, 1995; Reim and Leber, 1992; Reim and Becker, 1995).

(Bhattacherjee et al., 1979; Rochels et al., 1982; Kulkarni and Srinivasan, 1983;
Rochels, 1984; Reim and Leber, 1992; Becker et al., 1995; Reim et al., 1997). In
the corneal stroma, alkali hydrolyzed matrix proteins (Whikehart et al., 1991) into
smaller peptides, which showed leucotaxis and antigenicity (Pfister et al., 1993).
They collectively induced an inflammatory response following chemical injuries
(Haseba et al., 1991; Thiel et al., 1988).

Cytokines and Growth Factors in Cornea and Tears

Cytokines and growth factors play an important part in health and disease. Many
reports appeared on cytokines in ocular cells and tissues. Normal tears contain rather
high amounts of two important growth factors: epidermal growth factor (EGF)
enhances the regeneration of the corneal epithelium. It stimulates proliferation of
epithelial cells and fibroblasts. Transforming growth factor β (TGF-β) is a kind of
antagonist to EGF. It inhibits proliferation of corneal epithelium. Presumably, both
growth factors are responsible for homeostasis of the surface epithelium (Table 9.4;
Mishima et al., 1991; Kruse and Tseng, 1994;).

In experimental alkali burns with 0.5 or 0.1 N NaOH, interleukin IL-1α appeared
in the cornea on the first day after the injury and reaches maximum levels on days 3
to 7. IL-6 comes later and peaks on day 7. The levels of IL-1 and IL-6 were dependent
on the concentration of the NaOH used in these experiments (Sotozono et al., 1997;
Sotozono and Kinoshita, 1998). Interestingly, in severe burns by 1 N NaOH, IL-8 was
found in the corneas, appearing after 3 d and remaining on rather high levels for several

Table 9.4   Cytokines in Tears

EGF → regeneration of epithelium
TGFbeta 2 → inhibits proliferation
TNFalpha, in inflammation
Many others, but presumably released from damaged surface epithelia

Note: Cytokines and growth factors in tears influencing the corneal epithelium (Mishima et al., 1991; Kruse and Tseng, 1994; Sotozono and Kinshita, 1998).

weeks, inducing infiltration of polymorphonuclear leukocytes and corneal vascularization. Recently, IL-1 and IL-6 were analyzed in human corneal buttons obtained at corneal grafts for various diseases (Becker et al., 1995). In the inflammatory corneas, high levels of IL-1 and IL-6 were found (Figure 9.6). In relation to clinical diagnoses, including some severe chemical injuries, cytokine levels in the human corneal buttons showed clearly that higher interleukin levels were associated with inflammatory disease. In beginning disease, IL-1 was increased; later IL-6 reached highest levels.

The results of cytokine levels in human corneas are in agreement with clinical observations known for many years. Immediately after a chemical or thermal injury, the affected tissues, being necrotic, were free of cells. However, rather early polymorphonuclear leukocytes (PMNs) were activated and invaded the damaged tissues. Later, macrophages, plasma cells, and subsequently lymphocytes followed (Reim et al., 1980), which enhanced and maintained inflammation, to a large extent by continuous release of cytokines and superoxide radicals (Becker et al., 1994), which induced all of the problems listed in Table 9.3.

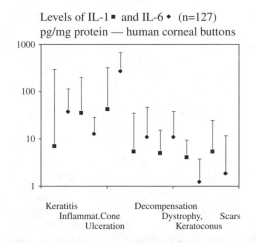

Figure 9.6   Interleukin-1β (IL-1) and Interleukin-6 (IL-6) in human corneal buttons from keratoplasty. Total number of cases: 127. The logarithmic ordinate shows the concentrations found in pg/mg extractable protein. The symbols represent the median, squares stand for IL-1, rhombs for IL-6. The error bars demonstrate the 75% percentiles. In the abscissa, the diagnoses of the cases were indicated corresponding to the position of the symbols (Becker et al., 1995). Inflamed corneas revealed very high levels of IL-1 and IL-6. The levels in the uninflamed, quiete corneas were lower by an order of magnitude.

Chemical Alteration of Extracellular Matrix

Collagen and proteoglycans withstand largely to chemical agents. Therefore, corneal stroma and sclera, the envelopes of the eyeball, remained intact. However, chemical agents changed the molecular structure of the extracellular matrix: collagen shrunk. Consequently, the axial length of the globes often decreased (Reim and Kuckelkorn, 1995) and the anterior segments became too narrow at corneal grafting and for a swelling lens.

The abovementioned small peptides produced by alkaline hydrolysis in the corneal stroma not only induced further disease by their antigenicity, but also changed the chemical structure of the extracellular matrix (Whikehart et al., 1991; Pfister et al., 1993).

Four to six weeks after the burn, proteolytic enzymes became activated and degraded corneal collagen and proteoglycans (Gnädinger et al., 1969). These activities induced corneal ulceration and anterior segment melting (Figure 9.4; Dohlman, 1971; Reim, 1982; Reim and Leber, 1992; Reim et al., 1993).

Stem Cell Insufficiency

Stem cells are cell populations of epithelia that are arrested in their cell cycle. They form the reservoir of dividing cells necessary for regeneration of defects (Cotsarelis et al., 1989). In the cornea, stem cells are located in the basal epithelium of the limbus, in the transition zone from conjunctiva to cornea (Kruse, 1996). It forms deep folds there. The base of the epithelial folds is well vascularized (Hogan et al., 1971). Stem cells do not show characteristic morphological criteria on histological examination, but some biochemical features (Zieske et al., 1992), e.g., high ATP levels, high activities of some enzymes of the energy producing metabolism, expression of cytokeratin 19 and vimentin (Lauweryns et al., 1993), and lack of cytokeratins 3 and 12, otherwise typical for corneal epithelium.

Enzyme Activities and Metabolites on the Ocular Surface

When surface epithelia of the eye were mildly and moderately damaged, glucose and lactate were released and increased in tears. Lactate levels were elevated to twice the normal values, and glucose was elevated up to five times the normal values (Reim et al., 1982). Also, after ocular surface trauma, enzymes were found in the ocular surface fluid, initially cellular enzymes, after some days, lysosomal enzymes. The N-acetylglucose aminidase was assayed as a marker enzyme (Reim and Leber, 1992). It appeared together with metalloproteinases (Gnädinger et al., 1969). Even in cases of mild and moderate eye burns and in atopic conjunctivitis, the release of this enzyme to the surface fluid reached five to ten times the normal activities (Figure 9.7; Reim et al., 1992).

In severe chemical injuries, when deep porcelain white ischemia had occurred, stem cells of the corneal epithelium were destroyed. In these regions of the limbal circumference, the corneal epithelium became insufficient to regenerate. This

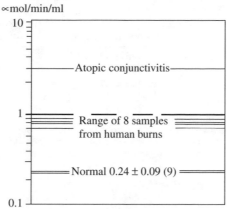

Figure 9.7   Activity of N-acetylglucose aminidase (NAcGA, E.C.3.2.1.50) in human tears collected from nine human cases with eye burns stage I and II and an atopic patient. Please note that the ordinate is in logarithmic scale! The enzyme activity (µMol/min/ml) increased considerably in surface diseases.

condition induced persistent epithelial defects (Thoft, 1982; Reim and Kuckelkorn, 1995). After 3 to 4 weeks varying superficial corneal ulcers appeared (Reim et al., 1984; Reim, 1982). During this time, the ischemic conjunctiva became necrotic and melted. Ischemic sclera was exposed. With the inflammatory response, the adjacent healthy conjunctiva was heavily infiltrated by leukocytes and formed proliferation tissue, which released high activities of lysosomal enzymes, such as matrix-metallo proteinases (MMPs) and the marker enzyme N-acetylglucose aminidase (NAcGA) (Reim, 1982; Reim and Leber, 1992; Reim et al., 1993). This condition was clinically marked with corneo-scleral ulceration, 4–6 weeks post trauma (Reim, 1987a, 1987b).

If the proliferation tissue proceeded too slowly to cover the ischemic sclera and the denuded corneal stroma, the tissues were melted by the MMPs (Figure 9.4). If proliferation tissue proceeded faster, the ischemic region and the cornea were covered with highly vascularized proliferation and scar tissue.

Early surgical intervention with Tenon plasty and protection of the corneal surface prohibited or healed corneo-scleral ulceration and thereby saved the eyes (Reim and Teping, 1989; Reim et al., 1992; Kuckelkorn et al., 1995, 1997).

Changes of the Contents of Na^{1+}, K^{1+}, Cl^{1-}, and SO_4^{2-}

Changes of electrolyte levels were another aspect of pathophysiology (Schrage et al., 1993; Fischern et al., 1998). In the corneal stroma, after experimental alkali burns, sodium (Na^{1+}), chloride (Cl^{1-}), and sulfate (SO_4^{2-}) were decreased when the denuded stroma was rinsed four times daily with saline (Table 9.5; Schrage et al., 1996; Langefeld et al., 1997; Fischern et al., 1998). When balanced salt solution (BSS) was used, the decrease of electrolytes was less severe. However, the severe loss of sulfate after the burn could not be restituted by rinsing.

Table 9.5   Stroma of Rabbit Cornea, µMol/g H$_2$O, mean ± SD

EDXA	Normal (n = 20)	Alkali Burn, Denuded, Rinsed for 16 Days, 4× daily with 0.9% NaCl (n = 8)
Na	125 ± 42	90 ± 11
Cl	123 ± 25	65 ± 15
S	105 ± 21	24 ± 4
P	12 ± 4	22 ± 22
Ca	3 ± 3	1 ± 3

Note: Changes of the levels of some electrolytes in the corneal stroma after alkali burn. The denuded stroma was rinsed with saline, four times daily for 16 days. Na, Cl, and especially S were decreased, P increased (Fischern et al., 1998).

Calcification and Contamination

Moreover, when eyes denuded from epithelium were rinsed with phosphate buffer, or if they were treated with eye drops containing phosphate buffer as solvent or phosphate salts of drugs, such as prednisolone phosphate, rapid corneal calcification was observed in clinical patients and in model experiments (Table 9.6, Figures 9.8–9.10; Reim et al., 1997; Schrage et al., 1988). In addition, human corneal buttons obtained from burnt eyes on keratoplasty, as well as conjunctival samples, revealed a remarkably high contamination by various metals and minerals (Schrage at el., 1988; Schirner et al., 1991, 1995). These contaminations were explained on one hand by impurities in the test materials and on the other hand by secondary introduction of particles with ophthalmic solutions used in topical therapy on the denuded stroma surface (Reim et al., 1997).

Scarring

In many cases, the ulcerations did not perforate. Then, proliferation tissue covered the whole anterior eye segment and transformed it into shrinking scars. This induced symblephara, that the motility of the globe was restricted (Reim and Saric, 1986; Reim, 1987a), or the globe was totally immobilized. Healing of these cases

Table 9.6   Stroma of Rabbit Cornea, µMol/g H$_2$O, Mean ± SD

EDXA	Normal (n = 20)	Alkali Burn, Denuded, Rinsed for 16 Days, 4× Daily with Phosphate Buffer (n = 8)
Na	125 ± 42	105 ± 22
Cl	123 ± 25	88 ± 33
S	105 ± 21	28 ± 4
P	12 ± 4	623 ± 307
Ca	3 ± 3	435 ± 198

Note: Changes of the levels of some electrolytes in the corneal stroma after alkali burn and rinsing with isotonic phosphate buffer, four times daily for 16 days. Na, Cl, and especially S were decreased, but P and Ca were largely increased. Clinically, calcification of the cornea was observed (Schrage, 1997; Fischern et al., 1998; Haller, 2001).

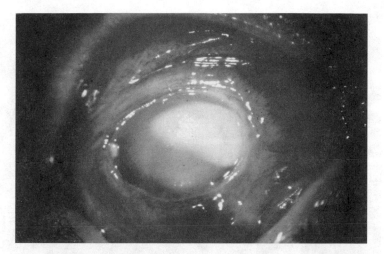

Figure 9.8   Left eye of a 16-year-old boy six months after a most severe chemical injury. In this accident, a highly alkaline etching fluid used to work on electronic parts spilled into both eyes of the patient. In this case, a severe inflammatory response had developed and remained for years. The conjunctiva-like proliferation tissue surrounding the cornea was swollen and very hyperemic. The cornea was devoid of epithelium. It showed extended ulceration especially in its marginal parts and was generally thinned. The upper right cornea showed white calcification. To save the eye from melting, a keratoplasty was performed. The excised cornea was examined with electron dispersive x-ray analysis method (EDXA) (see Figures 9.9 and 9.10).

was severely complicated by the inflammatory reaction, which often recurred when surgical rehabilitation was attempted. As this condition was extremely difficult to be restored, the primary goal of therapy must be to achieve a transparent cornea and to avoid its neovascularization as well as epibulbar and palpebral scars as much as possible (Figure 9.11).

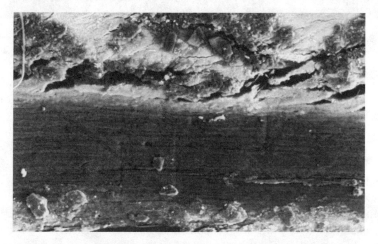

Figure 9.9   Scanning electron microscopy (SEM) on a cross section of the cornea seen in Figure 9.8. Magnification ×200. The upper part shows calcification, the lower one parallel corneal lamellae (Schrage et al., 1988, 1993, 1996).

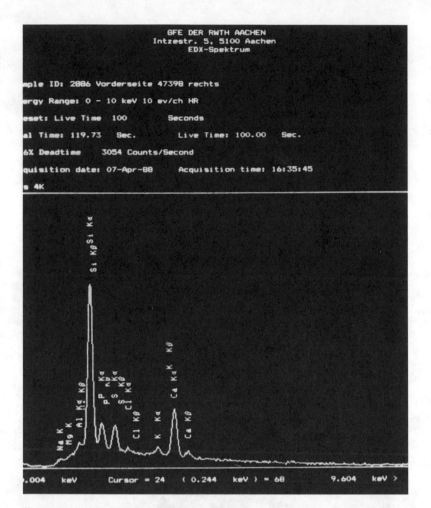

Figure 9.10 Electron dispersive x-ray analysis (EDXA) of the calcified cornea as demonstrated in Figures 9.8 and 9.9. The spectra of the x-rays backscattered at scanning electron microscopy (SEM) showed as expected high peaks for calcium (Ca) and phosphorus (P). But the most prominent peak from this sample was emitted from silicon (Si). Thus, EDXA revealed an unexpected high contamination of the cornea by silicone, which might have explained the severe and longstanding inflammatory response in this case (Schrage et al., 1988, 1993, 1996).

ASPECTS OF REPAIR

Healthy corneal epithelium is well equipped for defense. Minor trauma may be visible with the confocal rather than with the slit lamp microscope. However, invisible trauma is apt to cause alteration of corneal metabolism and cytokine activities. Microtechnique of analyses allows examination of single corneas and samples containing only a few cells. Therefore, analyses of metabolites such as ATP and lactate showed impaired cell vitality. Cytokines and enzyme activities in the cornea and on the ocular surface inform on cell responses to trauma and disease.

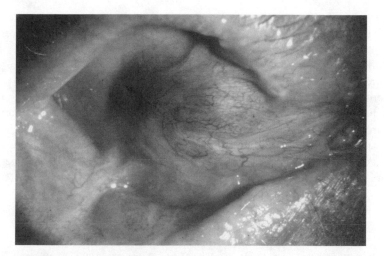

Figure 9.11 Eye of a 42-year-old male 2 years after severe lime burn. Heavy scar formation could not be prohibited. The cornea was covered with thick highly vascularized proliferation tissue. The conjunctiva developed strong scars between the globe and the lids, reducing eye motility. The conjunctival scars also deformed the lid margins. The hyperemic, red scar tissue showed that the inflammatory response had not subsided after 2 years. The eye was practically blind and had bad prognoses for surgical rehabilitation.

The denuded corneal stroma is an exposed unprotected tissue and needs special attention. EDXA (Schrage et al., 1993) revealed alterations of elements and electrolytes in the corneal stroma. If the epithelium is defect, it is not only the clinically visible edema that hurts the cornea, but also rapid and severe changes in the concentrations of sodium, potassium, chloride, sulfate, and lactate.

The understanding of pathophysiology in chemical and thermal injuries of the ocular surface is still incomplete and needs further improvement.

Alterations of cell biology in eye burns are beginning to be understood. Recently, the role of some growth factors and cytokines was explored (Sotozono and Kinoshita, 1998). The significance of keratocytes was just realized (Redbrake et al., 1997; Salla et al., 1995; Møller-Pedersen et al., 1998). The use of corticosteroids to inhibit the inflammatory reaction is still controversial (Chung and Fagerholm, 1987). The experience with cytostatic drugs to reduce conjunctival and Tenon's tissue proliferation is limited. New compounds to modulate cell biological factors are under investigation.

The findings, that rinsing fluids and eye drop solvents influenced concentrations of stromal electrolytes, suggested a search for fluid compositions that will be able to maintain a physiological environment for the ocular surface and the denuded stroma, which is apt to avoid corneal calcification and the loss of sulfate from the stromal matrix (Schrage et al., 1996).

At present, for first aid in chemical injuries, the buffered, hyperosmolar Diphoterine® (from Prevor, Paris) seemed to be useful. Aside from a nonphosphate buffer, it contains an amphoteric molecule with the capacity to bind anions and cations. Following first aid, for further rinsing, sterile water or saline may be as good as balanced salt solution for ophthalmological applications (BSS), or Ringer's lactate solution (Kompa et al., 2000). In continued rinsing, hypo-osmolar solutions removed soluble caustic material and contaminations from the stroma (Schrage et al., 1996).

In addition, medical therapy is imperative to suppress inflammatory responses and thereby prevent sequels of chemical and thermal injuries. However, surgical treatments like peridectomy, necrosectomy, Tenon plasty, corneal and conjunctival grafts, limbal and amniotic membrane transplantation, artificial epithelium, and keratoprotheses are indispensable and definitely improve results. Retrospective evaluation of results gave insight into problems and complications and gave evidence of chances for many patients with severely burned eyes that would have been lost 15 years ago and earlier (Kuckelkorn et al., 1997; Reim and Kuckelkorn, 1995).

References

Becker, J., Salla, S., Dohmen, U., Redbrake, C., and Reim, M. (1995) Explorative study of interleukin levels in the human cornea, *Graefes Arch. Clin. Exp. Ophthalmol.*, 233, 766–771.

Becker, J., Salla, S., Redbrake, C., Kuckelkorn, R., and Reim, M. (1991) The role of superoxide radicals in the inflammation of the anterior eye segment, *Doc. Ophthalmol.*, 77, 110–111.

Becker, J., Salla, S., Redbrake, C., Schrage, N.F., and Reim, M. (1994) Survival of corneal grafts after severe burns of the eye, *Ocular Immunol. Inflammation*, 2, 199–205.

Bhattacherjee, P., Kulkarni, P.S., and Eakins, K.E. (1979) Metabolism of arachidonic acid in the rabbit ocular tissues, *Invest. Ophthalmol. Vis. Sci.*, 18, 172–178.

Chung, J. and Fagerholm, P. (1987) Stromal reaction and repair after corneal alkali wound in rabbit: a quantitative microradiographic study, *Exp. Eye Res.*, 45, 227–237.

Cotsarelis, G., Cheng, S., Dong, G., Sun, T., and Lavker, R. (1989) Existence of slow cycling limbal epithelial basal cells that can be preferentially stimulated to proliferate. Implications on epithelial stem cells, *Cell*, 57, 201.

Dohlman, C. (1971) The function of the corneal epithelium in health and disease, *Invest. Ophthalmol. Vis. Sci.*, 10, 383–407.

Fischern, T., Lorenz, U., Burchard, W.G., Reim, M., and Schrage, N.F. (1998) Changes in the mineral composition of the rabbit cornea after alkali burns, *Graefes Arch. Klin. Exp. Ophthalmol.*, 236, 553–558.

Frantz, A., Salla, S., and Redbrake, C. (1998) A sensitive assay for the quantification of glucose and lactate in the human cornea using a modified bioluminscence technique, *Graefes Arch. Clin. Exp. Ophthalmol.*, 236, 61–64.

Gipson, I.K., Spurr-Michaud, S., Tisdale, A., and Keough, M. (1989) Reassembly of anchoring structures of corneal epithelium during wound repair in the rabbit, *Invest. Ophthalmol. Vis. Sci*, 30, 425–434.

Gnädinger, M., Itoi, M., Slansky, H.H., and Dohlman, C. (1969) The role of collagenase in the alkali-burned cornea, *Am. J. Ophthalmol.*, 68, 478–483.

Haller, W. (2001) Therapeutische Beeinflussung der Hornhautelemente nach Verätzung, doctoral thesis, Faculty of Medicine, Technical University (RWTH), Aachen, 93 p.

Haseba, T., Nakazawa, M., Kao, C., Murthy, R., and Kao, W. (1991) Isolation of wound specific cDNA clones from a cDNA library prepared with mRNAs of alkali burnt rabbit corneas, *Cornea*, 10, 322–329.

Hennighausen, U., Schmidt-Martens, F.W., and Reim, M. (1972) Metabolitspiegel und Enzymaktivitäten des Energie liefernden Stoffwechsels im regenerierenden Corneaepithel, *Ber. Dtsch. Ophthalmol. Ges.*, 71, 95–99.

Hogan, M.J., Alvarado, J.A., and Wedell, J.E. (1971) *Histology of the Human Eye. An Atlas and Textbook.* Saunders, Philadelphia, London, Toronto.

Hughes, W.J. (1946) Alkali burns of the eye. II. Clinical and pathological course, *Arch. Ophthalmol.*, 36, 189–214.

Kilp, H. (1974) Einfluß von Kontaktlinsen auf Metabolite und Hydratation der Kaninchenhornhaut, *Graefes Arch. Klin. Exp. Ophthalmol.*, 190, 275–280.

Kilp, H. and Heisig, B. (1975) Veränderungen der Glukose- und Laktatkonzentrationen in Tränenflüssigkeiten des Kaninchen auf mechanische Reizung und Kontaktlinsentragen, *Graefes Arch. Klin. Exp. Ophthalmol.*, 193, 259–267.

Kompa, S., Wüstemeyer, H., Neitzel, N., and Schrage, N. (2000) Spülung bei Verätzung - Wirkung unterschiedlicher Osmolaritäten auf intrakameralen pH, Hornhautquellung und Osmolarität, *Ophthalmologe*, 97 Suppl, 11.

Kruse, F. (1996) Die Stammzellen des Limbus und ihre Bedeutung für die Regeneration der Hornhautoberfläche, *Ophthalmologe*, 93, 633–643.

Kruse, F. and Tseng, S. (1994) Transformierender Wachstumsfaktor beta 1 und 2 hemmen die Proliferation von Limbus- und Hornhautepithel, *Ophthalmologe*, 91, 617–623.

Kuckelkorn, R., Kottek, A., Schrage, N., Redbrake, C., and Reim, M. (1995) Langzeitergebnisse mit Tenonplastik behandelter schwerverätzter Augen, *Ophthalmologe*, 92, 445–451.

Kuckelkorn, R., Redbrake, C., and Reim, M. (1997) Tenonplasty: A new surgical approach for the treatment of severe eye burns, *Ophthalmic Surg. Lasers*, 28, 105–110.

Kulkarni, P.S. and Srinivasan, B.D. (1983) Synthesis of slow reacting substance-like activity in rabbit conjunctiva and anterior uvea. *Invest. Ophthalmol. Vis. Sci.*, 24, 1079–1085.

Langefeld, S., Reim, M., Redbrake, C., and Schrage, N.F. (1997) The corneal stroma: an inhomogeneous structure, *Graefes Arch. Clin. Exp. Ophthalmol.*, 235, 480–485.

Lauweryns, B., Van den Oord, J.J., De Vos, R., and Missotten, L. (1993) A new epithelial cell type in the human cornea, *Invest. Ophthamol. Vis. Sci.*, 34, 1983–1990.

Mishima, H., Nakamura, M., Murakami, J., Nishida, T., and Otori, T. (1991) TGF-beta regulates actions of EGF, Interleukin-6 and fibronectin on the functions of corneal epithelial cells, *Invest. Ophthalmol. Vis. Sci.*, 32 suppl, 954.

Møller-Pedersen, T., Li, H.F., Petroll, W.M., Cavanagh, H.D., and Jester, J.V. (1998) Confocal microscopic characterization of wound repair following photorefractive keratectomy, *Invest. Ophthalmol. Vis. Sci.*, 39, 487–501.

Morley, N. and McCulloch, C. (1961) Corneal lactate and pyridine nucleotides with contact lenses, *Arch. Ophthalmol.*, 66, 379–382.

Pfister, R., Haddox, J., and Sommers, C. (1993) Alkali-degraded cornea generates a low molecular weight chemoattractant for polymorphonuclear leukozytes, *Invest. Ophthalmol. Vis. Sci.*, 34, 2297–2304.

Redbrake, C., Salla, S., Vonderhecken, M., Sieben, P., and Reim, M. (1997) Gewebezustand humaner Hornhäute vor und nach Organkultur—Einfluß der Todesursache des Spenders, *Ophthalmologe*, 94, 573–577.

Reim, M. (1972) Warum ist die Cornea durchsichtig?—Über Physiologie, Biochemie und Stoffwechsel der Cornea, *Ber. Dtsch. Ophthalmol. Ges.*, 71, 58–77.

Reim, M. (1982a) The clinical significance of proteolytic enzymes and glycosidases in corneal disease, in *Asian Pacific Acad. Ophthalmol. Bangkok*, Laetiangtong, T. and Chotibutr, S., Eds., Phickanes Press, Bangkok, pp. 342–346.

Reim, M. (1982b) Die Bedeutung des Limbus für die Ernährung der Cornea, in *Limbusprobleme*, Doden, W., Eds., F Enke, Stuttgart, pp. 1–6.

Reim, M. (1987a) Zur Behandlung schwerster Verätzungen und Verbrennungen der Bindehaut, *Fortschr. Ophthalmol.*, 84, 65–69.

Reim, M. (1987b) Zur Pathophysiologie und Therapie von Verätzungen, *Fortschr. Ophthalmol.*, 84, 46–54.

Reim, M. (1992a) Chirurgische Anatomie, Physiologie, Biochemie sowie Fragen der Inlay-Technik, *Ophthalmologe*, 89, 109–118.

Reim, M. (1992b) The results of ischemia in chemical injuries, *Eye*, 6, 376–380.

Reim, M., Bahrke, C., Kuwert, T., and Kuckelkorn, R. (1993) Investigation of enzyme activities in severe burns of the anterior eye segment, *Graefes Arch. Clin. Exp. Ophthalmol.*, 231, 308–312.

Reim, M. and Becker, J. (1995) Cell protection in the anterior segment of the alkali burnt eye, in *Cell and Tissue Protection in Ophthalmology*, Schmidt, K.H., Ed., Hippokrates Verlag, Stuttgart, pp. 49–55.

Reim, M. et al. (1976) The redox state of the glutathione in the bovine corneal epithelium, *Graefes Arch. Klin. Exp. Ophthalmol.*, 201, 143–148.

Reim, M., Beil, K.H., Kammerer, G., and Krehwinkel, S. (1982) Influence of systemic ascorbic acid treatment on metabolite levels after regeneration of the corneal epithelium following mild alkali burns, *Graefes Arch. Klin. Exp. Ophthalmol.*, 218, 99–102.

Reim, M., Boeck, H., Krug, A., and Venske, G. (1972) Aqueous humour and cornea stroma metabolite levels under various conditions, *Ophthalmic Res.*, 3, 241–250.

Reim, M., Cattepoel, H., Bittmann, K., and Kilp, H. (1969) Methodische und physiologische Aspekte bei der statistischen Auswertung von Metabolitspiegeln in verschiedenen Kompartimenten der vorderen Augenabschnitte, *Graefes Arch. Klin. Exp. Ophthalmol.*, 177, 355–368.

Reim, M., Foerster, K.H., and Cattepoel, H. (1970) Some criteria of the metabolism in the donor cornea, paper presented in the *XXI. Concil Ophthalmol. Int. Mexico City*, Solanes, M.P. Eds., Excerpta Medica, Amsterdam, pp. 728–733.

Reim, M., Kaufhold, F.M., Kehrer, T., Kuckelkorn, R., Kuwert, T., and Leber, M. (1984) Zur Differenzierung der Therapie bei Verätzungen, *Fortschr. Ophthalmol.*, 81, 583–587.

Reim, M., Kottek, A., and Schrage, N. (1997) The cornea surface and wound healing, *Prog. Retinal Eye Res.*, 16, 183–225.

Reim, M. and Kuckelkorn, R. (1995) Verätzungen und Verbrennungen der Augen, *Akt. Augenheilk.*, 20, 76–89.

Reim, M. and Leber, M. (1992) N-acetylglucose aminidase activity in cornea-scleral ulceration following severe eye burns related to individual patients, *Cornea*, 12, 1–7.

Reim, M., Leber, M., and Kaufhold, F.M. (1982) Normale und pathologische Bestandteile der Tränen des Bindehautsekretes, *Neues Opt. J.*, 20, 375–382.

Reim, M., Meyer, D., and Cattepoel, H. (1967) Über die Bedeutung des Frierstopverfahrens für den in vivo Status der Metabolite im Corneaepithel, *Graefes Arch. Clin. Exp. Ophthalmol.*, 174, 97–102.

Reim, M., Overkämping, B., and Kuckelkorn, R. (1992) Zweijährige Erfahrungen mit der Tenonplastik, *Ophthalmologe*, 89, 524–530.

Reim, M. and Saric, D. (1986) Treatment of chemical burns of the anterior eye segment with macromolecular sodium hyaluronate (Healon), in *Viscoelastic Materials: Basic Science and Clinical Application*, Rosen, E.S., Ed., Pergamon Press, London, pp. 41–52.

Reim, M., Schmidt, F., and Meyer, D. (1966) Die Metabolite des Energie liefernden Stoffwechsels in der Hornhaut verschiedener Säugetiere, *Ber. Dtsch. Ophthal. Ges.*, 67, 164–171.

Reim, M. and Schmidt-Martens, F.W. (1982) Treatment of burns of the anterior eye segment, paper presented in the *XXIV Concil Ophthalmol. Int. San Francisco*, Maumenee, E., Ed., J.P. Lippincott, Philadelphia, pp. 1063–1066.

Reim, M., Schmidt-Martens, F.W., Hö rster, B., and Scheidhauer, E. (1980) Morphologische und biochemische Befunde bei experimentellen Verätzungen mit Alkali, *Ber. Dtsch. Ophthalmol. Ges.*, 77, 749–759.

Reim, M., Seidl, M., and Brucker, K. (1978) Accumulation of ascorbic acid in the corneal epithelium, *Ophthalmic Res.*, 10, 135–139.

Reim, M. and Teping, C. (1989) Surgical procedures in the treatment of most severe eye burns, *Acta Opthalmol. Suppl.*, 67, 47–54.

Ringvold, A., Anderssen, E., and Kjønniksen, I. (1998) Ascorbate in the corneal epithelium of diurnal and nocturnal species, *Invest. Ophthalmol. Vis. Sci.*, 39, 2774–2777.

Rochels, R. (1984) Animal experiment studies on the role of inflammation mediators in corneal neovascularisation, *Doc. Ophthalmol.*, 57, 215–262.

Rochels, R., Busse, W., Hackelbusch, R., and Knieper, P. (1982) Prostaglandin-Konzentrationsbestimmung im Kammerwasser nach der Bindehaut-Hornhautverätzung: Korrelation biochemischer, funktioneller und morphologischer Befunde, *Fortschr. Ophthalmol.*, 80, 145–147.

Rohen, J.W. (1977) Die Hornhaut. Der präcorneale Film, in *Augenheilkunde in Klinik und Praxis*, Francois, J. and Hollwich, F., Eds., G. Thieme: Stuttgart, pp. 1.1–1.57.

Roper-Hall, M.J. (1965) Thermal and chemical burns, *Trans. Ophthalmol. Soc. U.K.*, 85, 631.

Salla, S., Redbrake, C., Becker, J., and Reim, M. (1995) Remarks on the vitality of the human cornea after organ culture, *Cornea*, 14, 502–508.

Salla, S., Redbrake, C., and Frantz, A. (1996) Employment of bioluminescence for the quantification of adenosine phosphates in the human cornea, *Graefes Arch. Clin. Exp. Ophthalmol.*, 234, 521–526.

Schirner, G., Schrage, N., Salla, S., and Reim, M. (1995) Conjunctival tissue examination in severe eye burns: a study with scanning electron microscopy and energy-dispersive x-ray analysis, *Graefes Arch. Clin. Exp. Ophthalmol.*, 233, 251–256.

Schirner, G., Schrage, N.F., Salla, S., Teping, C., Reim, M., Burchard, W.G., and Schwab, B. (1991) Silbernitratverätzung nach Crede'scher Prophylaxe. Eine röntgenanalytische und rasterelektronenmikroskopische Untersuchung, *Klin. Mbl. Augenheilk.*, 199, 283–291.

Schrage, N. (1997) *Elemente in der Cornea*, Habilitationsschrift, faculty of medicine, Technical University (RWTH), Aachen, p. 90.

Schrage, N.F., Benz, K., Beaujean, P., Burchard, W.G., and Reim, M. (1993) A simple empirical calibration of energy dispersive x-ray analyses (EDXA) on the cornea, *Scanning Microscopy*, 7, 881–888.

Schrage, N.F., Flick, S., Redbrake, C., and Reim, M. (1996) Electrolytes in the cornea: a therapeutic challenge, *Graefes Arch. Clin. Exp. Ophthalmol.*, 94, 492–495.

Schrage, N.F., Lorenz, U., von Fischern, T., and Reim, M. (1994) The microtrephine—a new diagnostic tool for obtaining corneal biopsies, *Acta Ophthalmologica*, 72, 384–387.

Schrage, N.F. and Reim, M. (1996) Der Mikrotrepan: experimentelle Erfahrungen, erste klinische Anwendung, *Klin. Mbl. Augenheilk.*, 209, 132–137.

Schrage, N.F., Reim, M., and Burchard, W.G. (1988) Untersuchungen an schwerstverätzten Corneae nach Langzeittherapie unter besonderer Beachtung von partikulären Rückständen aus Trauma und Therapeutika, *Beitr. Elektronenmikroskop. Direktabb. Oberfl.*, 21, 465–472.

Sotozono, C., He, J., Matsumoto, Y., Kita, M., Imanishi, J., and Kinoshita, S. (1997) Cytokine expression in the alkali burned cornea, *Curr. Eye Res.*, 16, 670–676.

Sotozono, C. and Kinoshita, S. (1998) Growth factors and cytokines in corneal wound healing, in *Corneal Healing Responses to Injuries and Refractive Surgeries*, Nishida, T., Ed., Kugler Publications, the Hague, pp. 29–40.

Thaer, A.A. and Geyer, O.C. (1997) Die Anwendung der konfokalen Spalt-Scanning-Mikroskopie auf die in vivo-Untersuchung der Kornea-Mikrostruktur im Zusammenhang mit dem Tragen von Kontaktlinsen, *Contactologica*, 19, 158–177.

Thiel, H., Richter, U., Zierhut, M., and Müller, C. (1988) Immunreaktionen der Bindehaut und Hornhaut nach schweren Verätzungen des äußeren Auges, *Klin. Mbl. Augenheilk.*, 193, 565–571.

Thoft, R. (1978) Chemical and thermal injury, *Int. Ophthalmol. Clin.*, 19, 243–256.

Thoft, R. (1982) Indications for conjunctival transplantation, *Ophthalmology*, 95, 335–339.

Thoft, R. and Friend, J. (1978) Functional competence of the regenerating ocular surface epithelium, *Invest Ophthalmol. Vis. Sci.*, 17, 134–139.

Thoft, R.A. and Friend, J. (1975) Biochemical aspect of contact lens wear, *Am. J. Ophthalmol.*, 80, 139–145.

Turss, R. and Schebitz, H. (1972) Die Bedeutung des Kammerwassers und der Randschlingengefäße für die Ernährung der Hornhaut, *Ber. Dtsch. Ophthalmol. Ges.*, 71, 87–91.

Whikehart, D.R., Edwards, W.C., and R.P.R. (1991) Sorption of sodium hydroxide by type I collagen and bovine corneas, *Cornea*, 10, 54–58.

Zieske, J.D., Bukusoglu, M., and Yankaukas, M.A. (1992) Characterisation of a potential marker of corneal epithelial stem cells, *Invest. Ophthalmol. Vis. Sci.*, 33, 143–153.

CHAPTER 10

Evaluation and Refinement of the Bovine Cornea Opacity and Permeability Assay

John L. Ubels, James D. Paauw, and Phillip L. Casterton

CONTENTS

INTRODUCTION

Because of limitations of the standard Draize rabbit eye irritation test, as well as an increasing demand to reduce animal use in toxicology, an alternative ocular toxicological method known as the bovine cornea opacity and permeability (BCOP) assay has been developed. The test, originally developed by Muir (1984) nearly two decades ago, involves clamping a bovine cornea between two saline-filled chambers and measuring transmittance of white light through the cornea using measurements of voltage from a photocell before and after chemical exposure. Gautheron, et al. (1992) refined the assay and demonstrated that the test results were consistent with the historical data of the Draize test. Casterton et al. (1996) later introduced the determination of opacity using spectrophotometer absorbance measurements at 570 nm and a corneal holder modification with removable end windows that allowed direct application of test materials to the corneal surface.

Although improvements have been made to the BCOP protocol, to gain regulatory acceptance, the assay must be able to distinguish between irreversible damage and temporary loss of transparency caused by increased corneal hydration due to chemical exposure. One of the goals of our experiments was to examine the role of changes in corneal hydration in increasing opacity. By comparing opacity data generated by maximum hydration of the cornea to opacity data after exposure to chemicals, tissue damage induced by chemical exposure can be determined.

In addition to the necessity of mechanistic determination of corneal damage, the BCOP should be further refined to more directly imitate realistic ocular exposure times and generate data more predictive of human response. Since the current BCOP protocol calls for a 10-min exposure, and nonclinical incidents of exposure are typically shorter, we examined the effect of limiting exposure time to 30 sec and 1 min on ocular irritancy.

Because the endothelial cell layer is essential to corneal function and transparency, the condition of these cells after chemical exposure should be examined to predict recovery from corneal exposure. Two compounds that cause a similar change in opacity may cause substantially different effects on endothelial cells despite being rated at the same toxicity level by the BCOP. In our experiments, endothelial cell damage was assessed by endothelial staining with Alizarin Red S and trypan blue.

Finally, it is important that the BCOP be able to distinguish corneal damage caused by experimental technique from that induced by chemical exposure. Since the currently used BCOP holder causes visible wrinkling in the cornea, opacity measurements may be skewed. Also, wrinkling itself directly damages the monolayer of endothelial cells. Because of this disadvantage to the BCOP, a goal of ongoing studies is to design a new cornea holder that prevents wrinkling and thus does not damage the epithelial or endothelial cell layers.

METHODS

The protocol for the hydration study has been previously described in detail (Ubels et al. 1998). Corneas were mounted either intact, with epithelium removed, or with both epithelium and endothelium removed in minimum essential medium (MEM) (Sigma Chemical Company, St. Louis, Missouri) or deionized (DI) water and incubated for 3 h at either 35°C or 4°C. After incubation an 8 mm corneal button was removed and weighed. The tissue was dried and reweighed to determine hydration as mg H_2O/mg dry weight. Absorbance readings were made at 570 nm.

To determine effects of various test substances on hydration, as well as the effect of hydration on opacity, several compounds were applied to the corneal epithelium for 10 min as per the BCOP protocol. After 3 h incubation in MEM at 35°C, hydration and A_{570}, absorbance at a wavelength of 570 nm, were measured.

Corneas were mounted according to the BCOP protocol and incubated in MEM for 15 min. The epithelial layers of the corneas were then exposed to test substances for either 30 sec or 1 min and were incubated for 3 h (Ubels et al. 2000). The A_{570} was measured for each cornea, and these values were compared to those obtained previously for 10-min exposures (Casterton et al. 1996). Corneal hydration was measured as previously described. After 3 h incubation, the endothelial layers were stained with trypan blue (Sigma) and Alizarin Red S (Sigma) as described by Ubels

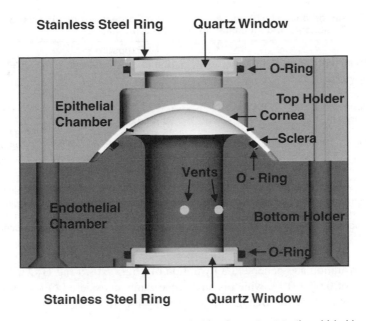
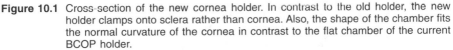

Figure 10.1 Cross-section of the new cornea holder. In contrast to the old holder, the new holder clamps onto sclera rather than cornea. Also, the shape of the chamber fits the normal curvature of the cornea in contrast to the flat chamber of the current BCOP holder.

et al. (2000). An 8 mm button was removed from the center of the cornea and placed endothelial-side up in the depression of a hanging drop slide. The corneas were examined by light microscopy and photographed.

Because the currently used corneal holder involves clamping an oval-shaped cornea between the flat surfaces of two chambers, we designed a new holder to accommodate the shape of the bovine cornea (Ubels et al., 2002). Measurements were made of the dimensions of the bovine cornea, and an improved holder was developed by computer-aided design using the ProEngineer program (Parametric Technologies Corporation, Waltham, Massachusetts). A prototype was built using a Selective Laser Sinterstation (Figure 10.1) (DTM Corporation, Austin, Texas). The prototype was tested by performing the BCOP protocol with control corneas. Corneas were removed from bovine eyes and mounted in the holder. MEM was added to the two chambers and A_{570} readings were made at 15 min and 3 h. The endothelial cell layers were stained with trypan blue and Alizarin Red S and photographed using light microscopy.

RESULTS

The hydration level of the intact untreated cornea after 3 h incubation was 3.86 ± 0.34 mg H_2O/mg dry weight with an average A_{570} of 0.05 ± 0.03. Removal of the epithelium caused an increase in hydration to 6.27 ± 0.47 mg H_2O/mg dry weight with only a minimal increase in absorbance to 0.11 ± 0.03. Removal of both epithelium and endothelium and incubation in water at 4°C was designed to cause

Table 10.1 Absorbance at 570 nm (A_{570}) of Bovine Corneas Exposed to Various Treatments and Incubated in MEM for 3 h

Treatment	Exposure			
	None	10 min	1 min	30 sec
Intact, 35°C, MEM	0.05 ± 0.03	—	—	—
w/o Epi, 35°C, MEM	0.11 ± 0.03	—	—	—
w/o Epi/Endo, 4°C, H_2O	0.67 ± 0.13	—	—	—
Isopropanol	—	0.59 ± 0.08	0.23 ± 0.04	0.24 ± 0.07
Acetone	—	1.38 ± 0.22	1.07 ± 0.21	0.87 ± 0.25
30% TCA	—	1.43 ± 0.08	2.28 ± 0.20	1.96 ± 0.06
1% NaOH	—	1.69 ± 0.22	1.28 ± 0.29	0.36 ± 0.19
30% SLS	—	0.095 ± 0.03	0.48 ± 0.28	0.21 ± 0.11

Note: Intact is untreated cornea incubated in MEM. w/o Epi is cornea with epithelium removed, not exposed to chemical, and incubated in MEM for 3 h. w/o Epi/Endo is cornea with both epithelium and endothelium removed, not exposed to chemical, and incubated in H_2O at 4°C. Values are mean ±SD, n = 5–10. (Data cited from Ubels et al. [2000]. With permission of Elsevier Science.)

maximal hydration and generated a hydration of 16.33 ± 0.79 mg H_2O/mg with an absorbance of 0.67 ± 0.13, which is still in the range considered to represent only moderate irritation by the BCOP (Table 10.1 and Figure 10.2).

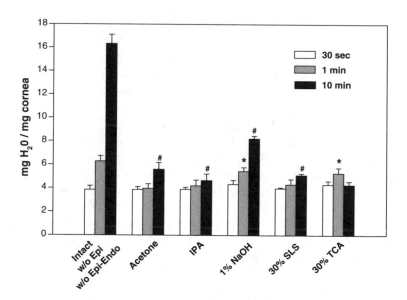

Figure 10.2 Corneal hydration (mg H_2O/mg cornea) following exposure to test substances for 30 sec, 1 min, or 10 min and incubation in MEM for 3 h. Intact is untreated cornea incubated in MEM. w/o Epi is cornea with epithelium removed, not exposed to chemical, and incubated in MEM for 3 h. w/o Epi-Endo is cornea with both epithelium and endothelium removed, not exposed to chemical, incubated in H_2O at 4°C. Mean ±SD, n = 5. Values for intact, without Epi, and without Epi-Endo were all significantly different from each other. 30-sec values and unmarked 1-min values are not different than intact value. # Significantly different than 30-sec and 1-min values within group. * Significantly different than 30-sec and 10-min values within group. (ANOVA and Dunnett's test, $P \leq 0.05$). (Data cited from Ubels et al. [2000]. With permission of Elsevier Science.)

Corneas exposed to four out of five test substances had lower hydration values for 30-sec and 1-min exposures than corneas exposed for 10 min. Only corneas exposed to 30% trichloroacetic acid (TCA) did not exhibit a difference between 10-min and shorter exposures. There was no difference in corneal hydration between a 30-sec and a 1-min exposure to acetone, isopropyl alcohol (IPA), or 30% sodium lauryl sulfate (SLS). A difference did result between corneal hydration measurements taken after 1-min exposure and those after 30-sec for exposure to 1% NaOH and 30% TCA (Figure 10.2). Although the hydration value for corneas with epithelium removed was higher than the values for corneas exposed to acetone or TCA for 10 min, the absorbance for these corneas was lower than in those exposed to acetone or TCA.

The absorbance of corneas exposed to acetone decreased with decreased time of exposure. The A_{570} dropped by over half for corneas exposed to IPA for 30 sec compared to 10 min exposures. Corneas undergoing a 30-sec 1% NaOH exposure had absorbance readings of less than a third of those measured for corneas treated with a 1-min exposure. Corneas treated with 30% TCA showed a lower absorbance after 30 sec than those exposed for 1 min. The 10-min readings for corneas treated with 30% TCA and 30% SLS, however, were lower than the 1-min readings for corneas exposed to these compounds (Table 10.1).

Mounting of corneas in the standard BCOP cornea holders caused approximately 20% of the endothelial cell layer to be damaged (Figure 10.3). The staining pattern corresponded to the wrinkles caused by the holders. In contrast, when mounted in the new holder (Figure 10.1), virtually none of the endothelial layer was damaged after 3-h incubation in MEM (Figure 10.3).

DISCUSSION

Several conclusions can be drawn from the hydration study (Ubels et al. 1998). First, when the corneal hydration increases to a level of 6.3 mg H_2O/mg dry weight in the absence of epithelium (Figure 10.2), the A_{570} increases to only 0.1 (Table 10.1). An absorbance of 0.1 is generally interpreted in the BCOP assay as indicative of a cornea that is only slightly damaged. Because loss of epithelium generates substantial edema and the absorbance reading indicates only minor damage, the absorbance alone is insufficient for determination of corneal damage. Because of this lack of correlation between hydration and absorbance, we propose that a hydration endpoint measurement be added to the BCOP protocol.

Second, exposure of corneas to some compounds caused high absorbance readings but relatively low levels of corneal hydration. Isopropanol (IPA), for example, caused an absorbance of 0.59 compared to 0.1 for corneas with epithelium removed, while the hydration level of corneas exposed to IPA was only 4.66 compared to 6.27 for corneas with epithelium removed (Table 10.1 and Figure 10.2). This indicates that damaged corneas may have hydration levels lower than what would be predicted from the A_{570} reading. This further supports the lack of a reliable correlation between absorbance and hydration. Absorbance levels in excess of that predicted from increased corneal hydration suggest chemical damage to the corneal tissue, rather

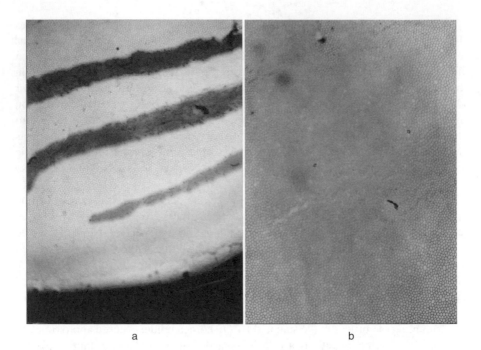

a   b

Figure 10.3 Corneal endothelial cell layers stained with Alizarin Red S and trypan blue. Twenty percent of the endothelial layer is damaged after mounting in the old corneal holder (left), and none of the endothelial layer is damaged after mounting in the new holder (right). The streaks of damaged cells exhibited after mounting in the old holder are characteristic of wrinkling caused by the holder. Magnification 35×. (Reproduced from Ubels et al. [2002]. With permission of Elsevier Science.)

than a decrease in transparency due to corneal edema. Such damage may be irreversible. Hydration measurements coupled with absorbance readings may provide a better indication of the mechanism of corneal damage.

Although corneas exposed to IPA, acetone, or 1% NaOH exhibited absorbance increases with increased exposure time, this is not a general rule (Table 10.1). For some compounds, such as 30% TCA, even a   reduced exposure time results in maximal irritation measurements.   Interestingly, some compounds, such as 30% SLS, cause a higher A_{570} at shorter exposure times than at 10 min. The reason for this is believed to be that at 1 min, damaged epithelial cells increase corneal opacity and thus produce higher absorbance readings. At 10 min, however, the surfactant property of SLS effectively removes the epithelial layer and those cells do not contribute to opacity. This indicates that in some instances the 10-min exposure may lead to an underestimation of irritancy if opacity alone is considered. We propose that for novel substances shorter exposure times be used in addition to the 10-min exposure to more accurately determine ocular damage.

Mounting of corneas in the newly designed holders involves placing the corneal epithelial side down into the anterior chamber of the holder. The posterior, endothelial chamber is then put in place such that it touches only sclera and prevents damage to the corneal endothelium. Using the new holder completely eliminated the corneal wrinkling commonly exhibited by the standard BCOP holders. Figure 10.2 indicates that the new design does prevent endothelial damage. With this new holder, endothelial damage induced by chemical exposure can be determined. Since endothelial cells are essential to proper corneal function, loss of endothelial cells could result in irreversible damage. We propose that endothelial staining using the new holder design be added to the BCOP protocol to strengthen the conclusions that can be made from the test.

ACKNOWLEDGMENTS

The authors thank Aileen Erickson, Christopher Kreulen, Rosanne Pruis, Justin Sybesma, and Dennis Kool for their contributions to the research reviewed in this paper.

REFERENCES

Casterton, P.L., Potts, L.F., and Klein, B.D. (1996) A novel approach to assessing eye irritation using the bovine corneal opacity and permeability test, *J. Toxicol. Cut. Ocular Toxicol.*, 15, 147–163.

Gautheron, P., Dukic, M., Alix, D., and Sina, J.F. (1992) Bovine corneal opacity and permeability test: an in vitro assay of ocular irritancy, *Fundam. Appl. Toxicol.*, 18, 442–449.

Muir, C.K. (1984) A simple method to assess surfactant-induced bovine corneal opacity *in vitro*: preliminary findings, *Toxicol. Lett.*, 22, 199–203.

Ubels, J.L., Erickson, A.M., Zylstra, U., Kreulen, C.D., and Casterton, P.L. (1998) Effect of hydration on opacity in the bovine corneal opacity and permeability (BCOP) assay, *J. Toxicol. Cut. Ocular Toxicol.*, 17, 197–220.

Ubels, J.L., Paauw, J.D., Casterton, P.L., and Kool, D.J. (2002) A redesigned corneal holder for the bovine cornea opacity and permeability assay that maintains normal corneal morphology, *Toxicol. in Vitro,* 16, 621–628.

Ubels, J.L., Pruis, R.M., Sybesma, J.T., and Casterton, P.L. (2000) Corneal opacity, hydration and endothelial morphology in the bovine cornea opacity and permeability assay using reduced treatment times, *Toxicol. In Vitro,* 14, 379–386.

CHAPTER 11

Corneal Organ Culture for Ocular Toxicity Test of Commercial Hair Care Products

Fu-Shin X. Yu and Ke-Ping Xu

CONTENTS

INTRODUCTION

Commercial products, whether drugs, cosmetics, or bulk chemicals, are subject to a variety of tests that are usually performed on animals to determine any potential adverse effects. Among the routinely performed tests is one designed to evaluate the test substance's potential to cause eye irritation or injury: the Draize test (Draize et al., 1944). The Draize test and its numerous modifications have remained the accepted method for evaluating ocular toxicity for more than five decades (Symposium Proceedings, 1996). It has, however, been subject to much criticism for its inhumane treatment to animals as well as the irreproducibility of the subjective scoring procedure. Therefore, there is a great need for minimizing the use of animals in chemical toxicity tests and developing a mechanistically based *in vitro* testing system (Symposium Proceedings, 1996).

Several promising systems for ocular toxicity test are used (Gautheron et al., 1992) or are currently under development, including using immortalized cell lines (Kruszewski et al., 1997; Ward et al., 1997), human corneal equivalents constructed from cell lines (Griffith et al., 1999) and confocal microscopy examination of stroma cell death (Jester et al., 1998a,b). We recently reported the use of a simple corneal organ culture system as an *ex vivo* model to assess ocular irritancy potential of test chemicals (Xu et al., 2000). Using two surfactants, sodium dodecyl sulfate (SDS) and benzalkonium chloride (BAK), we investigated alterations of corneal epithelial permeability and DNA-binding activity of stress-response transcription factors AP-1 and NF-κB caused by these surfactants at the concentrations known to cause different levels of ocular irritation. We observed that the degree of surfactant-induced tight junctions (TJ) disruption and the extent of small molecular penetration measured by surface biotinylation is correlated to *in vivo* irritancy measurements as determined by the Draize test. Using DNA-binding activity of AP-1 and NF-κB as indicators of cellular stress response, we demonstrated that surfactants at concentrations causing minimal to mild ocular irritation increased DNA-binding activity, which indicates epithelial stress response. The surfactants at concentrations causing severe ocular irritancy induced a decrease in DNA-binding activity, indicating destruction of epithelium. Thus, corneal organ culture, coupled with measurements of chemical-induced corneal epithelial barrier disruption and transactivation of stress-related genes, may be used as a mechanistically based alternative to *in vivo* animal testing.

To confirm the usefulness of this model, we evaluated three hair care products in a double-blind manner. We found that shampoos that are moderately irritating caused breakdown of the epithelial barrier and alteration of AP-1 and NF-κB DNA-binding activities, while a minimally irritating hair care product had no effects on cultured corneas. These results indicate the value of the system as an alternative for the *in vivo* Draize test.

METHODS

Corneal Organ Culture

Bovine eyes were obtained from a local abattoir and transported to the laboratory on ice in a moisture chamber. Corneal-scleral rims, with approximately 4 mm of the limbal conjunctiva present, were excised and rinsed in sterilized phosphate buffered saline (PBS). The excised corneas were placed epithelial-side down into a sterile "cup." The endothelial corneal concavity was then filled with minimum essential medium (MEM) containing 1% agarose and 1 mg/ml rat tail tendon collagen maintained at 42°C. This mixture was allowed to gel. Cornea along with its supporting gel was inverted and then transferred to a 35-mm diameter dish. The culture medium (about 2 ml) was added dropwise to the surface of central cornea until the limbal conjunctiva was covered, leaving the epithelium exposed to the air (Foreman et al., 1996, Xu et al., 2000).

Culture Treatment

Three hair care products, termed GA, GB, and GC, were applied directly or diluted with MEM first and then applied dropwise onto the center surface of the cornea. After discrete time intervals, the treated corneas were washed 3–5 times by dipping into PBS solution and then processed for either cell surface biotin labeling or epithelial nuclear extraction.

Surface Biotinylation-Tight Junction Permeability Assay

Cultured corneas were wetted with freshly made 1 mg/ml sulfo-NHS-LC-biotin (Pierce Chemicals, Rockford, IL) in Hank's balanced salt solution containing 1 mM CaCl$_2$ and 2 mM MgCl$_2$ (Chen et al., 1997). After a 30-min incubation, the surface-labeled corneas were rinsed with PBS, embedded in OCT, frozen in liquid nitrogen, and sectioned on a cryostat at a thickness of 6 μm. The sections were fixed with ice cold acetone and labeled with rhodamine-avidin D in PBS containing 1% bovine serum albumin (BSA) for 1 h. The slides were mounted and examined under a Nikon Eclipse E-800 fluorescence microscope equipped with a Spot digital camera.

Electrophoretic Mobility Shift Assay (EMSA)

To prepared cell extracts for EMSA, the epithelial cells were removed from cultured bovine corneas exposed to hair care products under a dissection microscope with a scalpel blade. Cells from each cornea were resuspended in 100 μl of extracting buffer (20 mM Hepes-KOH at pH 7.9, 1 mM dithiothreitol [DTT], 1 mM ethylene-diamine-tetraacetic acid [EDTA], 200 mM KCl, 20% glycerol, 0.1 mM phenylme-thylsulfonyl fluoride [PMSF], 0.1% NP40) and incubated with periodic agitation at 4°C for 1 h. Protein concentration was determined using micro BCA protein assay reagent kit (Pierce Chemical Co.). The oligonucleotide, CGCTTGATGAGTCAGC-CGGAA, for AP-1 binding and the oligonucleotide, AGCTTCAGAGGGGATTTC-CGAGAGG, for NF-κB binding, were labeled using T4 polynucleotide kinase and [γ-^{32}P] ATP. For detection of AP-1 and NF-κB DNA-binding activities, ^{32}P-labeled oligonucleotides were incubated with a 5 μg of epithelial extracted proteins and the reaction mixture was subjected to EMSA assay as described by Xu et al. (2000).

RESULTS AND DISCUSSION

We have used a corneal organ culture model to assess epithelial responses to surfactants, and our results indicated that the combination of corneal organ culture and measurements of corneal epithelial permeability and DNA-binding activity of stress-response transcription factors following surfactant exposure has the potential to be used as a mechanistically based alternative to *in vivo* animal testing (Xu et al., 2000). To validate the usefulness of the system, in this report we evaluated ocular toxicity of three hair care products, termed GA, GB, and GC.

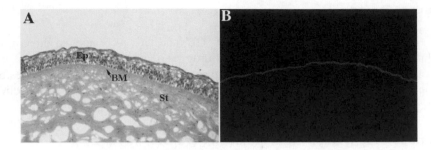

Figure 11.1 Biotin surface labeling to visualize epithelial barrier. Cultured bovine cornea was incubated with sulfo-NHS-LC-biotin for 30 min and then embedded in OCT, snap-frozen, and sectioned (6 μm). Cryostat sections (8 μm) were (A) stained directly with hematoxylin to reveal corneal morphology (B) or incubated with rhodamine-avidin D to visualize the bound biotin. The rhodamine staining represents biotiny-lation of accessible surface of normal bovine cornea and linear staining at the corneal surface indicates functional epithelial TJ barrier in cultured corneas. Ep, epithelium; BM, basement membrane; St, stroma that consists of fibroblasts. A and B are mirror orientations of the same corneal sections.

We first assessed disruption of epithelial tight junction induced by these hair care products in cultured bovine corneas. Mammalian corneal epithelia consist of several layers of cells (Figure 11.1A) (Gipson and Sugrue, 1994). A basement membrane lies immediately beneath the basal lamina of the corneal epithelium and the underlying stroma is composed of many lamellae of collagen fibers with flattened fibroblasts lying between adjacent lamellae. Using sulfo-NHS-LC-biotin that covalently cross links to proteins, we demonstrated the impermeable nature of the cornea (Figure 11.1B). In normal cornea only the outermost surface of epithelium was continually labeled with biotin, as indicated by a fluorescent line on the apical layer of the cornea epithelium, which suggests that the cornea under normal culture condition is impermeable to 500 kD sulfo-NHS-LC-biotin. Thus, as *in vivo,* the cultured corneas possess a fully functional barrier that prevents free passage of molecules and microorganisms into cell layers (Goodenough, 1999).

Chemicals causing eye irritation are likely to affect corneal epithelial integrity and cause breakdown of barrier function. Consistent with this hypothesis, we observed that the surface-labeling pattern is altered by two hair care products, GA and GB (Draize score 37.8 and 57.4, respectively, moderately irritating; Grant et al., 1992) when they were either applied directly or diluted first and then applied onto the center of the cultured corneas (Figure 11.2). We chose a short exposure time (2 min) to mimic *in vivo* accidental exposure to ocular irritants, which are usually removed quickly by tears and blinking. Treatment of cultured cornea with nondiluted GA for 2 min resulted in heavy labeling of the entire epithelium, while EP staining revealed the loss of epithelial cells. At lower concentration (25%), GA caused breakdown of epithelial tight junction, evidenced by labeling of epithelial cell layers and penetration of biotin into stroma. Thus, GA primarily caused disruption of surface labeling and the intensity of disruption was related to its concentration. Incubation of undiluted GB led to the penetration of biotin into the underlying layers of epithelium (primarily the basal layer) and faint labeling of the stroma, while EP staining suggested no loss of epithelium. Incubation of 25% GB for 2 min led to

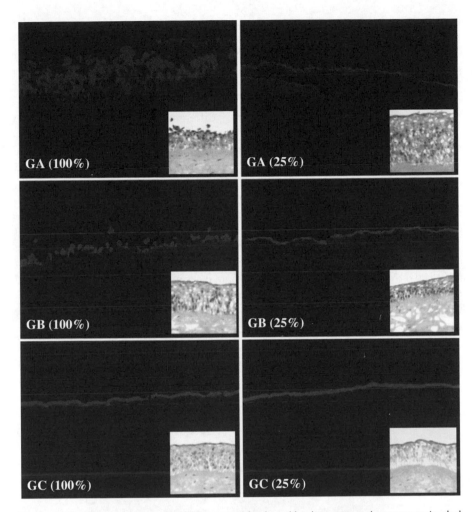

Figure 11.2 Tight junction permeability assay of cultured bovine corneas in response to challenge of three hair care products. Corneas in culture were treated with 100%, 50% (not shown), and 25% chemicals, and TJ permeability of corneal epithelium was assessed by surface biotinylation as described in Figure 11.1. Inserts: corneal sections stained directly with hematoxylin to reveal corneal morphology. Note: extended biotinylation of the corneal surface caused by GA and GB exposure in a concentration dependent manner. However, no disruption of TJ was observed in GC treated cornea.

visible disruption of surface labeling and labeling of multiple epithelial layers and the stroma. Unlike GA and GB, corneas exposed to GC (Draize score 14.2, minimally irritating) exhibited minimal disruption of surface biotinylation when undiluted GC was used and no apparent effects when 1:4 dilution was used (Figure 11.2). Taken together, our results suggest that hair care product–induced alteration of surface labeling was consistent with irritancy potential of these consumer products as determined by the *in vivo* Draize test. Furthermore, surface biotinylation of cultured cornea is an effective way to evaluate TJ permeability and, after a large number of chemicals with known ocular toxicity are tested, to grade the ocular toxicity of surfactant-based consumer products and other chemicals.

We also assess the alteration of NF-κB DNA-binding activity caused by the hair care products in the corneal epithelial cells. Disruption of TJs would allow chemicals to diffuse into deeper epithelial layers where sense neurons reside, causing "irritation" and epithelial cell stress-responses. It is generally believed that most toxicologically relevant outcomes require not only differential gene expression, but also differential expression of multiple genes (Farr and Dunn, 1999). Activated transcription factors coordinately modulate target gene expression via binding to the specific DNA sequences located in the promoter or enhancer. AP-1 (Karin et al., 1997) and NF-κB (Janssen et al., 1995; Pinkus et al., 1996) are well-characterized stress-response transcription factors known to transactivate a large number of stress-response genes and therefore fit the profile of indicators of stress-induced gene expression. In this study, NF-κB DNA-binding activity in response to chemical challenge of cultured corneas was measured using electrophoretic mobility shift assay (EMSA) with extracts from epithelial cells. Figure 11.3 showed alteration of NF-κB DNA-binding activity following hair care product challenges to cultured corneas. There was one major shifted band observed in untreated corneal epithelial cells. Increase in GA concentration led to a decrease in AP-1 DNA-binding activity

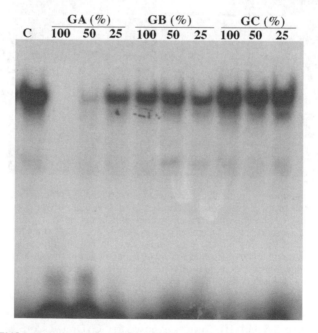

Figure 11.3 EMSA analysis of NF-κB DNA-binding activity in bovine corneal epithelial cells in response to consumer product challenge. Panels showed cultured corneas were treated with different concentrations of three hair care products for 5 min, untreated cells were used as control (C). The corneas were then cultured for 10 min without the presence of the chemicals. Cell extracts from corneal epithelial cells treatment were probed with ^{32}P-labeled AP-1 (upper panel) or NF-κB (lower panel) consensus oligonucleotide. EMSA experiments were repeated two times, and gels presented in the figure are from a representative set.

in a dose-dependent manner: 50% GA reduced NF-κB DNA-binding activity to 10% of the control, and 100% GA induced in almost undetectable NF-κB activity. Furthermore, a 65% decrease in DNA-binding activity was noted when the cultured cornea was exposed to GB for 5 min. There was not much difference in AP-1 DNA-binding activity between untreated control and cornea treated with GC. Taken together, although the mechanisms for regulating NF-κB activity in cells are very complex, we observed changes in NF-κB activity in the cultured cornea in response to consumer product challenges and the concentration-dependent response of epithelial cells to these chemical complexes correlated to toxicity as determine by the Draize test (Xu et al., 2000). Here, the observed reduction of NF-κB activity in the cultured cornea in response to hair care product challenges could be due to decreased viability that affects activation (NF-κB) either by chemical influence directly or secondary to decreased number of viable cells. Nevertheless, our results demonstrate a causal relationship between alteration of NF-κB activities and ocular toxicity, which suggests that NF-κB binding activity may serve as a specific and quantifiable toxicological end point for ocular irritation potential of test chemicals.

By comparison of GA-, GB-, and GC-induced alterations in epithelial permeability and AP-1 and NF-κB-DNA binding activity with the average Draize test scores (37.8, 57.4, and 14.2 for GA, GB, and GC, respectively), the results indicated that the degrees of the alterations induced by these products are in good agreement with the results of *in vivo* testing.

In summary, our aim has been to develop an *ex vivo* model to assess ocular irritancy potential of test chemicals using a simple corneal organ culture system. Using three hair care products, GA, GB, and GC, we observed that the degree of shampoo-induced TJ disruption and the extent of small molecular penetration measured by surface biotinylation correlated to *in vivo* irritancy measurements as determined by the Draize test, and we demonstrated that chemicals at concentrations causing ocular irritancy induced a decrease in DNA-binding activity, which indicates destruction of epithelium. Thus, corneal organ culture, coupled with measurements of chemical-induced corneal epithelial barrier disruption and transactivation of stress-related genes, represents a suitable *ex vivo* model as an alternative to the *in vivo* Draize test for evaluating ocular irritation potential for consumer products.

REFERENCES

Chen, Y., Merzdorf, C., Paul, D.L., and Goodenough, D.A. (1997) COOH terminus of occludin is required for tight junction barrier function in early Xenopus embryos, *J. Cell Biol.,* 138, 891–899.

Draize, J.H. and Woodard, G.H.O.C. (1944) Method for the study of irritation and toxicity of substances applied topically to the skin and mucous membrane, *J. Pharmacol. Exp. Ther.,* 82, 377–389.

Farr, S. and Dunn, R.T. (1999) Concise review: gene expression applied to toxicology, *Toxicol. Sci.,* 50, 1–9.

Foreman, D.M., Pancholi, S., Jarvis, E.J., McLeod, D., and Boulton, M.E. (1996) A simple organ culture model for assessing the effects of growth factors on corneal re-epithelialization, *Exp. Eye Res.,* 62, 555–564.

Gautheron, P., Dukic, M., Alix, D., and Sina, J. (1992) Bovine corneal opacity and permeability test: an *in vitro* assay of ocular irritancy, *Fundam. Appl. Toxicol.*, 18, 442–449.

Gipson, I. and Sugrue, S. (1994) Cell biology of the corneal epithelium, in *Principles and Practice of Ophthalmology*, Albert D. and Jakobiec, F., Eds., Philadelphia, WB Saunders, pp. 3–16.

Goodenough, D.A. (1999) Plugging the leaks, *Proc. Natl. Acad. Sci. U.S.A.*, 96, 319–321.

Grant, R.L., Yao, C., Gabaldon, D., and Acosta, D. (1992) Evaluation of surfactant cytotoxicity potential by primary cultures of ocular tissues: I. Characterization of rabbit corneal epithelial cells and initial injury and delayed toxicity studies, *Toxicology*, 76, 153–176.

Griffith, M., Osborne, R., Munger, R., Xiong, X., Doillon, C.J., Laycock, N.L., Hakim, M., Song, Y., and Watsky, M.A. (1999) Functional human corneal equivalents constructed from cell lines [see comments], *Science*, 286, 2169–2172.

Janssen, Y.M., Barchowsky, A., Treadwell, M., Driscoll, K.E., and Mossman, B.T. (1995) Asbestos induces nuclear factor kappa B (NF-kappa B) DNA-binding activity and NF-kappa B-dependent gene expression in tracheal epithelial cells, *Proc. Natl. Acad. Sci. U.S.A.*, 92, 8458–8462.

Jester, J.V., Li, H.F., Petroll, W.M., Parker, R.D., Cavanagh, H.D., Carr, G.J., Smith, B., and Maurer, J.K. (1998a) Area and depth of surfactant-induced corneal injury correlates with cell death, *Invest. Ophthalmol. Vis. Sci.*, 39, 922–936.

Jester, J.V., Petroll, W.M., Bean, J., Parker, R.D., Carr, G.J., Cavanagh, H.D., and Maurer, J.K. (1998b) Area and depth of surfactant-induced corneal injury predicts extent of subsequent ocular responses, *Invest. Ophthalmol. Vis. Sci.*, 39, 2610–2625.

Karin, M., Liu, Z., and Zandi, E. (1997) AP-1 function and regulation, *Curr. Opin. Cell Biol.*, 9(2), 240–246.

Kruszewski, F.H., Walker, T.L., and DiPasquale, L.C. (1997) Evaluation of a human corneal epithelial cell line as an *in vitro* model for assessing ocular irritation, *Fundam. Appl. Toxicol.*, 36, 130–140.

Pinkus, R., Weiner, L.M., and Daniel, V. (1996) Role of oxidants and antioxidants in the induction of AP-1, NF-kappaB, and glutathione S-transferase gene expression, *J. Biol. Chem.*, 271, 13422–13429.

Symposium Proceedings (1996) Replacing the Draize eye irritation test: scientific background and research needs, *J. Toxicol. Cut. Ocular Toxicol.*, 15, 211–234.

Ward, S.L., Walker, T.L., and Dimitrijevich, S.D. (1997) Evaluation of chemically induced toxicity using *in vitro* model of human corneal epithelium, *Toxicol. in vitro*, 11, 121–139.

Xu, K.P., Li, X.F., and Yu, F.S. (2000) Corneal organ culture model for assessing epithelial responses to surfactants, *Toxicol. Sci.*, 58, 306–314.

CHAPTER 12

Human Corneal Equivalents
for *In Vitro* Testing

May Griffith and Erik Suuronen

CONTENTS

INTRODUCTION

In this chapter, we review the development of tissue-engineered human corneas and associated structures for use as possible *in vitro* alternatives to ocular irritancy testing in animals. At present, tests of potential ocular toxicity are measured using the Draize or LVET (low volume eye test) rabbit ocular irritancy tests (Daston and Freeberg, 1991). The reliability and pertinence of results obtained from non–human-specific tissues remain questionable. This and the push for a ban on live animal testing has necessitated the development of alternatives for safety, efficacy, and toxicology testing of drugs and consumer products.

Our team (Griffith, Watsky, Osborne, and others) had previously developed a collagen-glycosaminoglycans based stabilized matrix that served as a scaffold for the construction of an *in vitro* tissue equivalent of the human cornea (Griffith et al., 1999). These human corneal equivalents comprised all three main layers of the cornea (stratified epithelium, stroma with keratocytes, and endothelial monolayer) and mimicked human corneas in key physical and physiological functions. Cells for

0-8493-1528-X/03/$0.00+$1.50

125

each of the tissue layers were isolated from the individual cellular layers of human eye bank corneas. In order to maintain a continuous supply of cells for research purposes, and also for homogeneity for repeatability in testing, corneal cell lines were developed by extending their life spans using viral genes that retarded or inhibited normal senescence.

DEVELOPMENT OF CELL LINES AND CONSTRUCTION OF CORNEAS

Corneal cell lines with extended life spans were developed by transfection (Kingston et al., 1997) of genes from SV40 large T antigen coding regions (Bryan and Reddel, 1997), adenovirus E1A (Quinlan, 1994), and human papilloma virus (HPV) 16 E6E7 region (Halbert et al., 1991, 1992; Rhim et al., 1998) into low passage primary cells from each of the three main layers of the cornea. Prior to use in the corneal equivalents, cell lines were screened for morphological, biochemical (protein and mRNA markers), and electrophysiological similarities to freshly dissociated or low passage cultured corneal cells obtained from post mortem human corneas. The goal was to identify lines with functional properties similar to normal cells for use in the corneal equivalents. Constructions using cell lines with appropriate ion channel activities yielded the most successful corneal equivalents.

Corneal equivalents were constructed in inserts as described by Griffith et al. (1999). Briefly, a collagen-chondroitin sulfate substrate was cross-linked with 0.02% to 0.04% gluteraldehyde and then treated with glycine to remove excess gluteraldehyde. This synthesized tissue matrix provided the scaffold to which cells were added. Stromal cells were mixed into the matrix and epithelium or endothelium cells were layered on top or below. Successful constructs were achieved with either epithelium or endothelium being seeded onto the insert first. Once the epithelium was confluent, the corneal equivalent was maintained at an air–liquid interphase to allow differentiation into multilayers. The corneal equivalents were allowed to differentiate for 2 weeks and were then tested for key physical and physiological functions. The equivalent corneal tissue was found to be suitable for ocular testing because it mimicked the human cornea in important functional characteristics such as morphology, biochemical marker expression, transparency, ion and fluid transport, and gene expression.

CHANGES IN CORNEAL TRANSPARENCY IN RESPONSE TO CHEMICALS

To evaluate the potential of the corneal equivalent as a model for testing of chemicals for ocular irritancy potential, we had exposed excised rabbit corneas, human eye bank corneas, and corneal equivalents to chemical agents. We demonstrated opacification within the treatment zone of all three types of corneas in response to potentially irritating chemicals that could be quantified on a custom instrument (Priest and Munger, 1998). Changes in transparency (light transmission) of the corneal equivalents in response to a panel of six chemicals that ranged from mild to harsh were comparable to those observed in *ex vivo* human and rabbit corneas (Griffith et al., 1999). The corneal equivalents demonstrated an active response to different grades of injury, an important functional characteristic of human corneas. The responses and trends observed were comparable to those seen in rabbit corneas and human corneas.

CHANGES IN GENE EXPRESSION IN RESPONSE TO CHEMICAL EXPOSURE

We used reverse transcription–polymerase chain reaction (RT-PCR) to examine relative changes in gene expression in corneal equivalents in response to injury and compared these with changes observed in excised human eye bank corneas. Corneas and corneal equivalents were exposed to an aqueous solution of 5% sodium dodecyl sulfate (SDS), a surfactant that causes mild to moderate injury to the cornea (Draize et al., 1994; Griffith et al., 1980). Exposure of corneas to SDS resulted in differential increases in mRNA levels in the different genes examined (*c-fos*, cytokines *IL-1*, *IL-6*, *bFGF* and *VEGF*, and type I collagen) whose products have roles in corneal wound healing (Griffith et al., 1999). Although similar trends were observed in both fabricated corneas and eye bank corneas, the former showed greater sensitivity, indicated by more marked increases in mRNA expression. One possibility is that the eye bank corneas had undergone storage for up to 48 h. In addition, all the healthiest eye bank corneas are used for transplantation and were therefore not available for our study.

DEVELOPMENT OF RELATED TISSUES

The present cornea gives quantifiable changes in transparency and gene expression, indicating different degrees of cellular damage in response to toxic stimuli. However, it provides no indications of sensitivity, pain, or potential neurotoxicity. For future testing of potential drug and chemical sensitivity, innervated corneal equivalents are being developed. Modification of the biopolymeric matrix of the stroma rendered the matrix conducive for the in-growth of neurites from sensory ganglia such as the dorsal root ganglia (DRG) that were cocultured with the corneal equivalents (Figure 12.1). Neurites extended through the stroma and into the epithelium.

In summary, we report the development of human corneal equivalents that reproduce key physical and physiological functions of human corneas, including cell phenotype, transparency, pump function, and gene expression. The immortalization, electrophysiology, matrix engineering, and casting method allow cellular layers to be grown into useful simulations of human corneas. An immediate application is for use in toxicology testing, particularly in light of proposed bans on live animal testing and the need for more accurate modeling of human tissues.

The innervated cornea could potentially be further developed into a model that could be used for sensitivity testing. This technology also provides a strong basis

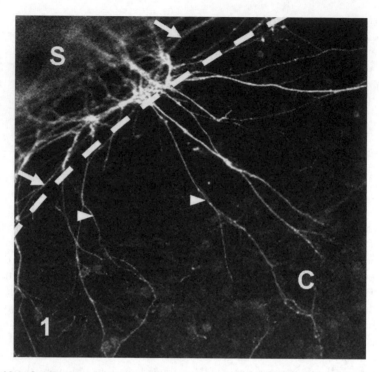

Figure 12.1 Confocal image of a corneal equivalent with surrounding sclera containing chick embryonic dorsal root ganglion (not shown). Neurites, labeled with nerve-specific antineurofilament antibody are seen traveling through the sclera (S) parallel to the corneal periphery and branching into the cornea (C). White dashed line, corneal periphery; arrows, parallel neurites; arrowheads, branching neurites.

for the development of low rejection rate, implantable temporary or permanent cornea replacements.

REFERENCES

Bryan, T.M. and Reddel, R.R. (1997) SV40-induced immortalization of human cells, *Crit. Rev. Oncog.,* 5, 331–357.

Daston, G.P. and Freeberg, F.E. (1991) Ocular irritation testing, in *Dermal and Ocular Toxicology,* Hobson, D.W., Ed., CRC Press, Boca Raton, 509–539.

Draize, J.H., Woodard, G., and Calvery, H.O. (1994) Methods for the study of irritation and toxicity of substances applied topically to the skin and mucous membranes. *J. Pharmacol. Exp. Ther.,* 82, 377–390.

Griffith, J.F., Nixon, G.A., Bruce, R.D., Reer, P.J., and Bannan, E.A. (1980) Dose-response studies with chemical irritants in the albino rabbit eye as a basis for selecting optimum testing conditions for predicting hazard to the human eye, *Toxicol. Appl. Pharmacol.,* 55, 501–513.

Griffith, M., Osborne, R., Munger, R., Xiong, X., Doillon, C.J., Laycock, N.L.C., Hakim, M., Song, Y., and Watsky, M.A. (1999) Functional human corneal equivalents constructed from cell lines, *Science,* 286, 2169–2172.

Halbert, C.L., Demers, G.W., and Galloway, D.A. (1991) The E7 gene of human papilloma-virus type 16 is sufficient for immortalization of human epithelial cells, *J. Virol.,* 65, 473–478.

Halbert, C.L., Demers, G.W., and Galloway, D.A. (1992) The E6 and E7 genes of human papillomavirus type 6 have weak immortalizing activity in human epithelial cells, *J. Virol.,* 66, 2125–2134.

Kingston, R.E., Chen, C.A., Okayama, H., and Rose, J.K. (1997) Introduction of DNA into mammalian cells, in *Current Protocols Molecular Biology,* Ausubel, F.M. et al. Eds., Wiley, New York, 9.0.1–9.1.11.

Priest, D. and Munger, R. (1998) A new instrument for monitoring the optical properties of corneas, *Invest. Ophthalmol. Vis. Sci.,* 39, S352.

Quinlan, M.P. (1994) Enhanced proliferation, growth factor induction and immortalization by adenovirus E1A 12S in the absence of E1B, *Oncogene,* 9, 2639–2647.

Rhim, J.S., Tsai, W.P., Chen, Z.Q., Chen, Z., Van Waes, C., Burger, A.M., and Lautenburger, J.A. (1998) A human vascular endothelial cell model to study angiogenesis and tumorigenesis, *Carcinogenesis,* 19, 673–681.

CHAPTER 13

The EpiOcular Prediction Model: A Reproducible *In Vitro* Means of Assessing Ocular Irritancy

Mitchell Klausner, Patrick J. Hayden, Bridget A. Breyfogle,
Kristen L. Bellavance, Melissa M. Osborn, Daniel R. Cerven,
George L. DeGeorge, and Joseph Kubilus

CONTENTS

INTRODUCTION

An accurate, reproducible *in vitro* means of replacing the Draize rabbit eye test (Draize et al., 1944) has remained elusive despite extensive validation studies to test possible *in vitro* alternatives. The Comite des Associations Europeenes de l'Industrie de al Parfumerie, des Produits Cosmetiques et de Toilette (COLIPA) international validation study investigated ten alternative methods and concluded that none of the methods could be deemed a valid replacement for the Draize eye irritation study although three methods (the fluorescein leakage test, red blood cell assay classification model, and the tissue equivalent assay) were found to be either reliable or relevant (Brantom et al., 1997). Similarly, the European Commission/British Home Office (EC/HO) international validation study investigated nine *in vitro* test methods and concluded that none of the methods met the desired performance criteria and that the methods could not be used to predict ocular irritancy, with the possible exception of predicting the irritancy of surfactants (Balls et al., 1995). Despite the disappointing results from these validation studies, industry successfully employs alternative methods for in-house purposes to identify potential eye irritants (Spielmann, 1997).

It has been suggested that one of the reasons for the successful internal use of alternative methods by individual companies is that in-house testing may be restricted to products or materials within narrow ranges of chemistry (Spielmann, 1997). Thus, it seems logical to approach validation of alternative methods by first demonstrating that a method is predictive for a specific class of materials. The current study investigates the use of an organotypic tissue model to predict the ocular irritancy potential of water-soluble, nonalcohol materials.

With the long-term goal of developing a validated *in vitro* assay system to replace Draize ocular testing, a prediction equation has been developed so that a "predicted" Draize score could be computed based on an EpiOcular MTT assay results. In order to evaluate the reliability and relevance of the prediction model, the 95% prediction intervals (PI) were determined (Brantom et al., 1997). The prediction model was used to compare *in vitro* and *in vivo* results for a variety of consumer products.

MATERIALS AND METHODS

EpiOcular (OCL-200) Tissue Source

The EpiOcular tissue model is prepared using proprietary manufacturing techniques in which normal human neonatal foreskin keratinocytes, derived from a single donor, are grown under standardized conditions to produce a highly uniform, reproducible cornea-like tissue. The keratinocytes are expanded in monolayer culture and harvested using trypsinization according to standard techniques described in literature available from Clonetics Corporation (La Jolla, CA), the commercial vendor from which the keratinocytes were obtained. Single cell suspensions of keratinocytes are aliquoted into 10-mm ID Millicell® polycarbonate (PCF) cell culture inserts (Millipore Corporation, Bedford, MA); polycarbonate Nunc cell culture inserts (Naperville, IL) also serve as suitable substrates. The inserts are placed in a 37°C, 5% CO_2 incubator and cultured at the air–liquid interface, i.e., only the basal side of the cell culture inserts is exposed to the medium. The culture medium is Dulbecco's modified eagle's medium (DMEM), to which a proprietary mixture of nutrients, growth factors, and hormones has been added; all media are serum free. After approximately 1 week of culture, the cell culture inserts containing the stratified tissue are placed atop agarose gels in a 24-well plate. This 24-well plate is hermetically sealed ("packaged") and shipped for commercial sale or stored at 4°C for 24 to 72 hr prior to testing. For commercial purposes, these packaged tissues are shipped every Monday on wet ice (ca. 4°C) via overnight express delivery.

All EpiOcular tissues used throughout the studies described herein were taken from standard lots of EpiOcular tissue that otherwise would have been used for commercial sale. The tissue was packaged as if for shipment and then stored for at least 24 hr at 4°C to simulate the wet ice shipping and storage procedures used for commercial product.

Histology

EpiOcular tissue samples were fixed in 10% formalin (room temperature, overnight) and cut from cell culture inserts using an 8-mm diameter dermal punch and cuticle scissors. Following dehydration in a graded series of ethanol, tissue samples were paraffin embedded, sectioned, and stained with hematoxylin and eosin (H&E). Light microscopy was performed using a Nikon Diaphot fitted with Hoffman modulation optics. A cornea from a white New Zealand rabbit, which was the unneeded byproduct of ophthalmic eye research at the Eye Research Institute (Boston, MA), was processed in an identical manner for comparison purposes.

TISSUE VIABILITY ASSAY—MTT ET-50 METHOD

Preequilibration of Tissue

After storage at 4°C, cultures were removed from the packages and reequilibrated to 37°C by placing them in six-well plates containing 0.9 ml per well of assay media (supplied with OCL-200 EpiOcular tissue model kit) for 1 hr. After 1 hr, the medium was replaced with fresh assay medium and tissues were dosed with test material.

Preparation of Test Articles

In order to handle materials for which the chemical nature and potential ocular irritancy is unknown, the specific gravity (SG) of liquid test materials is determined.

Materials that have a SG greater than 0.95 were diluted to 20% with ultrapure water and then applied; non–water-soluble materials were applied as a paste, which was made by mixing equal masses of the material and ultrapure water. Materials that have a SG less than 0.95 (for example, alcohols, alcohol-containing formulations, or many organic chemicals) are not discussed in this paper. The method used to determine SG was to pipette 100 µl of material into a tared container on an analytical balance, determine the mass, and repeat the procedure using 100 µl of ultrapure water. Both test material and ultrapure water were allowed to equilibrate to room temperature for 1 hr. A ratio of the masses (mass of test article divided by the mass of ultrapure water) gives the SG of the test article.

Application of Test Article to EpiOcular Tissue

If the SG was determined to be >0.95, the test article was diluted to 20%; materials of SG < 0.95 were not included in these studies. After dilution, 100 µl of the test material were applied evenly to the surface of the EpiOcular tissue. Free-flowing liquids were pipetted onto the surface of the EpiOcular tissue, and viscous materials were applied with a positive displacement pipette. Solids were prepared by making a 1:1 (wt/wt) slurry (solid/ultrapure H_2O); 200 mg of the slurry was spread evenly over a flat end of an applicator pin with a circular area of 0.50 cm², and the applicator pin was then inverted and placed gently in contact with the EpiOcular apical surface (the applicator pin was left in place for the duration of the exposure).

Exposure Times

All test materials were treated as unknowns. Three consecutive time points from the series, 1, 5, 20, 60, and 240 min were chosen for each test article as follows. An initial 20-min exposure of the test material ($N = 2$ tissue) was used to determine the exposure times, which would bracket 50% viability. For instance, if the initial 20-min dose resulted in less than 30% viability, additional exposure times of 1 and 5 min were used; if the 20-min exposure resulted in greater than 90% viability, 60- and 240-min exposure times were added; alternatively, if the 20-min exposure gave viabilities of 30 to 90%, additional time points of 5 and 60 min were used. The choice of additional time points based on the viability after a 20-min exposure is summarized in Table 13.1.

Typically, testing on a test material was performed on a single day by visually estimating the MTT assay viability of the 20-min exposure. This visual estimate was made 20 to 30 min after the rinsed tissue was placed into the MTT solution by

Table 13.1 Choice of Additional Exposure Times Based on the Viability of the Initial 20-Min Exposure

Viability after 20-min exposure	Additional exposure times (min)
90%	60, 240
<90% but > 30%	5, 60
<30%	1, 5

comparing the color of the tissue to that of concurrent negative controls. In some instances, testing was performed on subsequent days by choosing time points based on actual viabilities resulting from the 20-min exposure. By using the 20-min exposure time results to choose additional time points, the exposure time needed to reduce the viability to 50% (i.e., the effective time 50 [ET-50]) can be interpolated while using a minimum number of tissue samples. In all cases, the viability resulting from the original 20-min time point was included in the calculation of the ET-50.

Exposure Conditions

For all exposures of 5 min or longer, tissues were incubated with the test article at 37°C and 5% CO_2; exposures of less than 5 min were performed in the lab at room temperature and ambient atmospheric conditions.

Removal of Test Article from EpiOcular Tissue

After each exposure time was complete, the test materials were rinsed off the EpiOcular tissues by submerging the tissue culture insert at least three times in a beaker containing phosphate buffered saline (PBS) and then decanting. Additional PBS rinse/decant cycles were performed if there was any evidence that the test article had not been completely removed. After rinsing was complete, the tissue was submerged in 5.0 ml of assay media in a 12-well plate for 10 min to ensure complete removal of the test article. Tissue viability was then determined using the MTT assay.

Tissue Viability: MTT Assay

The viability of the EpiOcular tissue was determined using the MTT tissue viability assay. The MTT assay was performed as follows: after removal of the test material by rinsing with PBS, cultures were placed in 300 μL of DMEM containing 1 mg/ml solution of MTT dye (3-(4,5-dimethyl-2-thiazoyl)-2,5-diphenyl tetrazolium bromide) for 3 hr at 37°C, 5% CO_2; MTT is taken up by viable cells and reduced by mitochondrial dehydrogenases to form a purple formazan. Since only viable cells with functioning mitochondria will perform this reaction, the amount of colored formazan produced has been shown to be proportional to the number of viable cells (Mosmann, 1983). After 3 hr, the purple formazan dye was extracted overnight (or for a minimum of 2 hr with shaking) using 2.0 ml of isopropyl alcohol and the formazan extract was quantified by measuring the absorbance (A) at 570 nm using an E-MAX 96-well plate reader (Molecular Devices, Menlo Park, CA). The number of viable cells was normalized as a percent of the negative control cultures (solvent vehicle only) that have been loaded with MTT and extracted in an identical manner. The percentage of viable cells remaining was determined using the equation:

$$\% \text{ viability} = OD \text{ (treated culture)}/OD \text{ (control)}$$

The percentage viability was calculated using the average optical density reading from duplicate cultures treated in an identical manner.

Calculation of Effective Time 50 (ET-50)

Mathematical interpolation was used to determine an ET-50 value using the equation:

$$V = a + b \log t$$

where V = percentage viability, t = time in minutes, and a and b are constants that can be determined by using the viability data for two different exposure times of the test article to the tissue. In all testing, interpolation was performed using two exposure times that bracketed 50% viability. Alternatively, if viability at the lowest exposure time (1 min) was less than 50%, the ET-50 was set to 1.0 min; if the viability at the longest exposure time (240 min) exceeded 50%, the ET-50 was set to 240 min. For testing of ultramild materials, this maximum exposure time used was 48 hr (2880 min); if the viability after exposure for 48 hr exceeded 50%, the ET-50 was set to 2880 min.

Determination of Prediction Model

Draize data were available for 19 water-soluble materials in the ECETOC database (Bagley et al., 1992). Also, Draize data for an additional 40 cosmetic or personal care products/ingredients were made available to MatTek by commercial companies interested in the development of a data-set for EpiOcular. All 59 materials are listed in Table 13.2. An ET-50 for the 59 materials was determined using the procedures described above. For materials with Draize scores at a specified concentration, a solution of the specified concentration was made up prior to determination of the SG and the solution was used neat or diluted to 20% depending on the SG. All materials were tested at least twice using two different lots of EpiOcular tissue.

An average ET-50 for the various materials was determined, and the Draize score was plotted versus log (ET-50). Linear regression routines in the graphics program Slidewrite Version 5.0 (Advance Graphics Software, Encinitas, CA) were used to find the best fit to these data to determine a prediction equation.

Testing of Prediction Model

Draize scores for various consumer and personal care products, including five shampoos, six hand/face/body soaps, five laundry detergents, four dishwashing liquids, and four skin lotions were made available to MatTek Corporation by MB Research Laboratories (Spinnerstown, PA). All materials were off-the-shelf products available at retail stores. Each ET-50 was determined as outlined above in at least two separate lots of EpiOcular. Using each ET-50, predicted Draize scores were calculated and an average predicted Draize score was computed for each material. Subsequently, the *in vitro* predicted Draize score was plotted versus the actual Draize scores, the data were fitted to the line predicted Draize = actual Draize ($y = x$), and a correlation coefficient, r, was determined.

Table 13.2 *In Vitro* and *In Vivo* **Data Used to Generate the Prediction Model;** *In Vitro* **Data from EpiOcular ET-50 Determinations;** *In vivo* **Data from ECETOC Database or Commercial Sources**

#		Conc. tested	ET-50 (min)	Draize (MMAS)
1	Benzalkonium chloride (10%)	2.0%	1.07	108.0
2	Benzalkonium chloride (5%)	1.0%	1.0	83.8
3	Benzalkonium chloride (1%)	0.2%	5.9	45.3
4	Cetyl pyridinium bromide (10%)	2.0%	9.0	89.7
5	Cetyl pyridinium bromide (1%)	0.2%	30.1	36.0
6	Cetyl pyridinium bromide (0.1%)	0.02%	240.0	2.7
7	Glycerol	20.0%	240.0	1.7
8	Sodium hydroxide (10%)	2.0%	1.0	108.0
9	Sodium hydroxide (1%)	0.2%	2.3	25.8
10	Propylene glycol	20.0%	240.0	1.3
11	Sodium dodecyl sulfate (30%)	6.0%	2.1	60.5
12	Sodium dodecyl sulfate (15%)	3.0%	5.1	59.2
13	Sodium dodecyl sulfate (3%)	0.6%	9.0	16.0
14	Trichloro acetic acid (30%)	6.0%	1.0	106.0
15	Trichloro acetic acid (3%)	0.6%	155.1	6.7
16	Triton X-100 (10%)	2.0%	2.5	68.7
17	Triton X-100 (5%)	1.0%	5.3	33.1
18	Triton X-100 (1%)	0.2%	36.7	1.7
19	Tween 20 (100%)	20.0%	240.0	4.0
20	Body/hand wash	20%	9.1	32
21	Body/hand wash	20%	14.8	35
22	Eye gel/colorant	20%	240	0
23	Eye gel/colorant	20%	240	2
24	Face/body wash	20%	240	2
25	Face/body wash	20%	6.5	25
26	Face/body wash	20%	10.2	40
27	Hand/body lotion	20%	240	2
28	Hand/body lotion	20%	240	2
29	Hand/body lotion	20%	240	3
30	Shampoo—baby	20%	30.8	10
31	Shampoo—baby	20%	25.7	18
32	Conditioner	20%	240	2
33	Shampoo—regular	20%	6.0	30
34	Shampoo—regular	20%	8.7	35
35	Na_2-ricinoleadmido MEA sulfosuccinate	20%	108.9	0
36	Sodium trideceth sulfate	20%	2.5	33
37	Cetrimonium chloride	20%	116.9	6.67
38	Stearalkonium chloride	20%	240	14
39	Cocamide DEA	20%	240	0
40	Disodium cocoamphodipropionate	20%	11.2	15.3
41	Surfactant blend	20%	19.2	6.0
42	Surfactant blend	20%	40.4	2.67
43	Final formulation shampoo	20%	26.1	4.0
44	Final formulation shampoo	20%	29.1	12.5
45	Final formulation shampoo	20%	4.2	32.7
46	Final formulation shampoo	20%	9.3	31.6
47	Final formulation shampoo	20%	9.0	34.4

(continued)

Table 13.2 (continued) *In Vitro* and *In Vivo* Data Used to Generate the Prediction
Model; *In Vitro* Data from EpiOcular ET-50 Determinations; *In vivo* Data
from ECETOC Database or Commercial Sources

#		Conc. tested	ET-50 (min)	Draize (MMAS)
48	Final formulation shampoo	20%	31.0	3.9
49	Final formulation shampoo	20%	63.1	3.5
50	Final formulation shampoo	20%	47.1	8.3
51	Final formulation shampoo	20%	29.4	6.57
52	Final formulation shampoo	20%	42.1	4.8
53	Hydro-alcohol (hair spray) solution	20%	84.1	6.0
54	10% fatty alcohol ethoxylate	20%	189	3.5
55	Eye makeup remover (surfactant sol.)	20%	240	0
56	Lactic acid (3% solution)	20%	240	0
57	Oleic acid	20%	240	2
58	Skin care emulsion	20%	240	0
59	Body spray	20%	240	0

Quality Control Testing

Each weekly lot of EpiOcular tissue is tested using the common surfactant, Triton
X-100 (Sigma Chemical Company, St. Louis, MO). One hundred microliters of a
0.3% solution of Triton X-100 in ultrapure water (12 to 18 MOhm) are applied to
duplicate EpiOcular tissues ($N = 2$) for 5, 20, and 60 min; in addition, 100 µL of
ultrapure water are applied to triplicate tissues for 60 min to serve as the negative
control. The intralot variability of the tissue was assessed by determining an average,
standard deviation, and coefficient of variation (CV = 100 × standard deviation/aver-
age) for each of these timed applications; in addition, the CVs were averaged to
compute an average CV for the entire lot. The interlot variability was assessed by
computing the ET-50 for each tissue lot and then by comparing each ET-50 for
Triton X-100 from all EpiOcular tissue lots produced during the calendar years
1996–2000. Finally, the average MTT OD for the negative control tissues and the
resultant CV were determined.

Interlaboratory Testing

Tissues from a single production lot were packaged and shipped to the Procter
and Gamble Company (Cincinnati, OH) and the Institute for In Vitro Sciences
(Gaithersburg, MD). In addition, tissue from the same EpiOcular lot was retained
at MatTek and stored at 4°C for 48 hr prior to testing. Results from the two
laboratories and from MatTek's laboratory were compared for the positive control,
Triton 0.3% X-100, and for two additional materials from the ECETOC database
(Bagley et al., 1992): (a) 30% sodium dodecyl sulfate (SDS) and (b) 1.0% benzalkonium chloride (BAK). Note: As per the procedures described above, 6% SDS and
0.2% BAK were the actual concentrations tested in the three labs. Dose response
curves were constructed using $N = 3$ tissues, and an ET-50 was determined in each
lab for each of the three materials. As with the database testing, reproducibility of

the testing results was assessed by calculating averages, standard deviations, and coefficients of variation for each of the materials tested. In addition, a coefficient of variation was determined for each of the time points tested in each laboratory and an average CV was calculated for the laboratory. Finally, the ET-50 for each material from the three labs was compared.

Testing of Ultramild Materials

The method used to test very mild materials, i.e., those to which the Draize test was insensitive (MMAS < 1), differed from the method described above in two key aspects: (a) the materials were applied neat regardless of the SG and (b) exposure times were extended up to 48 hr. The ET-50 was determined as previously described using the MTT tissue viability assay.

RESULTS

Histological Characterization of the EpiOcular Tissue Model

Cross sections of H&E stained EpiOcular tissue and a rabbit cornea are shown in Figure 13.1. The structures are of equal thickness and consist of a cuboidal layer of basal cells with additional layers of flattened cells. There is no evidence of a granular or cornified layer, as would be seen with fully differentiated keratinocytes cultured at the air–liquid interface (Regnier et al., 1990; Mak et al., 1991; Boelsma et al., 2000). Cells on the apical surface of both tissues are squamous and show elongated nuclei.

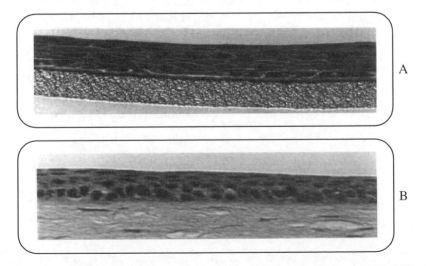

Figure 13.1 Hematoxylin and Eosin (H&E) stained histological cross sections of (A) EpiOcular tissue model and (B) rabbit cornea epithelium and underlying stroma. Tissues were fixed in 10% formalin, embedded in paraffin, and stained with H&E. Final magnification 360×.

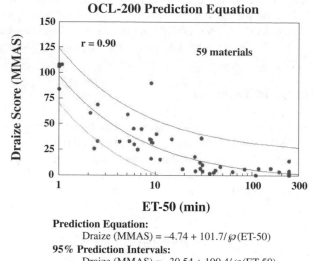

Prediction Equation:
    Draize (MMAS) = –4.74 + 101.7/℘(ET-50)
95% Prediction Intervals:
    Draize (MMAS) = –30.54 + 100.4/℘(ET-50)
    Draize (MMAS) = 21.07 + 102.9/℘(ET-50)

Figure 13.2 Graphical depiction of *in vivo* and *in vitro* data used to derive the prediction equation. All materials tested that had specific gravity >0.95 were diluted to 20% in ultrapure water. If actual ET-50 exceeded 240 min, ET-50 was set equal to 240 min. If ET was less than 1 min, ET-50 was set to 1 min.

Determination of Prediction Model

The chemical name or product category, the respective ET-50, and the Draize score for the materials used to construct the prediction equation are given in Table 13.2. ET-50 and Draize scores are plotted in Figure 13.2. The optimal fit for the prediction equation was determined to be

$$\text{Draize (MMAS)} = -4.74 + 101.7/\sqrt{\text{ET-50}}$$

where the ET-50 is expressed as $1 \leq \text{ET-50} \leq 240$ min.

The 95% confidence intervals for the prediction equation (95% prediction interval) are

$$\text{Upper limit: Draize MMAS} = 21.07 + 102.9/\sqrt{\text{ET-50}}$$

$$\text{Lower limit: Draize MMAS} = -30.54 + 100.4/\sqrt{\text{ET-50}}$$

Testing of Prediction Model

Table 13.3 shows predicted and actual Draize scores for the final formulation cosmetic/personal care products used to test the utility of the prediction model. A graphical comparison of the actual Draize and predicted Draize scores is shown in Figure 13.3. The ability to correctly predict the *in vivo* Draize scores was assessed

Table 13.3 EpiOcular Prediction Model Testing: Comparison between *In Vivo* and *In Vitro* Predicted Draize

	Code		Product	Predicted Draize	Actual Draize (MMAS)
1	10599	A	Body wash	14.6	16.7
2	10599	B	Body wash	31.3	44.7
3	10599	C	Dishwashing liquid	51.3	38.3
4	10599	D	Hand soap liquid	28.0	24.7
5	10599	E	Dishwashing liquid	25.2	39.3
6	10599	F	Facial soap	15.6	9.3
7	10599	G	Dishwashing liquid	50.8	39.0
8	10599	H	Dishwashing liquid	60.5	50.3
9	10599	I	Laundry detergent	37.3	37.3
10	10599	J	Laundry detergent	1.8	0.7
11	10599	K	Laundry detergent	33.4	37.7
12	10599	L	Dishwashing liquid	96.9	37.7
13	10599	M	Shampoo	6.5	4.0
14	10599	N	Shampoo	32.9	41.7
15	10599	O	Shampoo	8.4	3.3
16	10599	P	Hand soap liquid	18.1	13.3
17	10599	Q	Skin lotion	1.8	0.7
18	10599	R	Shampoo	46.9	33.7
19	10599	S	Skin lotion	1.8	0.0
20	10599	T	Shampoo	39.3	37.7
21	10599	U	Body wash	41.2	33.0
22	10599	V	Laundry detergent	1.8	0.7
23	10599	W	Laundry detergent	39.9	44.0
24	10599	X	Skin lotion	1.8	0.7

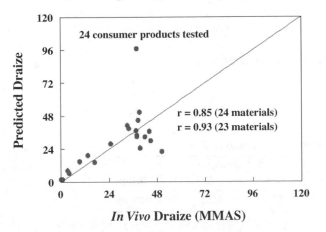

Testing of OCL-200 Prediction Model
In Vivo (MMAS) vs. Predicted Draize

Figure 13.3 Comparison of predicted and actual Draize scores for consumer products including: shampoos (5), face/body soap (6), dishwashing liquids (4), laundry detergents (5), and skin lotions (4). The predicted Draize scores were calculated based on the ET-50 using the prediction equation shown in Figure 13.2.

Table 13.4 EpiOcular QC Testing Results for Positive (0.3% Triton X-100) and
Negative (ultrapure water) Controls

Calendar Year	Tissue Lots	Triton ET-50 (min)	Neg. Control (OD)	Avg. Lot CV (%)
2000	60	23.1±6.0	1.441	5.5
1999	84	22.6±5.0	1.433	5.6
1998	85	25.2±5.6	1.354	5.5
1997	81	22.9±4.7	1.343	5.4
1996	47	24.9±6.3	1.274	5.2

by calculating the correlation coefficient, r, for the line actual Draize = predicted
Draize ($y = x$). The value of r was determined to be 0.85; however, if one of the
laundry detergents whose Draize score was overpredicted by EpiOcular was
excluded from the regression line, the correlation coefficient rises to $r = 0.93$.

Quality Control Results: 1996–2000

A summary of quality control data for calendar years 1996 through 2000 is
presented in Table 13.4. The yearly average for the positive control, 0.3% Triton X-
100, has remained stable, ranging from 22.9 to 25.2 min (1997 and 1998, respectively). The negative control has varied between an optical density of 1.274 to 1.441
(1996 and 2000, respectively). The variability within tissue lots has been extremely
low. In all years, the average lot CV was less than 6%.

Interlaboratory Reproducibility

The ET-50 for each of the three materials tested in the three laboratories is shown
in Table 13.5. For all three materials, interlaboratory reproducibility was good—coefficients of variation for the ET-50 were less than 10%. In addition, tissues within
given lots of tissue were highly reproducible as evidenced by the average coefficient
of the variation in each lab, which was less than 10%.

Testing of Ultramild Materials

The ET-50 for a broad range of concentrations of benzalkonium chloride (BAK)
and sodium dodecyl sulfate (SDS) are shown in Table 13.6 and Figure 13.4. At

Table 13.5 Results of Interlaboratory Testing

Laboratory:	ET-50 (mins): BAK	SDS	Triton	Intralaboratory Reproducibility Avg. CV (%)
P&G:	5.75	3.12	25.40	7.75
IIVS:	6.39	3.30	26.59	7.14
MatTek:	5.97	3.72	29.75	9.56
Average:	6.04	3.38	27.24	
Std. Dev.:	0.32	0.31	2.25	
CV:	5.36	9.19	8.26	

Table 13.6 ET-50 for Ultramild Materials for Which the
Draize Test Is Insensitive

In Vivo Concentration	Draize (MMAS)	ET-50 (min)
Benzalkonium chloride (BAK)		
10.00%	108.0	1.1
5.00%	83.8	1.0
1.00%	45.3	5.9
0.30%	8.67	28.9
0.10%	0	212.7
0.03%	0	2053.0
Sodium dodecyl sulfate (SDS)		
30.00%	60.5	2.1
15.00%	59.2	5.1
3.00%	16.0	9.0
1.00%	0.67	29.5
0.30%	0	740.1
0.10%	0	1938.3

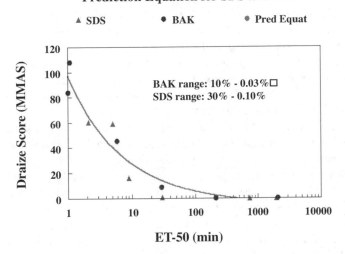

**Comparison of ET-50, Draize Score, and□
Prediction Equation for SDS and BAK**

▲ SDS   ● BAK   ● Pred Equat

BAK range: 10% - 0.03%□
SDS range: 30% - 0.10%

Figure 13.4 Use of EpiOcular to differentiate between very mild materials that cannot be distinguished by the *in vivo* Draize test (MMAS < 1.0).

concentrations of 0.1% BAK and 1.0% SDS, the Draize score drops below 1.0 and hence the Draize test cannot distinguish between lower concentrations of these surfactants. However, as shown in Table 13.6, EpiOcular tests reveal a dramatic difference in ET-50 below these concentrations. Thus, *in vitro* EpiOcular testing can be used to characterize materials that are too mild for the Draize test to distinguish. The EpiOcular test is sensitive at concentrations threefold and tenfold (for BAK and SDS, respectively) below the concentration at which the Draize score is ≤1.0.

DISCUSSION

A great deal of time, effort, and resources have been expended in attempting to develop a nonanimal means of determining the ocular irritancy potential of materials that may come in contact with the human eye. A large number of *in vitro* alternatives to the Draize eye test have been developed, and although industry uses such tests for internal purposes, no *in vitro* system has been validated for regulatory purposes. The EpiOcular tissue model described herein consists of cultured human epithelial cells that have been induced, using specially formulated media, to form a stratified cornea-like epithelium. Mechanistically, the EpiOcular tissue model is more relevant to the *in vivo* condition than many of the other proposed *in vitro* assays (e.g., cells in monolayer culture or in suspension). In addition, it has similarities to the ZK1200 tissue model, formerly offered by Advanced Tissue Sciences (La Jolla, CA), which was an *in vitro* alternative that met one of the two performance criteria in the COLIPA international validation study (Brantom et al., 1997).

The dilution method described herein represents an alternative to the neat testing method previously published (Stern et al., 1998). The dilution method is restricted to water soluble ingredients and formulations, whereas the neat method has no such restriction. The dilution method allows the calculation of an approximate Draize score by use of the prediction equation, whereas the neat method allows categorization into one of four irritation classifications. Both methods appear to have a high degree of success in appropriately predicting the ocular irritation of materials exposed to the human eye.

Reproducibility from individual tissue-to-tissue as well as from lot-to-lot is an extremely important characteristic of any toxicological system. For toxicological experiments to be meaningful, identical exposures should give a reproducible response (intralot reproducibility) in the model. In addition, in order to compare the relative toxicity of materials over a long time period, a reproducible system (interlot reproducibility) is required. Quality control data presented herein demonstrate a high degree of both lot-to-lot and intralot reproducibility.

Excellent intralot reproducibility has been observed for EpiOcular tissue. The intralot variability can be assessed by the average lot CVs, which are <6% (Table 13.4). The intralot reproducibility has important economic implications since low variability between tissues means the use of $n = 2$ tissues is justified. Thus, three exposure times using $n = 2$ tissues are sufficient to accurately determine an ET-50 and calculate a predicted Draize score.

In relation to the lot-to-lot reproducibility of the EpiOcular test method, pass/fail criteria have been established such that the positive control for each tissue lot must be within ±2 standard deviations of the 1996 average (see Table 13.4). Quality control (QC) testing of the EpiOcular tissue is performed both prior to shipment and after 1 day of storage at 4°C. The preshipment QC results (data not shown) have been found to be predictive of the postshipment/poststorage results shown in Table 13.4. Thus, screening of tissue properties prior to shipment avoids shipment of tissue that will not meet QC parameters. Pretesting has kept the percentage of failed lots below 5%.

Regarding the use of the dilution protocol presented here, it is understood that some dilution of the test materials will occur *in vivo* due to the tear film present on the cornea and as a result of tearing or other discharges resulting from instillation of the test material into the conjunctival sac (as per Draize test method). In addition, initial test results with the EpiOcular tissue model showed that relatively mild materials, such as baby shampoos with Draize scores of 15 or below, gave an ET-50 below 10 min. Thus, in order to more closely mimic *in vivo* Draize exposure conditions and to increase the range of *in vitro* scores, the dilution protocol was developed. Whether dilution of the test article due to the tear film and/or tearing will result in a 20% dilution is difficult to assess. Nonetheless, the dilution protocol appears to satisfactorily correlate *in vivo* and *in vitro* results for a broad variety of water-soluble materials.

The specific gravity cutoff was chosen to exclude alcohol-containing formulations since short chain alcohols (e.g., ethanol and isopropanol) are known to be overpredicted when the testing conditions and prediction equation heretofore described are used. Thus, an alternate protocol for alcohol-containing formulations has been explored. Initial results for a limited number of ethanol containing formulations ($N = 12$) demonstrate that a protocol using 10 µL of the undiluted ethanol-containing formulations gives ET-50 values that allow a reasonably reliable estimate of the Draize score (unpublished data). Additional protocol optimization may be necessary for alcohol-containing materials as well as for organic, non–water soluble materials. Nonetheless, the prediction model here presented appears to be reproducible and reliable for predicting *in vivo* eye irritation and represents an initial step toward the desirable goal of reducing or, if possible, eliminating the use of animal Draize eye testing.

The data presented for ultramild materials demonstrate the potential use of the EpiOcular model to classify materials that are designed to be in contact with, or to be in near proximity to, the eyes. For ophthalmic solutions, materials applied to eyelashes or eyelids, or materials applied to facial skin near the eyes, the tolerable level of ocular irritation is below that which is measurable by the Draize test. Similar levels of irritation are required for many baby care products. It has been reported that another popular *in vitro* test for ocular irritancy, the bovine corneal opacity and permeability test (BCOP), is insensitive/unreliable in the mild and submild range of ocular irritancy (Chamberlain et al., 1997). Thus, the ability of EpiOcular to differentiate between formulations of mild or sub-Draize irritancy is important and represents an improvement upon both the Draize and BCOP methodologies.

ACKNOWLEDGMENTS

The authors gratefully acknowledge the participants in the interlaboratory reproducibility study: Rosemarie Osborne and Dee Roberts of the Proctor and Gamble Company (Cincinnati, OH) and John Harbell, Hans Raabe, and Greg Mun of the Institute for In Vitro Sciences (Gaithersburg, MD).

REFERENCES

Bagley, D.M., Botham, P.A., Gardner, J.R., Holland, G., Kreiling, R., Lewis, R.W., Stringer, D.A., and Walker, A.P. (1992) Eye irritation: reference chemicals data bank, *Toxicol. In Vitro,* 6, 487–491.

Balls, M., Botham, P.A., Bruner, L.H., and Spielmann, H. (1995) The EC/HO international validation study on alternatives to the Draize eye irritation test, *Toxicol. In Vitro,* 9, 871–929.

Boelsma, E., Gibbs, S., Faller, C., and Ponec, M. (2000) Characterization and comparison of reconstructed skin models: morphological and immunohistochemical evaluation, *Acta Derm. Venereol.,* 80, 82–88.

Brantom, P.G., Bruner, L.H., Chamberlain, M., De Silva, O., Dupuis, J., Earl, L.K., Lovell, D.P., Pape, W.J.W., Uttley, M., Bagley, D.M., Baker, F.W., Bracher, M., Courtellemont, P., Declercq, L., Freeman, S., Steiling, W., Walker, A.P., Carr, G.J., Dami, N., Thomas, G., Harbell, J., Jones, A.J., Pfannenbecker, U., Southee, J.A., Tcheng, M., Argembeaus, H., Castelli, D., Clothier, R., Esdaile, D.J., Itigake, H., Kasai, Y., Kojima, H., Kristen, U., Larnicol, M., Lewis, R.W., Marenus, K., Moreno, O., Peterson, A., Rasmussen, E.S., Robies, C., and Stern, M. (1997) A summary report of the COLIPA international validation study on alternatives to the Draize rabbit eye irritation test, *Toxicol. In Vitro,* 11, 141–179.

Chamberlain, M., Gad, S.C., Gautheron, P., and Prinsen, M.K. (1997) IRAG working group—Organotypic models for the assessment/prediction of ocular irritation, Interagency Regulatory Alternatives Group, *Food Chem. Toxicol.,* 35, 23–37.

Draize, J.H., Woodard, G., and Calvery, H.O. (1944) Methods for study of irritation and toxicity of substances applied topically to the skin and mucous membranes, *J. Pharmacol. Exp. Therapeutics,* 82, 377–390.

Mak, H.W., Cumpstone, M.B., Kennedy, A.H., Harmon, C.S., Guy, R.H., and Potts, R.O. (1991) Barrier function of human keratinocytes grown at the air-liquid interface. *J. Investigative Dermatol.,* 96, 323–327.

Mosmann, T. (1983) Rapid colorimetric assay for cellular growth and survival: application to proliferation and cytotoxicity assays, *J. Immunol. Methods,* 65, 55–63.

Regnier, M., Asselineau, D., and Lenoir, M.C. (1990) Human epidermis reconstructed on dermal substrates *in vitro*: an alternative to animals in skin pharmacology, *Skin Pharmacol.,* 3, 70–85.

Spielmann, H. (1997) Ocular irritation, in *In Vitro Methods in Pharmaceutical Research,* Castell, J.V. and Gomez-Lechon, M.J., Eds., Academic, London, pp. 265–287.

Stern, M., Klausner, M., Alvarado, R., Renskers, K., and Dickens, M. (1998) Evaluation of the EpiOcular™ tissue model as an alternative to the Draize eye irritation test, *Toxicol. In Vitro,* 12, 455–461.

CHAPTER 14

Three-Dimensional Construct of the Human Corneal Epithelium for *In Vitro* Toxicology

D.H. Nguyen, Roger W. Beuerman, Bart DeWever, and Martin Rosdy

CONTENTS

INTRODUCTION

The corneal epithelium, comprising five or six layers of differentiated ectodermal cells, protects the cornea and contributes to its optical properties (Lemp, 1987; Beuerman and Pedroza-Schmidt, 1996). Injury to the cornea presents a substantial threat to vision (Gasset et al., 1974; Clayton et al., 1985; Osgood et al., 1990). Thus, determining the risk of corneal injury from exposure to chemicals — both at home and in the workplace — is of critical importance.

The Draize test has been used as a standard method to evaluate the potential ocular toxicity of industrial and household chemicals, such as those used in cosmetics and soaps, for many years. However, problems with the Draize test, such as inaccuracy and nonspecificity, have prompted development of more reliable evaluation methods. Newer models include eye organ culture, primary cultures, and immortalized cultures of corneal epithelial cells from humans and other species (Nardone and Bradlaw, 1983; Dawson and Mustafa, 1985; Grant et al., 1992; Kahn et al., 1993; Halenda et al., 1998). Various parameters of epithelial physiology, such as electrical resistance, have also been correlated with the concentrations of some toxic materials (Burstein and Klyce, 1977; Kruszewski et al., 1997). These alternative methods also have several disadvantages, however, including quality control, low throughput, and relationship to normal structure and function of the human cornea.

The use of cultured cells for this purpose is attractive if the cells can be produced in quantity and in a standardized fashion. Immortalized cell lines can be used to replicate important properties of the ocular cells or tissues when primary cultures are not practical or not available (Araki-Sasaki et al., 1995; Nguyen et al., 1999). Reconstituted human epithelial constructs have been reported to allow routine screening of cosmetic ingredients for assessment of eye irritation (Doucet et al. 1998, 1999). The purpose of the present study was to examine the properties of the three-dimensional corneal tissue construct in conjunction with an immortalized human corneal epithelial cell (IHCEC) line and to test the response of the cells in the construct to benzalkonium chloride, a cationic surfactant commonly used as a preservative in ocular medications and cosmetics. We found that this three-dimensional human corneal epithelial cell construct provides a quality controlled, reproducible, and rapid *in vitro* test system that can be used for preliminary large-scale screening of potential corneal irritants and toxic compounds.

MATERIALS AND METHODS

Three-Dimensional Corneal Epithelial Cell Constructs

Immortalized human corneal epithelial cells (IHCEC) were placed in an inert, permeable polycarbonate insert (Nunc A/S, Roskilde, Denmark) and cultivated at the air-liquid interface in a chemically defined medium for 7 d. The three-dimensional constructs were shipped overnight to the LSU Eye Center in New Orleans, Louisiana, from the SkinEthic Laboratories in Nice, France. Upon arrival, the constructs were aseptically removed and placed in six-well culture plates containing 500 µl of maintenance medium supplied by SkinEthic. The cultures were allowed to equilibrate in a humidified incubator at 37°C for 24 hr, after which the medium was removed and replaced with fresh medium.

Histology

Constructs were transferred to six-well plates filled with a solution containing 2% glutaraldehyde and 1% paraformaldehyde in a 0.1 *M* sodium cacodylate buffer (pH 7.4) containing 0.02% picric acid at 37°C (Beuerman and Pedroza-Schmidt 1996). The fixative solution was also pipetted into the interior of the constructs. Specimens were washed in 0.1 M sodium cacodylate overnight, postfixed in osmium tetroxide, dehydrated in a graded ethanol series, and embedded in plastic resin (Eponate 12, Ted Pella, Redding, CA). Ultrathin sections (70 nm) were stained for contrast with uranyl acetate and lead citrate (Ultrastainer, LKB, Bromma, Sweden) and viewed using a transmission electron microscope (EM10 C/A; Zeiss). Thick plastic sections (1 μm) were stained with toluidine blue for light microscopy and photography.

In Vitro Toxicology Assay

The effects of benzalkonium chloride were tested by pipetting 30 μl of a 0.1, 0.01, or 0.001% stock solution of the preservative in phosphate-buffered saline (PBS) directly onto the constructs in six-well culture plates. Benzalkonium chloride is a reference chemical for eye irritation testing as designated by the European Centre for Ecotoxicology and Toxicology of Chemicals. Control constructs received either vehicle alone (30 μl of PBS, pH 7.4) or no additional material. Six separate constructs were used for each experimental condition. After 24 hr of incubation, constructs were frozen, fixed for light and transmission electron microscopy, or processed for Western blot analysis.

Western Blot Analysis

The three-dimensional constructs were lysed with 150 μl of ice-cold buffered PBS containing Triton X-100 (10%), sodium deoxycholate (5%), sodium dodecyl sulfate (1%), leupeptin (0.5 μg/ml), EDTA (1 mM), pepstatin A (1 μg/ml), aprotinin (1 μg/ml), and phenylmethylsulfonyl fluoride (PMSF) (200 μM) for 15 min. The lysate was transferred to a centrifuge tube and the polycarbonate insert was removed using a No. 11 scalpel blade and transferred to the same centrifuge tube. Cultures were combined in groups of two. The combined specimens were mechanically processed using a disposable pestle (Kontes Glass Co., Vineland, NJ) and centrifuged at 4°C for 10 min at 5000 rotations per minute (rpm). Total protein was determined by UV spectrophotometry and estimated using the A260/A280 correction ratio (Robyt and White, 1990).

Western blots were carried out as previously described (Nguyen et al., 1999). Samples (25 μg) of the protein lysates were denatured by heating in equal volumes of 2× Laemmli buffer (4× buffer for the less concentrated protein samples), separated on 6, 7.5, or 10% polyacrylamide gels, and transferred to nitrocellulose membranes (Hybond-ECL; Amersham, Piscataway, NJ). Controls consisted of IHCEC cultured for 4 weeks, human donor corneal epithelial cells scraped from a pair of donor corneas obtained from the Central Florida Lions Eye and Tissue Bank within 24 hr of death, or rabbit lacrimal gland.

The membranes were subjected to 100 V for 75 min in an ice bath, then blocked in 5% powdered milk overnight, and incubated with various primary antibodies for 1 hr per antibody at room temperature: biochemical analysis — AE1 and AE3 (1:500)

(Boehringer Mannheim Group Roche, Basel, Switzerland), cornea-specific 64 kDa AE5 (1:500) (Research Diagnostics, Inc., Flanders, NJ), and laminin (1:500) (Calbiochem, San Diego, CA); toxicology analysis-phosphospecific mitogen-activated protein kinase (MAPK) (1:250) (Santa Cruz Biotechnology, Inc., Santa Cruz, CA). The membranes were then incubated with a horseradish peroxidase (HRP)-conjugated secondary antibody (1:1000) (antimouse HRP, Santa Cruz Biotechnology). Determination of reactivity was carried out using electrochemical luminescence (ECL) detection reagents and visualized on x-ray film (Hyperfilm, Amersham).

RESULTS

Histologic Characteristics of the Three-Dimensional Corneal Epithelial Constructs

Histologically, the three-dimensional constructs of IHCEC resembled the stratified cellular organization of human corneal epithelium (Figure 14.1). The nonkeratinized superficial cells were flattened in the plane of the construct. The outer membranes of these cells were thrown into microvilli a few microns in length. Cells in all layers exhibited a well-developed cytoskeletal network and were attached to adjacent cells by desmosomes (Figures 14.2 and 14.3). Cells of the intermediate layer displayed more lateral cytoplasmic extensions than those in the basal layer, similar to wing cells in human corneal epithelium. Mean thickness of the constructs was 60 μm ± 7 μm (±SE; $n = 6$), similar to that of normal human corneal epithelium.

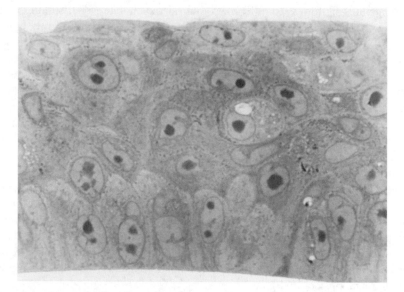

Figure 14.1 Light micrograph of a plastic section from a construct after 24 hr equilibration at 37°C. The tissue organization reveals a stratified appearance with columnar basal cells, defined wing cells, and flattened superficial cells. Toluidine blue and basic fuchsin, original magnification 160×.

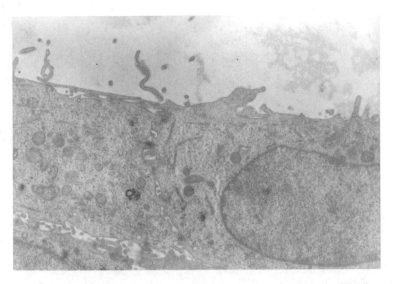

Figure 14.2 Transmission electron micrograph of the construct after 24 hr equilibration at 37°C. The superficial cells give rise to numerous villus processes. The nucleus is oriented parallel to the surface. Some small, spot-like junction arrangements are seen between cells at the surface. Desmosomes are present between adjacent cells. Original magnification 12,600×.

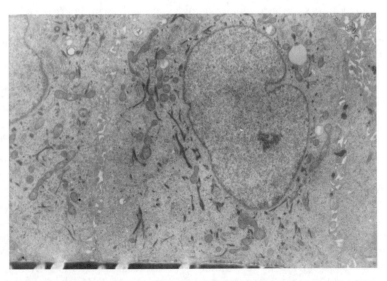

Figure 14.3 Transmission electron micrograph of basal cells of the three-dimensional construct. The nucleus of the basal cell is upright. Within the cell, there is an extensive cytoskeletal network. Mitochondria surround the nucleus and desmosomes join adjacent cells. Original magnification 10,000×.

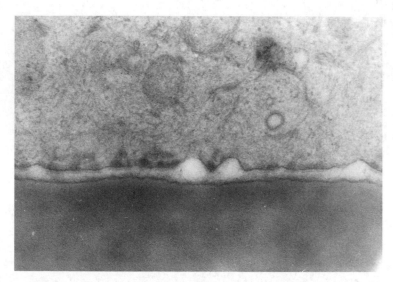

Figure 14.4 High-power transmission electron micrograph of the basal membrane of a basal cell revealing numerous mature hemidesmosomes. Also visible are the components of the hemidesmosomes: the intracellular membrane placode, filaments radiating through the membrane, and the typical band in what would be the lamina lucida. The amorphous band at the bottom is the polycarbonate support membrane of the construct. Original magnification 75,000×.

The basal cell layer consisted of a single layer of columnar cells whose basal membranes rested on the insert (Figures 14.1 and 14.3). At the ultrastructural level, the basal membranes revealed mature hemidesmosomes with internal placodes and filaments radiating through the cell membrane (Figure 14.4). The cytoplasm of the columnar cells was filled with mats of filaments and sparse mitochondria were located around the nucleus.

Biochemical Characteristics of the Three-Dimensional Corneal Epithelial Constructs

The three-dimensional constructs were assessed for immunoreactivity to the epithelial cell-specific keratins, a group of water-insoluble proteins that form the major components of the cytoskeletal complex. Keratins are divided into acidic and basic subfamilies and are found together in pairs. The characterization of specific keratins present in the human corneal epithelium by immunoblotting using the AE1 and AE3 monclonal antibodies has been reported (Tseng et al., 1992). As shown in the Western blots, the expression pattern of AE1 for the constructs was similar to that for IHCEC cultured for 4 weeks (Figure 14.5A). Expression of AE3 for the three-dimensional constructs was similar to the expression patterns seen in cultured IHCEC and freshly obtained human donor corneal epithelial cells (Figure 14.5B). Western blots using the AE5 antibody, a marker of corneal differentiation, showed positive immunoreactivity to a 64 kDa protein, indicating that the epithelial cells of the three-dimensional construct expressed cornea-specific keratin 3 (Figure 14.6).

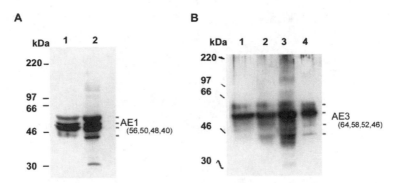

Figure 14.5 Western blots of the acidic (AE1) and the basic (AE3) keratin family in the three-dimensional construct: A. The reactivity pattern for AE1 in the three-dimensional construct (Lane 1) is similar to that of immortalized human corneal epithelial cells (IHCEC) cultured for 4 weeks (Lane 2). B. The reactivity pattern for AE3 (Lane 1) is similar to that of cultured IHCEC at 1 week (Lane 2) and 2 weeks (Lane 3) and human donor corneal epithelial cells obtained within 24 hr after death (Lane 4). The molecular weights of several cytokeratin isoforms recognized by the respective antibodies are indicated below under AE1 and AE3, respectively.

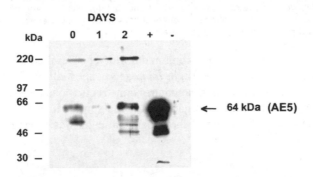

Figure 14.6 Western blot of the 64 kDa cornea-specific keratin AE5 in the three-dimensional construct. Lanes show the construct on Day 0 (immediately upon arrival), Day 1 (24 hr equilibration at 37°C), and Day 2 (48 hr at 37°C), as well as the fresh human donor corneal epithelial cell positive control (+) and the rabbit lacrimal gland negative control (−).

In vivo, corneal epithelial cells are anchored via hemidesmosomes to the underlying structure called the basal lamina. These mechanical attachments are responsible for holding the epithelium tight to the stroma. Laminin and collagen IV are prominent extracellular components of the basal lamina and are synthesized by corneal epithelial cells. In this study, Western blot (Figure 14.7) showed two bands, one at 220 kDa and one at 440 kDa, indicating that the epithelial cells in the three-dimensional construct synthesized laminin. Connexin-43, a protein component of the gap junction, was also present in these three-dimensional constructs (not shown).

Response to Benzalkonium Chloride

Benzalkonium chloride, which is commonly used as a preservative in ophthalmic solutions in concentrations from 0.004 to 0.1%, may increase epithelial

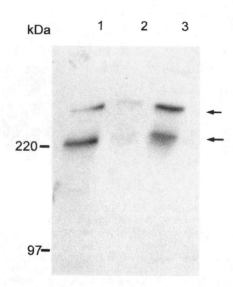

Figure 14.7 Western blot of laminin in the three-dimensional construct. One band is seen at 220 kDa and another at 440 kDa. Lane 1, three-dimensional construct; Lane 2, fresh human corneal donor epithelial cells from cadaver eyes; Lane 3, immortalized human corneal epithelial cells cultured for 4 weeks.

permeability. The effects of benzalkonium chloride at several concentrations were determined after 24-hr exposure. Light microscopy showed no differences in the vehicle (PBS) control and the normal control constructs (not shown). With 0.001% benzalkonium chloride, cellular organization was similar to that of the controls, although some minor sloughing of the superficial cells was seen (Figure 14.8A).

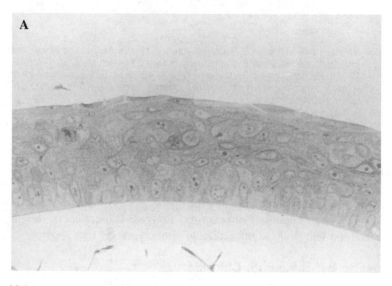

Figure 14.8 Light micrographs of the three-dimensional construct showing cellular damage after treatment with benzalkonium chloride for 24 hr. (A) 0.001%; (B) 0.01%; (C) 0.1%. Original magnification 126×.

(continued)

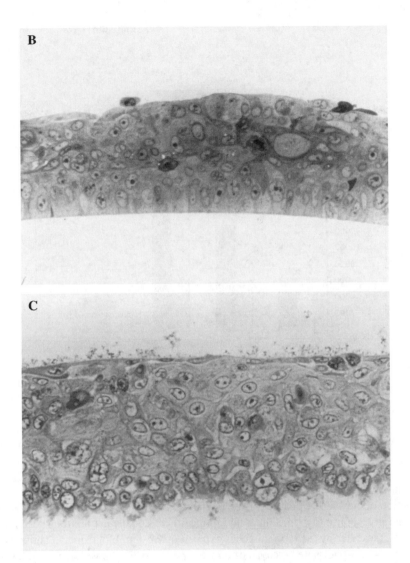

Figure 14.8 (continued) Light micrographs of the three-dimensional construct showing cellular damage after treatment with benzalkonium chloride for 24 hr. (A) 0.001%; (B) 0.01%; (C) 0.1%. Original magnification 126×.

With 0.01% benzalkonium chloride, the organization of the constructs was similar to that of the constructs treated with 0.001% benzalkonium chloride, although the amount of cellular debris was greater (Figure 14.8B). Transmission electron microscopy showed remnants of superficial cells and increased vesiculation (not shown). With 0.1% benzalkonium chloride, the effect was severe (Figure 14.8C). Cellular damage was clearly evident and the constructs were completely separated from the basal membrane; there was much more vacuolation and the nuclei appeared pyknotic.

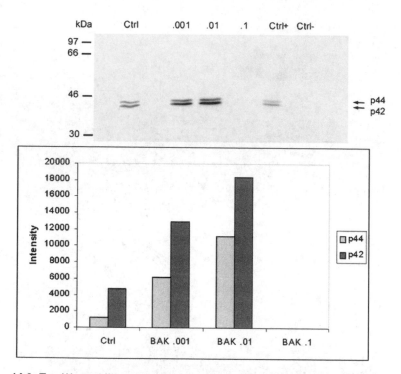

Figure 14.9 Top: Western blot analysis for phosphorylated (active) p42/p44 mitogen-activated protein kinase (MAPK) after treatment with benzalkonium chloride. Positive control (Ctrl +), epidermal growth factor-stimulated A431 cells. Negative control (Ctrl –), unstimulated A431 cells. Bottom: The histogram shows the increase in intensity level (activity) of p42/p44 with increasing concentrations of benzalkonium chloride (BAK). The absence of activity with 0.1% benzalkonium chloride is likely due to cell death resulting from toxic insult.

The effects of benzalkonium chloride were further characterized by examining the induction of the MAPK pathway. Both p42 and p44 MAPK are activated by phosphorylation in response to extracellular and intracellular signals that are transduced to the nucleus, thus altering the types of genes expressed. Western blot using an antibody that recognizes phosphorylated (activated) p42 and p44 MAPK showed increased levels of activated p42 and p44 with both 0.001% and 0.01% benzalkonium chloride, compared with the vehicle control (Figure 14.9). With the highest concentration (0.1%), however, the levels of p42 and p44 decreased below the control level, possibly due to the loss or death of cells as shown by transmission electron microscopy. These results suggest that the constructs may be able to demonstrate an incremental response to environmental stress, in this case benzalkonium chloride in concentrations up to 0.01%.

DISCUSSION

In this study, we demonstrated similarities between the three-dimensional IHCEC construct and normal human corneal epithelium in terms of the overall morphology and thickness (about 60 μm). The stratified appearance of the columnar basal cells and the wing cells overhanging the rounded surfaces of the basal cells was similar to the organization of epithelial tissue *in vivo*. Remarkably, the cultured construct cells produced mature hemidesmosomes along the basal membrane of the basal cells, and filaments were seen to radiate from the internal membrane placodes of the hemidesmosomes. These mechanical attachments were functional to some extent because 0.1% benzalkonium chloride affected their integrity, allowing the support membrane to fall away. This suggests an additional effect of this preservative that has not been previously noted.

Immunoreactivity to 64 kDa keratin 3 indicates that the cells of the construct retain this cornea-specific differentiation marker, i.e., IHCEC in the construct retain the ability to synthesize keratin and to differentiate as corneal epithelial cells (Kruse and Tseng, 1994). The advantage of using this immortalized cell line may be found in the method used to immortalize the cells. The immortalizing vector was an amphotropic retroviral vector (LXSN16E6E7) that contained the E6 and E7 genes of human papillomavirus (Halbert et al., 1991). This approach has also been used to produce an immortalized lacrimal gland epithelial cell line that expressed transferrin receptor and was able to express protein in response to pharmacological stimulation (Nguyen et al., 1999).

The surfactant benzalkonium chloride has been used as a preservative in cosmetics and ophthalmic medications for many years. The toxic effects of this and other surfactants, including corneal damage and delayed wound healing, are well known (Scaife, 1985; Green et al., 1989). The effects of benzalkonium chloride on epithelial cell morphology and physiology have been verified in numerous studies (Gasset et al., 1974; Burstein and Klyce, 1977; Clayton et al., 1985). However, the thrust of these studies has been to identify benzalkonium chloride-related problems in an effort to develop safer preservatives rather than as a means of evaluating models suitable for testing the toxic potential of chemical additives.

It is not yet clear whether the three-dimensional constructs will support combined studies on morphology, physiology, and molecular expression. However, as the constructs can be produced in large numbers, cross-validation may be expected. Another potential advantage of the constructs is the ability to distinguish cellular and molecular markers of toxic effects. Commonly used toxicity markers, such as neutral red staining and the MTT assay, may work well *in vivo*, but may not be useful in predicting tissue recovery or in identifying the cellular mechanisms activated by the toxic stress. In this study, the intracellular signal transduction pathway MAPK was shown to be activated by benzalkonium chloride. This suggests that cellular stress responses were initiated; however, verification will require parallel studies using whole eyes and other stress-activated signal pathways at early time points with comparison to scores from the Draize test. Nevertheless, this cell-based strategy could provide a new approach to predicting the severity of injury as well as the ability to heal after chemical insult.

Engineered constructs such as those used in this study provide substrate reliability and the opportunity to standardize testing to facilitate broad comparisons between laboratories. This could result in the development of a data base of chemical responses. As with *in vitro* tests in general, finding the parameters that describe coarse measures of the response is not difficult. However, further work is required to develop and refine these measures and improve their ability to increase our understanding of the capacity for healing and the return to the normal state after exposure to a toxic event.

ACKNOWLEDGMENTS

This study was supported in part by U.S. Public Health Service grants EY12416, EY04074, and EY02377 (departmental core grant) from the National Eye Institute, National Institutes of Health, Bethesda, Maryland, and an unrestricted departmental grant from Research to Prevent Blindness, Inc., New York, New York.

REFERENCES

Araki-Sasaki, K., Ohashi, Y., Sasabe, T., Hayashi, K., Watanabe, H., Tano, Y., and Handa, H. (1995) An SV40-immortalized human corneal epithelial cell line and its characterization, *Invest. Ophthalmol. Vis. Sci.*, 36, 614–621.

Beuerman, R.W. and Pedroza-Schmidt, L. (1996) Ultrastructure of the human cornea, *Microsc. Res. Tech.*, 33, 320–335.

Burstein, N.L. and Klyce, S.D. (1977) Electrophysiologic and morphologic effects of ophthalmic preparations on rabbit cornea epithelium, *Invest. Ophthalmol. Vis. Sci.*, 16, 899–911.

Clayton, R.M., Green, K., Wilson, R.M., Zehir, A., Jack, J., and Searle, L. (1985) The penetration of detergents into adult and infant eyes: possible hazards of additives to ophthalmic preparations, *Food Chem. Toxicol.*, 23, 239–246.

Dawson, M. and Mustafa, A.F. (1985) Use of cultured human conjunctival and other cells to assess the relative toxicity of six local anaesthetics, *Food Chem. Toxicol.*, 23, 305–308.

Doucet, O., Lanvin, M., and Zastrow, L. (1998) A new *in vitro* human epithelial model for assessing the eye irritation potential of formulated cosmetic products, *In Vitro Mol. Toxicol.*, 11, 273–283.

Doucet, O., Lanvin, M., and Zastrow, L. (1999) Comparison of three *in vitro* methods for the assessment of the eye-irritating potential of formulated cosmetic products, *In Vitro Mol. Toxicol.*, 12, 63–76.

Gasset, A.R., Ishii, Y., Kaufman, H.E., and Miller, T. (1974) Cytotoxicity of ophthalmic preservatives, *Am. J. Ophthalmol.*, 78, 98–105.

Grant, R.L., Yao, C., Gabaldon, D., and Acosta, D. (1992) Evaluation of surfactant cytotoxicity potential by primary cultures of ocular tissues: I. Characterization of rabbit corneal epithelial cells and initial injury and delayed toxicity studies, *Toxicology*, 76, 153–176.

Green, K., Johnson, R.E., Chapman, J.M., Nelson, E., and Cheeks, L. (1989) Surfactant effects on the rate of rabbit corneal epithelial healing, *J. Toxicol.-Cut. Ocular Toxicol.*, 8, 253–269.

Halbert, C.L., Demers, G.W., and Galloway, D.A. (1991) The E7 gene of human papilloma virus type 16 is sufficient for immortalization of human epithelial cells, *J. Virol.*, 65, 473–478.

Halenda, R.M., Grevan, V.L., Hook, R.R., and Riley, L.K. (1998) An immortalized hamster corneal epithelial cell line for studies of the pathogenesis of Acanthamoeba keratitis, *Curr. Eye Res.*, 17, 225–230.

Kahn, C.R., Young, E., Lee, I.H., and Rhim, J.S. (1993) Human corneal epithelial primary cultures and cell lines with extended life span: *in vitro* model for ocular studies, *Invest. Ophthalmol. Vis. Sci.,* 34, 3429–3441.

Kruse, F.E. and Tseng, S.C. (1994) Retinoic acid regulates clonal growth and differentiation of cultured limbal and peripheral corneal epithelium, *Invest. Ophthalmol. Vis. Sci.,* 35, 2405–2420.

Kruszewski, F.H., Walker, T.L., and DiPasquale, L.C. (1997) Evaluation of a human corneal epithelial cell line as an *in vitro* model for assessing ocular irritation, *Fundam. Appl. Toxicol.,* 36, 130–140.

Lemp, M.A. (1987) Recent developments in dry eye management, *Ophthalmology,* 94, 1299–1304.

Nardone, R.M. and Bradlaw, J.A. (1983). Toxicity testing with *in vitro* systems: I. Ocular tissue culture, *J. Toxicol.-Cut. Ocular Toxicol.,* 2, 81–98.

Nguyen, D.H., Beuerman, R.W., Halbert, C.L., Ma, Q., and Sun, G. (1999) Characterization of immortalized rabbit lacrimal gland epithelial cells, *In Vitro Cell. Dev. Biol. Anim.,* 35, 198–204.

Osgood, T.B., Ubels, J.L., Smith, G.A., and Dick, C.E. (1990) Evaluation of ocular irritancy of hair care products, *J. Toxicol.-Cut. Ocular Toxicol.,* 9, 37–51.

Robyt, J.F. and White, B.J. (1990) *Biochemical Techniques: Theory and Practice,* Waveland Press, Inc., Prospect Heights, IL, pp. 232–233.

Scaife, M.C. (1985) An *in vitro* cytotoxicity test to predict the ocular irritation potential of detergents and detergent products, *Food Chem. Toxicol.,* 23, 253–258.

Tseng, S.C.G., Jarvinen, M.F., Nelson, W.G., Huang, J.-W., Woodcock-Mitchell, J., and Sun, T.-T. (1982) Correlation of specific keratins with different types of differentiation: monoclonal antibody studies, *Cell,* 30, 361–372.

CHAPTER 15

The Human Corneal Epithelial HCE-T TEP Assay for Eye Irritation: Scientific Relevance and Summary of Prevalidation Study Results

Sherry L. Ward, Maximo Gacula, Jr., and Henry F. Edelhauser

CONTENTS

INTRODUCTION

New alternative test methods to the Draize rabbit eye irritation test must be able to meet the performance expectations of a formal validation study. International organizations have provided specific criteria that are to be met for test method validation in their published guidelines (Balls et al., 1995a; OECD, 1996; NIEHS, 1997).

Three conditions must be satisfied for a new toxicological test method to be considered valid, the scientific relevance, the predictive relevance, and the reliability of the new test method (NIEHS, 1997; Worth and Balls, 2001). The preferred development of a new test method would include strategically planning the test method development, prevalidation, and validation so that all conditions for its validation are fulfilled by the completion of the interlaboratory validation study. However, test methods in the process of validation at this time were developed before the formal validation processes defined by the European Center for the Validation of Alternative Methods (ECVAM), the OECD, and the Interagency Coordinating Committee on the Validation of Alternative Methods (ICCVAM) were finalized. Therefore, the flexibility that has been proposed for the validation processes (NIEHS, 1997; Worth and Balls, 2001) favors the continued evaluation of scientifically relevant methods that are likely to be useful replacements or adjuncts to current toxicity test methods.

This chapter describes two essential steps in the validation process, establishing the scientific relevance of a new test method, and the prevalidation of the test method. These components of the validation process are described for the HCE-T TEP assay, a human corneal epithelial cell-based assay that was developed as an *in vitro* alternative method to the Draize rabbit eye irritation test (Kahn and Walker, 1993; Kahn et al., 1993; Kruszewski et al., 1995, 1997).

SCIENTIFIC RELEVANCE

Background and Rationale for the Development of the HCE-T TEP Assay

The HCE-T TEP test method was developed at the Gillette Medical Evaluation Laboratories (GMEL) in 1992–1993 as an *in vitro* test method used to evaluate the ocular irritation potential of water-soluble chemicals and formulations (Kahn and Walker, 1993; Kahn et al., 1993; Kruszewski et al., 1995, 1997). The HCE-T TEP assay measures the dose-dependent effect of a test material on the subsequent fluorescein transepithelial permeability (TEP) across stratified cultures of human corneal epithelial cells (the HCE-T cell line).

The HCE-T TEP assay is performed using cultures of human corneal epithelial cells (the 10.014 HCE-T cell line). There are numerous reasons why the use of a cell line is preferable to the use of primary cells or tissues for the development of *in vitro* toxicological assays. Problems with the use of primary cells include biological variability, possible infectious agent contamination, and lack of availability. These problems are particularly evident when it comes to the use of human ocular surface epithelial cells, which are frequently difficult to obtain and do not survive long in culture. On the other hand, well-characterized cell lines provide a readily available source of cells that can be used for the development of reproducible *in vitro* test methods.

A number of human corneal epithelial cell lines were developed and characterized by GMEL scientists between 1991 and 1993. The 10.014 HCE-T cell line was developed by transfection (the insertion of viral genes) of primary cultures of human corneal epithelial cells (HCE) with the SV40 large T antigen plasmid RSV-T (Kahn et al., 1993; Kahn and Rhim, July 1998; Walker and Kahn, September 1997). The resulting cell lines were characterized using a number of criteria to determine their comparability to primary HCE cells, including cell morphology, calcium-mediated modulation of morphology, keratin expression, cytokine release, lactate production, metalloproteinase expression, and the ability to form stratified cultures that develop a measurable epithelial permeability barrier and express tight junctions (Kahn et al., 1993; Kahn and Walker, 1993; Kruszewski et al., 1995; Ward et al., 1995, 1997a, 1997b, 2002a; Clothier et al., 2000). Research findings in other laboratories have also confirmed the retention of corneal epithelial phenotype by the 10.014 HCE-T cell line (Braunstein et al., 1999; Kurpakus et al., 1999; Burbach et al., 2001; Chen and Hazlett, 2001; Song et al., 2001). HCE-T cells are not immortalized, but do have an extended life span relative to primary HCE cells (2 to 5 passages for HCE cells versus approximately 20 passages for 10.014 HCE-T cells), thereby providing a readily available source of human corneal epithelial cells for *in vitro* toxicological studies. The production of a second HCE-T cell line, the 2.040 HCE-T cell line, that has properties similar to those of the 10.014 HCE-T cell line (unpublished observations), indicates that comparable cell lines can be developed to support their continued use in the HCE-T TEP assay. Several HCE-T cell lines, including the 10.014 HCE-T cell line, are available from the American Type Culture Collection (ATCC) in Manassas, VA.

For the HCE-T TEP assay, the HCE-T cells are grown on permeable collagen membranes where they develop into multilayered cell cultures that resemble the structure of the corneal epithelium (Ward et al., 1997b), the most anterior tissue of the human cornea that faces the tear film. These *in vitro* cultures of stratified HCE-T cells are called the HCE-T model. The bottom layers of HCE-T cells are immersed in cell culture medium and the top layer faces the air, so they are described as grown at the air–liquid interface (Figure 15.1A). This type of culture format promotes the development of multiple cell layers (stratification) and the formation of junctions between the cells, which are normal processes that corneal epithelial cells undergo as they proliferate and differentiate.

One of the major functions of an epithelial tissue is to form a border between different biological environments, thus providing both a protective role and a selective permeability barrier (Mackay et al., 1991). At the ocular surface, the corneal epithelium forms a barrier to protect the eye from the external environment. The intact corneal epithelium forms a tight barrier that is impermeable to the small molecular weight fluorescent dye, sodium fluorescein (Maurice, 1967; Norn, 1970). Thus, the technique of vital staining of the cornea by fluorescein can be used by ophthalmologists to identify ocular surface epithelial defects.

The stratified cultures of the HCE-T model develop an epithelial barrier function, which is relatively impermeable to fluorescein. Disruption of the epithelial barrier function in the HCE-T model by a chemical irritant can be measured by its increased permeability to sodium fluorescein (Ward et al., 1997b; Kruszewski et al., 1997). Chemical irritants have likewise been found to disrupt the impermeability of the intact human cornea to fluorescein (Marsh and Maurice, 1971). Since disruption of

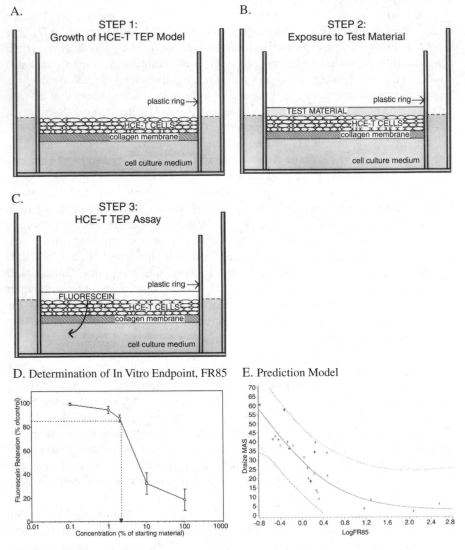

Figure 15.1 The three major steps in the execution of the HCE-T TEP assay (A–C), a typical dose-response curve (D), and the prediction model (E).

the corneal epithelial barrier is one of the earliest biological events that occurs in chemical-induced eye irritation (Maurice, 1955; 1967), it has been identified as a parameter that should be predictive of the ocular irritation potential of chemicals and other eye irritants (Tchao, 1988; Ward et al., 1997b).

The HCE-T TEP assay provides a means to measure the transepithelial permeability (TEP) of the multilayered corneal epithelial cultures to sodium fluorescein after their exposure to increasing doses of a test material. The HCE-T TEP assay consists of three major steps: (1) development and growth of the HCE-T cultures (Figure 15.1A), (2) exposure of the cultures for 5 min to different concentrations of a test material (Figure 15.1B), and (3) evaluation of test material effects on the permeability of the cultures to sodium fluorescein (Figure 15.1C). By measuring the amount of fluorescein that passes through the cultures into the basal media, the HCE-T TEP assay provides a quantitative measure for the dose-dependent effect of a test material on the HCE-T cell cultures. The results can be plotted as a dose-response curve (Figure 15.1D). The endpoint for the *in vitro* assay, the log FR85, is obtained from the dose-response curve. The FR85 is the concentration of test material associated with 85% fluorescein retention (FR) relative to the control cultures. The FR85 was empirically determined to be the endpoint that provided optimal correlation to Draize eye irritation data (Kruszewski et al., 1997).

A prediction model contains an algorithm that defines the quantitative relationship between the data derived from a new test method and the data from the reference method (Bruner et al., 1996; Holzhutter et al., 1996; Archer et al., 1997). The reference method for the HCE-T TEP assay is the Draize rabbit eye irritation test (Draize et al., 1944). A prediction model for the HCE-T TEP assay was developed by statistical modeling of the relationship between the *in vitro* TEP data and the *in vivo* historical Draize maximum average score (MAS) test data for 29 water-soluble surfactants and surfactant-containing formulations (Figure 15.1E). The prediction model can be used to determine a predicted Draize score (MAS) for a test material by using the toxicity test result from the HCE-T TEP assay (the assay endpoint, log FR85). The calculations for the assay have been described in detail by Kruszewski et al. (1997). The log FR85 values from the HCE-T TEP assay for a set of water-soluble chemicals and formulations were also shown to correlate with other Draize tissue scores, such as the corneal score (CS), the conjunctival score, and the iris score (Kruszewski et al., 1997).

Scientific Basis for the HCE-T TEP Assay

The standard method accepted by regulatory agencies for determining the eye irritation potential of a substance has been the Draize rabbit eye irritation test (Draize et al., 1944). The original test has been modified to use three to six animals, and various modified versions are specified by different regulatory agencies (reviewed in Chan and Hayes, 1994, pp. 608–611; DiPasquale and Hayes, 2001, p. 886). In general, a small amount of test material (0.1 ml or 100 mg) is placed in the conjunctival sac of one eye of a specified number of albino rabbits. The ocular reaction to the test material is determined and graded at various scoring intervals according to responses in the cornea, the conjunctiva, and the iris. In a standard grading scheme the total irritation is ranked on a scale of 0 to 110, the corneal responses comprise 80/110 points, the conjunctival responses 20/110 points, and the iris responses 10/110 points. Toxicologists feel comfortable with the continued use of this method because of its familiarity and because of the large database of information available. However, considerable differences exist between the rabbit and the human eye, which has led many to question the use of the Draize test for the prediction of the human ocular response (Beckley, 1965; Beckley et al., 1969; Gershbein and McDonald, 1977; Green et al., 1978; Walker, 1985; ILSI AAT, 1996). Problems with the reproducibility of Draize test results have also been a concern, for example, as demonstrated by the large intralaboratory and interlaboratory variability in Draize test results that were reported in the study of Weil and Scala (1971).

The major similarities and differences between the Draize rabbit eye irritation test method and the HCE-T TEP assay, and their endpoints, are listed in Table 15.1.

The corneal response to an eye irritant is the primary ocular response that needs to be assessed by a Draize alternative method. Human ocular exposures to chemicals and consumer products usually occur as an accidental splash onto the anterior surface of the globe. The eye is designed to protect itself from these types of splashes by the eye lid, a physical barrier, by tearing to wash out noxious substances, and by the epithelium covering the entire anterior portion of the globe, another physical barrier. The cornea, however, as the most anterior ocular tissue, is the most likely to be exposed to a substance during an accidental exposure. In addition to the protective barrier function provided to the eye, the cornea also serves as the transparent port for the entry of light to the retina (Smolin and Thoft, 1987; Albert and Jakobiec, 1994). Corneal damage could lead to opacity and decreased vision. Thus, injury to the cornea has been designated the appropriate significance of 73% of the total Draize score (80 maximum corneal score out of 110 maximum total score).

The corneal epithelium, as the outermost layer of the cornea, serves as a functional barrier to toxicant entry into the eye (Daston and Freeberg, 1991; Hackett and McDonald, 1991). The corneal epithelium is a stratified tissue composed of five to six cell layers. The surface cells are connected by tight junctions, and additional desmosomal intercellular junctions exist throughout the remaining cell layers (Figure 15.2). These multiple cell layers and intercellular adhesions provide the protective barrier of the ocular surface. The outer tight junction of the corneal epithelium is the primary junction to regulate epithelial permeability. The intercellular adhesions and tight junctions are organized in a tissue-specific manner, providing a unique type and degree of barrier function by the corneal epithelium (Mackay et al., 1991; Hamalainen et al., 1997).

An understanding of the structure and physiology of the cornea is essential to the development of appropriately structured *in vitro* corneal models. The cornea is composed of three cellular layers: the outermost corneal epithelium; the stroma, which is interspersed with fibroblast-type cells called keratocytes; and the single cell layer of the corneal endothelium, which provides the interface with the aqueous humor of the anterior chamber. The three cellular layers of the cornea provide a differential permeability barrier to the penetration of compounds into the eye, which is at least partially based upon the partitioning behavior of a particular compound (DeSantis and Patil, 1994). The epithelium provides the barrier to the penetration of hydrophilic substances into the cornea, while the stroma and endothelium provide most of the barrier to the penetration of more lipophilic substances. These physiologic properties of the cornea provide the biological rationale for using an *in vitro* model of the corneal epithelium to evaluate surfactant-induced corneal effects.

Both the rabbit and the human cornea have been shown to respond similarly to surfactant ocular exposures. Berry and Easty (1993) showed that corneal effects in isolated rabbit and human eyes were similar after exposures to an anionic (sodium dodecyl sulfate) and a nonionic (Tween 20) surfactant. However, other

Table 15.1 Similarities and Differences in the Endpoint Measured in the HCE-T TEP Assay and in the Draize Eye Irritation Test

Test Species	Test Tissue	Exposure Route	Exposure Time	Concentration Tested	Endpoint Measured	Mechanism of Tissue Damage
Human (in vitro)	Corneal epithelium	Superficial to cell cultures	5 min	5 concentrations with highest equal to that evaluated in Draize test	Concentration of test material causing 15% of fLuorescein to penetrate through the corneal epithelium (FR85)	Cytotoxicity and junctional disruption in the corneal epithelium
Rabbit (in vivo)	Ocular surface (cornea, conjunctiva and iris)	Superficial to eye	Until washed out by blinking and tearing (<5 min)	Concentration defined by toxicologist (neat or diluted)	Cornea: area of damage and opacity Conjunctiva: chemosis, redness and discharge Iris: degree of effect	Area of corneal damage is related to epithelial cytotoxicity and junctional disruption; opacity is related to penetration of test material into stroma. Conjunctiva damage similar to cornea—epithelial toxicity and penetration. Iris—material has penetrated to cause more severe damage.

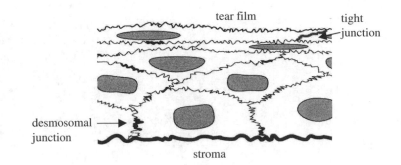

Figure 15.2 Cross-sectional diagram of the human corneal epithelium. A drawing illustrating the multiple cell layers, the apical tight junctions, and the intercellular desmosomal junctions of the corneal epithelium.

substances, such as ethanol and acetone, showed species-specific corneal effects. These results support the biological relevance of using Draize rabbit eye test data as the reference method for a human corneal cell-based *in vitro* test method for the evaluation of surfactants and surfactant-based test materials. These findings could also explain why some other chemical classes showed a lower correlation between the Draize data and the HCE-T TEP assay data (Kruszewski et al., 1997). Other considerations, such as the large variabilities observed between animals and between laboratories with Draize eye test data (Weil and Scala, 1971), still make the Draize eye irritation test less than optimal as the reference method for the development of new test methods.

Recent studies in one laboratory indicate that ocular injury from surfactants results in cell death, and that the extent of cell death may be predictive of the degree of ocular irritation (Jester et al., 1998). Previous studies in this lab demonstrated that the ocular irritation produced by surfactants of increasing irritancy is related to increased area and depth of corneal injury (Jester et al., 1996; Maurer et al., 1997, 1998b). They found that slight to mild irritants produced injury mostly to the ocular surface epithelium, while the damage from moderate to severe irritants showed increasingly greater depths of injury through the corneal stroma. Severe irritants also caused corneal endothelial cell damage. Thus, a corneal epithelial model is appropriate for the evaluation of slight and mild irritants and for moderate irritants when dilutions of the materials are evaluated. This conclusion is supported by the results obtained in evaluating surfactant exposures using the stratified HCE-T model. The HCE-T TEP assay has also been able to identify severe eye irritants, but an insufficient number have been evaluated to determine the accuracy and precision of the results.

Reproduction of the biological characteristics of the corneal surface was taken into consideration during the development of the HCE-T model. The HCE-T model consists of a multilayered culture of HCE-T human corneal epithelial cells grown on a permeable collagen membrane at the air–liquid interface. Culture of the HCE-T cells on permeable membranes at the air–liquid interface in medium containing an elevated concentration of calcium (1.15 mM) induces the cells to stratify and differentiate, forming a tissue with a well-developed barrier function. Barrier

A   B

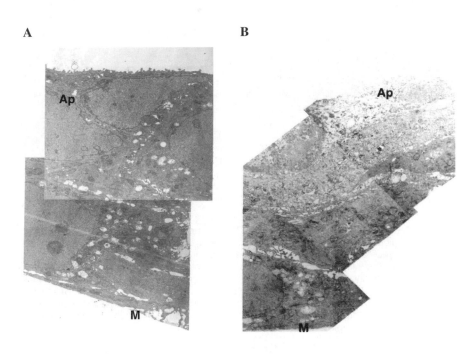

KGM   0.01% BAC

Figure 15.3 Cross sections of stratified HCE-T cultures visualized by transmission electron microscopy following 5-min superficial exposures to (A) cell culture medium (KGM) (5000×); and (B) 0.01% benzalkonium chloride (BAC) (6000×). Ap = apical surface of the culture; M = collagen membrane. [Photos contributed by S.D. Dimitrijevich.]

function in the HCE-T model can be measured by the ability of the cultures to restrict the permeation of sodium fluorescein (measured as transepithelial permeability to fluorescein; TEP) and to develop tight junctions (measured as transepithelial electrical resistance; TER) (Kahn and Walker, 1993; Kruszewski et al., 1995, 1997; Ward et al., 1995, 1997b).

Ultrastructural analysis of the HCE-T model illustrates its comparability to the human corneal surface (Ward et al., 1995, 1997a, 1997b) (Figures 15.3 and 15.4). The surface cell layers in the cornea (Mackay et al., 1991) and in the HCE-T model are composed of flattened, squamous epithelial cells that contain the tight junctions responsible for regulation of paracellular permeability in this tissue. The middle and basal cell layers of the HCE-T model express numerous desmosomal intercellular junctions.

The cross-section photomicrographs shown in Figure 15.3 illustrate the effect of the chemical toxicant benzalkonium chloride (BAC) on the cells of an HCE-T culture. Figure 15.3A shows a cross section from an untreated 6-day HCE-T culture. BAC (0.01%) was cytotoxic to the superficial cells in another HCE-T culture, as shown by the lack of intracellular content in the surface cell of the photomicrograph (Figure 15.3B). The epithelial cells in the BAC-treated culture also appear to have some edema, indicated by their plump appearance and by the increased intercellular spaces. Physiological assessment of the cultures showed that 0.01% BAC caused

A   B

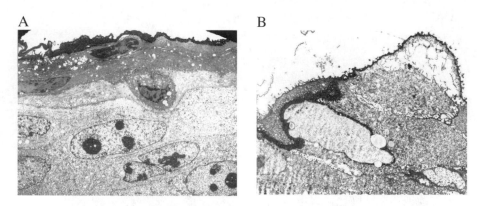

Figure 15.4 Cross sections of stratified HCE-T cultures, visualized by transmission electron microscopy, which were fixed in a special buffer to retain the mucin layer. The dark-stained surface material is the mucin produced by the corneal epithelial cells. (A) A continuous layer of mucin is found on the surface of a differentiated culture (maintained at the air–liquid interface in serum-free medium containing 1.15 mM calcium) in which the TER is high (tight junctions are intact); and (B) mucin is found between the cells in this non-differentiated culture (maintained submerged in serum-free medium containing 0.15 mM calcium) in which the TER is low (tight junctions not intact).

less than 10% overall cytotoxicity (MTT assay), only slightly increased the fluorescein permeability of the cultures (decreased TEP), but significantly damaged the tight junctions (decreased TER) (Ward et al., 1997b).

Another similarity between the HCE-T cultures and the *in vivo* corneal surface is the production of mucin by the corneal epithelial cells, and its localization at the surface of the intact cornea and on the surface of the HCE-T cultures (Ward et al., 1997a) (Figure 15.4). Mucin is a component of the tear film that is produced by corneal and conjunctival epithelial cells, as well as the goblet cells of the conjunctiva (Inatomi et al., 1995). The functions of mucin at the ocular surface are to facilitate spreading of the aqueous portion of the tear film and to serve as a protective covering for the surface of the eye. The apical mucin layer modulates the local environment of the surface epithelia and plays a role in the cells interaction with exogenous substances (DeSantis and Patil, 1994). Perturbation of the tight junctions in the HCE-T model was accompanied by a disruption in the protective apical mucin layer, and mucin was then found between the lower cell layers (Ward et al., 1997a) (Figure 15.4). These results are similar to observations reported with the rabbit cornea (Ubels et al., 1995; Edelhauser et al., 1998).

The multiple cell layers and intercellular junctions of the HCE-T model, like those of the corneal surface, provide a protective barrier that cannot be modeled by the monolayer cell cultures typically used for *in vitro* toxicological assays (Ward et al., 1997b). The multilayered epithelial cultures of the HCE-T model have been shown to be more resistant than monolayer cultures of the same cells to chemical (Ward et al., 1997b) and protein toxicant (Ward et al., 1995) damage. These findings support the biological relevance of using a differentiated, three-dimensional corneal epithelial cell model for the development of a Draize alternative test method.

Fluorescein permeability, as a measure of barrier disruption in epithelial cultures, was originally proposed as a model to evaluate potential chemical toxicity to the eye by Tchao (1988). The original fluorescein leakage assay used monolayer cultures of Mandin-Darby canine kidney epithelial cells (MDCK cells). The MDCK cell fluorescein leakage assay is a useful screen for eye irritants (Shaw et al., 1990, 1991). Although studies are ongoing, fluorescein permeability across monolayer MDCK cultures has not demonstrated sufficient correlation to the Draize test to warrant its recommendation for validation (Balls et al., 1995b; Gettings et al., 1996; Bradlaw et al., 1997; Brantom et al., 1997; Zanvit et al., 1999). Tight junction disruption in MDCK cultures appears to occur simultaneously with increased fluorescein permeability (personal communication, R. Clothier, 1997). Tight junction disruption, however, is only part of the mechanism of barrier function disruption when it occurs at the ocular surface. In the stratified human corneal epithelium the multiple cell layers, tight junctions, and other intercellular junctions act to retard fluorescein penetration into the corneal stroma (Araie and Maurice, 1987). The same mechanisms are responsible for fluorescein retention by HCE-T cultures. The data shown in Figure 15.5 illustrate this point. Chemical exposures disrupted the tight junctions (TER) before fluorescein impermeability (TEP) was perturbed in the HCE-T model (Ward et al., 1997b) (Figure 15.5). In the same experiments, recovery in the ability of the cultures to retain fluorescein was found to be independent of recovery in TER. Thus, although the MDCK fluorescein leakage assay is useful as a screen, it does not contain all of the tissue-specific features needed to reproduce the irritant response at human ocular surface.

The experimental data and the scientific literature reported here support the conclusion that the HCE-T TEP assay is a test method that is biologically and mechanistically based, and thus should provide a good model for the human corneal response to eye irritants.

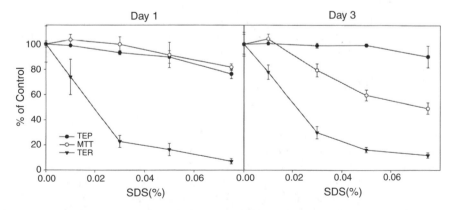

Figure 15.5 Three assays were used to evaluate the dose-dependent effects of sodium dodecyl sulfate (SDS) on HCE-T cultures on the day of treatment (day 1), and 48 hr later (day 3). TEP, transepithelial permeability to fluorescein; TER, transepithelial electrical resistance; MTT, cell viability assay using the MTT dye [3-(4,5-dimethylthiazol-2-yl)-2,5-diphenyl tetrazolium bromide]. Each dose is represented by triplicate cultures, and the error bars are the standard deviations.

The Mechanism of Action of Fluorescein TEP in the Test System Compared to the Human Eye

One of the primary responses that occur upon superficial ocular exposure to an irritating material is disruption of the corneal epithelial barrier function. Barrier disruption can be measured by the loss of fluorescein impermeability across the corneal epithelium, both in the human eye and in the HCE-T model. As explained in the previous section, this is due to the similarity in the cellular mechanisms involved in the maintenance of barrier function in the *in vivo* corneal epithelium and in the stratified HCE-T cultures.

Transepithelial fluorescein permeability has been shown to be a useful indicator of the integrity of the *in vivo* corneal epithelial barrier (Maurice, 1967; Maurice and Singh, 1986; Burstein, 1984). Vital staining of the human cornea, using sodium fluorescein, is a standard technique used by ophthalmologists to assess damage to the corneal epithelium. Sodium fluorescein is a small (367 molecular mass), brightly fluorescent, and yellowish-green colored molecule. The sodium salt of fluorescein is water-soluble, shows negligible binding to the intact ocular surface, and is considered to be nontoxic (Maurice, 1967), which are properties that make sodium fluorescein a useful molecule for ophthalmologic use. In solution, the colored fluorescein can be quantitated by measuring either absorbance or fluorescence, with peak absorption at 490 nm, and peak emission at 520 nm (Maurice, 1967). The permeability of fluorescein in the human corneal epithelium (in one subject) was reported to be 1.5×10^{-5} cm/hr, which is significantly less than that measured for the corneal endothelium (1.0×10^{-2} cm/hr) (Maurice, 1967). Those findings demonstrate the significant role of the corneal epithelium as the major barrier to the penetration of water-soluble drugs and compounds, including sodium fluorescein, into the eye.

The *in vivo* corneal epithelial barrier to fluorescein has been determined by measuring the loss of fluorescein from the tear film and its appearance in the anterior chamber (Maurice, 1955, 1967; de Kruijf et al., 1987). An instrument called a scanning fluorophotometer is used to evaluate the permeation of fluorescein into the anterior chamber of the eye (Edelhauser and Green, 1997). A review of this procedure is beyond the scope of this chapter. It is worthy to note, however, that the procedure is limited by the resolution of the instrument and by other methodological problems, so that a large population needs to be evaluated to determine effects among treatment groups (Joshi et al., 1996; McNamara et al., 1997). These technical difficulties with fluorophotometry make it unlikely that the correlation of *in vivo* fluorophotometry data to the *in vitro* HCE-T TEP assay would be feasible. However, the principle underlying the two techniques is the same.

Corneal permeability to fluorescein is a measure of cellular damage manifested as cytotoxicity and junctional disruption to the corneal epithelium (Araie and Maurice, 1987; McCarey and Reaves, 1995). Epithelial cell damage and junctional disruption are early events that occur during chemical-induced human eye irritation (Ramselaar et al., 1988; Gobbels and Spitznas, 1992; Grant and Schuman, 1993; McCarey and Reaves, 1997; Jester et al., 1998; Maurer et al., 1998b). A recently proposed classification scheme for human chemical-induced eye injury that was developed by a group of ophthalmic researchers has identified corneal epithelium as one of the first ocular tissues to be affected by superficial chemical exposure (Maurer et al., 1998a; Blazka et al., 2002). The classification scheme indicates that the degree of corneal epithelial injury increases with the overall severity of chemical injury to the eye, until the epithelium is totally destroyed. Likewise, in the HCE-T model, ocular surface epithelial barrier disruption as measured by altered fluorescein permeability occurs quickly upon superficial toxicant exposure. Fluorescein permeability, epithelial cell cytotoxicity, and disruption of intercellular adhesions/junctions increase in a dose-dependent manner with chemical exposure (Ward et al., 1997b; Figure 15.5). Since the TEP assay provides a measure of the integrity of the HCE-T epithelial barrier, it is analogous to the *in vivo* event of epithelial barrier disruption that can be measured by increased epithelial permeability to fluorescein following chemical exposure.

A retrospective evaluation of the fluorescein staining data for rabbit eyes following exposure to surfactant-containing formulations, which was collected during the Cosmetic Toiletries and Fragrance Association (CTFA) Phase III Study (Gettings et al., 1996), demonstrates that corneal fluorescein staining correlates well with the Draize score data collected from the same animals (Figure 15.6). The same formulations were evaluated using the HCE-T TEP assay. The relationship between the *in vivo* fluorescein staining data at 24 hr versus the *in vitro* log

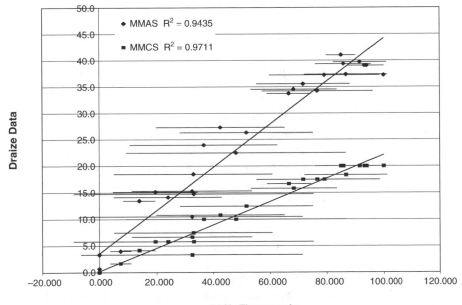

Figure 15.6 Fluorescein staining data from rabbit eyes following surfactant-containing formulation exposure correlates well with Draize tissue score data (modified maximum average score, MMAS and modified maximum average corneal score, MMCS) from the same animals. The error bars are the standard deviations; n = 5–6 rabbits evaluated per Draize test; and n = 2–4 rabbits evaluated for fluorescein staining at 24 hr. [Data from Gettings et al., 1996.]

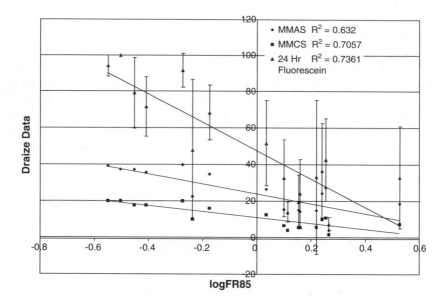

Figure 15.7 The relationship between the *in vivo* 24-hour fluorescein staining data and the *in vitro* log FR85 values for the subset of the CTFA formulations that are represented in the HCE-T TEP assay Prediction Model. The error bars are the standard deviations; $n = 2$ TEP assays; $n = 5$–6 rabbits per Draize test; and $n = 2$–4 rabbits per fluorescein data.

FR85 values for the CTFA formulations, which are part of the HCE-T TEP assay prediction model, is shown in Figure 15.7. These results demonstrate (1) the relationship between fluorescein staining of the rabbit cornea and the Draize scores (Figure 15.6) and (2) the relationship between the *in vivo* fluorescein staining and the *in vitro* HCE-T TEP assay (Figure 15.7). The fluorescein staining data are available along with the standard Draize score data for the surfactant-containing formulations evaluated in the CTFA Phase III Study (Gettings et al., 1996). Unfortunately, fluorescein data are not available for many of the materials evaluated with the Draize test, and sufficient materials with fluorescein data were not available for use in test method validation.

The results reported in the ophthalmology and toxicology literature for surfactant exposures of the human and rabbit eye support the use of fluorescein permeability as an appropriate measure for surfactant-induced eye irritation. Marsh and Maurice (1971) observed that human eyes treated with nonionic detergents showed perturbation of epithelial fluorescein permeability at concentrations just slightly less than those that produced marked eye irritation. On the other hand, in two different experiments that compared the responses of human and rabbit eyes to superficial applications of benzalkonium chloride (BAC), the rabbit eyes were found to be more sensitive than human eyes treated with the same surfactant concentrations (Burstein, 1984; Buehler and Newmann, 1964). These observations led Burstein (1984) to conclude that "measurements of ocular permeability and surface damage are not directly transferable from rabbits to humans." His results, however, only indicate that the rabbit eye overpredicted the human ocular response to the cationic surfactant BAC. Preliminary HCE-T TEP assay data obtained at GMEL for several cationic surfactants, including BAC, showed that they also were underpredicted in the *in vitro* assay relative to the Draize test (unpublished observations).

This review of the scientific literature and the results with the HCE-T model and the HCE-T TEP assay led us to conclude that the mechanistic basis of fluorescein impermeability/permeability in the HCE-T model is analogous to the mechanism of fluorescein impermeability/permeability in the *in vivo* corneal epithelium. Fluorescein impermeability in the HCE-T model is due to the biological relevance of the stratified corneal epithelial cultures, with their analogous multiple cell layers, tight junctions, and other intercellular adhesions that are responsible for the impermeability of the epithelium to fluorescein. Surfactants perturb the impermeability of the *in vivo* corneal epithelium and the HCE-T model by the same mechanism—cytotoxicity and junctional disruption to the superficial cells that increases in a dose-dependent manner. Thus, the test system (the HCE-T TEP assay) and the human eye (the species of interest) share a similar mechanism for fluorescein impermeability in the undamaged tissues, and a similar mechanism for the increase in fluorescein permeability observed after superficial exposure to surfactants.

PREVALIDATION STUDY RESULTS

As one of the steps in the validation process, the HCE-T TEP assay was evaluated in a prevalidation study. Prevalidation has been defined as "the process during which a standardized test protocol is evaluated for use in validation studies. Based on the outcome of those studies, the test protocol may be modified or optimized for use in further validation studies" (ICCVAM, 1999).

The prevalidation study and its results are only briefly summarized here and will be published in greater detail elsewhere (Ward et al., 2003b).

Purpose for the HCE-T TEP Assay

For the Prevalidation Study, the HCE-T TEP assay was evaluated for its ability to predict the eye irritation potential of water-soluble surfactant-containing formulations within the range of irritation referenced by a Draize MAS of 0 to 61 (or Draize total corneal score of 0 to 38). The goals of the interlaboratory prevalidation study were to develop an optimized protocol for validation of the test method, to demonstrate the method's transferability to other laboratories, and to provide a preliminary assessment of the reliability and the relevance of the HCE-T TEP assay *for its stated purpose.*

Study Structure

The study consisted of the evaluation of five surfactant-containing formulations by three laboratories, with each material tested four times in each laboratory for a total of 60 TEP assays (20 assays per laboratory). The three laboratories participating in the study were the Gillette Medical Evaluation Laboratories (GMEL) in Gaithersburg, MD; the Institute for In Vitro Sciences (IIVS) in Gaithersburg, MD; and the U.S. Army Edgewood Chemical and Biological Command (ECBC) in Aberdeen Proving Ground, MD. Testing was conducted as a double-blind procedure where a third party packaged, coded, and distributed the test materials to each laboratory. The prevalidation study was not fully good laboratory practice (GLP) compliant, but all laboratories conducted assays and recorded data using GLP-based practices. The testing laboratories were trained by GMEL staff in the performance of all procedures, and each laboratory performed a set of "training" assays to demonstrate their proficiency with the assay before initiation of the study. Test materials were selected for the study that had good quality, historical reference method data. The five test materials were water-soluble, surfactant-based, consumer product formulations, which spanned the range of eye irritation from nonirritating to severe (see Table 15.2). Two of the formulations were Gillette product formulations, and three were CTFA Phase III formulations (Gettings et al., 1996). Two of the test materials are classified as negative (nonirritants), two as positive (irritants), and one as indeterminate using the Federal Hazardous Substances Act (FHSA) guidelines (FHSA, 1979).

Data Analysis

Before the beginning of the study, a prediction model (PM) was developed by the statistical modeling of the relationship between the *in vitro* TEP data and the historical *in vivo* Draize MAS data for 26 water-soluble surfactants and surfactant-containing formulations (Figures 15.1E and 15.8). This model is described by the equation: Draize MAS $= [a/(1 + \exp (b(\log \mathrm{FR}85 - c)))] + d$, which is a four-parameter logistic curve with parameter estimates of $a = 98.116$, $b = 1.525$, $c = -0.588$, and $d = 0.426$. The generalized correlation coefficient, R, for the MAS PM plot is 0.876, and the outer dashed lines represent the 95% confidence intervals.

The dose-response data from each TEP assay are plotted as fluorescein retention (FR) (percentage of control) versus the log of the concentration (percentage of initial test material concentration) (Figure 15.1D). The log FR85 is the concentration of test material where the HCE-T cultures retain 85% of the fluorescein relative to control cultures and is the endpoint from the dose-response curve that is used for correlation with the reference method data. The TEP assay endpoint, the log FR85, was used to define the predicted *in vivo* Draize MAS for the material evaluated in each assay by using this prediction model. Prediction models were also developed using the Draize corneal score (CS) and the corneal opacity score (COS), which were used to obtain the predicted CS and predicted COS for each test material.

Test method performance was evaluated by (1) evaluating the fit of the HCE-T TEP assay data within the 95% confidence intervals of the established prediction model and (2) by comparing the irritation classification for each test material determined by the *in vivo* Draize test to that determined by the HCE-T TEP assay. The irritation classifications can be used to calculate the performance statistics

Table 15.2 Prevalidation Study Test Materials and Draize Data

Product Type	Conc. Tested[a]	Surfactant Ingredients	Percent Formula (w/w)	Surfactant Class	Draize Scores[b]	FHSA Class[c]
Bubble bath	2.5%	sodium laureth sulfate cocamidopropyl betaine	25.0 5.0	anionic amphoteric	MAS 4.8 CS 0.0 COS 0.0	–
Hair conditioner	100%	stearalkonium chloride ceteth-24 dimethyl stearamine glyceryl stearate	1.14 1.0 0.67 0.44	cationic nonionic cationic nonionic	MAS 14.2 CS 0.0 COS 0.0	–
Cleansing gel	100%	cocoamphodiacetate sodium nonoxynol-6-phosphate quaternium-26 PEG-120-methyl glucose dioleate	15.0 6.0 1.5 1.5	amphoteric anionic cationic nonionic	MAS 22.0 CS 10.0 COS 0.5	–/+
Shampoo 1	100%	sodium lauryl sulfate disodium laureth sulfosuccinate butylene gylcol lauramide DEA	25.0 15.0 5.0 0.5	anionic anionic non onic nonionic	MAS 37.8 CS 20.0 COS 1.0	+
Shampoo 2	100%	ammonium lauryl sulfate lauramide DEA ethoxydiglycol hydroxypropyl methylcellulose	12.0 2.0 0.4 0.15	anionic nonionic — —	MAS 57.4 CS 38.0 COS 2.0	+

[a] Concentration used in Draize test, and initial concentration for dilution in TEP assay.
[b] MAS is the maximum average score; CS is the corneal score; COS is the corneal opacity score.
[c] Federal Hazardous Substances Act (FHSA) classifications: –, negative; +, positive; –/+ repeat test (FHSA, 1979).

(including test method sensitivity and specificity) for a test method using a 2×2 contingency table analysis (Cooper et al., 1979; ICCVAM, 1999). However, a data set of only five test materials did not provide a sufficient sample size for this type of analysis.

Several methods were used to assess the repeatability, or within (intra-) laboratory variability, and the reproducibility, or between (inter-) laboratory variability. All methods resulted in the same conclusions, and only the results from the coefficient of variation (CV) analysis will be shown here.

Results

One method for evaluating the performance of a new toxicity test method is to determine whether the new test results follow the algorithm of the existing prediction model. The lab average assay results for all five test materials fell within the 95% confidence intervals (CI) of the MAS PM; 55/60 of the individual assays (Figure 15.8). The lab average results for four out of five materials fell within the 95% CI of the corneal score (CS) PM; and five out of five materials fell within the 95% CI of the corneal opacity score (COS) PM (not shown). Another type of statistical analysis used to determine data relationships, a chi-square analysis, showed significant relationship between irritation classification obtained by the MAS PM and classification obtained by the Draize test ($p < 0.001$).

A second way to evaluate test method performance is by comparing the irritation classification for each test material determined by the reference method (Draize test) to that determined by the new test method (TEP assay). All five materials were correctly classified as irritant or nonirritant by the TEP assay relative to their classification by the Draize test (Table 15.3). The irritation classifications for each test material, based on the four classes assigned by Kay and Calandra (1962), are shown in Table 15.4. These irritation classifications were in agreement for four of the five test materials. The most irritating material, shampoo 2, was underpredicted by the TEP assay by one classification level in all three laboratories.

The statistical analyses showed no significant differences in both between-laboratory and within-laboratory variability for the five test materials (not shown). The coefficient of variation (CV) for the between-laboratory predicted MAS results were 3 to 16% (Table 15.5). A discussion of the statistical analysis for test method reliability will be presented in greater detail elsewhere (Ward et al., 2003b).

Conclusions

The prevalidation study results provide a preliminary assessment of test method performance, and intralaboratory and interlaboratory assay variability.

The results indicate that the HCE-T TEP assay (1) is transferable to other laboratories, (2) has acceptable intralaboratory and interlaboratory variability when performed by trained staff following the designated protocol, (3) demonstrated good performance in predicting the Draize scores for five surfactant-containing

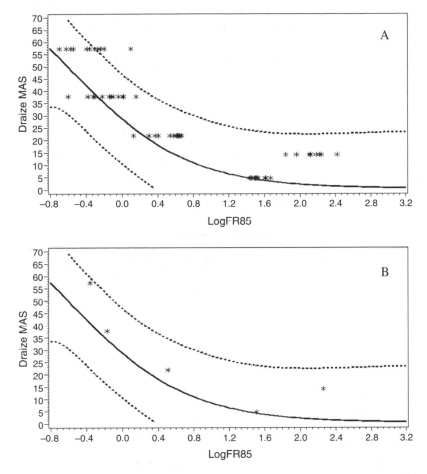

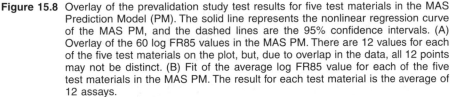

Figure 15.8 Overlay of the prevalidation study test results for five test materials in the MAS Prediction Model (PM). The solid line represents the nonlinear regression curve of the MAS PM, and the dashed lines are the 95% confidence intervals. (A) Overlay of the 60 log FR85 values in the MAS PM. There are 12 values for each of the five test materials on the plot, but, due to overlap in the data, all 12 points may not be distinct. (B) Fit of the average log FR85 value for each of the five test materials in the MAS PM. The result for each test material is the average of 12 assays.

formulations in three laboratories, and (4) has good potential for use in making risk assessment decisions for the ocular irritation potential of surfactant-containing formulations.

The HCE-T TEP assay demonstrated good predictive capability (performance), and acceptable within and between laboratory assay variability in this preliminary assessment. Therefore, the management team recommended the HCE-T TEP assay for evaluation in a larger interlaboratory validation study where its performance will be further assessed. The results of the prevalidation study for the HCE-T TEP assay were reported to the ICCVAM Ocular Toxicity Working Group (OTWG) in January 2001 (Gillette, 2001).

Table 15.3 The Nonirritant/Irritant Classification of the Five Test Materials as Determined by the Draize Test and by the HCE-T TEP Assay

Test Material	Draize Score Classification[a]	TEP Assay MAS PM[b]	TEP Assay CS PM[b]	TEP Assay COS PM[b]
Bubble bath	1	1	1	1
Hair conditioner	1	1	1	1
Cleansing gel	2	2	2	1
Shampoo 1	2	2	2	2
Shampoo 2	2	2	2	2

[a] Draize classification was the same across the MAS, CS, and COS scores, except for the cleansing gel which was an irritant by the MAS and CS, but a nonirritant by the COS.
[b] Draize scores for the classifications: nonirritant MAS ≤ 15; nonirritant CS < 5; nonirritant COS < 0.667.
Note: Draize maximum average score, MAS; corneal score, CS; corneal opacity score, COS.

Table 15.4 Average HCE-T TEP Assay Results for Five Test Materials in Three Laboratories; The Predicted MAS and Class from the TEP assay Are Compared to the Draize MAS and Class for Each Test Result

Test Material	Draize MAS[a]	Draize Class[b]	Predicted MAS[a]	Predicted Class[b]
Bubble bath	4.8	1	4.20	1
Hair conditioner[c]	14.2	1	1.82	1
Cleansing gel	22.0	2	16.15	2
Shampoo 1	37.8	3	34.62	3
Shampoo 2	57.4	4	41.18	3

[a] MAS, maximum average score.
[b] The four classification cutoffs for MAS are based on the scheme proposed by Kay and Calandra (1962): MAS 0–15, minimal (class 1); MAS 15.1–25, mild (class 2); MAS 25.1–55, moderate (class 3); MAS > 55, severe (class 4).
[c] Hair conditioner was less water soluble than other test materials, which may account for its underprediction when it was diluted.

SUMMARY

This chapter describes for the HCE-T TEP assay the results for two of the essential steps in the validation process, establishing the scientific relevance of the new test method and the prevalidation of the method.

A new toxicity test method to evaluate human eye irritation potential must be relevant to the biological and toxicological processes that occur when a chemical or chemical mixture makes contact with the human ocular surface. The scientific relevance of the HCE-T TEP assay was defined using results obtained from a number of different experiments conducted using the test system and with relevant supporting information from the ophthalmologic research literature. The HCE-T TEP assay achieves biological relevance by combining a model of the human corneal surface with a test method that has a mechanistic relationship to human eye irritation. The experimental data and the scientific literature reported here support the conclusion that the HCE-T TEP assay is a test method that is biologically and mechanistically based, and thus should provide a good model for the human corneal response to eye irritants.

Table 15.5 Variability in the Draize MAS Compared to the Predicted MAS for the HCE-T TEP Assay Prevalidation Study Data

Test Material	Intralab CV (%) for Draize MAS[a]	Intralab CV (%) for Predicted MAS[b]	Interlab CV (%) for Predicted MAS[c]
Bubble bath	22.82	9.94	6.03
		10.06	
		4.94	
Hair conditioner[d]	19.67	33.19	15.59
		15.80	
		54.09	
Cleansing gel	53.24	17.50	15.10
		3.01	
		25.90	
Shampoo 1	10.31	12.54	12.49
		21.21	
		20.42	
Shampoo 2	8.32	14.60	2.83
		14.62	
		29.49	

[a] Evaluated using five to six animals from one lab.
[b] Evaluated using four replicates per lab for three labs.
[c] Results from three testing labs.
[d] Hair conditioner was less water soluble, which may account for its greater variability when it was diluted.
Notes: Intralab is the within lab variability (repeatability); interlab is the between lab variability (reproducibility). Coefficient of variation, CV; maximum average score, MAS.

A prevalidation study was conducted to evaluate the performance of the HCE-T TEP assay for the prediction of the ocular irritation potential of surfactant-based formulations. The test method was transferred to other laboratories, and the results of the interlaboratory assessment suggest that the HCE-T TEP assay is a reliable and relevant method for the prediction of the eye irritation potential of surfactant-containing formulations.

REFERENCES

Albert, D.M. and Jakobiec, F.A. (1994) *Principles and Practice of Ophthalmology,* Vol. 1, W.B. Sauders Company, Philadelphia.

Araie, M. and Maurice D. (1987) The rate of diffusion of fluorophores through the corneal epithelium and stroma, *Exp. Eye Res.,* 44, 73–87.

Archer, G., Balls, M., Bruner, L.H., Curren, R.D., Fentem, J.H., Holzhutter, H.-G., Liebsch, M., Lovell, D.P., and Southee, J.A. (1997) The validation of toxicological prediction models, *Alt. Lab. Anim.,* 25, 505–516.

Balls, M., Blaauboer, B.J., Fentem, J.H., Bruner, L., and Combes, R.D. (1995a) Practical aspects of the validation of toxicity test procedures. The report and recommendations of the ECVAM workshop 5, *Alt. Lab. Anim.,* 23, 129–147.

Balls, M., Botham, P.A., Bruner, L.H., and Spielmann, H. (1995b) The EC/HO international validation study on alternatives to the Draize eye irritation test, *Toxicol. In Vitro,* 9, 871–929.

Beckley, J.H. (1965) Comparative eye testing: man versus animal, *Toxicol. Appl. Pharmacol.,* 7, 93–101.

Beckley, J.H., Russell, T.J., and Rubin, L.F. (1969) Use of the rhesus monkey for predicting human response to eye irritants, *Toxicol. Appl. Pharmacol.,* 15, 1–9.

Berry, M. and Easty, D.L. (1993) Isolated human and rabbit eye: Models of corneal toxicity, *Toxic. In Vitro,* 7, 461–464.

Blazka, M.E., Casterton, P.L., Dressler, W.E., Edelhauser, H.F., Kruszewski, F.H., McCulley, J.P., Nussenblatt, R.B., Osborne, R., Rothenstein, A., Stitzel, K.A., Thomas, K., and Ward, S.L. (2003) Proposed new classification scheme for chemical injury to the human eye, in preparation.

Bradlaw, J., Gupta, K., Green, S., Hill, R., and Wilcox, N. (1997) Practical application of non-whole animal alternatives: summary of IRAG Workshop on eye irritation testing, *Food and Chem. Toxicol.,* 35, 175–178.

Brantom, P.G., Bruner, L.H., Chamberlain, M., DeSilva, O., Dupuis, J., Earl, L.K., Lovell, D.P., Pape, W.J.W., and Uttley, M. (1997) A summary of the COLIPA international validation study on alternatives to the Draize rabbit eye irritation test, *Toxicol. In Vitro.,* 11, 141–179.

Braunstein, S.G., Deramaudt, T.G., Rosenblum, D.G., Dunn, M.G., and Abraham, N.G. (1999) Heme oxygenase-1 gene expression as a stress index to ocular irritation, *Curr. Eye Res.,* 19, 115–122.

Bruner, L.H., Carr, G.J., Chamberlain, M., and Curren, R.D. (1996) Validation of alternative methods for toxicity testing, *Toxicol. In Vitro,* 10, 479–501.

Buehler, E.V. and Newmann, E.A. (1964) A comparison of eye irritation in monkeys and rabbits, *Toxicol. Appl. Pharmacol.,* 6, 701.

Burbach, G.J., Naik, S.M., Harten, B.J., Liu, L., Dithmar, S., Grossniklaus, H., Ward, S.L., Armstrong, C.A., Caughman, S.W., and Ansel, J.C. (2001) Interleukin-18 expression and modulation in human corneal epithelial cells, *Curr. Eye Res.,* 23, 64–68.

Burstein, N.L. (1984) Preservative alteration of corneal permeability in humans and rabbits, *Invest. Ophthalmol. Vis. Sci.,* 25, 1453–1457.

Chan, P.K. and Hayes, A.W. (1994) Acute toxicity and eye irritancy, in *Principles and Methods of Toxicology,* 3rd ed., Hayes, A.W., Ed., Raven Press, Ltd., New York pp. 579–647.

Chen, L. and Hazlett, L.D. (2001) Human corneal epithelial cell extracellular matrix perlecan serves as a site for Pseudomonas aeruginosa binding, *Curr. Eye Res.,* 22, 19–27.

Clothier, R., Orme, A., Walker, T.L., Ward, S.L., Kruszewski, F.H., DiPasquale, L.C., and Broadhead, C.L. (2000) A comparison of three cytotoxicity assays using the corneal HCE-T model, *Alt. Lab. Anim.,* 28, 293–302.

Cooper, J.A., Saracci, R., and Cole, P. (1979) Describing the validity of carcinogen screening tests, *Br. J. Cancer,* 39, 87–89.

Daston, G.P. and Freeberg, F.E. (1991) Ocular irritation testing, in *Dermal and Ocular Toxicology, Fundamentals and Methods,* Hobson, D.W., Ed., CRC Press, Inc., Boca Raton, FL, pp. 509–539.

de Kruijf, E.J.F.M., Boot, J.P., Laterveer, L., van Best, J.A., Ramselaar, J.A.M., and Oosterhuis, J.A. (1987) A simple method for determination of corneal epithelial permeability in humans, *Curr. Eye Res.,* 6, 1327–1334.

DeSantis, L.M. and Patil, P.N. (1994) Pharmacokinetics, in *Havener's Ocular Pharmacology,* 6th ed., Mauger, T.F. and Craig, E.L., Eds., Mosby, St. Louis, MO, pp. 34–37.

DiPasquale, L.C. and Hayes, A.W. (2001) Acute toxicity and eye irritancy, in *Principles and Methods of Toxicology,* 4th ed., Hayes, A.W., Ed., Taylor and Francis, Philadelphia, pp. 853–916.

Draize, J.H., Woodward, G., and Calvery, H.O. (1944) Methods for the study of irritation and toxicity of substances applied topically to the skin and mucous membranes, *J. Pharmacol. Exp. Ther.*, 82, 377–390.

Edelhauser, H.F. and Green, K. (1997) Workshop on *in vitro* versus *in vivo* models for ocular toxicity testing, in *Advances in Ocular Toxicology.*, Green, K. et al., Eds., Plenum Press, New York, pp. 207–259.

Edelhauser, H.F., Rudnick, D.E., and Axar, R.G. (1998) Corneal epithelial tight junctions and the localization of surface mucin, *Adv. Exp. Med. Biol.*, 438, 265–271.

FHSA (Federal Hazardous Substances Act) (1979) Regulations under the Federal Hazardous Substances Act, Chapter II, Title 16, Code of Federal Regulations.

Gershbein, L.L. and McDonald, J.E. (1977) Evaluation of the corneal irritancy of test shampoos and detergents in various animal species, *Food Cosmet. Toxicol.*, 15, 131–134.

Gettings, S.D., Lordo, R.A., Hintze, K.L., Bagley, D.M., and Casterton, P.L. (1996) The CTFA Evaluation of Alternatives Program: an evaluation of *in vitro* alternatives to the Draize Primary Eye Irritation Test. (Phase III) Surfactant-based formulations, *Food Chem. Toxicol.*, 34, 79–117.

Gillette Prevalidation Study (January 2001) Prevalidation study results for the HCE-T TEP assay background review document, Submission to the ICCVAM Ocular Toxicity Working Group.

Gobbels, M. and Spitznas, M. (1992) Corneal epithelial permeability of dry eyes before and after treatment with artificial tears, *Ophthalmology*, 99, 873–878.

Grant, W.M. and Schuman, J.S. (1993) *Toxicology of the Eye*, 4th ed., Charles C Thomas, Springfield, IL.

Green, W.R., Sullivan, J.B., Hehir, R.M., Scharpf, L.G., and Dickinson, A.W. (1978) *A Systematic Comparison of Chemically Induced Eye Injury in the Albino Rabbit and Rhesus Monkey*, The Soap and Detergent Association, New York.

Hackett, R.B. and McDonald, T.O. (1991) Eye irritation, in *Dermatotoxicology*, 4th ed., Marzulli, F.N. and Maibach, H.I., Eds., pp. 749–815.

Hamalainen, K.M., Konturri, K., Auriola, S., Murtornaki, L., and Urtti, A. (1997) Estimation of pore size and pore density of biomembranes from permeability measurements of polyethylene glycols using an effusion-like approach, *J. Controlled Release*, 49, 97–104.

Hotzhutter, H.-G., Archer, G., Dami, N., Lovell, D.P., Saltelli, A., and Sjostrom, M. (1996) Recommendations for the application of biostatistical methods during the development and validation of alternative toxicological methods, *Alt. Lab. Anim.*, 24, 511–530.

ICCVAM (Interagency Coordinating Committee on the Validation of Alternative Methods) (1999) *ICCVAM Submission Guidelines*, url: http://iccvam.niehs.nih.gov/docs/guidelines/subguide.htm.

Inatomi, T., Spurr-Michaud, S., Tisdale, A.S., and Gipson, I.K. (1995) Human corneal and conjunctival epithelia express MUC1 mucin, *Invest. Ophthalmol. Vis. Sci.*, 36, 1818–1827.

ILSI, AAT (International Life Sciences Institute, Technical Committee on Alternatives to Animal Testing) (1996) Replacing the Draize eye irritation test: scientific background and research needs, *J. Toxicol Cut Ocular Toxicol.*, 15, 211–234.

Jester, J.V., Maurer, J.K., Petroll, M., Wilkie, D.A., Parker, R.D., and Cavanagh, H.D. (1996) Application of *in vivo* confocal microscopy to the understanding of surfactant-induced ocular irritation, *Toxicol. Pathol.*, 24, 412–428.

Jester, J.V., Li, H.-F., Petroll, M., Parker, R.D., Cavanagh, H.D., Carr, G.J., Smith, B., and Maurer, J.K. (1998) Area and depth of surfactant-induced corneal injury correlates with cell death, *Invest. Ophthalmol. Vis. Sci.*, 39, 922–936.

Joshi, A., Maurice, D., and Paugh, J.R. (1996) A new method for determining corneal epithelial barrier to fluorescein in humans, *Invest. Ophthalmol. Vis. Sci.,* 37, 1008–1016.

Kahn, C.R. and Rhim, J.S. (July 28, 1998) U.S. patent 5,786,201.

Kahn, C.R. and Walker, T.L. (1993) Human corneal epithelial cell lines with extended lifespan: transepithelial permeability across membranes formed *in vitro, Invest. Ophthalmol. Vis. Sci.,* 34, 1010.

Kahn, C.R., Young, E., Lee, I.H., and Rhim, J.S. (1993) Human corneal epithelial primary cultures and cell lines with extended life span: *in vitro* model for ocular studies, *Invest. Ophthalmol. Vis. Sci.,* 34, 3429–3441.

Kay, J.H. and Calandra, J.C. (1962) Interpretation of the eye irritation test. *J. Soc. Cos. Chem.,* 13, 281–289.

Kruszewski, F.H., Walker, T.L., Ward, S.L., and DiPasquale, L.C. (1995) Progress in the use of human ocular tissues for *in vitro* alternative methods, *Comments on Toxicol.,* 5, 203–224.

Kruszewski, F.H., Walker, T.L., and DiPasquale, L.C. (1997) Evaluation of a human corneal epithelial cell line as an *in vitro* model for predicting ocular irritation, *Fundam. Appl. Toxicol.,* 36, 130–140.

Kurpakus, M.A., Daneshvar, C., Davenport, J., and Kim, A. (1999) Human corneal epithelial cell adhesion to laminins. *Curr. Eye Res.,* 19, 106–114.

Mackay, M., Williamson, I., and Hastewall, J. (1991) Cell biology in epithelia, *Adv. Drug Deliv. Rev.,* 7, 313–338.

Marsh, R.J. and Maurice, D.M. (1971) The influence of non-ionic detergents and other surfactants on human corneal permeability, *Exp. Eye Res.,* 11, 43–48.

Maurer, J.K., Li, H.-F., Petroll, W.M., Parker, R.D., Cavanaugh, H.D., and Jester, J.V. (1997) Confocal microscopic characterization of initial changes of surfactant-induced eye irritation occurring to the rabbit, *Toxicol. Appl. Pharmacol.,* 143, 291–300.

Maurer, J.K., McCulley, J.P., Edelhauser, H.F., and Nussenblatt, R.B. (1998a) A proposed new classification scheme for chemical injury to the human eye, *Invest. Ophthalmol. Vis. Sci.,* 39, S83.

Maurer, J.K., Parker, R.D., and Carr, G.J. (1998b) Ocular irritation: microscopic changes occurring over time in the rat with surfactants of known irritancy, *Toxicol. Pathol.,* 26, 217–225.

Maurice, D. (1955) Influence on corneal permeability of bathing with solutions of differing reaction and tonicity, *Brit. J. Ophthalmol.,* 39, 463–473.

Maurice, D.M. (1967) The use of fluorescein in ophthalmological research, *Invest. Ophthalmol. Vis. Sci.,* 6, 464–477.

Maurice, D.M. and Singh, T. (1986) A permeability test for acute corneal toxicity, *Toxicol. Lett.,* 31, 125–130.

McCarey, B.E. and Reaves, T.A. (1995) Noninvasive measurement of corneal epithelial permeability, *Curr. Eye Res.,* 14, 505–510.

McCarey, B.E. and Reaves, T.A. (1997) Effect of tear lubricating solutions on *in vivo* corneal epithelial permeability, *Curr. Eye Res.,* 16, 44–50.

McNamara, N.A., Fusaro, R.E., Brand, R.J., Polse, K.A., and Srinivas, S.P. (1997) Measurement of corneal epithelial permeability to fluorescein. *Invest. Ophthalmol. Vis. Sci.,* 38, 1830–1839.

NIEHS (National Institute of Environmental Health Sciences) (1997) Validation and regulatory acceptance of toxicological test methods: A report of the ad hoc Interagency Coordinating Committee on the Validation of Alternative Methods (NIH Publication No. 97–3981), NIEHS: Research Triangle Park, NC. URL: http://ntp-server.niehs.nih.gov/htdocs/ICCVAM/ICCVAM.html or http://iccvam.niehs.nih.gov/docs/guidelines/validate.pdf.

Norn, M.S. (1970) Micropunctate fluorescein vital staining of the cornea, *Acta Ophthalmol.,* 48, 108–118.

OECD (Organization for Economic Co-operation and Development) Environment Directorate, Chemicals Group and Management Committee (1996) Final Report of the OECD Workshop on Harmonization of Validation and Acceptance Criteria for Alternative Toxicological Test Methods (ENV/MC/CHEM/TG(96)9), OECD, Paris, France.

Ramselaar, J.A.M., Boot, J.P., van Haeringer, N.J., van Best, J.A., and Oosterhuis, J.A. (1988) Corneal epithelial permeability after instillation of ophthalmic solutions containing local anaesthetics and preservatives, *Curr. Eye Res.,* 7, 947–950.

Shaw, A.J., Clothier, R.H., and Balls, M. (1990) Loss of transepithelial impermeability of a confluent monolayer of Mandin-Darby canine kidney (MDCK) cells as a determinant of ocular irritancy potential, *Alt. Lab. Anim.,* 18, 145–151.

Shaw, A.J., Balls, M., Clothier, R.H., and Bateman, N.D. (1991) Predicting ocular irritancy and recovery from injury using Mandin-Darby canine kidney cells, *Toxicol. In Vitro,* 5, 569–571.

Smolin, G. and Thoft, R.A. (1987) *The Cornea: Scientific Foundations and Clinical Practice,* 2nd ed., Little, Brown and Company, Boston.

Song, P.I., Abraham, T., Park, Y., Zivony, A., Harten, B., Edelhauser, H.F., Ward, S.L., Armstrong, C.A., and Ansel, J.C. (2001) The expression of functional LPS receptor proteins CD14 and toll-like receptor 4 in human corneal cells, *Invest. Ophthalmol. Vis. Sci.,* 42, 2867–2877.

Tchao, R. (1988) Trans-epithelial permeability of fluorescein *in vitro* as an assay to determine eye irritants, in *Alternative Methods in Toxicology. Progress in In Vitro Toxicology,* Vol. 6. Goldberg, A.M., Ed., Mary Ann Liebert, Inc., New York, pp. 271–283.

Ubels, J.L., McCartney, M.D., Lantz, W.K., Beaird, J., Dayalan, A., and Edelhauser, H.F. (1995) Effects of preservative-free artificial tear solutions on corneal epithelial structure and function, *Arch. Ophthalmol.,* 113, 371–378.

Walker, A.P. (1985) A more realistic animal technique for predicting human eye response, *Food Chem. Toxicol.,* 23, 175–178.

Walker, T.L. and Kahn, C.R. (September 30, 1997) U.S. patent 5,672,498.

Ward, S.L., Gleich, G.J., Dimitrijevich, S.D., Kruszewski, F.H., Walker, T.L., and Trocme, S.D. (1995) The barrier properties of an *in vitro* human corneal epithelial model are not altered by eosinophil major basic protein or eosinophil cationic protein, *Invest. Ophthalmol. Vis. Sci.,* 36, S699.

Ward, S.L. et al. (1997a) Corneal epithelial mucin and ultrastructure expressed by stratified cultures of a transfected human corneal epithelial cell line, *Invest. Ophthalmol. Vis. Sci.,* 38, S284.

Ward, S.L., Walker, T.L., and Dimitrijevich, S.D. (1997b) Evaluation of chemically-induced toxicity using an *in vitro* model of human corneal epithelium, *Toxicol. In Vitro,* 11, 121–139.

Ward, S.L., Dimitrijevich, S.D., Trocme, S.D., and Gleich, G.J. (2003a) Cytotoxic Effects of Eosinophil MBP and ECP on an In Vitro Human Corneal Epithelium, in preparation.

Ward, S.L., Gacula, M., Jr., Cao, C., DiPasquale, L., Edelhauser, H., Kruszewski, F., Valdes, J., Walker, T., and Hayes, A.W. (2003b) Prevalidation study results for the human corneal epithelial fluorescein transepithelial permeability assay for eye irritation, the HCE-T TEP assay, *J. Toxicol Cut. Ocular Toxicol.,* submitted.

Weil, C.S. and Scala, R.A. (1971) Study of intra- and inter-laboratory variability in the results of rabbit eye and skin irritation test, *Toxicol. Appl. Pharmacol.,* 19, 276–360.

Worth, A.P. and Balls, M. (2001) The importance of the prediction model in the validation of alternative tests, *Alt. Lab. Anim.,* 29, 135–143.

Zanvit, A., Meunier, P.-A., Clothier, R., Ward, R., and Buiatti-Tcheng, M. (1999) Ocular irritancy assessment of cosmetics formulations and ingredients: fluorescein leakage test, *Toxicol. In Vitro,* 13, 385–391.

PART III

Dermal Testing Alternatives

HARRY SALEM AND SIDNEY A. KATZ

In this section, the five chapters present recent developments in dermal testing alternatives. A summary of the progress for the validation of tests to measure skin corrosion, irritation, sensitization, and phototoxicity is provided by Robert Bronaugh. Denise Sailstad has reviewed the mechanisms of contact hypersensitivity and the basic protocols used to detect sensitizing agents with special emphasis on the local lymph node assay as an alternative to methods using guinea pigs. Robert Zendzian and Michael Dellarco present a case study on the validity of *in vitro* methodology in relation to the *in vivo* process using matched *in vitro* and *in vivo* dermal adsorption studies of acetochlor in the rat. Melissa Fitzgerald, Vera Morhenn, Stacey Humphrey, Nirmala Jayakumar, and Lawrence Rheims describe a molecular diagnostic assay for distinguishing between allergic contact dermatitis and irritant contact dermatitis based on mRNA profiles. Patrick Hayden, Seyoum Ayehunie, G. Robert Jackson, Sarah Kupfer, Thomas Last, Mitchell Klausner, and Joseph Kubilus present data on intralot and interlot reproducibility for a differentiated human dermal epithelial tissue model, describe a new model composed of both keratinocytes and melanocytes, and survey applications to irritation, phototoxicity, and corrosivity.

CHAPTER 16

Alternative Methods
for Dermal Toxicity Testing

Robert L. Bronaugh

CONTENTS

INTRODUCTION

Progress is being made in the validation of alternative tests for dermal toxicity testing. A brief summary of recent progress is provided for the validation of tests to measure skin corrosion, irritation, sensitization, and phototoxicity. Current efforts to validate an *in vitro* percutaneous absorption method are discussed.

SKIN CORROSION

Two methods have recently been validated for the measurement of skin corrosivity by the European Centre for Validation of Alternative Methods (ECVAM, Fentem et al., 1998). Both the transcutaneous electrical resistance assay (TER, Oliver and Pemberton, 1986) and the Episkin® test were found to be acceptable for a wide range of chemical classes. They met all of the criteria of underprediction and overprediction and showed acceptable intralaboratory and interlaboratory reproducibility. Corrositex® was also evaluated in the study but was not usable for about 40% of the test chemicals. This test did not meet all the criteria for acceptability.

A proposed OECD testing strategy for corrosive chemicals was evaluated by using the test results for the 60 chemicals in the above validation study (Worth et al., 1998). The authors concluded that chemicals can be classified as corrosive or noncorrosive by the sequential application of three alternative methods: structure-activity relationships (where available), pH measurements, and either one of the above validated methods (TER or Episkin®). A finding of noncorrosivity in the tier test needs to be confirmed with a rabbit test.

In Vitro International asked the Interagency Coordinating Committee on the Validation of Alternative Methods (ICCVAM) to evaluate the usefulness of Corrositex® for skin corrosivity measurements. The ICCVAM peer-review panel concluded that in certain circumstances (use for U.S. Department of Transportation) Corrositex® could be used as a stand-alone assay. In other cases, the assay could be used as part of a tiered assessment strategy.

SKIN IRRITATION

Although a number of methods for skin irritation have been evaluated in cell culture and skin membrane preparations, no methods have as yet been validated. Skin irritation and the resulting inflammatory response is a complex process. Simulation of skin irritation is likely to be more difficult in an *in vitro* system than is simulation of the corrosivity response. The ECVAM skin irritation task force report concluded that human skin equivalent models should get high priority for ECVAM prevalidation studies (Botham et al., 1998). Furthermore, the report states that monolayer keratinocyte cultures are not suited for routine testing of chemicals because skin permeation is important in the irritation process and cannot be evaluated in cell cultures.

An ECVAM-sponsored prevalidation study was conducted during 1999 and 2000. The study compared the predictive capabilities of five test methods: Epiderm®, Episkin®, Prediskin®, the nonperfused pig ear model, and the mouse skin integrity function test (SIFT). Neither Prediskin nor the nonperfused pig ear model performed well enough to advance to phase III. The performance of Epiderm and Episkin in phase III did not meet the criteria set for a formal validation study. The SIFT test remains to be evaluated in phase III (Fentem et al., 2001).

SKIN SENSITIZATION

The local lymph node assay (LLNA) recently became the first test method validated by ICCVAM. The peer-review panel recommended the LLNA as a stand-alone alternative for contact sensitization provided that the protocol contained certain specific steps as outlined in the report (Anon., 1999). Although the LLNA requires the use of mice, fewer animals are needed than with an *in vivo* study. Furthermore, the mice have less discomfort since the assay only involves induction of sensitization.

SKIN PHOTOTOXICITY

The European Union (EU) and Colipa sponsored a prevalidation study beginning in 1992 that evaluated the accuracy of seven methods in measuring phototoxicity: photohemolysis test, histidine oxidation test, *Candida albicans* test, Solatex PI, Skin², Testskin, and the 3T3 mouse fibroblast test (neutral red uptake, NRU). The 3T3 NRU test was found to give the best correlation with *in vivo* data. The formal validation of the 3T3 NRU test was conducted in 1994–1995 by EU/COLIPA using 30 chemicals in 11 laboratories. The results were reproducible and correlated well with *in vivo* data (Spielmann et al., 1998). The ECVAM Scientific Advisory Committee and the European Commission (EC) concluded that the 3T3 NRU test was validated and ready to be considered for regulatory acceptance. The EC/SCCNFP (Scientific Committee for Cosmetics and Non-Food Products) has recently proposed that the 3T3 NRU method be the standard method for testing UV light absorbing cosmetic ingredients for phototoxic potential.

PERCUTANEOUS ABSORPTION

In vitro skin absorption values are used in exposure estimates of potentially hazardous topically applied chemicals. Local and/or systemic absorption may be of concern in the exposure estimate. Absorption data from *in vivo* human studies would be most relevant, but ethical considerations often require the use of *in vitro* methods to obtain human skin absorption data. *In vivo* animal absorption data are sometimes collected, but the problem of extrapolation to human absorption values remains. Animal absorption data are usually considered overestimates of absorption through human skin. If metabolism of the test compound is of interest, metabolism values from human skin would be most relevant for exposure assessments.

In vitro skin absorption studies have been conducted for over 30 yr with many studies reporting good correlations between *in vivo* and *in vitro* results. The *in vitro* skin model is probably more accurately referred to as an *ex vivo* system since the skin structure is intact and functions as a diffusional barrier to absorption in a similar manner in either the *in vivo* or *in vitro* study. The use of viable skin more closely simulates the *in vivo* situation and can provide useful information on metabolism during the percutaneous absorption process. We proposed a protocol for conducting an *in vitro* skin absorption study with viable human or animal skin (Bronaugh and Collier, 1991). Nonphysiological solubilizing agents could not be added to the receptor fluid to promote partitioning of the test compound into the receptor fluid. Absorption was defined as the sum of the receptor fluid and skin contents at the end of the study. Split-thickness human skin gave preferred absorption values by minimizing retention of absorbed material in skin. Although the protocol specifies the use of viable skin, nonviable skin should be sufficient when skin metabolism is not an issue. However, the barrier properties of skin must be shown to be intact. Protocols have also been proposed recently in Europe by the European Center for Ecotoxicology and Toxicology of Chemicals (ECETOC, 1993), the European Cosmetic Toiletry and Perfumery Association (COLIPA,

Macmillan, 1995), and the European Centre for the Validation of Alternative Methods (ECVAM, Howes et al., 1996).

Major areas of disagreement exist between our protocol and some or all of those prepared by the above European organizations. The issues are listed below:

Should skin contents of test material be summed with receptor fluid values to get total percutaneous absorption?

Should surfactants and organic solvents be allowed in receptor fluid, or should a physiological buffer be used?

Should the protocol require human or animal skin?

Should viable or nonviable skin be used?

Should full-thickness skin be allowed, or must a split-thickness preparation (dermatome/heat separation) be prepared?

A draft OECD protocol and guidance document has addressed these issues and is currently in the approval process.

REFERENCES

Anon. (1999) The marine local lymph node assay: a test method for assaying the allergic contact dermatitis potential of chemicals/compounds, NIH publication 99-449.

Botham, P.A., Earl, L.K., Fentem, J.H., Raged, R., and van de Sandt, J.J.M. (1998) Alternative methods for skin irritation testing: the current status, *Alt. Lab. Anim.*, 26, 195–211.

Bronaugh, R.L. and Collier, S.W. (1998) Protocol for *in vitro* percutaneous absorption studies, in *In Vitro Percutaneous Absorption: Principles, Fundamentals, and Applications,* Bronaugh, R.L. and Maibach, H.I., Eds. (1991). CRC Press, New York, pp 237–241.

ECETOC (1993) *Percutaneous Absorption, Monograph 20*, ECETOC, Brussels.

Fentem, J.H., Archer, G.E.B., Balls, M., Botham, P.A., Curren, R.D., Earl, L.K., Esdaile, D.J., Holzhutter, H.-G., and Liebsch, M. (1998) The ECVAM international validation study on *in vitro* tests for skin corrosivity. 2. Results and evaluation by the management team, *Toxicol. In Vitro,* 12, 483–524.

Fentem, J.H., Briggs, D., Chesne, C., Elliott, G.R., Harbell, J.W., Heylings, J.R., Portes, P., Roguet, R., van de Sandt, J.J.M., and Botham, P.A. (2001) A prevalidation study on *in vitro* tests for acute skin irritation: results and evaluation by the Management Team, *Toxicol. In Vitro,* 15, 57–93.

Howes, D. et al. (1996) Methods for assessing percutaneous absorption: The report and recommendations of ECVAM Workshop 13, *Alt. Lab. Anim.*, 24, 81–106.

Macmillan, R., Ed. (1995) *Cosmetic Ingredients: Guidelines for Percutaneous Absorption/Penetration*, Colipa, Brussels.

Oliver, G. J. A. and Pemberton, M.A. (1986) The identification of corrosive agents for human skin *in vitro. Food Chem. Toxicol.*, 24, 513–515.

Spielmann, H., Maibach, J., et al. (1998) The International EU/COLIPA *in vitro* phototoxicity validation study: results of phase II (blind trial), part 1: the 3T3 NRU Phototoxicity test, *Toxicol. In Vitro,* 12, 305–327.

Worth, A.P., Fentem, J.H., Balls, M., Botham, P.A., Curren, R.D., Earl, L.K., Esdaile, D.J., and Liebsch, M. (1998) An evaluation of the proposed OECD testing strategy for skin corrosion, *Alt. Lab. Anim.*, 26, 709–720.

CHAPTER 17

Allergic Contact Hypersensitivity:
Mechanisms and Methods*

Denise M. Sailstad

CONTENTS

* This manuscript has been reviewed by the U.S. Environmental Protection Agency and approved for publication. Approval does not signify that the contents necessarily reflect the view and policies of the Agency, endorsement or recommendation for use.

INTRODUCTION

The murine local lymph node assay (LLNA) was the first test method submitted to the Interagency Coordinating Committee on the Validation of Alternative Methods (ICCVAM) for consideration of its validation status. The LLNA is an *in vivo* mouse test developed for the detection of chemicals with potential for inducing allergic contact dermatitis (ACD)/contact hypersensitivity (CH) in humans and was proposed as an alternative test method to the guinea pig (GP) sensitization tests previously accepted by regulatory agencies in the United States and elsewhere.

The ICCVAM process and the value that this process offers to regulatory agencies, industry, and animal welfare concerns is significant. In addition, the role of researchers in the development of alternative testing methods is brought to fruition with the evaluation of these test methods (ICCVAM, 1997). This first ICCVAM endeavor was the evaluation of a method to assess contact sensitization potential of chemicals.

In order to appreciate the ICCVAM process for this first method to undergo review, a clear understanding of current test methods and mechanisms of hypersensitivity is essential. The purpose of this manuscript is to (1) provide background and mechanistic information on CH and (2) clarify the animal tests methods used for the detection of potential contact sensitizers.

PROCESS

ICCVAM and the LLNA Review

The framework for the ICCVAM goals and process was refined and tested with the first method evaluation, the LLNA (Figure 17.1; Sailstad et al., 2001).

Using the National Institutes of Health publication, *Validation and Regulatory Acceptance of Toxicological Test Methods: A Report of the ad hoc Interagency Coordinating Committee on the Validation of Alternative Methods* (ICCVAM, 1997) as a guide, G. Frank Gerberick (Procter and Gamble, U.S.), David A. Basketter (Unilever, U.K.), and Ian Kimber (Zeneca, U.K.) (sponsors) prepared a LLNA submission and requested that ICCVAM review the method. The sponsors specifically requested that the LLNA protocol be reviewed as an alternative (option) to the traditionally used GP tests for the assessment of ACD (and CH). At the time of the request for review, the status of the LLNA for regulatory use was only as a screen for ACD, whereby a positive response would be accepted and a negative LLNA response required additional guinea pig testing (OECD, 1993).

Based on the initial sponsor-submitted information, ICCVAM concluded that an evaluation of the LLNA had regulatory relevance and was an appropriate method for ICCVAM review. As with all reviews and initiatives managed through ICCVAM, information was necessary to evaluate the extent that specific ICCVAM criteria were addressed by the method. These include addressing animal use and welfare issues and economic issues, along with the promise for better assessment of human health (hazard identification).

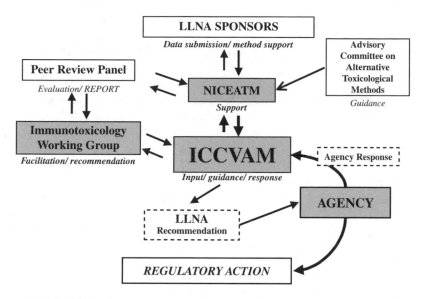

Figure 17.1 ICCVAM review process: the local lymph node assay. (Modified from Sailstad, 2000.)

ICCVAM established an expert working group composed of 18 U.S. government agency representatives to further evaluate the submitted materials and to aid in the peer-review process. This group was referred to as the Immunotoxicology Working Group or IWG. The purpose of the IWG was to provide leadership and guidance for the LLNA peer review and to provide recommendations to specific agencies following peer review. Specific tasks undertaken by the IWG included (1) the modification of the general ICCVAM test method submission guidelines for relevance to the method for the sponsor; (2) identification of potential peer review panel (PRP) candidates; (3) the development of evaluation guidance for the panel to use in their assessment of the LLNA to ensure that the ICCVAM validation and acceptance criteria were adequately addressed; (4) input for the panel meeting and report format; (5) preparation of a revised LLNA protocol that reflected the panel recommendations; (6) input and guidance to ICCVAM agencies on the strengths and limitations of the LLNA; and (7) assistance with aspects of implementation at the agency level.

Following selection of the panel experts, a PRP chair was selected and guidance materials were provided to the PRP along with the sponsors' submission package. The panel functioned independently, although the National Toxicology Program (NTP) Interagency Center for the Evaluation of Alternative Toxicological Methods (NICEATM) provided additional materials and data analyses as requested, and the IWG and ICCVAM cochairs were available for consultation. The panel consisted of 14 experts in immunology, allergy, dermatology, and biostatistics. Members were from a diverse professional background, including academia, industry, federal agencies, and clinical medicine. Additionally, three PRP members represented the international scientific community, one each from Denmark, Norway, and Japan. The LLNA review through the ICCVAM process is discussed elsewhere (ICCVAM, 1999; Sailstad et al., 2000; Dean et al., 2001).

BACKGROUND

Contact Hypersensitivity and Allergic Contact Dermatitis Test Methods

Traditionally, GP tests have been used to assess the ACD/CH potential of chemicals. These tests, used since 1935, have been important tools for pharmaceutical and chemical companies, as well as regulatory agencies (Klecak, 1996). However, the submission of a LLNA protocol to ICCVAM for consideration as an alternative to GP tests and the suggestion to use a murine system introduced a new approach to the evaluation of CH. The sponsors of the LLNA requested its evaluation as an alternative to the currently accepted GP tests, thus providing another method for the identification of CH potential of chemicals. The request and intended use of a new method must be clear and in this case, the sponsors were not requesting elimination of existing tests, but acceptance of the LLNA as an alternative method that could be used in lieu of the traditional GP test if desired and appropriate.

Background: An Example of the Dilemma of GP Tests

In 1988 work was initiated in the Experimental Toxicology Division (ETD) of The Environmental Protection Agency (EPA) as an interagency agreement with the Army to evaluate the allergic potential of three dyes (Sailstad et al., 1994). These dyes were used in M18 colored smoke grenades. There was concern for the individuals repeatedly exposed to these dyes in the manufacturing facilities and their potential to develop allergies or hypersensitivity to the chemicals. The nature of these dyes accelerated the investigation in our laboratory for availability, effectiveness, and practicality of methods to assess the sensitizing potential of chemicals.

Hypersensitivity is defined as excessive humoral or cellular response to an antigen, which can lead to tissue damage. The Army Dye Project required the evaluation of the asthma-like Type I hypersensitivity and the Type IV contact hypersensitivity responses.

Interaction between pulmonary and immunotoxicologists in ETD provided necessary experience to evaluate the pulmonary responses (bronchoconstriction) and cytophilic antibody formation from a repeated (dye) inhalation exposure and challenge system that was previously established.

However, the lack of expertise in the CH and ACD area required an extensive review of existing models and modification to meet the needs of dye assessment. The perplexing dilemma for CH/ACD assessment using traditional methods revolved around the method of assessment and mechanism of action along with the nature of these dyes. Traditional guinea pig tests for CH require the visual assessment of erythema. However, the topical application of these dyes caused a dramatic change in skin color to either a dark violet or deep red, potentially making visual assessment impossible. This initiated ETD interest in alternative methods to the guinea pig tests and eventually led to our involvement in the ICCVAM LLNA review process.

Mechanisms: Contact Hypersensitivity/Allergic Contact Dermatitis

The terms allergic contact dermatitis (ACD) or contact hypersensitivity (CH) can be used interchangeably. ACD or CH is a process of skin sensitization. While the most well-known contact sensitizer is probably poison ivy, CH is usually associated with workplace chemical exposure, becoming considerably important to occupational health. CH results from the repeated encounter of a contact allergen with the skin of a sensitized individual and is a common occupational health problem usually resulting from the exposure to low molecular weight (<3000) materials. CH develops in two phases (Figure 17.2; Selgrade et al., 2001).

Induction Phase

The first phase, sensitization (induction phase) originates upon epicutaneous application of a hapten. It is believed that haptens couple to carrier proteins on dermal and epidermal cells to become fully immunogenic. The dendritic cells within skin, Langerhans cells (LC), take up and process the antigen (hapten) and migrate to the regional draining lymph node where they present the antigen to lymphocytes.

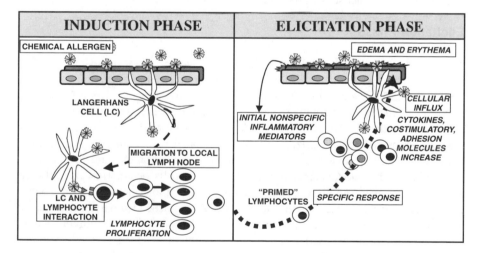

Figure 17.2 Illustration of contact hypersensitivity (CH) mechanisms: induction and elicitation phase. During the *induction phase* of CH, immature dendritic cells of the skin, called "Langerhans cells" (LC), effectively uptake and process the allergen. Simultaneously, epidermal keratinocytes and the LCs themselves release cytokine mediators which assist the LCs in the migration to the draining lymph node and maturation into effective antigen-presenting cells. In the lymph node, LC to T lymphocyte interactions occur, which is followed by lymphocyte proliferation. The proliferation results in "primed" effector lymphocytes which maintain a memory for the specific allergen. The *elicitation phase* of CH appears to involve two mechanisms of action. Initially, allergens cause direct cellular action releasing a series of nonspecific inflammatory mediators. These mediators are responsible for some of the cellular influx into the site of allergen challenge. Additionally, the "primed" lymphocytes are called into the area in a very specific response. These responses and the cytokines, costimulatory factors, and adhesion molecules act to produce the end results of erythema and edema. (Modified from Selgrade et al., 2001.)

Once antigen is effectively presented to lymphocytes within the lymph node, activation and rapid proliferation of these cells occurs. Cellular proliferation is considered a hallmark of the induction phase of CH and is the mechanistic basis for the LLNA.

The initial application of a sensitizing agent to the skin induces soluble factors such as cytokines that activate a cascade of events critical for sensitization (Kimber and Dearman, 1996). Epidermal keratinocytes secrete inflammatory cytokines that facilitate the maturation of LCs at the site of antigen application. Cytokines initially produced include interleukin (IL)-1β, IL-6, and IL-12 (Enk and Katz, 1992; Kimber and Dearman, 1996). LCs also produce cytokines in an autocrine self-regulatory fashion, all of which contribute to the LCs activation and migration to the draining lymph node (Kimber and Dearman, 1996).

During LC maturation, antigen presentation is enhanced through the expression of cell-surface molecules, including major histocompatibility complex (MHC) class I and II and adhesion and costimulatory molecules. Antigen presentation requires an increase in membrane ICAM-1 to facilitate association of antigen bearing Langerhans cells with the lymphocytes (Ullrich, 1995). Although T cells are thought to be the key effector cells in the development of CH, both T and B lymphocytes proliferate in response to contact sensitizers (Gerberick et al., 1997).

Elicitation Phase

Grabbe and Schwarz (1998) provide an excellent review of the events involved in the elicitation phase of CH. Following proliferation, T lymphocytes are considered "primed" and have a specific memory for the sensitizing agent. Upon subsequent exposure to the agent, an antigen-specific response occurs. This second phase is referred to as the elicitation phase. While events associated with the elicitation of CH are not as well characterized as those associated with induction, it is evident from histopathology that mast cell degranulation, vasodilation, and the influx of neutrophils and mononuclear and T (lymphocytes) cells occur. However, clinical manifestation, histopathology, and immunohistology of allergic and irritant contact dermatitis are virtually indistinguishable. CH is distinguished from irritation because it requires immunologic memory of a specific allergen. Thus, an individual must have been previously exposed or sensitized. Additionally, CH is a systemic response and will occur even at sites distal to the original site of sensitization. Erythema, edema, and pruritus are characteristics of the elicitation phase and occur 24 to 72 hr after epicutaneous application of the allergen (whereas irritant responses occur much sooner). These endpoints, especially the evaluation of erythema, are used in the guinea pig test methods.

Exposure of a sensitized individual to the relevant hapten triggers the same cytokine responses that occur following induction. Two theories have been used to describe subsequent events in the elicitation phase. One theory suggests that Ag-specific primed (memory) T cells, which carry skin homing receptors, are constantly patrolling throughout the skin. As with induction, Langerhans cells take up and process antigen. However, unlike induction, antigen is presented to these primed T cells in the skin (rather than the lymph node), triggering the local responses classically associated with CH. A recent theory suggests that the initial response to elicitation is a nonspecific inflammatory response triggered by the production of proinflammatory cytokines and mediators produced by the keratinocytes. These mediators activate local endothelial cells, attract other cells, and, as during induction, upregulate surface expression of MHC, costimulatory, and adhesion molecules on resident cells. It is also believed that cytokines play a stimulatory role in this process of CH (Grabbe and Schwarz, 1998).

In summary, CH/ACD, like other hypersensitivity responses, is characterized by an induction and an elicitation phase. Keratinocytes, Langerhans cells, and lymphocytes are important cellular components of CH. A number of cytokines, chemokines, and adhesion molecules are involved in the CH response. Additionally, each mechanistic component is important to the understanding of models used for the assessment of the potential for chemicals to produce ACD or CH.

TEST METHODS

Traditional Contact Hypersensitivity Tests—Guinea Pig

The GP has been identified as an animal model for CH for more than 65 yr. There are several guinea pig tests for the assessment of CH. These include the guinea pig maximization test (GPMT), the Buehler assay (BA), Freund's complete adjuvant test, split adjuvant, open epidermal, and Draize. The tests most commonly accepted and used by regulatory agencies are the GPMT and BA (Klecak, 1966).

While there are variations in the GP test methods, the GPMT and the BA are the most common (Figure 17.3; Sailstad, 2002). Both of these tests require 20 animals per test group. They rely on the sensitization and challenge phases, requiring about 1 month to perform and the visual assessment of the erythema response (Klecak, 1966).

The GPMT depends on the induction and elicitation phase of CH, requiring the repeated dermal sensitization of guinea pigs and then the evaluation of the challenge or elicitation response. This test is noted for its ability to detect weak sensitizers. It has also been criticized for giving false positive responses. This method also requires the use of potentially irritating Freund's complete adjuvant via intradermal injections. On day 21 there is a challenge exposure, which is visually assessed for erythema 24 hr later. The assessment of the challenge site is graded: no visual change = 1; patchy erythema = +; confluent erythema = ++; confluent erythema and edema = +++ (Klecak, 1966).

The BA is mechanistically similar to the GPMT; however, it does not require the use of adjuvant. It requires the use of an occluded patch for 3 weeks of sensitization exposure. The challenge is then applied on day 28 and visually assessed as the GPMT 24 hr later (Klecak, 1966).

In summary, these guinea pig tests require 1 month or longer to perform and can use as many as 20 guinea pigs per group. These tests require the induction and elicitation phase of the CH response. The endpoint measured for both GP methods is visual assessment (subjective) of erythema at the challenge site location. The

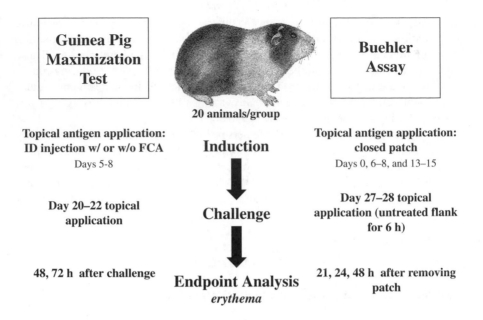

Figure 17.3 Guinea pig models. (Modified from Sailstad, 2002.)

visual assessment of erythema makes the evaluation of colored reagents such as dyes very difficult and vulnerable to subjectivity. While the GPMT has been classified as more "sensitive" than the BA, it has also been criticized for false positive responses and the deleterious affect that adjuvant has on the guinea pigs. Additionally, since the tests require both phases of CH, there is a certain amount of pain and distress caused by the edema and erythema that is associated with the elicitation phase (Sailstad, 2002).

The Local Lymph Node Assay (LLNA)—Murine

The LLNA as submitted to ICCVAM for review (Figure 17.4; Sailstad, 2002), using the induction phase of CH, measures the incorporation of ^{3}H-methyl thymidine (or ^{125}I-iododeoxyuridine) into proliferating lymphocytes in the draining lymph nodes of animals topically exposed to the test agent. The protocol specifies that the test agent be applied for three consecutive days to the dorsal portion of the ears of CBA mice. On day 6, the radioisotope is injected into the tail vein of each mouse. Five hours after the injection, the draining lymph node of each ear is excised and pooled for each animal. Depending upon the isotope selected, specific manipulation of the lymph node cells is performed followed by measurements from either B-scintillation counting or gamma counting. These values are expressed as disintegration per minute (dpm). While the majority of the data for the ICCVAM evaluation were analyzed from pooled animals per test group, individual animal data were also effective in the evaluation of chemical sensitization potential. The mean dpm for each test group is compared to the control group, and if the stimulation index (SI) of a test group is greater than or equal to threefold higher than the concurrent control,

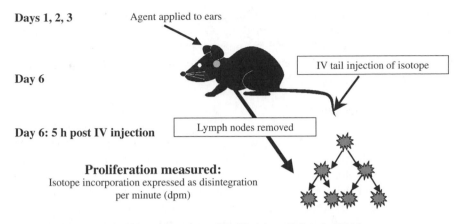

Days 1, 2, 3   Agent applied to ears

Day 6   IV tail injection of isotope

Day 6: 5 h post IV injection   Lymph nodes removed

Proliferation measured:
Isotope incorporation expressed as disintegration
per minute (dpm)

Figure 17.4 The local lymph node assay. (Modified from Sailstad, 2002.)

the test chemical is considered to be a sensitizer. Additionally, with the use of individual animal data, statistical analysis is possible (ICCVAM, 1999; Sailstad et al., 2000; Dean et al., 2001; Sailstad, 2002).

The LLNA sponsors proposed that this method provides specific advantages to the traditionally used GP tests: (1) objective endpoint of measurement, (2) reduction in the number of animals used, (3) reduction in cost and time of doing the test, and (4) reduction in distress to the animals. The ICCVAM PRP for the LLNA addressed these questions and provided the following summarized response. They agreed that the LLNA has several advantages over guinea pig test methods. The LLNA advantages include (1) quantitative data, (2) dose response assessment, (3) reduction of animal distress, (4) reduction in the number of animals needed, (5) potential for better cost effectiveness, (6) requires less time, (7) mechanistically based using the induction phase of sensitization, and (8) allows for future assay improvements and mechanistic studies (ICCVAM, 1999). In addition, the PRP endorsed the LLNA as a stand-alone alternative for contact sensitization in the hazard identification of chemicals with the potential for contact sensitization. However, they indicated that the following protocol modifications be accepted: (1) CBA female mice should be used exclusively until mouse strain and gender comparison studies are performed; (2) animals should be individually identified; (3) body weight data should be collected at the start and end of the study; (4) lymphocyte proliferation data should be collected at the level of individual animal, (5) statistical analysis should be performed; (6) a single dose of a sensitizer inducing a moderate response should be included as a concurrent positive control in each study; (7) ^{3}H-methyl thymidine or ^{125}I-iododeoxyuridine may be used in the LLNA; (8) evaluation of response should include a SI > 3, statistical significance, and dose response information; and (9) an illustration should be added to the protocol, indicating the nodes draining the exposure site that are to be collected. The panel also recommended that retrospective data audits be conducted on at least three of the intralaboratory and interlaboratory LLNA validation studies conducted by the sponsors. There were some limitations (or potential limitations) of the LLNA identified by the PRP. These are the evaluation of mixtures, metals, and irritants. The panel recommended that GP tests be used for the evaluation of such materials. The PRP concluded unanimously that the LLNA is a definite improvement with respect to animal welfare (i.e., refinement and reduction) over the accepted GPMT (ICCVAM, 1999).

Other Murine Systems

The result of the LLNA review and initial discussion of CH test models involved an enlightened, expansive discussion of CH test methods (Kimber, 1996a,b). This dialogue emphasized that there are other murine systems under development and there are potential advantages of these systems for the future. However, none of the other murine methods had the extensive level of research information and data that was offered by the LLNA submission to ICCVAM. These other tests were not ready for rigorous evaluation. Additionally, the emphasis of the ICCVAM peer review was on the evaluation of the LLNA, requiring a full focus on this procedure. Discussion of the other murine assays was therefore limited during the review process.

LLNA—*Ex Vivo*

Similar to the proposed LLNA, an *ex vivo* approach employs the induction phase of CH. Antigen is painted on the ears; however, the draining nodes are removed prior to the introduction of the tritiated thymidine. The lymph nodes are homogenized into a single cell suspension, and thymidine is added to the cell suspension and incubated. The endpoint proliferation that is measured occurs outside of the intact animal system. Conventional housing and disposal of nonradioactive carcasses from the *ex vivo* system would have clear advantages. Additionally, the technique of IV tail injections is not needed. There are also drawbacks. For example, sterile techniques must be used throughout and initial studies indicate that the sensitivity of this technique may be inferior to the *in vivo* LLNA. Additionally, limited data are available using this method.

Mouse Ear Swelling Test (MEST)

Another murine system, the mouse ear swelling test (MEST), depends upon both the elicitation response and induction phase of sensitization like the guinea pig tests. Mice are sensitized by the application of antigen on the abdomen or back. The challenge application is applied to the ears. The endpoint analysis of response is the measurement of edema as a change in ear thickness using calipers. This assay provides an objective endpoint and requires less time and cost than the traditional guinea pig assays. However, while there is promise for this assay, the amount of data available are limited, and results to date are somewhat variable (Kimber, 1996b). Additionally, the technical training required to perform mouse ear measurements can be extensive and may introduce another source of variability and subjectivity.

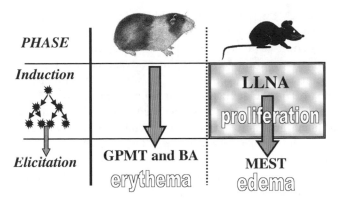

Figure 17.5 Contact hypersensitivity models and endpoint mechanisms.

SUMMARY OF ACD/CH ANIMAL MODELS

CH can be divided into two mechanistic phases, induction and elicitation. Methods that are available rely on these mechanisms (Figure 17.5) and the endpoint evaluation of the CH phase. Thus, the LLNA measures proliferation by the incorporation of a radioisotope, and the GPMT or BA measures erythema by visual assessment. Additionally, the MEST measures the edema produced by the antigen challenge.

FUTURE

Advantages of the murine system for the identification of potential contact sensitizing chemical go beyond the specific LLNA evaluated by ICCVAM. There are many immunochemicals and commercially available reagents for the mouse. Immunochemicals such as cytokines and other soluble components are readily available and correlate to the human factors. Additionally, the biology of the murine immune system is well understood, especially when compared to that of the guinea pig. These advantages should lead to additional advances in CH assessment. Other endpoints of CH using a LLNA approach may include another marker for proliferation (nonradioisotope) or identification of alterations in cytokine production. As data are collected for chemicals with CH potential, the ability to examine structure activity relations is enhanced. Some investigation has been conducted to examine the possibility of using the LLNA to examine low molecular weight respiratory sensitizers.

The future application of the LLNA is substantial, especially as other areas of science develop. The biotechnical advances made increase availability of these technologies for a better understanding of the mechanisms and process of CH, thus creating an environment where the potential for new more sensitive and specific endpoints of CH can be defined and measured. The ICCVAM evaluation of the LLNA provided the first step in the acceptance of new test methods for the future of CH evaluation.

The LLNA review by an ICCVAM-established independent peer review panel and their conclusions and findings concerning this new test method indicate that the LLNA has multiple advantages over the GP tests. Scientifically the LLNA uses an objective endpoint and provides a distinct advantage when colored materials are tested. Additionally, the reduction of the numbers of animals used and the reduction in distress to the animals is a significant animal welfare improvement. Based on these advantages, along with the recommended procedures, the LLNA was proposed as an alternative for GP tests. This level of endorsement accepts negative data without further animal testing. The ICCVAM endorsed the PRP's recommendations and sent their report to U.S. agencies. In turn, U.S. federal agencies associated with allergic contact dermatitis accepted the ICCVAM LLNA and recommendations. Individually agencies have worked with their guidelines to incorporate these changes to accept the LLNA. Following the ICCVAM review, the LLNA was endorsed internationally as the OECD also accepted the LLNA (with slight modifications to the ICCVAM protocol) as a stand-alone alternative to the GP test methods (OECD, 2002).

In summary, there are a number of mechanistic animal models that have been used to assess the potential for chemicals to produce allergic contact dermatitis. The guinea pig tests have been used for the longest period of time, whereas the murine models are relatively new. The more recent evaluation of murine models as alternatives to the guinea pig test led to the LLNA review. The LLNA has been extensively evaluated. Through review and acceptance by the ICCVAM, OECD, and U.S. federal agencies, the LLNA is a stand-alone alternative to GP test methods. The LLNA offers a variety of scientific and animal welfare advantages that indicate its use in most testing situations.

REFERENCES

Dean, J.H., Twerdok, L.E., Tice, R.R., Sailstad, D.M., Hattan, D.G., and Stokes, W.S. (2001) ICCVAM evaluation of the murine local lymph node assay. Conclusions and recommendations of an independent scientific peer review panel, *Regul. Toxicol. Pharmacol.*, 34, 258–273.

Enk, A.H. and Katz, S.I. (1992) Early molecular events in the induction phase of contact sensitivity, *Proc. Natl. Acad. Sci. U.S.A.*, 89, 1398–1402.

Gerberick, G.F. et al. (1997) Selective modulation of T cell memory markers CD62L and CD44 on murine draining lymph node cells following allergen and irritant treatment, *Toxicol. Appl. Pharmacol.*, 146, 1–10.

Grabbe, S. and Schwarz, T. (January 1998) Immunoregulatory mechanisms involved in elicitation of allergic contact hypersensitivity, *Immunol. Today*, 1, 37–44.

ICCVAM (Interagency Coordinating Committee on the Validation of Alternative Methods) (1997) Validation and regulatory acceptance of toxicological test methods: A report of the *ad hoc* Interagency Coordinating Committee on the Validation of Alternative Methods, NIH publication 97-3981, National Institute of Environmental Health Sciences, Research Triangle Park, NC.

ICCVAM (Interagency Coordinating Committee on the Validation of Alternative Methods) (1999) The murine local lymph node assay: a test method for assessing the allergic contact dermatitis potential of chemicals/compounds, NIH publication 99-4494, National Institute of Environmental Health Sciences, Research Triangle Park, NC.

Kimber, I. (1996a) The local lymph node assay, in *Dermatotoxicology,* 5th ed., Marzulli, F.N. and Maibach, H.I. Eds., Taylor and Francis, Washington, D.C., pp. 469–473.

Kimber, I. (1996b) Mouse predictive tests, in *Toxicology of Contact Hypersensitivity,* Kimber, I. and Maurer, T., Eds., Taylor and Francis, London, U.K., pp. 127–139.

Kimber, I. and Dearman, R.J. (1996) Contact hypersensitivity: immunological mechanisms, in *Toxicology of Contact Hypersensitivity,* Kimber, I. and Maurer, T., Eds., Taylor and Francis, London, pp. 4–25.

Klecak, G. (1966) Test methods for allergic contact dermatitis in animals, in *Dermatotoxicology,* 5th ed., Marzulli, F.N., and Maibach, H.I., Eds., Taylor and Francis, Washington, D.C., 437–459.

OECD (Organization for Economic Cooperation and Development) (1993) OECD guidelines for testing of chemicals, 406, skin sensitization, OECD, Paris.

OECD (Organization for Economic Cooperation and Development) (2000) Test guidelines for the testing of chemicals [skin sensitisation: Local Lymph Node Assay], Guideline 429 accepted April 24, 2002, OECD, Paris.

Sailstad, D.M. (2002) Murine local lymph node assay: an alternative test method for skin hypersensitivity testing, *Lab. Anim.,* 31, 36–41.

Sailstad, D.M., Topper, J.S., Doerfler, D.L., Qasim, M., and Selgrade, M.J.K. (1994) Evaluation of an Azo and Two Anthraquinone Dyes for Allergic Potential, *Fundam. Appl. Toxicol.,* 23, 569–577.

Sailstad, D.M., Hattan, D., Hill, R., and Stokes, W. (2000) The first method evaluation by the Interagency Coordinating Committee on the Validation of Alternative Methods (ICCVAM): the murine local lymph node assay (LLNA), in *Progress in the Reduction, Refinement and Replacement of Animal Experimentation,* Balls, M., van Zeller, A.-M., and Halder, M.E., Eds., Elsevier Science, Amsterdam, 428.

Sailstad, D.M., Hattan, D., Hill, R.N., and Stokes, W.S. (2001) ICCVAM evaluation of the murine local lymph node assay. The ICCVAM review process, *Regul. Toxicol. Pharmacol.,* 34, 249–257.

Selgrade, M.J.K., Germolec, D.R., Luebke, R.W., Smialowicz, R.J., Ward, M.D., and Sailstad, D.M. (2001) Immunotoxicity, in *Introduction to Biochemical Toxicology,* 3rd ed., Hodgson, E. and Smart, R.C., Eds., Wiley, New York, p. 595.

Ullrich, S.E. (1995) The role of epidermal cytokines in the generation of cutaneous immune reactions and ultraviolet radiation-induced immune suppression, *Photochem. Photobiol.,* 62, 389–401.

CHAPTER 18

Validating *In Vitro* Dermal Absorption Studies: An Introductory Case Study

Robert P. Zendzian and Michael Dellarco

CONTENTS

INTRODUCTION

The process of adding new testing procedures to regulatory processes follows three steps: test development, test validation, and test acceptance (Balls et al., 1990). Test development is the process of conceiving, designing, and making the test work as projected and convincing others that the test is worthy of entering the validation process. Test validation is the process of determining whether other laboratories can routinely perform the test and get the expected results. Test acceptance is the decision by individuals or agencies that the test can be routinely used for their specified purposes. These three steps should be followed whether the test is a new procedure or it is intended to replace or augment an established procedure. In practice, these steps are frequently incompletely performed and recorded, jumbled together, or performed out of order. Because of this failure to achieve a defined process, we are frequently left with accepted test procedures where instructions are incomplete or lacking and where we have no evidence that the results are consistent or accurately represent the process that we are observing. This has become particularly true in the general process of validating *in vitro* dermal absorption (dermal penetration) procedures and the development of *in vitro* dermal absorption test guidelines by the Organization for Economic Cooperation and Development (OECD) (Anon., 1996). This chapter focuses on the first step of the process, test development, and uses the reports on the dermal absorption of acetochlor submitted to the Office of Pesticide Programs (OPP), U.S. Environmental Protection Agency (EPA), to illustrate the standard for experimental design and reporting necessary to move from test development to test validation and ultimate acceptance. The studies were performed *in vivo* using the rat (Lythgoe and Jones, 1990), *in vitro* using the rat epidermal membrane preparation (Clowes and Scott, 1990a), and *in vitro* in the human epidermal membrane preparation (Clowes and Scott, 1990b).

METHODS FOR EVALUATION OF THE REPORTS

Study reports on the dermal absorption of acetochlor were submitted to OPP by a pesticide registrant in the process of reregistration of the pesticide acetochlor. The reports conform to the OPP requirements for study (test) reporting. OPP reporting requirements are in two parts: regulatory requirements and scientific requirements. Regulatory requirements apply to all study reports submitted to OPP. In general, they consist of requirements for and detailed composition of title page, statement of no data confidentiality claims (signed), good laboratory practice compliance statement (signed), quality assurance statement (signed), certification of data accuracy (signed), table of contents, summary, and body of report. The signatures required are those of the individuals responsible for each particular aspect of the study. These requirements are specified in the federal register (CFR 40 parts 150 to 189) and have the force of law. The scientific requirements for reporting vary to some extent with the type of study. The requirements for dermal absorption studies are specified in the Guideline for Dermal Absorption of Pesticides (Zendzian, 1994). In general, they consist of the following: identification and properties of the test compound, vehicle, and experimental animal; the experimental design; animal husbandry, observations, and preparation for dosing; dose preparation, dose application, and protection of the application site; handling during exposure; and termination, sample collection, and sample analysis. All data generated during the study must be reported, usually in appendices, and the results discussed with summary tables or illustrations. The reports of the acetochlor studies satisfied all of these data reporting requirements.

The studies were judged scientifically acceptable. In each study the following criteria for a dermal absorption study were met:

1. The test material was radiolabeled (with ^{14}C) in such a manner as to permit the quantitative tracing of it and/or its metabolites.
2. The test material was dissolved/suspended in a vehicle, which mimicked that of field exposure.
3. The test material was applied quantitatively as mass per unit area of application site.
4. The application site was prepared in a standard manner.
5. The application site was protected against disturbance or loss of the test material.

6. At the end of the exposure period, the application site was washed with a water solution of soap/detergent to mimic human washing.
7. All components of the test system were collected and analyzed separately so as to obtain a complete material balance of dose distribution.
8. The portion of the dose in the skin/epidermal membrane and the portion that had passed through it was determined.
9. At least four individual animals/membrane samples were used for each dose-exposure tested.

In each study, radiolabeled acetochlor (^{14}C-phenyl) was the tracer diluted with unlabeled acetochlor where necessary to make up the dose. It was applied in a use formulation. Doses applied were as follows: 3.0, 42, 270, and 2934 μg/cm^2 *in vivo* rat and 3.02, 47.3, 318, and 3095 μg/cm^2 *in vitro* rat and human. Exposure durations were 0.5, 1, 2, 4, 10, and 24 hr for the rat *in vivo* and *in vitro* and 2, 10, and 24 hr for the human *in vitro*. The doses and durations of exposure were judged sufficiently similar to allow comparison of the experimental results.

In particular, the evaluation determined that the test material applied in each study was identical, the doses were essentially identical, and common exposure durations were used. Thus, one can compare and contrast the entry into and passage through the skin/membrane in the three test systems.

MATERIALS AND METHODS OF THE INDIVIDUAL STUDIES

Dose preparation was as follows. Dose preparation was the same in the three studies. (Lythgoe and Jones, 1990; Clowes and Scott, 1990a,b).

The four dose levels corresponding to the formulation concentrate (768 mg acetochlor/ml) and three aqueous dilutions thereof, nominally 1/10, 1/70 and 1/1000. For each preparation, the required amount of a methanol stock solution of [^{14}C]-labeled acetochlor was transferred to a glass vial and the solvent evaporated under a stream of nitrogen. The amount of unlabeled acetochlor required to give the appropriate specific activity was added to the vial and mixed with the radiolabeled material. The required blank formulation was then added and allowed to mix with the acetochlor. Finally, the required amount of deionized water was added and the suspension mixed by stirring. In the case of the 1/1000 dilution, which contained no unlabeled acetochlor, this procedure was followed by sonication for 10 minutes to assist dispersion.

Dose solutions were sampled and analyzed, for radioactivity and concentration of acetochlor, before, during, and after dosing. Animal preparation, dosing, and sample collection for the rat *in vivo* study of Lythgoe and Jones (1990) were as follows:

Approximately 24 hours before dosing the fur from the shoulders and back of each rat was shaved. After several hours, the condition of the shaved skin was examined and only animals with undamaged skin were retained in the study. The shaved area of the skin was washed with acetone to remove sebum and two 25.5 mm internal diameter, 3 mm thick nitrile rubber 'O' rings were glued to the skin surface, one behind each shoulder, using cyano-acrylate glue. The internal surface of skin encompassed by each ring was approximately 5 cm². A Queen Ann plastic collar was secured around the neck of each animal and the rats transferred to individual stainless steel metabolism cages.

Using a 25 μl capacity positive displacement pipette, and disposable polypropylene tips, 20 μl of dose suspension was applied to the skin surface within one 'O' ring and was spread over the 5 cm² application area using the side and end of the pipette tip, which was retained for analysis.

The applied suspension was allowed to dry. The application site was then protected by applying cyano-acrylate glue around the surface of the 'O' ring and superimposing a second similar rubber '0' ring covered with a fine permeable nylon gauze (100 μm bolting cloth) glued to the surface of the ring with Bostik. For the 1/1000 dilution experiment, the nylon gauze was replaced with an active charcoal filter pad. This dosing procedure was then repeated for the second application site. Radioactivity in/on the pipette tips was determined for dose quantization. Animals were returned to the metabolism cages and urine and feces collected for the duration of exposure.

At 0.5, 1, 2, 4, 10 and 24 hours, four acceptable rats were selected and were anaesthetized with FLUOTHANE vapor. Animals with detached or badly damaged protective rings were deemed unacceptable and were excluded from the study.

For each rat, the nylon gauze or carbon filters covering both application sites were detached and retained in a single vial. The skin surface was carefully washed with a 3% aqueous solution of Teepol-L using cotton wool swabs. The skin surface was then rinsed with water, which was also recovered on cotton wool swabs. All swabs used to wash each animal were retained in a single vial and were retained for radioactivity analysis.

A blood sample was taken by cardiac puncture and the animal sacrificed. Residual urine was removed from the bladder and added to the urine collection.

The rubber 'O' rings were detached from the skin surface and were retained in the same vial as the nylon gauze covers for subsequent solvent extraction. The rubber 'O' rings from the 1/1000 dilution experiment were retained and extracted in a separate vial. The skin encompassing both application sites was then removed and transferred to a single vial for each animal.

The residual carcass was retained for analysis.

For each rat in the formulation concentrate (707 mg/g), 1/10 aqueous dilution (76.9 mg/g), and 1/70 aqueous dilution (11.7 mg/g), the following samples were analyzed: skin wash, protective cover, skin (application site), urine, feces, cage wash, and carcass. For the 1/1000 aqueous dilution (0.763 mg/g), the rubber 'O' rings and carbon filter were analyzed separately.

The epidermal membrane used in these studies were prepared as follows (Clowes and Scott, 1990a):

Rats were killed when they were 27 or 28 days of age (weight 70–100 g) by FLUOTHANE anesthesia followed by cervical dislocation and fur from the dorso-lumbar region removed using animal clippers, ensuring that the skin was not damaged. The clipped area of skin was excised and any subcutaneous fat removed. The skins were soaked for 16–20 hours in 1.5 M sodium bromide, then the epidermis was carefully peeled from the dermis.

Each epidermal membrane was given an identifying number and stored on aluminum foil in a freezer (at −20°C) until used. Epidermal samples were used within 7 days of preparation.

Percutaneous absorption was studied as follows (Clowes and Scott, 1990a):

Glass diffusion cells in which the epidermis forms a horizontal membrane separating donor (outer) and receptor chambers were used for measuring skin absorption.

2.54 cm² of epidermal surface was available for absorption and all experiments were conducted at 30°C. Receptor solutions were stirred.

The volume of the chamber was not specified. The integrity of the membrane was assessed as follows:

Initially, the integrity of all epidermal membranes was established by measurement of their permeability to tritiated water. Membranes displaying permeability coefficients of 3.0×10^{-3} cm hr^{-1} or greater were regarded as 'damaged' and rejected. Tritiated water was desorbed from the membranes by careful washing of the donor receptor chambers with saline. The donor chamber was left open to the atmosphere overnight and approximately 0.5 ml saline was left in the receptor chamber to maintain a high relative humidity.

Percutaneous absorption of [^{14}C]-acetochlor was assessed as follows:

A measured volume of 50% v/v ethanol:water was placed into the receptor chambers of the cells. The [^{14}C]-acetochlor formulations were applied to the membranes at a rate of 4 µl/cm² (10.2 ul per cell to give acetochlor dose rates of 3095 µg/cm², 318 µg/cm², 47.3 µg/cm² and 3.02 µg/cm².

The applications were spread over the skin surface using individual loops of silicone rubber tubing (0.5 mm id) which were analyzed for radioactivity after use.

At the designated times (0.5, 1, 2, 4, 10 and 24 hours) the exposure was terminated by removal of the donor chamber and the receptor solution. The receptor solution was sampled and the remainder discarded. The empty receptor chamber was rinsed with 5 ml of fresh receptor fluid and the rinsing discarded. The donor chamber was placed in a 50 ml beaker and soaked in 5 ml fresh receptor fluid for at least 0.5 hr before a sample (50 µl) was taken for analysis. Residual donor material was removed from the exposed surface of the epidermis by rinsing with 5 ml aliquot of 3% w/v TEEPOL-L in water until the radioactivity in the rinse was less than 100 cpm in a sample (50 µl) of the 5 ml rinse. The rinsings were combined and the total volume recorded. A sample (50 µl) was analyzed by liquid scintillation counting.

Each epidermis membrane, whilst still attached to the receptor chamber, was placed in a 50 ml glass beaker and 25 ml of Soluene 350 added to cover the epidermis. When the epidermis sample had dissolved, a 1 ml sample was added to Hionic-Flour in a glass scintillation vial and analyzed by liquid scintillation counting.

The following describe the preparation of skin samples, dose administration, and sample collection for the human *in vitro* study (Clowes and Scott, 1990b):

Abdominal whole skin (dermis and epidermis) was obtained post mortem from subjects of varying ages. Female samples were used as the more densely haired male samples were less likely to give intact epidermal membranes after separation. The epidermis was removed from the dermis by immersion of the whole skin in water at 60°C for 45 seconds followed by gently teasing the epidermis free. The epidermal membranes were given unique identifying numbers and stored on tin foil in a freezer until required. Epidermis samples were used within 7 days of preparation.

Glass diffusion cells in which the epidermis forms a horizontal membrane separating donor (outer) and receptor chambers were used for measuring skin absorption. 2.54 cm^2 of epidermal surface was available for absorption and all experiments were conducted at 30°C. Receptor solutions were stirred.

Volume for the receptor chamber was not specified.

Initially, the integrity of all epidermal membranes was established by measurement of their permeability to tritiated water.

In this study membranes displaying permeability coefficients of 1.5×10^{-3} cm hr^{-1} or greater were regarded as 'damaged' and rejected.

Tritiated water was desorbed from the membranes by careful washing of the donor receptor chambers with saline. The donor chamber was left open to the atmosphere overnight and approximately 0.5 ml saline was left in the receptor chamber to maintain a high relative humidity.

A measured volume of 50% v/v ethanol:water was placed into the receptor chambers of the cells. The [^{14}C]-acetochlor formulations were applied to the membranes at a rate of 4 µl cm^{-2} to give acetochlor dose rates of 3095 µg cm^{-2}, 318 µg cm^{-2}, 47.3 µg cm^{-2}, and 3.02 µg cm^{-2}.

The applications were spread over the skin surface using individual loops of silicone rubber tubing (0.5 mm id) which were analyzed for radioactivity after use.

At the designated times (2, 10 and 24 hours) the exposure was terminated by removal of the donor chamber and the receptor solution. The receptor solution was sampled and the remainder discarded. The empty receptor chamber was rinsed with 5 ml of fresh receptor fluid and the rinsing discarded. The donor chamber was placed in a 50 ml beaker and soaked in 5 ml fresh receptor fluid for at least 0.5 hr before a sample (50 μl) was taken for analysis. Residual donor material was removed from the exposed surface of the epidermis by rinsing with 5 ml aliquots of 3% w/v TEEPOL-L in water until the radioactivity in the rinse was less than 100 cpm in a sample (50 μl) of the 5 ml rinse. The rinsings were combined and the total volume recorded. A sample (50 μl) was analyzed by liquid scintillation counting.

Each epidermal membrane, whilst still attached to the receptor chamber, was placed in a 50 ml glass beaker and 25 ml of SOLUENE 350 added to cover the epidermis. When the epidermal sample had dissolved, a 1 ml sample was added to HIONIC-FLOUR in a glass scintillation vial and analyzed by liquid scintillation counting.

RESULTS OF THE STUDIES

The study reports were reviewed by the first author and a review, called a data evaluation report (DER), was written for each report. The DERs summarized the study reports, in particular, material tested, experimental design, methods of dose preparation, dosing, animal handling, sample collection, and sample analysis. The data generated in the studies were summarized in tabular form. Summary results of the studies are presented in Tables 18.1, 18.2, and 18.3 from the DERs. Owing to rounding, numbers may not add up.

Table 18.1 summarizes the results from the rat *in vivo* study. The samples analyzed provide a complete material balance of dose distribution in the rats. One can follow entry into the skin, passage through the skin into the systemic compartment, and excretion. The amount absorbed is the sum of acetochlor in the urine, feces, cage wash, and carcass. Of particular importance is the quantity and percent of dose in the washed skin and absorbed. The quantity in the washed skin shows little change with increased duration of exposure. However, the quantity in the washed skin does increase with dose but the percent does not increase. The percent in the skin decreases between 3 μg/cm^2 and 42 μg/cm^2 but is similar for the doses of 42, 270, and 2934 μg/cm^2. The quantity absorbed increases with increasing duration of exposure and with increasing dose. In contrast, the percent absorbed increases with increasing duration of exposure but decreases with increasing dose. This pattern is typical of a chemical that is approaching saturation in passage through the skin.

Table 18.2 summarizes the results of the rat *in vitro* study. Here the dose distribution of concern is wash, skin, and absorbed. The quantity in the washed skin shows no increase with duration of exposure but does increase with increasing dose. The percent of dose in the skin is similar for all four doses. The quantity absorbed increases with increasing duration of exposure and with increasing dose. The percent absorbed increases with increasing duration of exposure but is similar for the doses of 3.02, 47.3, and 318 μg/cm^2. The percent absorbed decreases between doses of 318 and 3095 μg/cm^2, indicating that the high dose is on the saturation portion of the absorption curve.

Table 18.1 Acetochlor *In Vivo* (Mean dose distribution as µg equivalents of acetochlor per cm². Mean of four male rats.)

Exposure (hr)	Wash	Cover	Carbon Filter	Skin µg/cm²	Skin %	Urine	Feces	Cage Wash	Carcass	Absorbed µg/cm²	Absorbed %
3 µg/cm²											
0.5	0.22	0.2	0.1	0.1	4.00	<0.01	<0.001	<0.001	0.1	0.1	3.79
1	2.2	0.2	0.1	0.2	6.00	<0.01	<0.001	<0.001	0.1	0.1	4.28
2	2.0	0.2	0.2	0.2	7.17	<0.01	<0.001	<0.001	0.2	0.2	7.32
4	1.8	0.2	0.3	0.2	7.93	0.02	<0.001	0.01	0.3	0.3	9.93
10	1.2	0.3	0.4	0.3	9.63	0.2	0.01	0.01	0.4	0.6	19.55
24	0.9	0.4	0.7	0.4	12.53	0.5	0.2	0.02	0.2	0.9	31.37
42 µg/cm²											
0.5	34.1	3.0	—	1.4	3.18	<0.004	0.001	<0.01	1.7	1.7	3.95
1	32.3	3.2	—	1.3	2.99	<0.02	0.001	0.01	2.5	2.5	5.98
2	34.9	4.1	—	1.2	2.78	<0.02	0.005	0.3	1.8	1.9	4.38
4	31.1	4.9	—	1.2	2.81	0.2	0.003	0.01	3.6	3.9	9.24
10	22.1	5.6	—	1.2	2.66	2.1	0.3	0.4	7.0	9.8	23.06
24	15.1	8.1	—	0.9	1.83	5.5	2.1	0.6	4.4	12.6	29.64
270 µg/cm²											
0.5	212.0	24.2	—	9.2	3.40	<0.01	<0.01	<0.04	12.9	12.9	4.79
1	204.9	21.7	—	8.7	3.21	<0.02	<0.01	<0.05	15.1	15.2	5.63
2	216.9	23.7	—	13.3	4.91	<0.02	<0.01	<0.05	8.1	8.2	3.03
4	218.5	21.0	—	8.7	3.21	0.7	<0.01	<0.06	12.3	13.0	4.83
10	190.4	28.2	—	10.8	3.99	3.5	0.1	0.56	21.1	25.2	17.52
2934 µg/cm²											
0.5	2571.9	285.9	—	74.2	2.53	<0.1	<0.3	<0.4	40.3	40.9	1.39
1	2175.7	405.4	—	95.2	3.24	0.2	<0.3	<0.2	150.9	153.04	5.22
2	2322.7	355.2	—	98.9	3.37	<0.5	0.1	<0.6	98.5	99.6	3.39
4	2260.1	502.7	—	93.3	2.18	2.3	0.1	<1.1	74.8	78.3	2.67
10	2261.4	435.5	—	88.3	3.01	15.2	0.2	1.6	114.3	131.3	4.47
24	1788.9	627.2	—	86.0	2.92	97.1	47.9	8.4	216.7	369.9	12.61

a *Absorbed* is sum of urine, feces, cage wash, and carcass.

Source: Lythgoe, 1990a.

Table 18.2 Acetochlor *In Vitro* (Mean dose distribution *in vitro* dermal absorption in rat skin. Mean of four to seven skin samples. Results presented as µg/cm².)

Exposure (hr)	Absorbed µg/cm²	%	Wash	Skin µg/cm²	%	Donor	Loop	Total Recovered
				3.02 µg/cm²				
0.05	0.41	13.68	1.73	0.11	3.60	0.08	0.55	2.89
1	0.82	27.12	1.32	0.11	3.77	0.04	0.44	2.73
2	1.14	37.78	0.95	0.12	3.84	0.03	0.50	2.73
4	1.37	45.30	0.80	0.09	2.98	0.05	0.43	2.75
10	2.15	71.19	0.17	0.08	2.52	0.01	0.59	2.99
24	2.12	70.13	0.13	0.08	2.75	0.02	0.41	2.77
				47.3 µg/cm²				
0.5	2.02	4.27	25.6	1.09	2.30	1.41	1.03	31.1
1	3.90	8.25	28.2	1.17	2.47	0.97	1.02	35.3
2	10.3	21.78	18.7	1.46	3.09	0.57	1.25	32.2
4	16.0	33.83	13.6	1.08	2.28	0.58	1.38	32.7
10	20.7	43.76	7.1	1.00	2.11	0.78	0.98	30.6
24	28.7	60.68	2.9	0.79	1.73	0.14	1.21	33.7
				318 µg/cm²				
0.5	6.58	2.07	283	12.9	4.06	10.5	13.4	325
1	21.4	6.73	383	16.6	5.22	14.3	16.7	452
2	33.4	10.50	261	28.1	8.84	19.4	8.25	350
4	80.9	25.44	262	16.2	5.09	4.41	11.6	375
10	182	57.23	158	22.6	7.11	5.59	11.6	379
24	246	77.36	67	14.4	4.53	5.52	13.3	347
				3095 µg/cm²				
1	17	0.55	2411	143	4.62	311	118	2999
2	104	3.36	3146	187	6.04	313	138	3858
4	137	4.43	2103	111	3.59	316	161	2828
10	264	8.53	2344	196	6.33	294	156	3253
24	757	24.46	1598	202	6.53	182	127	2866

Note: The 0.5-hr exposure was not performed at the high dose.

Source: Clowes and Scott, 1990a.

Table 18.3 summarizes the results of the human *in vitro* study. The same four doses were used, but the durations of exposure were limited to 2, 10, and 24 hr due to the limited availability of human skin. Again the dose distribution of concern is wash, skin, and absorbed. The quantity in the washed skin does not increase with increasing duration of exposure, but it does with increasing dose. The percent of dose in the washed skin is similar for increasing duration of exposure but decreases with increasing dose. The quantity of dose absorbed increases with increasing duration of exposure for doses of 3.02, 47.3, and 318 µg/cm² but is similar for the doses of 318 and 3095 µg/cm², indicating saturation of absorption at the two high doses.

Overall the quantity and percent of dose entering and passing through the rat skin *in vitro* is greater than that entering and passing through the human skin *in vitro*.

Table 18.3 Acetochlor *In Vitro* (Mean dose distribution in vitro dermal absorption in human skin. Mean of six skin samples. Results expressed as µg/cm².)

Exposure (hr)	Absorbed µg/cm²	%	Wash	Skin µg/cm²	%	Donor	Loop	Total Recovered
			3.02 µg/cm²					
2	0.015	0.486	2.36	0.273	9.04	0.035	0.359	3.04
10	0.074	2.44	2.61	0.271	9.98	0.136	0.194	3.28
24	0.261	8.63	1.54	0.092	3.03	0.098	0.244	2.24
			47.3 µg/cm²					
2	0.140	0.296	34.2	1.89	3.99	3.12	2.61	41.9
10	1.70	3.59	30.4	4.43	9.37	3.86	2.31	42.7
24	3.63	7.68	26.2	1.63	3.45	2.80	3.09	37.4
			318 µg/cm²					
2	0.816	0.256	239	18.9	5.94	70.4	22.4	352
10	5.69	1.79	221	12.1	3.82	91.8	15.8	347
24	43.6	13.7	245	18.2	5.72	62.3	15.8	384
			3095 µg/cm²					
2	4.57	0.148	2796	51.5	1.67	772	260	3884
10	22.4	0.722	2057	80.5	2.60	896	259	3314
24	32.5	1.05	1669	38.4	1.24	671	217	2628

Source: Clowes and Scott, 1990b.

DISCUSSION

The studies were well designed, well performed, and well reported. They satisfied all of the OPP data reporting requirements. With the reports in hand, any properly equipped laboratory could repeat the studies and determine whether the results are reproducible. That is, other laboratories could perform the test validation step. However, there remains one small question: Should the procedure enter the validation step? The studies were carefully designed to produce comparable *in vivo* and *in vitro* data at the same four doses and the same six durations of exposure in the rat and at the same four doses and three matching durations of exposure *in vitro* in the human. How do the results match? In order to enter the test validation step, the test developers must present matching results from matched *in vivo* and *in vitro* tests.

The percent of dose absorbed *in vivo* and *in vitro* in the rat and the ratio *in vitro* to *in vivo* are presented in Table 18.4. To be acceptable, the ratio of *in vitro* to *in vivo* should approximate one for all doses and durations of exposure. The ratios of *in vitro* rat to *in vivo* rat, for each dose, are plotted in Figure 18.1 as ratio against duration of exposure. The data clearly show that this particular *in vitro* procedure in the rat overestimated dermal absorption in the majority of doses and exposure durations with the greatest error in the lower doses. The ratio varies inconsistently with dose and duration of exposure. There is no common factor which would indicate

Table 18.4 Comparison of the Percent Absorbed *In Vitro* and *In Vivo* in Rat Skin; Data Are from Tables 18.1 and 18.2

Dose (µg/cm²)	0.5	1.0	2.0	4.0	10.0	24.0
			Exposure Duration (hr)			
3.0 *in vivo*	3.8	4.3	7.3	9.9	19.5	31.4
3.02 *in vitro*	13.7	27.1	37.8	45.3	71.2	70.1
42.5 *in vivo*	4.0	6.0	4.4	9.2	23.1	29.6
47.3 *in vitro*	4.3	8.2	21.8	33.8	43.8	60.7
270 *in vivo*	4.8	5.6	3.0	4.8	9.3	17.5
318 *in vitro*	2.1	6.7	10.5	25.4	57.2	77.4
2934 *in vivo*	1.4	5.2	3.4	2.7	4.5	12.6
3095 *in vitro*	—	0.6	3.4	4.4	8.5	24.5
			Ratio *in Vitro/in Vivo*			
3.02/3.0	3.6	6.3	5.2	4.6	3.7	2.2
47.3/42.4	1.1	1.4	5.0	3.7	1.9	2.1
318/270	0.4	1.2	3.5	5.3	6.2	4.4
3095/2934	—	0.1	1.0	1.6	1.9	1.9

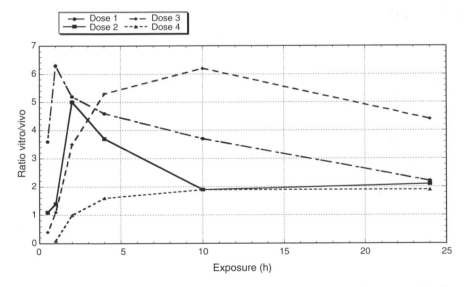

Figure 18.1 The ratio of the *in vitro* absorption to the *in vivo* absorption with exposure duration in the rat. Dose ratios 1, 2, 3, and 4 are in order of low dose ratio to high dose ratio. Data are from Table 18.4.

a systematic error in the *in vitro* procedure. This indicates that the procedure may not be correctable. The data strongly show that the procedure is not ready to enter the test validation step.

We have no human *in vivo* data to compare with the human *in vitro* data and so cannot directly assess its validity. However, the point has been raised that even if *in vitro* data do not match *in vivo,* one may compare rat and human *in vitro* data to obtain

Table 18.5 Comparison of the Percent Absorbed *In Vitro* in Rat and Human Epidermal Membrane Preparations; Data Are from Tables 18.2 and 18.3

Dose (μg/cm²)	2.0	10.0	24.0
	Exposure Duration (hr)		
3.03 rat	37.8	71.2	70.1
human	0.49	2.44	8.63
47.3 rat	21.8	43.8	60.7
human	0.30	3.59	7.68
318 rat	10.5	57.2	77.4
human	0.26	1.79	13.7
3095 rat	3.4	8.5	24.5
human	0.15	0.72	1.05
	Ratio Rat/Human		
3.03	77.1	29.2	8.1
47.3	72.7	12.2	7.9
318	40.4	32.0	5.6
3095	22.7	11.8	23.3

a rat to human absorption conversion factor. It is generally accepted that rat skin is more permeable to chemicals than human, in the order of three to five times more permeable. A conversion factor would enable one to convert rat dermal toxicity data to human dermal toxicity. The percent of dose absorbed *in vitro* in the rat and in the human epidermal membrane preparation and their ratio are presented in Table 18.5. The ratios of *in vitro* rat to *in vitro* human, for each dose, are plotted in Figure 18.2 as ratio against

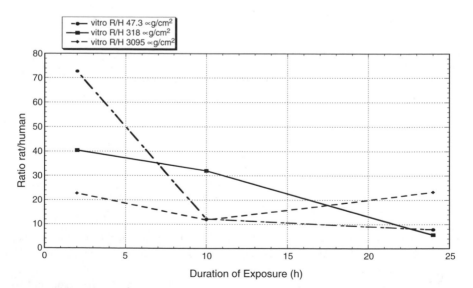

Figure 18.2 The ratio of the rat *in vitro* absorption to the human *in vitro* absorption with exposure duration. Dose ratios 1, 2, 3, and 4 are in order of low dose ratio to high dose ratio. Data are from Table 18.5.

duration of exposure. This particular procedure does not provide a single conversion factor or anything even approaching a factor. The ratio of rat to human varies from 0.5 to 77.1 and shows no evidence of a pattern either with duration of exposure or with dose. This variation and its magnitude strongly argue that the procedure is not correctable. Again the procedure is not ready to enter the test validation step.

Based on this data set, the isolated epidermal membrane preparation is not ready for the test validation or the test acceptance steps. At this time it appears that additional developmental work is necessary on the procedure to determine if it can be revised to produce comparable data. The variation and inconsistency of the comparable data strongly indicate that the procedure is not correctable.

REFERENCES

Anon. (May 1996) Draft, OECD Guideline for the Testing of Chemicals, Proposal for a New Guideline, Dermal Delivery and Percutaneous Absorption: *in vitro* Method, Paris, OECD.

Balls, M., Blaaiboer, B., Brusick, D., et al. (1990) Report and recommendations of the CAAT/ERGATT workshop on the validation of toxicology test procedures, *Alt. Lab. Anim.*, 18, 313–337.

Clowes, H.M. and Scott, R.C. (1990a) Acetochlor: *in vitro* percutaneous absorption through Sprague Dawley rat epidermis from formulation WF1301, ICI Central Toxicology Laboratory, report number JVI1348, CTL/P3067, MRID 41963311, available from Public Docket and Freedom of Information Office, Field Operations Division (7506C) Office of Pesticide Programs, U.S. Environmental Protection Agency, 401 M St., Washington, D.C. 20460.

Clowes, H.M. and Scott, R.C. (1990b) Acetochlor: *in vitro* percutaneous absorption through human epidermis from formulation WF1301, report number CTL/P/3068, JVI1348, MRID 41963312, available from Public Docket and Freedom of Information Office, Field Operations Division (7506C) Office of Pesticide Programs, U.S. Environmental Protection Agency, 401 M St., Washington, D.C. 20460.

Lythgoe, R.E. and Jones, B.K. (1990) Acetochlor: *in vivo* percutaneous absorption study in the rat, ICI Central Toxicology Laboratory, report number CTL/P/3088, URO295MRID 41778301 (03), available from Public Docket and Freedom of Information Office, Field Operations Division (7506C) Office of Pesticide Programs, U.S. Environmental Protection Agency, 401 M St., Washington, D.C. 20460.

Zendzian, R.P. (1994) Guideline for Dermal Absorption of Pesticides (PB95–148616: National Technical Information Service, Front Royal Rd., Springfield, VA 22161).

CHAPTER 19

A Molecular Diagnostic Approach to Irritant or Allergic Patch Testing Using the DermPatch

Melissa M. Fitzgerald, Vera B. Morhenn, Stacey B. Humphrey, Nirmala Jayakumar, and Lawrence A. Rheins

CONTENTS

BACKGROUND

Elucidation of the molecular events that lead to irritant contact dermatitis (ICD) or allergic contact dermatitis (ACD) in human skin will be helpful in developing mechanistic toxicological assays that permit the reduction, refinement, or replacement of animals in product safety testing. The first alternative toxicological test approved by ICCVAM was a mechanistic test, the murine local lymph node assay (MLLNA), which replaced the guinea pig maximization test in 1999. The MLLNA measures lymphocyte proliferation through ^{3}H-methyl thymidine uptake in the draining lymph nodes of animals topically exposed to the test article. Since the test is based on events occurring during the induction phase of allergic contact dermatitis,

Table 19.1 Skin Cytokins (adapted from Gerberick et al., 1998)

Cytokines	Constitutive or inducible expression in		
	Langerhans cells	Keratinocytes	Fibroblasts
IL-1α	−	+	+
IL-1β	+	−	+
IL-3	−	+	
IL-6	+	+	+
IL-7	−	+	−
IL-8	−	+	+
IL-10	−	+	−
IL-12	−		+
IL-15			+
G-CSF	−	+	+
M-CSF	−	+	−
GM-CSF	−	+	+
TGF-α	−	+	−
TGF-β	+	+	+
TNF-α	−	+	−
MIP-1α	+	−	−
MIP-1β	+	+	−
IP-10	−	+	+

the animal does not have to develop and suffer from an allergic skin reaction. Compared with the guinea pig maximization assay, the MLLNA reduces the number of animals by half, and the testing time from 6 weeks to 1 week. A limitation of the MLLNA is difficulty in detecting strong irritants and difficulty in discerning contact allergy induced by metals. The ICCVAM recommended that future improvements to the MLLNA should include alternative endpoints such as cytokine production (National Toxicology Program, 1999).

Cytokines are glycoproteins that induce and regulate cell growth, division, differentiation, and movement. In addition, cytokines have been shown to be involved in inflammatory reactions and other disease states. The role of cytokines in dermatotoxicology has been reviewed by Gerberick et al. (1998). Table 19.1 shows the various cell types that are capable of producing cytokines in the skin.

Table 19.2 compares cytokine profiles for irritant versus allergic contact dermatitis obtained from studies using skin biopsies or cell cultures. Although a number of cytokines appear to be upregulated in the two types of contact dermatitis, it is not yet clear what markers distinguish ICD from ACD, or whether different profiles will result across chemical classes of irritants or allergens. When using reverse transcriptase polymerase chain reaction (RT-PCR) to amplify mRNA obtained from punch biopsies, the cellular source of the mRNA is unclear, since the skin tissue contains both dermal and epidermal cells. The dose of an irritant can influence the cytokine profile; a dose dependent increase in IL-8 and IL-1 has been observed for the irritant sodium lauryl sulfate using a human skin equivalent model (Ponec and Kempenaar, 1995). Gene expression profiles are likely to vary depending on the delay between the sampling time and the time of initial contact with a substance. Finally, genetic variation across individuals will also influence gene expression profiles in the skin in human clinical studies of ICD and ACD.

Table 19.2 mRNA Cytokine Profiles from Human Skin Biopsy or Human Cell Samples

	ACD	ICD
TNF-α	increased	increased
IFN-γ	increased	increased
IL-2	increased	increased
GM-CSF	increased	increased
IL-1α (human cells)	dependent on allergen	increased
IL-1β (human cells)	increased	increased
IL-4	increased	not determined
IL-6	increased	not determined
IL-10	increased	no change
IL-12 p35 (human cells)	no change	no change
IL-12 p40 (human cells)	increased	no change

Source: Adapted from Wakem and Gaspari, 2000.

A thorough review of the mechanisms of ICD and ACD was written by Wakem and Gaspari (2000). Table 19.3 summarizes salient features of ICD and ACD. Although their mechanisms appear to be similar, it may be possible to discern fundamental differences between ICD from ACD at the molecular level by gene expression profiling studies.

Reviews of methods for testing the irritation and sensitization potential of substances have been prepared by Maibach and co-workers (Marzulii and Maibach, 1998; Patil et al., 1998; Bashir and Maibach, 2000). Both the Draize test for predicting skin irritation and the modified Draize test for determining skin sensitization potential are based on visual grading scales. However, it is frequently difficult to distinguish irritant from immunological reactions of the skin either clinically or by routine histological examination (Table 19.4).

In human clinical studies using patch tests with selected irritants and allergens, we have obtained mRNA encoding cytokines from epidermal cells isolated with a noninvasive adhesive tape stripping methodology, the DermPatch (Morhenn et al., 1999). Gene expression profiles of skin cells obtained with the DermPatch can be

Table 19.3 Mechanisms of Irritant versus Allergic Contact Dermatitis

Feature	Allergic	Irritant
Chemical agents	low molecular weight, lipid soluble	acids, alkalies, surfactants, solvents, oxidants, enzymes
Concentration of the agent	less critical	more critical
Genetic predisposition	++++	++
Sensitization and lag period	necessary	not necessary
Trigger	interaction of antigen with primed T cells	damage to keratinocytes
Cytokine release	++++	+++
T-cell activation	early ++++	later ++++
Mast-cell activation	++	++
Langerhans' cells	increased	decreased
Eicosanoid production	++	++

Source: Adapted from Marks and DeLeo.

Table 19.4 Clinical and Histological Aspects of Contact Dermatitis

Feature	Allergic	Irritant
Itch	++++ (early)	+++ (late)
Pain, burning	++	++++ (early)
Erythema	++++	++++
Vesicles	++++	+
Pustules	+	+++
Hyperkeratosis	++	+++
Fissuring	++	++++
Sharp demarcation	yes	yes
Reaction delay after contact	days	minutes to hours
Spongiosis	++++	++++
Dermal edema	++++	++++
Necrotic keratinocytes	++++	++++
Ballooning degeneration	+	+++
Lymphocytic infiltrate	++++	++++
Neurotrophilic infiltrate	+	+++

Source: Adapted from Marks and DeLeo.

analyzed by standard molecular biology techniques such as the ribonuclease protection assay (RPA), quantitative reverse transcriptase polymerase chain reaction (Q-RT-PCR), or gene array technology.

MATERIALS AND METHODS

Tape Stripping and Extraction of Total RNA

The use of tape stripping to remove small quantities of epidermis was initially described by Wolf (1939). Later the technique was modified to remove the upper layers of the epidermis in rodents in an attempt to isolate Langerhans cells (Streilein et al., 1982). We have used the tape stripping technique to isolate epidermal cell fragments. Using this method, one can isolate small amounts of RNA, DNA, protein, or lipids from one and the same skin harvesting procedure. Skin cells were removed using D-Squame® tape (CuDerm, Dallas, TX) to strip the skin's cell layers. The skin was stripped multiple times with the tape to obtain epidermal fragments. The first three tape strips were discarded, and the subsequent 20 tape strips were extracted. Each tape was then placed in an RNase-free Eppendorf® tube containing 0.5 ml of Tri Reagent (Molecular Research Center, Inc.; Cincinnati, OH). RNA from tapes used at the same skin site was extracted with and pooled in the same aliquot of Tri Reagent. The RNA then was extracted by vortexing and centrifuging the tape(s) in the Eppendorf® tube.

Ribonuclease Protection Assay

The RPA has been described by Gilman (1991). This assay makes use of the fact that mRNA at one point in its life cycle exists as a single stranded molecule. At this stage, the mRNA of interest can be "protected" by allowing it to bind to a labeled antisense molecule that has been prepared previously. At this stage, allowing the hybridization of the single stranded mRNA that encodes, for example, the mRNA sequence for IL-4 with its labeled antisense construct, results in the formation of a double stranded RNA molecule that has now become resistant to the enzyme RNAse. Thus, when RNAse is added to the suspension of total RNA, this enzyme will only digest the nonprotected single stranded mRNA molecules leaving only the double stranded, e.g., labeled mRNA for IL-4 intact. Then, to prevent further digestion, the RNAse is destroyed by incubation with proteinase K. To identify which mRNA has been protected, the double stranded mRNA for IL-4 is then unwound and converted back to its single-stranded state by heating the mixture at 90°C. Finally, the labeled mRNA, e.g., IL-4, is identified using a standard polyacrylamide sequencing gel.

The RPA not only identifies small quantities of mRNA but, at the same time, it quantitates the amount of the mRNA present in a given cell suspension. This is accomplished by adding labeled antisense molecules for the so-called "housekeeping" genes, e.g., the mRNA for glyceraldehyde phosphate dehydrogenase (GAPDH). GAPDH is vital in performing many cellular functions, and thus relatively large quantities of this enzyme are produced in the cell at all times. Therefore, the total amount of GAPDH produced in a cell does not fluctuate greatly over a given time period, and the amount of mRNA for GAPDH per cell remains relatively constant. Thus, the quantity of mRNA for GAPDH in each lane can be used as a marker for the total amount of RNA in the tissue isolated, i.e., the amount of cellular material, that originally was present in the tape stripped sample.

Induction of Erythematous Reactions on the Skin

We induced ICD or ACD reactions using standard prognostic testing techniques. Briefly, dibutyl squarate (2%) in acetone was applied for 48 hr under occlusion to the upper arm to induce the ACD reaction (Marzulli and Maibach, 1974). After about 14 d, the dibutyl squarate (2%) was reapplied to elicit the immune-mediated reaction. In the same individual, application of 0.2 ml of sodium lauryl sulfate (SLS) (Fisher Scientific, San Diego, CA) (0.5% in distilled water) to the contralateral upper arm for 72 hr under occlusion was used to generate the ICD. The tape stripping was performed 48 hr after elicitation of the ACD and 72 hr after induction of the ICD. The total RNA isolated from each sample was used directly for the RPA using the RiboQuant® Multi-Probe RNase protection assay system without prior determination of the amount of total RNA by, e.g., measurement of the optical density. Undigested probes for the cytokine(s) were run parallel with samples on standard acrylamide sequencing gels and used to identify digested cytokine messages. Gels containing digested RNA bands were exposed to a phosphor screen (Molecular Dynamics, Inc., Sunnyvale, CA).

RESULTS

We recently have used probes for the cytokines interleukin-4 (IL-4), interleukin-8 (IL-8), interleukin-9 (IL-9), interleukin-13 (IL-13), the proteins gamma-interferon (γIFN), and inducible nitric oxide synthase (iNOS), as well as the housekeeping genes L32, GAPDH for hybridization to RNA samples obtained from several individuals (Streilein et al., 1982). By RPA analysis, the mRNA for the cytokines IL-4 and Il-13 could be clearly identified in three of the five subjects, only in the skin samples obtained by tape stripping of the sites demonstrating an ACD. Similarly, the mRNA for γIFN was observed for the ACD skin site in two of the five subjects. Both the ICD and the ACD reactions clearly demonstrated bands for IL-8. IL-9 and iNOS were observed in all of the skin samples, including control sites that were not patched.

DISCUSSION

We have shown that small amounts of mRNA can be extracted from the skin fragments obtained by tape stripping human skin. We have established that certain cytokine patterns appear to be specific for ACD versus ICD. Recently, a group of investigators has demonstrated differences in the mRNA expression of proteins in skin biopsies obtained from ACD and ICD using *in situ* hybridization (Flier et al., 1999). These authors demonstrated clearly that only skin cells taken from ACD but not from normal skin or ICD expressed the mRNA for HLA-DR antigen as well as ICAM-1. These two proteins are known to be induced by γIFN on keratinocytes both *in vivo* and *in vitro*.

In addition to being noninvasive, an advantage of the DermPatch approach to gene expression profiling of the skin is that cells isolated by tape stripping are thought to be predominantly epidermal cells. The epidermis is comprised of keratinocytes in various stages of differentiation, along with a small number of other cell types such as Langerhans cells. In ICD, keratinocytes are the first cell types to be damaged by the irritating substance after it passes through the stratum corneum. Keratinocytes are involved in the signaling pathways that initiate the inflammatory cascade that eventually leads to infiltration of mononuclear cells, swelling, and damage to the underlying dermis. In the induction phase of ACD, after the antigen encounters the Langerhans cells, the keratinocytes signal the Langerhans cells to migrate to the local lymph nodes. The role of the keratinocyte in cutaneous irritation and sensitization has been recently reviewed (Coquette et al., 2000). In attempting to differentiate ICD from ACD by gene expression profiles, selectively sampling epidermal cells by adhesive tape stripping may be a simpler approach than taking biopsy samples, which contain both dermis and epidermis.

The technique we describe here can be expanded to sample a larger set of gene probes by preparing cDNA from the mRNA sample using a reverse transcriptase reaction, amplifying the cDNA, and applying the resulting cDNA pool to a gene array such as the Sigma cytokine array. Preliminary results obtained by our laboratory (unpublished data) indicate that sufficient quantities of high quality mRNA for gene array experiments can be obtained by the DermPatch adhesive tape stripping methodology. The use of gene arrays in carefully designed human clinical studies will be essential for establishing a consistent set of markers to distinguish ICD from ACD.

REFERENCES

Bashir, S. J. and Maibach, H. I. (2000) Methods for testing the irritation and sensitization potential of drugs and enhancers, in *Biochemical Modulation of Skin Reactions, Transdermals, Topicals, Cosmetics,* Kydonieus, A.F. and Wille, J.J., Eds., CRC Press, Boca Raton, pp. 45–60.

Coquette, A., Berna, N., Poumay, Y., and Pittelkow, M.R. (2000) The keratinocyte in cutaneous irritation and sensitization, in *Biochemical Modulation of Skin Reactions, Transdermals, Topicals, Cosmetics,* Kydonieus, A.F. and Wille, J.J., Eds., CRC Press, Boca Raton, pp. 125–143.

Gerberick, G.F., Sikorski, E.E., Ryan, C.A., and Limardi, L.C. (1998) Use of cytokines in dermatotoxicology, in *Dermatotoxicology Methods,* Marzulli, F.N. and Maibach, H.I., Eds., Taylor and Francis, Washington, D.C., pp. 187–206.

Flier, J., Boorsma, D.M., Bruynzeel, D.P., van Beek, P.J., Stoof, T.J., Scheper, R.J., Willemze, R., and Tensen, C.P. (1999) The CXCR3 activating chemokines IP-10, Mig, and IP-9 are expressed in allergic but not in irritant patch test reactions, *J. Invest. Dermatol.,* 113, 574–578.

Gilman M. (1991) Ribonuclease protection assay, in *Current Protocols in Molecular Biology,* Ausubel, F. et al. Eds., New York, Greene Publishing and Wiley-Interscience, pp. 4.7.1–4.7.8

National Toxicology Program (February, 1999). The Murine Local Lymph Node Assay: A Test Method for Assessing the Allergic Contact Dermatitis Potential of Chemicals/Compounds, NIH publication 99-4494.

Marzulii, F.N. and Maibach, H.I. (1974) The use of graded concentrations in studying skin sensitizers: experimental contact sensitization in man, *Food Cosmet. Toxicol.,* 12, 219–227.

Marzulli, F.N. and Maibach, H.I. (1998) Test methods for allergic contact dermatitis in humans, in *Dermatotoxicology Methods,* Marzulli, F.N. and Maibach, H.I., Eds., Taylor and Francis, Washington, D.C., pp. 153–159.

Morhenn, V.B., Chang, E.-Y., and Rheins, L.A. (1999) A noninvasive method for quantifying and distinguishing inflammatory skin reactions, *J. Am. Acad. Dermatol.,* 41, 687–692.

Patil, S.M., Patrick, E., and Maibach, H.I. (1998) Animal, human, and *in vitro* test methods for predicting skin irritation, in *Dermatotoxicology Methods,* Marzulli, F.N. and Maibach, H.I., Eds., Taylor and Francis, Washington, D.C., pp. 89–114.

Ponec, M. and Kempenaar, J. (1995) Use of human skin recombinants as an in vitro model for testing the irritation potential of cutaneous irritants, *Skin Pharmaocol.,* 8, 49–59.

Streilein, J.W., Lonsberry, L.W., and Bergstresser, P.R. (1982) Depletion of epidermal Langerhans cells and Ia immunogenicity from tape-stripped mouse skin, *Exp. Med.,* 155, 863–871.

Wakem, P. and Gaspari, A.A. (2000) Mechanisms of allergic and irritant contact dermatitis, in *Biochemical Modulation of Skin Reactions, Transdermals, Topicals, Cosmetics,* Kydonieus, A.F. and Wille, J.J., Eds., CRC Press, Boca Raton, pp. 83–106.

Wolf, J. (1939) Die innere Struktur der Zellen des Stratum desquamans der menschlichen Epidermis, *A Mikr. Anat. Forscj.,* 46, 170.

CHAPTER 20

In Vitro Skin Equivalent Models for Toxicity Testing

**Patrick J. Hayden, Seyoum Ayehunie, G. Robert Jackson,
Sarah Kupfer-Lamore, Thomas J. Last, Mitchell Klausner,
and Joseph Kubilus**

CONTENTS

INTRODUCTION

Prior to human use of new cosmetic or therapeutic products, *in vivo* animal tests are often conducted in order to screen for safety and efficacy. However, modern product development processes are rendering animal testing increasingly expensive and impractical. Furthermore, the tenets of ethical animal testing call for practice of the three Rs of refinement, reduction, and replacement of animal tests. Therefore, a growing need exists for rapid and reliable *in vitro* methods for safety screening of new cosmetic formulations and lead candidates for topical therapeutics. This need is especially acute for cosmetic producers, who must produce safe and efficacious products, but whose consumers increasingly will not tolerate animal testing. For drugs and cosmetics intended for topical application to the skin, safety issues include irritation, sensitization, toxicity, and carcinogenicity. A further issue for topical products is their potential interaction with UV radiation to produce photoinduced irritation, sensitization, toxicity, or carcinogenicity.

Common methods of *in vitro* safety testing include the use of human cells grown in submerged monolayer cultures. However, the use of submerged monolayer cultures is not well suited for testing of many ingredients or finished products intended for topical application. For example, submerged cultures restrict the testing to materials that can be dissolved in aqueous media. Thus many oil-soluble ingredients or finished products such as creams, lotions, or powders cannot be adequately tested in submerged culture systems. Furthermore, submerged culture systems of skin cells do not possess differentiated functions and barrier properties of stratified skin tissues and thus do not accurately reflect the *in vivo* physiology of the skin.

Three-dimensional organotypic skin models, which overcome many of the shortcomings of safety testing in submerged monolayer skin cell cultures, are commercially available (MatTek Corp., Ashland, MA). These models are cultured at the air–liquid interface (ALI) and are more suitable for safety and efficacy testing of topical products. Among the safety issues that organotypic skin models can address are tissue damage (i.e., cell death by necrosis or apoptosis), irritation, and DNA damage caused by topical treatment or ultraviolet radiation. This paper will describe a variety of commercially available ALI cultures and present a survey of applications of these models for topical pharmaceutical and cosmetic product safety assessment.

AIR–LIQUID INTERFACE TISSUE CULTURES

ALI tissues are typically produced by seeding epithelial cells onto a microporous membrane contained in a specially designed tissue culture insert. Figure 20.1 shows a schematic representation of an ALI culture system. Cells are initially fed by exposing both the upper and lower surface of the membrane to culture medium. Following several days of completely submerged culture to allow a confluent cell layer to develop, medium is removed from the top surface of the membrane and subsequent feeding of the cells occurs by addition of fresh medium to the underside of the membrane only. The top surface of the cell layer is thus exposed to the

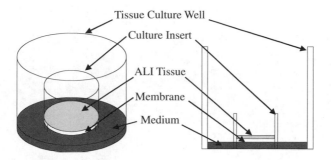

Figure 20.1 Schematic representation of the air–liquid interface (ALI) tissue culture technique.

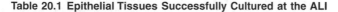

Table 20.1 Epithelial Tissues Successfully Cultured at the ALI

Skin equivalents[a]
  Keratinocytes only
  Keratinocytes plus fibroblasts[b]
  Keratinocytes plus melanocytes
  Keratinocytes plus Langerhans cells
Ocular corneal epithelium[a]
Tracheal/bronchial[a] epithelium
Tracheal/bronchial submucosal glands
Vaginal epithelium[a,b]
Gingival epithelium[a,b]

[a] Cultured at MatTek Corp.
[b] In development.

atmosphere. Continued ALI culture of epithelial cells eventually results in the formation of a differentiated, *in vivo*-like tissue (Bell et al., 1981).

A variety of ALI tissues including dermal, ocular, tracheal/bronchial, gingival, and vaginal epithelia tissues are produced by MatTek Corp (Table 20.1). All of these tissues are produced from normal human cells and are cultured in a completely defined, serum-free medium. Detailed characteristics of the EpiDerm (keratinocyte culture), MelanoDerm (keratinocyte/melanocyte coculture), ImmunoDerm (keratinocyte/Langerhans cell coculture), and EpiDerm-FT (keratinocyte/fibroblast coculture) products are described in detail below.

EpiDerm cultures are composed of normal human epidermal keratinocytes cultured on a collagen type I gel matrix. These tissues display a stratified, differentiated morphology with basal, spinous, granular, and stratum corneum layers evident. The well-developed stratum corneum and normal ceramide and lipid profile confers a barrier function that, although not equal to *in vivo* skin, is significant and reproducible. Figure 20.2A shows a histological cross section of EpiDerm tissue. Normal *in vivo*-like ultrastructure of EpiDerm's intercellular lamellar lipid sheets is demonstrated by transmission electron microscopy (Figure 20.2B).

Keratinocytes have also been cocultured with normal human melanocytes to produce the MelanoDerm product. These cocultures can be produced with melanocytes from donors of various skin types to achieve tissues with various degrees of pigmentation. Figure 20.3 shows a top view of MelanoDerm tissue produced with

(A)

(B)

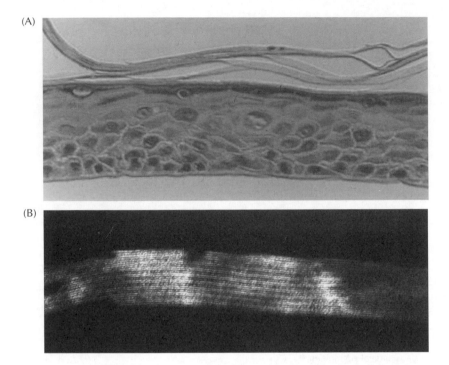

Figure 20.2 (A) Histological cross section of H&E stained EpiDerm-200. Magnification = 440×. (B) Transmission electron micrograph of ruthenium tetroxide stained intercellular lamellar lipid sheets (150,000×).

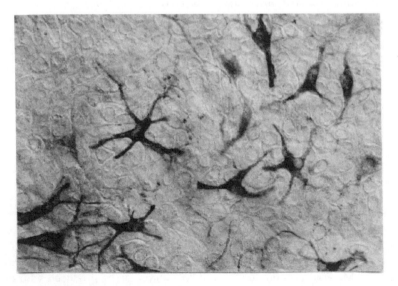

Figure 20.3 Top macroscopic view of MelanoDerm tissues containing normal human melanocytes derived from Black donor skin (400× magnification).

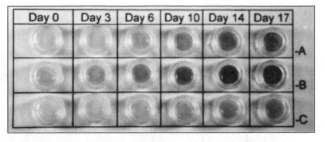

• **Asian (A)**

• **Black (B)**

• **Caucasian (C)**

Figure 20.4 Development of pigmentation in MelanoDerm tissue produced with melanocytes derived from various skin phototypes. The figure shows the top macroscopic view of tissue inserts. Day 0 indicates the day of shipment of a fully differentiated tissue. Pigmentation develops during additional culture of the fully differentiated tissue by the end user.

melanocytes from Black donors. Macroscopic pigmentation of cultures incorporating melanocytes from donors of different skin phototypes, demonstrating the expected levels of pigmentation, are shown in Figure 20.4. MelanoDerm tissues also exhibit macroscopic darkening or lightening in response to chemical or biochemical treatments, as well as melanosome transfer to keratinocytes (Seiberg, 2000a; Klausner, 2000; Seiberg, 2000b). For example, the tissues can be induced to darken by treatment with growth factors such as α-melanocyte-stimulating hormone (α-MSH) and β-fibroblast growth factor (β-FGF) (Figure 20.5). Alternatively, topical kojic acid treatment induces a lightening of MelanoDerm tissue (Figure 20.6). A quantitative melanin assay has also been developed to facilitate pigmentation studies (www.matTek.com). The lightening effect of topical kojic acid on development of pigmentation in MelanoDerm, as determined by the melanin assay, is shown in Table 20.2.

A model of normal human keratinocytes cocultured with normal human fibroblasts to produce a "full thickness" dermal/epidermal tissue (EpiDerm-FT) is also available. This tissue model possesses a dermal component composed of viable fibroblasts embedded in a collagen type I gel, as well as a fully differentiated epidermis (Figure 20.7). The full-thickness skin equivalents will facilitate investigation

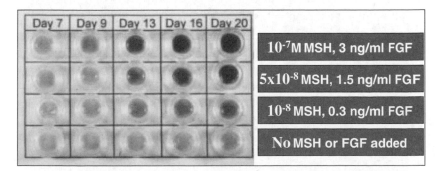

Figure 20.5 Pigmentation of MelanoDerm tissue (Black melanocytes) induced by α-MSH and β-FGF as shown by top macroscopic view of tissue inserts. Tissues were cultured in media containing the indicated concentrations of growth factors for up to 20 days following shipment of commercial MelanoDerm tissue.

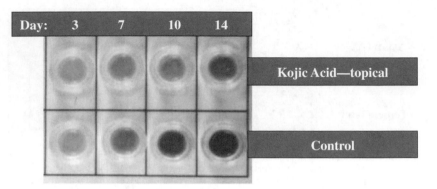

Figure 20.6 Lightening effect of topical kojic acid on MelanoDerm tissue. Tissues containing Black melanocytes were treated topically with 1% kojic acid for the indicated number of days (25 µl applied topically every other day). The top macroscopic view of the tissues reveals the visually observable lightening effect.

Table 20.2 Lightening of MelanoDerm Tissue by Topical Treatment with 1% Kojic Acid

Treatment	Melanin content (µg/tissue)	
	Day 10	Day 14
H_2O	19.9	35.3
1% kojic acid	11.4	18.3

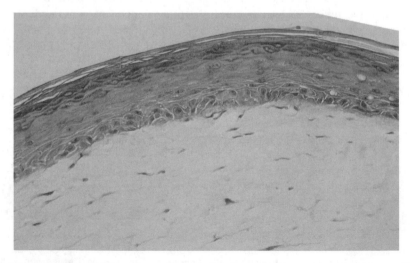

Figure 20.7 EpiDerm-FT tissue contains normal human fibroblasts cultured within a collagen type I dermal matrix. A fully differentiated epidermis derived from normal human keratinocytes is cultured on the top of the dermis.

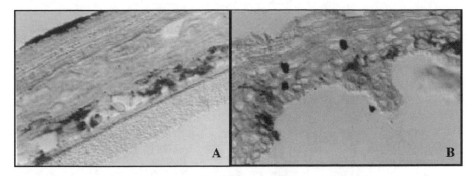

Figure 20.8 Immunohistochemical staining of HLA-DR on human Langerhans cells within (A) ImmunoDerm tissue and (B) excised human skin.

of cross-talk and interactions between the two cell types. Such interactions are believed to play important roles in phenomena such as photoaging and skin cancer.

Additionally, coculture models of human keratinocytes and Langerhans cells are currently in the development stage. Human Langerhans cell precursors obtained from cord blood are induced to differentiate into mature Langerhans cells by treatment with various hormones and cytokines. The cells obtained display all the hallmark features of Langerhans cells, including Birbeck granules and surface markers including HLA-DR (MHC class II). Immunohistochemical cross-sections comparing ImmunoDerm tissue to *in vivo* human skin show similar levels and location of Langerhans cells (Figure 20.8).

SURVEY OF USES AND ENDPOINTS

ALI cultures of epidermal tissues can be used for a variety of toxicological studies, including corrosivity, phototoxicity, irritation, melanogenesis, percutaneous absorption, and various drug metabolism and mechanistic studies. A brief survey of some of these uses is presented below.

Corrosivity

The EpiDerm model has been formally validated by The National Center for Documentation and Evaluation of Alternative Methods to Animal Experiments (ZEBET) as an alternative method for testing corrosivity of materials following topical exposure (Liebsch et al., 2000b). This protocol uses the MTT assay (Mosmann, 1983) to determine tissue viability after treatment of EpiDerm with topically applied materials. If tissue viability is <50% after 3 min exposure (compared to untreated controls), or if tissue viability is <15% after 60 min exposure, the material is labeled as corrosive (Liebsch et al., 2000b).

Phototoxicity

EpiDerm tissues have been successfully utilized for phototoxicity screening of topically applied products (Liebsch et al., 1997, 1999, 2000a; Jones et al., 2000). In

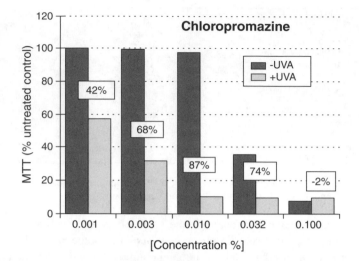

Figure 20.9 Phototoxicity of chlorpromazine. EpiDerm tissues were topically treated with the indicated concentrations of chlorpromazine and incubated overnight. On the following
day tissues were either irradiated with 6 J/cm² of UVA or kept in the dark. Tissues
were then rinsed, fed with fresh medium, and incubated overnight. Finally, tissue
viability was determined by the MTT assay. A decrease in tissue viability of 30% or
greater between the irradiated and nonirradiated tissues indicates a phototoxic effect.

fact, a phototoxicity protocol that uses the EpiDerm model has recently been prevali-
dated in multilaboratory studies sponsored by ZEBET (Liebsch et al., 1997, 1999,
2000a). The protocol compares the toxicity of topically applied treatments to EpiDerm
in the presence or absence of UVA-irradiation (Liebsch et al., 1997, 1999, 2000a).
Toxicity (loss of tissue viability) is measured by assessing mitochondrial reduction of
3-(4,5-dimethylthiazole-2-yl)-2,5-diphenyl tetrazolium bromide (MTT) (Mosmann
1983). A compound is considered phototoxic if a 30% or greater loss of viability is
observed in irradiated tissues compared to nonirradiated tissues. Figure 20.9 shows an
example of quantitative data obtained with the phototoxic compound chlorpromazine.

Irritation

A number of endpoints have been used with the EpiDerm model to screen for
contact irritation potential of topically applied treatments. These include tissue
viability (MTT assay), cytokine release by ELISA [interleukin-1α (IL-1α), interleu-
kin-1 receptor antagonist (IL-1ra), interleukin-8 (IL-8)], and prostaglandin release
by ELISA [prostaglandin E$_2$ (PGE$_2$)]. Several consumer product companies have
used EpiDerm to produce good correlations between these *in vitro* endpoints and *in
vivo* irritation (Koschier et al., 1995; Perkins et al., 1996; Earl et al., 1996; Botham
et al., 1998; Perkins et al., 1999; Warren et al., 1999; Bernhofer et al., 1995, 1999).

Melanogenesis

MelanoDerm tissue, which contains normal human melanocytes cocultured
with normal human keratinocytes, is finding increasing use for studies involving

melanogenesis and pigmentation studies (Seiberg et al., 2000a) and skin lightening (Klausner et al., 2000; Seiberg et al., 2000b) (Figures 20.3–20.6, Table 20.2).

Percutaneous Absorption

The barrier developed by EpiDerm and other *in vitro* skin equivalent tissues is significant but typically less than that of *in vivo* skin (Roguet et al., 1999). However, EpiDerm tissues can be successfully used for percutaneous absorption studies. For example, EpiDerm has been used in studies to evaluate permeation of benzoyl chloride in cosmetic products (Fares et al., 1995), to study electrotransport drug delivery technology (Daddona, 1996), and to measure permeation of chemicals such as lauric acid, caffeine, or mannitol (Roguet et al., 1999).

Drug Metabolism

Skin is known to contain phase I (oxidative) and phase II (conjugative) drug metabolizing enzymes (Mukhtar et al., 1992; Merk et al., 1996). To date, relatively few drug metabolism studies have been reported in skin equivalents. Characterization of drug metabolism capabilities of *in vitro* skin equivalents is currently incomplete. However, EpiDerm has been used to study metabolism of vitamin E (Nabi et al., 1998) and glutathione S-transferase activity (Roguet et al., 1999). *In vitro* skin equivalents will undoubtedly find expanded utility for cutaneous drug metabolism applications in the future.

MISCELLANEOUS STUDIES

As noted above, skin equivalent models can be used for a wide variety of mechanistic studies involving numerous endpoints. EpiDerm and similar skin equivalents have been used to study inflammatory mediators including cytokines (IL-1α, TNFα, IL-8) and prostaglandins (PGE$_2$) at the message or protein level. More recently, studies related to mediators of apoptosis (p53, p21, GADD, caspases) (Zhao et al., 1999; Hayden et al., 2000), angiogensis (e.g., vascular endothelial growth factor, placenta growth factor) (Rendl et al., 1999, 2000; Hayden et al., 2000), and photoaging (Martin et al., 2000) have been reported. EpiDerm has also been employed to study heat shock (Bowers et al., 1999) and the effects of chemical warfare agents (Rhoads et al., 1994). Further refinement of skin equivalent models and application of advances in genomics and proteomics should lead to expanded use of these models for study of a wide variety of cutaneous phenomena (see emerging uses below).

QUALITY CONTROL AND VALIDATION ISSUES

In order for *in vitro* epithelial tissues to be successfully used for safety assessment in the industrial product development process, they must first be validated. The

Interagency Coordinating Committee on the Validation of Alternative Methods (ICCVAM) has defined validation as establishment of reliability and relevance for a specific purpose (NIH publication 97-3981). In practical terms, this means that *in vitro* models must satisfy two important criteria: (1) they must be highly reproducible from batch to batch in terms of physical/biochemical properties and biological responses and (2) they must accurately predict the relevant *in vivo* outcome.

Although methods for culturing skin equivalents are well described in the literature, and skin equivalents are commonly produced by various academic and industrial laboratories, lot-to-lot reproducibility and performance of the tissues should not be taken for granted (Roguet et al., 1999; Boelmsa et al., 2000). Significant variability will lead to difficulties in achieving quantitative results and generally poor performance in the testing laboratory.

Therefore, the following quality control procedures are routinely performed to ensure lot-to-lot reproducibility and satisfactory performance of EpiDerm tissues in industrial safety assessment applications.

HISTOLOGICAL EVALUATION OF EACH TISSUE LOT

H&E cross sections of each tissue lot are evaluated in terms of number of cell layers and proper formation of appropriate tissue architecture. The tissue should consist of eight to twelve cell layers in thickness and display basal, spinous, and granular cell layers and a well-developed stratum corneum.

QUANTITATIVE ASSESSMENT OF FUNCTIONAL RESPONSE TO TOPICAL TRITON X-100 TREATMENT

A reproducible, quantifiable functional response is perhaps the most important attribute required for successful use of skin equivalents in safety assessment applications and is the most telling indicator of the reproducibility of a particular skin equivalent production process. Each lot of EpiDerm tissue is subjected to topical treatment with 1.0% Triton X-100 for various times up to 12 hr. The time required to reduce the viability of the tissues to 50% of control (ET50) is then determined by the MTT assay (Mosmann, 1983, www.MatTek.com http://www.MatTek.com). The ET50 provides an assessment of barrier function and overall robustness of tissue. The baseline ET50 (1.0% Triton X-100) for EpiDerm-200 was established in 1996. The ET50 of each new tissue lot must fall within two standard deviations of the baseline in order to be acceptable for delivery to customers. The average ET50 of EpiDerm-200 tissues produced each year for the past 6 years is shown in Table 20.3.

The quality control attributes listed above are important for ensuring reproducible functioning of *in vitro* skin equivalents in safety assessment applications and validation studies. Adherence to these criteria has allowed EpiDerm to be included in, and perform well in, recent European validation and prevalidation studies (Liebsch et al., 1997, 1999, 2000a,b). These procedures are also recommended by testing laboratories involved in validation of alternate *in vitro* methods (Cooper-Hannan et

Table 20.3 EpiDerm-200 Triton X-100 ET50 Database Summary

Year	EPI-200 Triton ET-50	EPI-200 Triton C.V.	Lots	Avg. C.V.
2000[a]	6.76	16.4	89	6.2
1999	6.75	18.2	146	5.7
1998	7.24	17.9	175	9.2
1997	6.78	15.9	228	9.9
1996	6.74	14.6	184	9.6
1995	6.65	77.8	112	4.9

[a] Through September 2000.

al., 1997; Harbell et al., 1997). Similar protocols were recently used by Roguet et al. (1999) and Boelsma et al. (2000) to evaluate a number of commercially available *in vitro* epidermal models including EpiDerm. The EpiDerm model performed favorably in these studies, highlighting the result of careful attention to quality control (Roguet et al., 1999; Boelmsa et al., 2000).

EMERGING APPLICATIONS OF ALI TISSUES

Gene Microarray Technology

Recently, gene expression microarray technologies have become widely available. These emerging technologies hold considerable promise for enabling greatly enhanced discovery and predictive potential from *in vitro* systems. Gene expression microarrays consisting of gene-specific DNA sequences bound to a solid matrix make it possible to simultaneously analyze hundreds or even thousands of gene expression changes (Eisen and Brown, 1999; Hegde et al., 2000; Lockhart and Winzeler, 2000; Celis et al., 2000). Gene array data analysis programs employing clustering techniques have been developed to facilitate the identification of predictive "fingerprint" patterns of gene expression caused by exposure to various chemical or environmental treatments (Brazma and Vilo, 2000; Sherlock, 2000). The power of this technology has already been demonstrated for classifications of cancerous tumors and identification of new tumor types (Eisen et al., 1998; Golub et al., 1999; Perou et al., 1999; Alon et al., 1999; Alizadeh et al., 2000), diseases such as atherosclerosis (Hiltunen et al., 1999; McCaffrey et al., 2000), and toxicology and drug screening applications (Rockett and Dix, 2000; Bartosiewicz et al., 2000). In these examples, analysis of several thousands of genes revealed a much smaller subset of genes that provide the required predictive information. Once discovered, these small subsets can be used for routine screening applications. In addition to allowing predictive classifications to be made, microarray gene expression profiling holds great promise for identifying mechanisms of cancer and other diseases, drug effects, and toxicity (Afshari et al., 1999; Lockhart and Winzeler, 2000; Celis et al., 2000; Nuwaysir et al., 1999).

ALI cultures of human skin equivalents are ideal systems for use with emerging microarray technologies. The ability to produce cocultures of keratinocytes with melanocytes, Langerhans cells, or fibroblasts and the fully differentiated nature of these tissues makes them far superior to monolayer cultures in terms of physical and bio-chemical similarity to *in vivo* skin. Furthermore, the human origin of the tissues avoids the problematic issue of cross-species extrapolation encountered with animal studies. Finally, the ability to add or remove cell types from *in vitro* tissues allows researchers to study the cellular origin of gene expression and the interplay between cell types.

This technology has recently been applied to studies with EpiDerm tissue (Hayden 2000). EpiDerm tissues were exposed to 175 mJ/cm^2 ultraviolet B (UVB) radiation. Sham-treated control tissues were also placed in phosphate-buffered saline (PBS) for an equivalent time but were not irradiated. Following irradiation, tissues were transferred back to fresh assay medium and incubated at 37°C in a 5% CO$_2$ atmosphere for various times prior to viability determination or RNA isolation. Total RNA was isolated by use of a commercially available kit (Atlas™ Pure Total RNA Isolation kit, Clontech Laboratories, Palo Alto, CA).

To analyze changes in gene expression, each RNA sample was converted to ^{32}P-labeled cDNA as specified in the Atlas™ cDNA expression array user manual (Clontech), and hybridized with Atlas™ human cancer cDNA expression array membranes containing 588 cancer-related cDNAs. Following probe hybridization, membranes were washed and exposed to x-ray film for 88.5 hr. Autoradiographs were digitized with a scanner and analyzed with AtlasImage™ 1.01 software (Clontech). A twofold difference in signal intensity between the test and control membranes was considered to represent significant differences in gene expression due to UVB treatment. A complete listing of genes included in the Atlas™ human cancer cDNA expression array can be obtained on the Clontech web site (www.Clontech.com http://www.Clontech.com).

The output of the computer analysis for the 6-hr timepoint is shown in Figure 20.10. Numerous RNA messages were either up-regulated or down-regulated by the UVB exposure. A partial listing of the differentially regulated messages from the 6-hr timepoint is given in Table 20.4. Many of the messages are for genes that have been previously reported to be altered by UVB irradiation, including several apop-tosis-related genes and DNA repair genes.

The array analysis also identified placenta growth factor (PlGF), a gene message that has not previously been reported to be up-regulated by UVB irradiation of epidermis. Placenta growth factor is a potent angiogenic factor of potentially great significance in relation to skin-related phenomena including wound healing and skin cancer (Lacal et al., 2000). Therefore, further experimentation was conducted to confirm the up-regulation of PlGF following UVB-irradiation of EpiDerm.

Placenta growth factor primer sequences (5′-GGCCCTGCTACCTGTTCTT-GGGCCTC-3′ and 5′-CCAGTACAAGCAAATGGCAAAGTGGAGGG-3′) were obtained from Clontech. Reverse transcription polymerase chain reaction (RT-PCR) was performed on total RNA isolated from UVB-irradiated (20 hr postirradiation) or nonirradiated control EpiDerm samples (EpiDerm RNA isolation protocol available from MatTek Customer Service, see www.MatTek.com http://www.MatTek.com). PCR conditions were as follows: melt temperature = 94°C, annealing temperature = 60°C, extension temperature = 72°C. By the 25th cycle, the expected PCR product (273 bp) was observed only in the irradiated sample (Figure 20.11). After 30 or 35 cycles, the 273 bp product was observable in both irradiated and control samples but was strongly up-regulated in the irradiated samples (Figure 20.11).

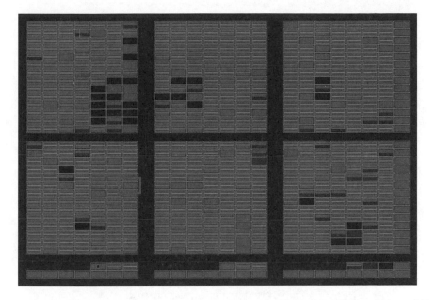

Figure 20.10 Changes in cancer-related gene expression following UVB-irradiation of Epi-Derm tissue. Atlas™ human cancer cDNA expression array analysis of gene expression changes induced in EpiDerm tissues 6 hr after irradiation with 175 mJ/cm² UVB.

Table 20.4 UVB-Irradiation of EpiDerm Tissue

WAF-1 (+)
MAP Kinase p38 (+)
Growth-arrest-specific protein (+)
c-Myc binding protein MM-1 (+)
TRAF-interacting protein (+)
Caspases (+)
Death-associated protein kinase (DAP kinase 1, +)
p53-induced protein (+)
GADD45 (+)
DNA excision repair protein ERCC1 (+)
DNA-repair protein XRCC1 (+)
Placenta growth factors 1+2 (+)
TIMP-1 (+)
T-plasminogen activator (+)
Rho GDP dissociation inhibitor 1 (+)
Endothelin 2 (–)
IL-6 (–)
Leukocyte interferon-inducible peptide (–)
60S ribosomal protein (–)

The above example illustrates the power of new gene array technology for discovery of novel information. Ongoing gene array experimentation by us and others will continue to provide important new information relevant to dermal biology.

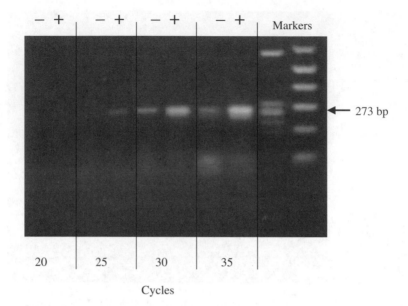

Figure 20.11   Induction of PlGF expression following UVB-irradiation of EpiDerm tissue. Agarose gel electrophoresis of products obtained by RT-PCR of total RNA isolated from EpiDerm tissue 20 hours following UVB-irradiation. (−) no irradiation. (+) UVB-irradiated. The expected PlGF PCR product is 273 bp.

High-Throughput ALI Tissue Formats

To enhance the utility of ALI tissues with modern high-throughput (HTP) and genomic technologies, new HTP ALI tissue formats and RNA isolation procedures have been developed. EpiDerm tissues can be produced in either 24-well (EpiDerm-224) or 96-well (EpiDerm-296) formats (Figure 20.12) (Hayden et al., 2000b). These new formats will facilitate robotic as well as manual HTP manipulation of ALI tissues.

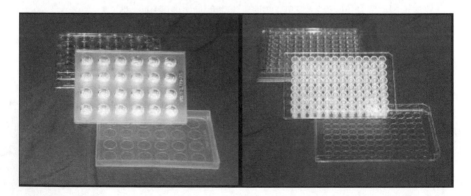

Figure 20.12   EpiDerm tissues cultured in 24 well (EpiDerm-224) or 96 well (EpiDerm-296) high throughput ALI formats. Each tissue has its own individual media reservoir to avoid cross-contamination of samples.

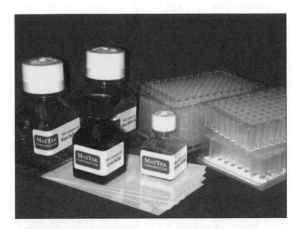

Figure 20.13   Total RNA-96 isolation kit designed for high throughput total RNA isolation from EpiDerm-296.

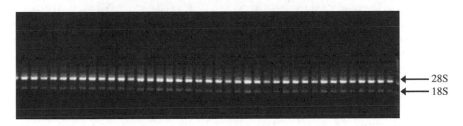

Figure 20.14   Agarose gel electrophoresis of total RNA isolated from EpiDerm-296 with the Total RNA-96 isolation kit. Average yield is approximately 10 μg DNA-free total RNA/EpiDerm-296 tissue.

A convenient kit has also been developed that allows for total RNA isolation in a 96-well format. The kit consists of buffers for lysis/binding, washing, and elution; DNAse reagents; a 96-well glass fiber filter binding plate; and 96-well plasticware for lysis, washing, DNAse, and elution operations (Figure 20.13). Briefly, EpiDerm-296 tissues are lysed and the lysate is transferred to the glass fiber filter binding plate. Contaminates are washed away and DNAse treatment is perform directly on the binding filters. Finally, purified total RNA is eluted ready for PCR, gene expression microarrays, or other uses. The procedure yields approximately 10 μg of high-quality, DNA-free total RNA/EpiDerm-296 tissue (Figure 20.14).

SUMMARY

In vitro skin equivalent models cultured at the air–liquid interface are now routinely available for safety assessment, product development, and basic research applications. Strict attention to quality control facilitates satisfactory performance of these tissues and validation of protocols for various industry applications. Emerging genomic and high-throughput applications will allow these models to make important contributions to modern safety assessment and product development efforts and reduce animal testing for these purposes.

ACKNOWLEDGMENTS

This work was supported by NIH grants 1 R43 ES10237-01 and R44 AR4303-03 and DOD grant DAMD17-00-C-0029.

REFERENCES

Afshari, C.A., Nuwaysir, E.F., and Barrett, J.C., (1999) Application of complementary DNA microarray technology to carcinogen identification, toxicology, and drug safety evaluation, *Cancer Res.,* 59, 4759–4760.

Alizadeh, A.A., Eisen, M.B., Davis, R.E., Ma, C., Lossos, I.S., Rosenwald, A., Boldrick, J.C., Sabet, H., Tran, T., Yu, X., Powell, J.I., Yang, L., Marti, G.E., Moore, T., Hudson, J., Lu, L., Lewis, D.B., Tibshirani, R., Sherlock, G., Chan, W.C., Greiner, T.C., Weisenburger, D.D., Armitage, J.O., Warnke, R., and Staudt, L.M. (2000) Distinct types of diffuse large B-cell lymphoma identified by gene expression profiling, *Nature,* 403, 503–511.

Alon, U., Barkai, N., Notterman, D.A., Gish, K., Ybarra, S., Mack, D., and Levine, A.J. (1999) Broad patterns of gene expression revealed by clustering analysis of tumor and normal colon tissues probed by oligonucleotide arrays, *Proc. Natl. Acad. Sci. U.S.A.,* 96, 6745–6750.

Bartosiewicz, M., Trounstine, M., Barker, D., Johnston, R., and Buckpitt, A. (2000) Development of a toxicological gene array and quantitative assessment of this technology, *Arch. Biochem. Biophys.,* 376, 66–73.

Bell, E., Ehrlich, H.P., Buttle, D.J., and Nakatsuji, T. (1981) Living tissue formed *in vitro* and accepted as skin equivalent tissue of full thickness, *Science,* 211, 1052–1054.

Bernhofer, L.P., Barkovic, S., Appa, Y., and Martin, K.M. (1999) IL-1α and IL-1ra secretion from epidermal equivalents and the prediction of the irritation potential of mild soap and surfactant-based consumer products, *Toxicol. in Vitro,* 13, 231–239.

Bernhofer, L., Juneja, C., and Martin, K. (1995) The use of Mattek epidermal equivalents for prediction of irritation potential, *J. Invest. Dermatol.,* 105, 874.

Boelmsa, E., Gibbs, S., Faller, C., and Ponec, M. (2000) Characterization and comparison of reconstructed skin models: morphological and immunohistochemical evaluation, *Acta Derm. Venerol.,* 80, 82–88.

Botham, P.A., Earl, L.K., Fentem, J.H., Roguet, R., and van de Sandt, J.J.M. (1998) Alternative methods for skin irritation testing: the current status, *Alt. Lab. Anim.,* 26, 195–211.

Bowers, W., Blaha, M., Alkhyya, A., Sankovich, J., Kohl, J., Wong, G., and Patterson, D. (1999) Artificial human skin: cytokine, prostaglandin, HSP70 and histological responses to heat exposure. *J. Dermatol. Sci.,* 20, 172–182.

Brazma, A. and Vilo, J. (2000) Gene expression data analysis, *FEBS Lett.,* 480, 17–24.

Celis, J.E., Khruhoffer, M., Gromova, I., Frederiksen, C., Ostergaard, M., Thykjaer, T., Gromova, P., Yu, J., Palsdottir, H., Magnusson, M., and Orntoff, T.F. (2000) Gene expression profiling: monitoring transcription and translation products using DNA microarrays and proteomics, *FEBS Lett.,* 480, 2–1.

Cooper-Hannan, R., Harbell, J.W., Coecke, S., Balls, M., Bowe, G., Cervinka, M., Clothier, R., Hermann, F., Klahm, I.K., de Lange, J., Liebsch, M., and Vanparys, P. (1997) ECVAM workshop report 37, *Alt. Lab. Anim.*, 27, 539–577.

Daddona, P. (1996) New drug delivery systems: validation of *in vitro* models, *Alt. Lab. Anim.*, 24, 111.

Earl, L.K., Hall-Manning, T.J., Holland, G.H., Irwin, A., McPherson, J.P., and Southee, J.A. (1996) Skin irritation potential of surfactant mixtures: using relevant doses in *in vitro* systems. *Alt. Lab. Anim.*, 24(Abstr. 73), 249.

Eisen, M.B. and Brown, P.O. (1999) DNA arrays for analysis of gene expression. *Meth. Enzymol.*, 303, 179–205.

Eisen, M.B., Spellman, P.T., Brown, P.O., and Botstein, D. (1998) Cluster analysis and display of genome-wide expression patterns, *Proc. Natl. Acad. Sci. U.S.A.*, 95, 14863–14868.

Fares, H.M., Chatterjee, S., and Hayward, M. (1995) *In vitro* permeation and irritation of benzoyl peroxide-containing products, paper presented at the American Association of Pharmaceutical Scientists 10th Annual Meeting, November., paper PDD 7352.

Golub, T.R., Slonim, D.K., Tamayo, P., Huard, C., Gaasenbeek, M., Mesirov, J.P., Coller, H., Loh, M.L., Downing, J.R., Caligiuri, M.A., Bloomfield, C.D., and Lander, E.S. (1999) Molecular classification of cancer: class prediction by gene expression monitoring, *Science*, 286, 531–537.

Harbell, J., Southee, J., and Curren, R.D. (1997) The path to regulatory acceptance of *in vitro* methods is paved with the strictest scientific standards, in *Animal Alternatives, Welfare and Ethics*, van Zutphen, L.F.M. and Balls, M., Eds., Elsevier Science, New York, pp. 1177–1181.

Hayden, P.J., Jackson, G.R., Jr., Klausner, M., and Kubilus, J. (2000b) Highly differentiated *in vitro* skin model for high-throughput screening of topical therapeutics, *Toxicol. Sci.*, 54(Abstr. 688), 146.

Hayden, P.J., Klausner, M., and Kubilus, J. (2000a) Changes in cancer-related gene expression in an *in vitro* human skin model following UVB-irradiation, *J. Invest. Dermatol.*, 114(Abstr. 449), 824.

Hegde, P., Qi, R., Abernathy, K., Gay, C., Dharap, S., Gaspard, R., Hughes, J.E., Snesrud, E., Lee, N., and Quackenbush, A. (2000) A concise guide to cDNA microarray analysis, *BioTechniques*, 29, 548–562.

Hiltunen, M.O., Niemi, M., and Yla-Herttuala, S. (1999) Functional genomics and DNA array techniques in atherosclerosis research, *Curr. Opin. Lipidol.*, 10, 515–519.

Jones, B.C., Raabe, H.A., Sizemore, A., Mun, G.C., Theophilus, E.H., and Dickens, M.S. (2000) Lack of phototoxicty of cosmetic formulations containing glycolic acid in an *in vitro* human skin model, *Toxicol. Sci.*, 54(Abstr. 1853), 394–395.

Klausner, M., Breyfogle, B., Neal, P., and Kubilus, J. (2000) Use of MelanoDerm™, an epidermal model containing functional melanocytes, for skin lightening studies, *J. Invest. Dermatol.*, 114(Abstr. 661), 859.

Koschier, F.J., Roth, R.N., Wallace, K.A., Curren, R.D., and Harbell, J.W. (1995) A comparison of three dimensional human skin models to evaluate the dermal irritation of selected petroleum products, paper presented at CAAT Symposium *In Vitro* Approaches to Contact Dermatitis, Baltimore, MD.

Lacal, P.M., Failla, C.M., Pagani, E., Odorisio, T., Schietroma, C., Falcinelli, S., Zambruno, G., and D'Atri, M. (2000) Human melanoma cells secrete and respond to placenta growth factor and vascular endothelial growth factor, *J. Invest. Dermatol.*, 115, 1000–1007.

Liebsch, M., Barrabas, C., Traue, D., and Spielmann, H. (1997) Development of a new *in vitro* test for dermal phototoxicity using a model of reconstituted human epidermis (EPIDERM™), *ALTEX*, 14, 165–174.

Liebsch, M., Traue, D., Barrabas, C., Spielmann, H., Gerberick, F., Cruse, L., Diembeck, W., Pfannenbecker, U., Spieker, J., Holzhütter, H.-G., Brantom, P., Aspin, P., and Southee, J.A. (1999) Prevalidation of the EpiDerm™ phototoxicity test, *Alt. Lab. Anim.*, 72, 301.

Liebsch, M., Traue, D., Barrabas, C., Spielmann, H., Gerberick, F., Cruse, L., Diembeck, W., Pfannenbecker, U., Spieker, J., Holzhütter, H.-G., Brantom, P., Aspin, P., and Southee, J.A. (2000a) Prevalidation of the EpiDerm phototoxicity test, *Toxicol. Sci.*, 54(Abstr. 1777), 379.

Liebsch, M., Traue, D., Barrabas, C., Spielmann, H., Uphill, P., Wilkins, S., McPherson, J., Wiemann, C., Kaufmann, T., Remmele, M., Holzhütter, H.-G., Brantom, P., Aspin, P., and Southee, J.A. (2000b) Prevalidation of the EpiDerm™ skin corrosivity test, *Alt. Lab. Anim.* 28, 371–401.

Lockhart, D.J. and Winzeler, E.A. (2000) Genomics, gene expression and DNA arrays, *Nature* 405, 827–835.

Martin, K.M., Lyte, P., Mazuruk, K., and Shapiro, S. (2000) Inhibition of UV induced MMP-1 in epidermal equivalents by antioxidants, *J. Invest. Dermatol.*, 114(Abstr. 309), 803.

McCaffrey, T.A., Fu, C., Du, B., Eksinar, S., Kent, K.C., Bush, H., Kreiger, K., Rosengart, T., Cybulsky, M.I., Silverman, E.S., and Collins, T. (2000) High-level expression of Egr-1 and Egr-1-inducible genes in mouse and human atherosclerosis, *J. Clin. Invest.*, 105, 653–662.

Merk, H.F., Jugert, F.K., and Frankenberg, S. (1996) Biotransformations in the skin, in *Dermatotoxicology*, Marzulli, F.N. and Maibach, H.I., Eds., Taylor and Francis, Washington, D.C., 61–73.

Mosmann, T. (1983) Rapid colorimetric assay for cellular growth and survival: application to proliferation and cytotoxicity assays, *J. Immunol. Meth.*, 65, 55.

Mukhtar, H. (1992) Cutaneous metabolism of xenobiotics and steroid hormones, in *Pharmacology of the Skin*, H. Mukhtar, Ed., CRC Press, Boca Raton, FL, p. 90–109.

Nabi, Z., Tavakkol, A., Soliman, N., and Polefka, T.G. (1998) Bioconversion of tocopheryl acetate to tocopherol in human skin organ culture models, *J. Invest. Dermatol.*, 110(Abstr. 1239), 679.

Nuwaysir, E.F., Bittner, M., Trent, J., Barrett, J.C., and Afshari, C.A. (1999) Microarrays and toxicology: the advent of toxicogenomics, *Mol. Carcinogens* 24,153–159.

Perkins, M.A., Osborne, R., Robinson, M.K., Rana, F., Ghassemi, A., and Hall, B. (1999) Comparison of *in vitro* and *in vivo* human skin responses to consumer products and ingredients with a range of irritancy potential, *Toxicol. Sci.* 48, 218–229.

Perkins, M.A., Osborne, R., Rana, F.R., Ghassemi, A., and Robinson, M.K. (1996) Comparison of *in vitro* and *in vivo* human skin responses to consumer products and ingredients with a range of irritancy potential, *The Toxicologist,* 30(Abstr. 864), 168.

Perou, C.M., Jeffrey, S.S., van de Rijn, M., Rees, C.A., Eisen, M.B., Ross, D.T., Pergamenschikov, A., Williams, C.F., Zhu, S.X., Lee, J.C., Lashkari, D., Shalon, D., Brown, P.O., and Botstein, D. (1999) Distinctive gene expression patterns in human mammary epithelial cells and breast cancers, *Proc. Natl. Acad. Sci. U.S.A.*, 96, 9212–9217.

Rendl, M., Mayer, C., Fischer, H., Pammer, J., Weninger, W., and Tschachler, E. (2000) Wounding upregulates vascular endothelial growth factor production by keratinocytes of *in vitro* reconstructed epidermis, *J. Invest. Dermatol.*, 114(Abstr. 636), 855.

Rendl, M., Mayer, C., and Tschachler, E. (1999) Topically applied lactic acid increases spontaneous secretion of vascular endothelial growth factor/vascular permeability factor (VEGF/VPF) by human reconstructed epidermis, *J. Invest. Dermatol.*, 112(Abstr. 614), 625.

Rhoads, L.S., Mershon, M.M., and Van Buskirk, R.G. (1994) A synthetic human epidermal model can differentiate acute from latent effects of the monofunctional mustard analogue 2-chloroethylethyl sulfide, *In Vitro Toxicol.*, 7, 69.

Rockett, J.C. and Dix, D.J. (2000) DNA arrays: technology, options and toxicological applications, *Xenobiotica*, 30, 155–77.

Roguet, R., Beck, H., Boelsma, E., Bracher, M., Faller, C., Harris, I., Lotte, C., Dreher, F., and Ponec, M. (1999) Testing and improvement of reconstructed skin kits in order to elaborate European standards: first results, *Alt. Lab. Anim.* 27, 333.

Seiberg, M., Paine, C., Sharlow, E., Andrade-Gordon, P., Costanzo, M., Eisinger, M., and Shapiro, S.S. (2000b) Inhibition of melanosome transfer results in skin lightening, *J. Invest. Dermatol.*, 115, 162–167.

Seiberg, M., Paine, C., Sharlow, E., Andrade-Gordon, P., Costanzo, M., Eisinger, M., and Shapiro, S.S. (2000a) The protease-activated receptor 2 regulates pigmentation via keratinocyte-melanocyte interactions, *Exp. Cell Res.*, 254, 25–32.

Sherlock, G. (2000) Analysis of large-scale gene expression data, *Curr. Opin. Immunol.*, 12, 201–205.

Warren, R., Sanders, L.M., Curtis, S.L., Wong, L.F., Zhu, C., Tollens, F.R., and Otte, T.E. (1999) Human *in vitro* and *in vivo* cutaneous responses to soap suspension: role of solution behavior in predicting potential irritant contact dermatitis, *In Vitro Mol. Toxicol.*, 12, 97.

Zhao, J.F., Thang, Y.J., Kubilus, J., Jin, X.H., Santella, R.M., Athar, M., Wang, Z.Y., and Bickers, D.R. (1999) Reconstituted 3-dimensional human skin as a novel *in vitro* model for studies of carcinogenesis, *Biochem. Biophys. Res. Commun.*, 254, 49–53.

PART IV

A Case Study in the Use of Alternatives to Determine the Mechanism of Sulfur Mustard Action

WILLIAM J. SMITH

Sulfur mustard is an alkylating agent that causes debilitating injuries when it contacts tissue. Its primary target tissues are skin, respiratory tract, and eyes. Even though sulfur mustard has been recognized as a chemical threat agent for more than 80 years, there is no available therapy for the mustard injury. The lack of therapy is, in large measure, due to the complex pathology that is induced by this agent. Numerous cellular and tissue alterations occur after exposure to mustard, and development of therapeutic measures requires understanding of those pathological processes most relevant to the observed tissue injuries. The U.S. Army Medical Research Institute of Chemical Defense (USAMRICD) has been tasked with defining the mechanisms of mustard-induced pathology and with using the understanding of these toxic mechanisms to develop medical countermeasures to protect U.S. citizens, both military and civilian, from the devastating effects of exposure to this insidious chemical threat agent.

In this section, nine chapters report on various models that have been employed to answer mechanistic questions about the toxicity of sulfur mustard and to evaluate candidate prophylactic and therapeutic compounds against mustard injury. Most of the research has used *in vitro* models to define toxic mechanisms, but, ultimately, evaluation of therapy for such a complex pathology must use a whole animal model to represent the full range of cytotoxic, histotoxic, and inflammatory processes manifested upon exposure to the agent. Fortunately, *in vitro* technologies can go a long way to reduce the number of animal used. The animal studies can then be focused on those candidate compounds most likely to provide success.

The papers presented provide a microcosm of drug development efforts by our institute and its collaborating laboratories. Two of the papers are focused on establishing toxicological screening models. One uses the single-cell protista, Tetrahymena, to evaluate the cytotoxic potential of mustard. Unfortunately, its direct application to a drug screening program is limited because it has a high resistance to *in vitro* concentrations of sulfur mustard, possibly due to its redundancy of genomic

DNA (Chapter 21, Platteborze and Smith). The other screening model studied is the human epidermal keratinocyte (HEK). HEK is the *in vitro* equivalent of the basal epidermal cell layer, which is believed to be the principal target cell of mustard in skin. Several indicators of cell death were evaluated in Chapter 24 (Kelly et al.) for ease of use in cytotoxicty screening

The HEK model is used in six of these papers to study genomic, biochemical, and cytoskeletal alterations induced by mustard. Schlager et al. (Chapter 23) evaluate the toxicogenomic changes that are indicative of inflammatory responses. Smith et al. (Chapter 22) look at a number of biochemical alterations, while Smith et al. (Chapter 26) demonstrate specific DNA responses that could affect the ability of HEK to undergo cytokinesis. Since epidermal–dermal separation is the hallmark of the mustard lesion in skin, Kelly et al. (Chapter 25) use several assays of proteolysis in HEK and isolated human lymphocytes to study the role of protease activity following *in vitro* mustard exposure and to define a model for evaluating antiprotease therapies. Knowing that inflammatory processes are critical to the full expression of the mustard lesion, Cowan et al. (Chapter 28) demonstrate mustard-induced expression of the cytokine IL-8 in mustard exposed HEK and establish this model as a useful screen for antiinflammatory therapies. Moving from the single-cell models to tissue interactions, Werrlein and Madren-Whalley (Chapter 27) use both isolated HEK and epidermal explant cultures to experimentally evaluate the nature of cytoskeletal elements such as keratins, integrins, and other adhesion complex components following mustard exposure both at the cellular and tissue levels.

Finally, the chapter by Smith et al. (Chapter 29) is a culmination of a large body of basic research and drug screening using *in vitro* and *in vivo* evaluations that have generated the proof of concept for a medical countermeasure against the vesicant agent sulfur mustard. This chapter summarizes the work of several laboratories and many investigators over more than 15 years. That research, of which the chapters presented here are but a mere sampling, has allowed us to unravel the complexities of mustard damage and to focus on key pharmacological strategies that are providing the framework for development of medical intervention for those individuals who become exposed to this debilitating chemical agent.

CHAPTER 21

Cellular Resistance of *Tetrahymena* to Sulfur Mustard

Peter L. Platteborze, James E. Sistrunk, and William J. Smith

CONTENTS

INTRODUCTION

Sulfur mustard (SM, bis-(2-chloroethyl) sulfide) is a potent alkylating agent that continues to be a threat as a chemical weapon. Research has shown that SM is highly reactive to many cellular nucleophiles, with DNA appearing to be a critical target. These alkylation events involve DNA strand breaks as well as the formation of intrastrand or interstrand cross-links (Papirmeister, 1991). The latter events are largely thought to cause the observed SM-induced reduction in DNA synthesis and subsequent interruption of the normal cell cycle (Emisson and Smith, 1997).

In humans exposed to SM, the first target of incapacitation is the eyes, followed by a latent period in which vesication occurs. Despite ocular injuries having been reported since World War I, the current lead therapies provide at best transient, symptomatic relief. A battery of candidate therapeutic compounds exists but has not been adequately tested as the current test model, standard Draize test (Draize et al.,

1944), and is cumbersome, labor-intensive, and expensive. These difficulties could be circumvented through the use of alternative *in vitro* models.

In this study the common freshwater, ciliated protozoan *Tetrahymena* was examined as an alternative *in vitro* model. Silverman et al. illustrated that this unicellular eukaryote is a suitable alternative model to ocular testing in rabbits by consistently showing that *in vitro* testing had equal or greater "irritancy" than *in vivo* testing for most chemicals (Silverman, 1983; Silverman and Pennisi, 1987). These bioassays were proven to be quick, reliable, sensitive, and inexpensive, aspects that made *Tetrahymena* an ideal candidate organism to begin an alternatives study.

MATERIALS AND METHODS

Cell Culture and SM Exposures

Tetrahymena pyriformis was the kind gift of John Kloetzel (University of Maryland, Baltimore County, Catonsville, MD). *Tetrahymena* were raised axenically in 0.8% (w/v) Carnation nonfat dry milk powder supplemented with 0.1% (w/v) yeast extract (Sigma, St. Louis, MO). Stock cultures were maintained in the dark at room temperature (RT) and used to seed new cultures, which were grown for 24 hr prior to testing. Cells were examined on a hemocytometer to observe their health and ensure they were in the logarithmic growth phase. All studies were conducted in the maintenance medium described above with one exception, the Coulter study, which was completed in keratinocyte growth medium (KGM, Clonetics Corp., San Diego, CA). SM was obtained from the U.S. Army Edgewood Chemical and Biological Center (Aberdeen Proving Ground, MD).

Stock SM was suspended in deionized water (with the one exception involving KGM as mentioned above) to a final concentration of 4 or 16 mM. This was followed by a 1:1 dilution and subsequent serial dilutions to the desired concentration. Upon dilution, SM was immediately added to a healthy *Tetrahymena* culture, mixed for ~10 sec on a vortex-action mixer, and placed on a rocking platform. The negative control was treated identically, but SM was absent from the culture medium and cells. At specific time points, a bacteriologic loopful of this mixture (~0.01 ml) was placed on a microscope coverglass and inverted into a depression slide and cells were examined for motility at 40× magnification. The motility pattern of the *Tetrahymena* (excluding speed of movement) was observed, evaluated, and quantified. Each low-power microscopic field contained approximately 25 to 60 organisms. Motility was estimated by making an approximate count of the total number of cells in the microscopic sample and the number of cells moving normally. Cells moving slower or faster than the controls were considered to be moving normally.

Coulter Counter Studies

Cells were examined with a Coulter (Hialeah, FL) ZM-1 particle counter. An aliquot (0.5 ml) of cell suspension was mixed with 20 ml of Coulter Isoton in an Accuvette and read on the counter. Cell number and average size were recorded.

RESULTS

Observations from SM exposures were based on multiple triplicate experiments. *Tetrahymena* cell viability was not affected by SM concentrations below 4.0 mM (Figure 21.1). At 15 min postexposure SM had no observable effect on cell viability at all concentrations analyzed. However, by 90 min, cells exposed to 8.0 mM SM had become sluggish, highly vacuolated, and rounded and had cytolysed. At 4.0 mM SM this effect was also observed but over a longer time; cell viability was 75% at 90 min postexposure, 50% at 24 hr, 35% at 48 hr, and 0% at 72 hr.

At SM concentrations between 0.5 and 2.0 mM, cell counts were comparable to positive controls at 15 and 90 min (Figure 21.2). However, at 24 hr the cell number had not changed, indicating cell division had ceased. By 48 hr cell division had resumed at comparable growth rates to positive control for those cells exposed to 0.5 to 1.0 mM. Cells exposed to SM below 0.5 mM behaved as the positive control.

Cell size was also examined by the use of a Coulter counter. Relative to the positive unexposed control, which remained unchanged, SM-treated cells had increased in size at 4 hr postexposure. This effect was linear at concentrations up to 1.0 mM: cell size had increased ~5% at 0.25 mM, ~10% at 0.5 mM, and ~15% at 1.0 mM. At 2.0 mM cells had decreased in size but this cell population was determined to not be alive. By 24 hr postexposure, viable cells had nearly regained their initial size.

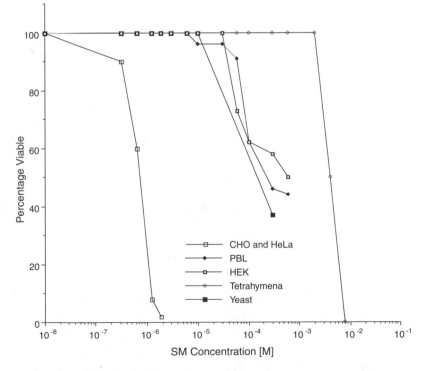

Figure 21.1 Cell viability vs. [SM]. Viability of six different cell lines was analyzed over a range of SM concentrations. Symbols are represented within the graph.

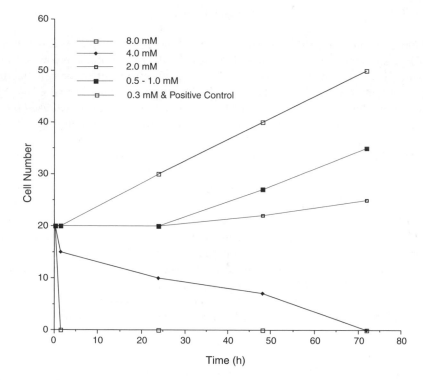

Figure 21.2 Effects of SM on cell number over time. The number of *Tetrahymena* was determined after exposure to a range of SM concentrations and over a period of 72
hr. Symbols are represented within the graph.

DISCUSSION

SM has been determined to be very toxic at low concentrations in all *in vitro*
systems examined to date. Cell systems examined include human epidermal keratinocytes (HEK), peripheral blood lymphocytes (PBLs), Chinese hamster ovary (CHO),
HeLa, and yeast (Roberts et al., 1971; Kircher and Brendel, 1983; Papirmeister et al.,
1991; Smith et al., 1991). *Tetrahymena* were anticipated to exhibit normal or heightened sensitivity to SM relative to these systems; however, they appear to have significant resistance since the present data clearly indicate survival in concentrations up to
4.0 m*M* SM. This phenomenal degree of insensitivity is exemplified relative to other
in vitro systems in Figure 21.1. *Tetrahymena* viability is initially affected by SM at a
concentration over 100× that of HEK, the current *in vitro* skin model. SM concentrations below 4.0 m*M* appeared to have no effect on cell viability, while exposure to
concentrations at or above 4.0 m*M* resulted in cell death. These high concentrations
may be sufficient to destroy outer membrane integrity and lead to cytolysis.

SM concentrations below 4.0 m*M* did have a significant impact on cell proliferation as shown in Figure 21.2. All cells exposed to concentrations above 0.3 m*M*
had cell division arrested for 24 hr but continued to grow in size. This unbalanced
cell growth is a characteristic of SM injury, and has been well documented in HEK
(Smith et al., 1999), albeit at a much lower concentration. This cellular response is

thought to be due to extensive DNA damage that severely impedes the normal replication. Subsequently, cellular mass accumulates in the form of increased cell volume, protein, and RNA content, but the cells fail to divide until the damaged DNA is sufficiently repaired. Cell division in SM-exposed *Tetrahymena* had resumed by 48 hr. At SM concentrations from 0.5 to 1.0 mM, these growth rates were nearly comparable to positive control.

In the presence of 8.0 mM SM, cells assumed a spherical shape and cytolysed within 15 to 90 min. The fact that this deformity in body shape was quickly followed by cytolysis suggests a sudden change in the cortical gel structure. Similar changes occur in *Tetrahymena* exposed to mercaptoethanol or the alklylating agent metepa, and both were attributed to alterations in the –SH, S-S balance, which is necessary for the maintenance of the cortical gel structure (Shivaji et al., 1964; Zimmerman, 1964). This explanation would also seem logical here, since SM, like all known alkylating agents, has an affinity for thiol groups (Papirmeister et al., 1991). The deviation in cell viability between the Coulter analysis [cell death at 2.0 mM SM] and all other studies is attributed to the former being conducted in cell culture medium. The salts present in keratinocyte growth medium could negatively affect the viability of this fresh water organism.

It is worthwhile to speculate on the reason(s) behind *Tetrahymena* resistance. As stated earlier, SM is highly genotoxic and resistance is likely to be coupled with an organism's ability to abrogate this. While *Tetrahymena* have the usual features of a eukaryotic cell (i.e., nucleus, compartmentalized organelles, mitochondria, etc.), they do have some unusual properties. The most obvious difference is that they exhibit nuclear dimorphism. That is to say, they have two nucleuses, a macronucleus and a micronucleus, which divide the labor of somatic and germline genetic functions (Prescott, 1994). The macronucleus (mac) is a large, polyploidy somatic nucleus that divides amitotically. It is the only DNA actively expressed during vegetative multiplication and is not transmitted to the sexual progeny. The mac consists of approximately 250 autonomously replicating species that are derived from the five micronucleus chromosomes (220 Mbp) by site-specific fragmentation immediately after meiosis. Tucked in a small pocket alongside the mac is the small, diploid micronucleus (mic). It is transcriptionally inert, divides mitotically, and functions as the cell's germline during meiotic recombination.

The observed cellular resistance to SM may in part be attributed to this nuclear dimorphic feature, specifically that the mac may be preferentially alkylated by SM, thereby leaving the mic's genetic integrity relatively intact. This is plausible since alkylating agents have been shown to preferentially target DNA that is being actively transcribed (Papirmeister et al., 1991). This site-specific targeting in the *Tetrahymena*'s mac has previously been observed with the alklylating agent methyl methane sulfonate (MMS) (Campbell and Romero, 1998). Even in the unlikelihood that there was a limited preference in DNA alkylation, the mac is stoichiometrically present at a tenfold greater concentration than the mic (Prescott, 1994; Marsh et al., 2000). Assuming that alkylations accumulate in the autonomously replicating species (i.e., mac), the resulting DNA damage may not significantly impair normal cellular homeostasis as each species exists on the average at 45 copies per cell. Thus, SM concentrations that are genotoxic to diploid mammalian cells may have a limited effect on *Tetrahymena*.

The limited effects observed on cellular proliferation may also in part be due to the quiescent mic's germline genetic integrity remaining intact after SM exposures. If these cells can undergo meiosis, the resulting daughter cells would only contain the relatively undamaged mic. This would naturally lead to the generation of an entirely new mac and the cells genetic integrity would remain fully intact.

Apart from this unusual genome organization, *Tetrahymena* also appear to have a more efficient DNA repair system than mammalian cells. Exposure to UV light or to MMS resulted in over a 100× increase in the mRNA for Rad51, the eukaryotic homolog of the *E. coli* recA recombinase (Campbell and Romero, 1998). Cells responded quickly to these insults; Rad51 levels were significantly increased at 30 min postexposure, the earliest time point examined. This significant degree of induction appears to be a unique response of *Tetrahymena*, as in other organisms only a two to tenfold induction has been observed. Unarguably, the induction of significant amounts of Rad51 directly contributes to the observed *Tetrahymena*'s heightened resistance to SM alkylation. It seems likely that sufficient levels of DNA repair enzymes accumulate during the 24 hr period of *Tetrahymena* cell arrest and the SM-induced damage is repaired. This eventually leads to the resumption of cell division.

Tetrahymena also have two other distinct characteristics that could contribute to the heightened SM resistance. They have powerful active transport mechanisms that could possibly discharge toxic metabolites and help maintain a healthy intracellular equilibrium and they do not undergo apoptosis. Programmed cell death has been shown to directly contribute to the low-dose toxicity of SM observed in mammalian cells.

The data presented in this short report indicate that *Tetrahymena* cannot successfully serve as an *in vitro* model for SM-induced ocular injury; however, they may prove an excellent choice model to study cellular resistance to SM. Owing to their size, rapid doubling, and ease of manipulation, *Tetrahymena* have historically served as an excellent model system for the investigation of many fundamental molecular and cellular mechanisms, including the discovery of ribozymes and telomeres. The increased resistance to SM cytotoxicity documented here may provide a useful tool to dissect specific mechanisms of SM toxicity that could be harder to observe in more sensitive models.

ACKNOWLEDGMENTS

The authors would like to thank Clarence Broomfield and Stephen Baskin for many insightful discussions.

REFERENCES

Campbell, C. and Romero, D.P. (1998) Identification and characterization of the RAD51 gene from the ciliate *Tetrahymena thermophila, Nucleic Acids Res.*, 26, 3165–3172.

Draize, J., Woodard, G., and Calvery, H. (1944) Methods for the study of irritation and toxicity of substances applied topically to the skin and mucous membranes, *J. Pharm. Exp. Ther.*, 82, 377–390.

Emisson, E. and Smith, W. (1997) Cytometric analysis of DNA damage in cultured human epithelial cells following exposure to sulfur mustard, *J. Am. Coll. Toxicol.,* 15, S9–S18.

Kircher, M. and Brendel, M. (1983) DNA alkylation by mustard gas in yeast strains of different repair capacity, *Chem. Biol. Interact.,* 44, 27–39.

Marsh, T.C., Cole, E.S., Stuart, K.R., Campbell, C., and Romero, D.P. (2000) Rad51 is required for propagation of the germinal nucleus in *Tetrahymena thermophila, Genetics,* 154, 1587–1596.

Papirmeister, B., Feister, A.J., Robinson, S.I., and Ford, R.D. (1991) *Medical Defense against Mustard Gas: Toxic Mechanisms and Pharmacological Implications,* Science Applications International Corporation, CRC Press, Boca Raton, FL.

Prescott, D.M. (1994) The DNA of ciliated protozoa, *Microbiol. Rev.,* 58, 233–267.

Roberts, J.J., Plant, J.E., Sturrock, J.E., and Crathorn, A.R. (1971) Quantitative aspects of the repair of alkylated DNA in cultured mammalian cells, *Chem. Biol. Interact.,* 3, 29–47.

Shivaji, S., Saxena, D.M., and Pillai, M.K. (1964) Mode of action of alkylating agents using a ciliate protozoan as a model system. III. Effects of metepa on cell division and DNA synthesis in the ciliate *Blepharism intermedium, Indian J. Exp. Biol.,* 16, 450–454.

Silverman, J. (1983) Preliminary finding on the use of protozoa (*Tetrahymena thermophila*) as a model for ocular irritation testing in rabbits, *Lab. Anim. Sci.,* 33, 55–59.

Silverman, J. and Pennisi, S. (1987) Evaluation of *Tetrahymena thermophila* as an *in vitro* alternative to ocular irritation studies in rabbits, *J. Toxicol. Cutaneous Ocular Toxicol.,* 6, 33–42.

Smith, W.J., Blank, J.A., Starner, R.A., Menton, R.G., and Harris, J. (1999) Effect of sulfur mustard exposure on human epidermal keratinocyte viability and protein content, in *Toxicity Assessment Alternatives: Methods, Issues, Opportunities,* Salem, H. and Katz, S.A., Eds., Humana Press, Totowa, NJ, 197–204.

Smith, W.J., Sanders, K.M., Gales, Y.A., and Gross, C.L. (1991) Flow cytometric analysis of toxicity by vesicating agents in human cells *in vitro, J. Toxicol. Cutaneous Ocular Toxicol.,* 10, 33–42.

Zimmerman, A.M. (1964) Effects of mercaptoethanol on the furrowing capacity of arbacia eggs, *Biol. Bull.,* 127, 345–352.

CHAPTER **22**

Studies of Cellular Biochemical Changes Induced in Human Cells by Sulfur Mustard

William J. Smith, Offie E. Clark III, Fred M. Cowan, Maura E. DeJoseph, Charisse Davenport, and Clark L. Gross

CONTENTS

INTRODUCTION

The mission of the U.S. Army Medical Research Institute of Chemical Defense (MRICD) includes basic research into the mechanisms of action of chemical threat agents. The results obtained from such studies are then used to define pharmacological intervention strategies to protect war fighters and civilians against injury by these agents. The cellular pharmacology team at the MRICD focuses its research on the active cellular and tissue pathogenic mechanisms active following exposure to sulfur mustard (2,2'-dichloroethyl sulfide, Army designation HD). This report presents some of the results of those studies and raises questions pertaining to models and procedures employed.

MATERIALS AND METHODS

Cell Cultures

HEK

Primary cultures of adult normal human epidermal keratinocytes (HEKs) were obtained from Clonetics Corporation (San Diego, CA). The cells were passaged into 75- or 150-cm² tissue culture flasks, maintained in Keratinocyte growth media (KGM, Clonetics), and grown to various confluencies. HEKs were exposed to either 50, 100, or 300 μM HD along with untreated controls. Postexposure incubation times were from 4 to 24 hr, after which cells were harvested by Trypsin/EDTA (Clonetics Corporation).

HeLa

HeLa cultures were maintained in 150-cm² culture flasks (Corning Glass Works, Corning, NY) in minimal essential medium (MEM) with 10% fetal calf serum (FCS) at 37°C and 5% CO_2.

When the cultures were 80 to 90% confluent, the medium was removed and replaced with a medium containing HD (0.1 to 100.0 μM) and the cells were incubated for 60 min in an approved fume hood at room temperature to remove any hazardous vapors. After 1 hr, the medium was removed and replaced with fresh MEM without HD to incubate an additional 0 to 23 hr. The cells were harvested by removing the medium and adding phosphate buffered saline containing trypsin and EDTA to the flask. The detached cells were pipetted into a conical centrifuge tube containing MEM with 10% FCS and Trypsin inhibitor solution (Clonetics, San Diego, CA). The cells were harvested via centrifugation at $250 \times g$ for 10 min. The supernate was removed and the cells suspended in 10 ml of 50 mM Tris buffer (pH 8.0) and 25 mM $MgCl_2$. The cultures were maintained on ice until the assay was initiated.

Lymphocytes

Blood was obtained from a normal human volunteer under an approved human use protocol. The blood was diluted with phosphate buffered saline (PBS) and EDTA (Sigma, St. Louis, MO), layered on a Percoll (d = 1.08), and centrifuged at 425 × g for 30 min at 20°C. The lymphocyte band was removed, collected, placed in a centrifuge tube, and then centrifuged at 250 × g for 20 min. Pellets were resuspended and washed with Tyrodes free with glucose, recentrifuged as above, and resuspended in RPMI-1640 (Sigma, St. Louis, MO).

DNA Isolation

Reagents

The following buffers and solutions were employed:

1. Lysis buffer—500 mM Na$_2$ EDTA, 10 mM Tris—HCl, 1% Lauroyl sarcosine.
2. TE buffer consisted of 10 mM Tris (Trizma Base), 1 mM Na$_2$ EDTA, pH 7.5.
3. 5× TBE Buffer—1× TBE in 90 mM Tris, 88 mM boric acid, 2 mM EDTA, pH 8.0.
4. Storage buffer—0.5 M EDTA, pH 8.0.
5. 10× React 3 Buffer—prepared as per manufacturer's instructions aliquoted in 1-ml volumes.
6. Proteinase K (stock) used 1 to 10 mg/ml in SDS.
7. RNase (stock) 10 mg/ml.
8. Not I restriction enzyme — 1000 units at 15 U/μl.
9. Phenyl methyl sulfonyl fluoride (PMSF) 40 mM stock solution, Isopropanol.
10. Sodium acetate—3 M solution prepared per manufacturers instructions, pH 7.0.

Phenol-Chloroform Extraction

HEKs were lysed in lysis buffer for 2 hr containing 144 μg/ml proteinase K. After 2 hr, 500 μg/ml of RNase A was added and incubated for 1 hr. Lysates were extracted with phenol/chloroform (1:1 mixture) using a volume equal to the volume of original aqueous solution. Phases were resolved for 2 min by microcentrifugation. The aqueous phase was removed and transferred to a new tube. 1/10 volume 3 M sodium acetate pH 7.0 and 2.5 volume ethanol was added to aqueous phase. Sample was incubated on ice for 10 min. Precipitate was collected by microcentrifugation for 10 min at 14,000 rpm. Five hundred microliters of 70% ethanol was added to pellet. DNA pellet was dried and then dissolved in 1 ml TE buffer, pH 8.0. DNA concentration was determined by OD 260, and purity was determined by 260/280 absorbance.

Commercial Kits

Kits for isolation of DNA from mammalian cells and tissue were obtained from Boehringer-Mannheim and used according to the manufacturer's directions.

Modified Kit Usage

The following modifications to the Boehringer kit were employed: the lysis buffer temperature was decreased from 65 to 37°C; the amount of proteinase K was doubled; the protein precipitation step was extended to overnight at –20°C.

Pulse Field Gel Electrophoresis (PFGE)

PFGE was run using 2% low-melt agarose and a 0.8% running gel. The gels were stained with 24.5 µl of SYBR green nucleic acid stain in 245 ml of 0.5× TBE buffer.

PARP Assay

The cell suspension was sonicated on ice with a microtip (setting of 50) in a Branwill Biosonik III sonicator by pulsing for 6 sec followed by 1 min of cooling. This step was repeated twice for maximal liberation of poly(ADP-ribose) polymerase (Sudhakar et al., 1979). The standard assay involved the addition of sample (50 µg wet weight of cells) to a reaction mixture (50 mM tris [pH 8.0] and 25 mM MgCl$_2$) with a final volume of 125 µl. The reaction mixture was incubated for 20 sec at 25°C and the reaction initiated by the addition of 15 µl of [Adenine-2,8-3H]-NAD (specific activity 60 mCi/mMol) at a final concentration of 100 µM NAD (NAD in excess). The reaction proceeded for 45 sec at 25°C and was terminated by the addition of 2 ml of 20% trichloroacetic acid (TCA). The sample was placed on ice for at least 30 min, and the resulting precipitate collected on 0.45-µM pore size filters (Whatman, Hillsboro, OR), washed with 10 ml of 20% TCA, rinsed with 20 ml of 95% ethanol, and dried. Radioactivity was determined by liquid scintillation spectrometry.

Calcium Measurement

Two types of HEK preparations were used: trypsinized/suspended and coverslip grown (Thermanox Coverslips, Nunc). The suspended HEK were at a concentration of 1.0 × 10^6/ml in KGM. The coverslip cell concentration was assumed to be approximately the same as the suspended cells. Both cell preparation types were loaded with 20 µM Fura-2 AM, the acetoxymethyl ester form (Molecular Probes). The cells were incubated in the dark for 45 min and then washed. The cells were transferred to a cuvette—either 1 ml suspended cells with 1 ml PBS or 1 coverslip in 2 ml PBS, depending on the experiment. A fluorometric scan was performed using an excitation ratio of 340:380 nm and 510 nm emission. A baseline was established for the cells and, as the scan continued to run, HD was added to the cuvette to a final concentration of 300 µM. The scan was carried out over 20 to 30 min.

Interleukin ELISA

Quantikine Elisa kits for human IL-1α, IL-1β, IL-6, and IL-8 were obtained from R&D Systems (Minneapolis, MN) and used according to manufacturer's directions.

Measurement of Fc and C1q Receptors

At 8 and 24 hr after HD exposure, adherent HEK were stained with fluorochrome conjugated monoclonal antibodies against the FcRIII (CD16), FcRII (CD32) (Pharmingen, San Diego, CA), or unconjugated antihuman C1q (Quidel, San Diego, CA), counterstained with fluorochrome conjugated antimouse IG (Pharmingen). Fluorescence intensity was judged microscopically on a Zeiss fluorescent microscope.

RESULTS

Our initial attempts at pulsed-field gel electrophoresis (PFGE) of HEK DNA following exposure to HD used the procedure described by Bentley et al. (1991) in which treated cells are placed in agarose plugs exposed to lysing buffers and then transferred to the gels. This step presumably would significantly reduce the time and handling for optimized analysis, but we could not detect DNA migration through the PFGE. To ensure that HEK DNA exhibited normal migration patterns through our PFGE, we used a commercial DNA isolation kit from Boehringer-Mannheim designed for mammalian cells and tissues. Although we obtained low yields of DNA, the purity of the isolates was insufficient as judged by the 260:280 nm ratio (must be >1.8). These results along with those of our other isolation attempts are listed in Table 22.1.

To validate the ability of the kits to isolate human DNA, we used human peripheral blood leukocytes (PBL) and obtained good yield recoveries with adequate purity. Using phenol/chloroform extraction of DNA, we also failed to generate decent yields of pure DNA from control HEK. We modified the kit procedure, as described in the methods, and ultimately yielded sufficient quantities of pure DNA from control HEK. This modified extraction procedure was then used on HD-exposed cells, and Table 22.2 shows the high yields and purities obtained.

Table 22.1 Problems Seen with DNA Isolation from HEK

Procedure	Date	Sample	Purity Level of DNA (260/280 Ratio)	DNA Yield (mg/ml)
Purification of HEK DNA using Boehringer Mannheim Kit for mammalian cells	8/4/98	Control	1.35	60
	8/18/98	Control	1.65	45
	8/24/98	Control	1.35	25
Purification of lymphocyte DNA using Boehringer Mannheim Kit for mammalian blood	9/2/98	Control	1.82	189
	9/8/98	Control	1.81	185
	9/29/98	Control	1.93	194
Phenol/chloroform extraction of HEK DNA	10/1/98	Control	1.22	60
	10/7/98	Control	1.35	33
	10/13/98	Control	1.47	67
Purification of HEK DNA using Boehringer Mannheim Kit for mammalian cells (modified procedure)	10/19/98	Control	1.90	94
	10/27/98	Control	1.86	93
	11/5/98	Control	1.86	98

Table 22.2 Purification of HEK DNA using Boehringer
Mannheim Kit for Mammalian Cells Exposed to
Sulfur Mustard (HD)

Date	Sample	Purity Level of DNA (260/280 Ratio)	DNA Yield
11/19/98	Control	1.81	122
	50 mM HD	2.10	163
	100 mM HD	1.89	150
	300 mM HD	1.82	199
11/26/98	Control	1.85	194
	50 mM HD	1.99	213
	100 mM HD	1.86	198
	300 mM HD	1.81	172
12/8/98	Control	1.98	183
	50 mM HD	1.96	179
	100 mM HD	1.91	176
	300 mM HD	1.86	199

Using PFGE, we observed that the standards and controls migrated as expected through the gels, but DNA from HEK exposed to 50, 100, and 300 μM failed to migrate from the origin 4 hr post-HD. Sonication of the DNA samples allowed them to fully migrate through the gels, but no obvious banding patterns were noted (data not shown).

HD increased PARP activity in both HeLa and HEK cells (Figure 22.1). In HeLa cells the maximal response of PARP was seen at 1 hr post-HD with 100 μM. PARP levels decreased but remained elevated over control for the next 6 hr, declined to control levels at 9 hr, and elevated again slightly at 24 hr post-HD. In HEK, the initial PARP response to HD was observed at 4 hr, followed by a decline and a maximal elevation at 24 hr. At 10 μM HD, both cell types demonstrated elevation of PARP at 4 hr, with recurrent elevations at 24 hr.

Our laboratory has never been able to convincingly demonstrate calcium elevations in HEK exposed to HD. We have primarily used passage 3 HEK from a commercial source as both trypsinized cells in suspension and adherent cells on coverslips. We have looked over a wide range of confluencies from 50 to 100%. Based on discussions with our colleagues at DRES, we undertook studies using passage 2 HEK. Using adherent cells on coverslips at any confluency or trypsinized cells that had been at <80% confluency, we once again failed to detect any change in intracellular calcium levels in HEK exposed to 300 μM HD. But, when we used passage 2 HEK grown to full confluency, trypsinized the cells, and exposed them as suspensions, we were able to detect a small, 19% elevation of intracellular calcium within 15 min of exposure (Figure 22.2).

Since the tissue response to HD is known to involve an inflammatory component, we attempted to define the inflammatory-related responses of HEK to *in vitro* HD exposure. Using immunofluorescent assays with commercial monoclonal antibodies, we were able to detect increased expression of receptors for the Fc region of immunoglobulin and receptors for the initiating sequence of the complement pathway, C1q (Table 22.3). In addition, using Elisa assays for human interleukins, we demonstrated significantly increased release of IL-1β, IL-6, and IL-8 in culture supernatant fluids at 24 hr after 300 μM HD. IL-8 was also significantly elevated at 50 and 100 μM (Figure 22.3).

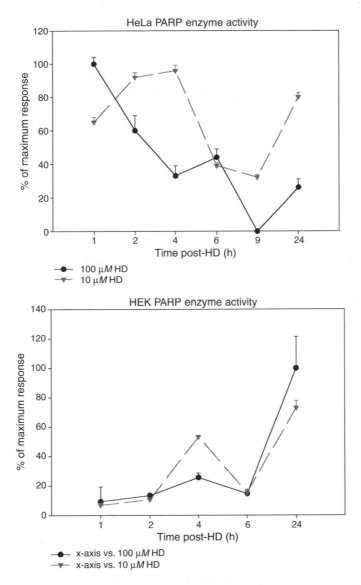

Figure 22.1 Time-dependent response of PARP activity following HD exposure of (top) HeLa cells and (bottom) HEK cells. Two concentrations of HD were used, 10 and 100 μ*M*, and PARP activities are presented as percent maximal response.

DISCUSSION

We encountered significant difficulties isolating pure DNA from both control and HD exposed cells. Although we have not seen similar difficulties reported in the literature, similar observations have been made at MRICD for years. After modification of Boehringer's kit procedure, we finally recovered good quantities of pure DNA. However, DNA from HD-treated HEK failed to migrate past the origin by PFGE

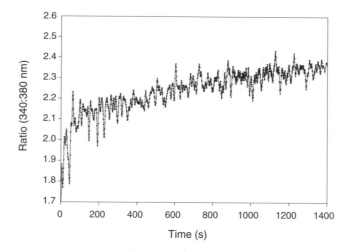

Figure 22.2 Increase in intracellular calcium in HEK (passage 2) exposed to 300 μ*M* HD as measured by 340:380 nm ratio of Fura-2 AM.

Table 22.3 Binding in HD-Exposed HEK[a]

Hrs post HD	Dose HD (μ*M*)			
C_1q	0	100	200	300
8	–	–	–	–
16	–	–	NT	++
24	–	+	+++	+++
CD32	**0**	**50**	**100**	**200**
8	–	+	+	+
24	–	+	++	+++

[a] + = weak; ++ = moderate; +++ = intense; NT = not tested. Grading of staining was judged visually by fluorescence microscope and HEK controls not exposed to HD were negative for fluorescence.

analysis. Sonication could release the DNA from whatever was holding it up, but this is not a desirable procedure when one is attempting to quantify strand breakage.

Since NAD+ depletion has been seen in all cells and tissues exposed to HD, it is a natural assumption that the depletion is caused by DNA strand break activation of PARP, which uses cellular NAD+ as a substrate. The data reported here demonstrate that two different epithelial cell types have separate kinetics of PARP response following HD exposure. The HeLa cells have an early (1 hr) maximal response, while HEK have their initial response at 4 hr, which may reflect the kinetics of DNA strand breakage in the different cell types. Both cell types show a rebound in PARP activity at 24 hr, which may be related to a secondary depletion in cellular NAD+ occurring around 24 hr postexposure (unpublished observation).

The calcium results are intriguing and raise serious questions about the *in vitro* models being used. While our normal culture conditions (passage 3 and less than 80% confluency) have never shown alterations of intracellular calcium levels following HD, using passage 2 cultures at 100% confluency gave results not inconsistent with those

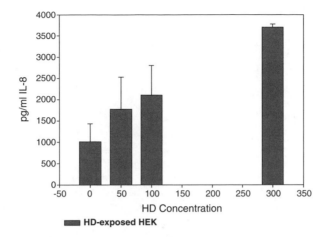

Figure 22.3 Concentration-dependent increase in the secretion of IL-8 from HEK exposed to HD.

reported by Hamilton et al. (1998). What are the optimal conditions of HEK growth as to passage number and confluency at time of exposure? Do HEKs *in vitro* mimic their *in vivo* counterparts in all biochemical responses to toxic agents? These questions must be addressed if the HEK model is to advance our knowledge of the HD injury.

The increased expression of Fc and C1q receptors along with IL-8 in HEK exposed to HD *in vitro* supports the concept of a primary role of basal epidermal cells in generation of an inflammatory response in tissue exposed to HD *in vivo*. We have seen histopathologic evidence of edema and induration in exposed tissue long before infiltrating inflammatory cells can be detected. The data presented here argue that the progenitor of the HD-induced inflammatory response may be skin keratinocytes with full presentation of the inflammatory damage being a combination of early and late events involving all components of the inflammatory response.

The human epidermal keratinocyte cell culture model has been, along with human PBL, a mainstay of cellular research into the mechanisms of action of HD. There are, however, many questions that must be addressed as we approach defining antivesicant countermeasures. We will never be permitted to expose humans to HD for research purposes because of its carcinogenic potential. Therefore, selection and optimization of *in vitro* and *ex vivo* models will be crucial to any long-term success.

REFERENCES

Bentley, K.L., Bieberich, C.J., and Ruddle, F.H. (1991) Pulsed-field electrophoresis: procedures, problems, and practicalities, in *Methods in Nucleic Acids Research*, CRC Press, Boca Raton, FL, ch. 7.

Hamilton, M., Dorandeu, F., McCaffery, M., and Sawyer, T. (1998) Modification of cytolsolic free calcium concentrations in human keratinocytes after sulphur mustard exposure, *Toxicol. In Vitro,* 12, 365–372.

Sudhakar, S., Tew, K.D., and Smulson, M.E. (1979) Effect of 1-methyl-1-nitrosourea on poly(adenosine diphosphate-ribose) polymerase activity at the nucleosomal level, *Cancer Res.,* 39, 1405–1410.

CHAPTER **23**

Human Keratinocyte Inflammatory Transcript Gene Activity Following Sulfur Mustard*

John J. Schlager, Kashif Ali, Hilma R. Benjamin, Claire F. Levine,
Douglas P. Avery, and James H. Clark

CONTENTS

INTRODUCTION

Human skin exposure to SM disrupts tissue homeostasis through covalent alkylation of cellular nucleophiles. Exposure to SM at a sufficient dose produces skin blisters at the epidermal-dermal junction (Papirmeister et al., 1991; Petrali and Ogesby-Megee, 1997). The specific cellular pathways affected by SM alkylation

* The opinions or assertions contained herein are the private views of the authors and are not to be construed as official or as reflecting the views of the Department of the Army or the Department of Defense.

leading to this loss of epidermal–dermal adherence, as well as the activated pathways producing the latent inflammation that forms large fluid-filled human skin blisters, have been difficult to elucidate. We were interested in using transcriptional analysis to identify the inflammatory or irritant components of SM exposure in cultured adult human epidermal keratinocytes (HEK). Two SM exposure concentrations were studied: a high dose at 200 µM SM (in 25 ml of medium), which is estimated to be equivalent to a skin blistering exposure, and a low dose at 25 µM SM, which is not sufficient to produce skin vesication but known to produce significant DNA damage (Smith et al., 1993; Hart and Schlager, 1997). The 25 µM SM concentration was used for comparison to the 200 µM SM exposure to distinguish the transcriptional events associated with cellular damage producing inflammation or blistering from those associated with DNA damage at a nonblistering exposure. Gene expression assays were performed with RNA isolated at 8 and 16 hr after SM exposure. This timeframe was chosen so that analyses would be within or precede the timeframe known for human SM skin blistering at 12 to 24 hr post-SM exposure (Papirmeister et al., 1991).

In this study two procedures were used to identify the SM-induced mRNA changes in HEK based on the assumption that a significant elicitation diversity of transcripts occurs following a SM exposure. In the first approach, mRNA transcripts were isolated at 16 hr from untreated HEK and from HEK treated with either 25 or 200 µM SM. The purified polyA mRNA was reverse transcribed into radiolabeled cDNA that was used to probe a blot containing 588 known transcriptionally regulated human genes. The second approach used a polymerase chain reaction (PCR) subtraction library generation technique (Diatchenko et al., 1996) to capture the predominant transcripts upregulated at 25 and 200 µM SM exposures at 8 and 16 hr. The subtraction library technique was performed to ensure isolation of any dominant inflammatory transcript not contained on the cDNA array blot. Although many more gene changes were found using both procedures, this report focuses on only the inflammation-associated transcripts identified by these techniques.

MATERIALS AND METHODS

Materials

The human Atlas™ 588 gene array, AtlasImage™ 1.5 software, PCR-select™ cDNA subtraction kit, and AdvanTAge™ PCR cloning kit containing the T/A cloning bacterial plasmid were obtained from Clontech (Palo Alto, CA). Superscript murine Moloney leukemia virus reverse transcriptase (MMLV) was obtained from Life Technologies (Gaithersburg, MD). SM was acquired from the U.S. Army Edgewood Research, Development, and Engineering Center (Aberdeen Proving Ground, MD). SM (6.35 mg) was aliquoted into 20-ml crimp-cap vials containing 10 ml keratinocyte growth medium (KGM) by the drug assessment agent dilution team and the solution immediately frozen in liquid nitrogen unmixed in two phases for storage at –80°C. All other chemicals and reagents used were obtained from Sigma Chemical (St. Louis, MO) unless otherwise stated.

Cell Culture and Exposure

HEKs from adult breast tissue (lot 4075, donor age 25) were obtained as cyropreserved first passage (P1) stocks of 5.0×10^5 cells/vial from Clonetics, Inc. (San Diego, CA). Cells were thawed and seeded at 2,500/cm² into 75 cm² flasks (Corning, Acton, MA). HEKs were grown in keratinocyte growth medium (KGM-D, Clonetics) to 70 to 80% density prior to trypsin detachment and reseeding at 2,500/cm² into 150 cm² flasks. Third passage flasks of HEK at 70% confluence were removed from the 37°C culture incubator and allowed to cool to room temperature prior to treatment. A frozen aliquot(s) of SM-KGM was thawed, and when the two liquid phases were apparent by noting the 10 µl SM droplet, a 4 mM SM solution was prepared by rapid liquid vortexing. This SM solution was placed immediately in an ice bath to slow the rate of hydrolysis during SM addition to cell medium. Three to five flasks per exposure condition were either left untreated (control) or exposed to 25 or 200 µM SM in 25 ml for both time points investigated.

RNA Preparation

At 8 and 16 hr, the medium was removed and the cells from both treated and control flasks were lysed with a buffer containing 4 M guanidium thiocynanate, 25 mM sodium citrate, 0.5% sodium sarcosine, pH 7.0. Total cellular RNA was isolated using the acid guanidium thiocynanate buffer/phenol/chloroform extraction method (Farrell, 1993). After phase separation and precipitation, the RNA samples were solubilized in guanidium buffer and stored frozen at –70°C until use. Just prior to cDNA preparation, the RNA was purified by polyA mRNA selection using a poly dT column (Qiagen, Valencia, CA). The purified mRNA was concentrated by ethanol precipitation in the presence of glycogen and dissolved in water for determining mRNA concentration using absorbance at 260 nm. These samples were used the same day for cDNA preparation.

Probing cDNA Array Blot

mRNA (0.5 µg) was radiolabeled with α^{32}P dATP using MMLV. The radiolabeled cDNA was purified away from unincorporated radionucleotides using gel columns (Clontech). The labeled cDNA from each treatment group and control was added to a hybridization buffer containing 1 mg of salmon sperm DNA, and the mixtures were used to expose three separate cDNA blots, which originated from the same production lot, for 16 hr at 68°C. The blots were rinsed three times with 2× SSC, 1% SDS, followed by two times with 0.1× SSC, 0.5% SDS prior to blot exposure to phosphorimage storage plates (Molecular Dynamics, Sunnyvale, CA). Images were captured using phosphorimaging at progressive screen exposures of 24, 72, and 192 hr (for example, see Figure 23.1) and scanned using ImageQuant software (Molecular Dynamics). Image data from all radioactivity measurements were analyzed using the Clontech AtlasImage 1.5 software. The abundance of individual gene transcripts was normalized by dividing by the sum of the total abundance of all gene transcripts on the blot. The quotient of normalized treated/control cell values was used for determination of induction or loss of a specific transcript (Tables 23.1 and 23.2).

Table 23.1 HEK Housekeeping Gene Transcripts at 16 Hr Following Sulfur Mustard

Gene Transcript	Gene Ratio[a]		
	Control Intensity[b]	25 µM SM	200 µM SM
14-3-3 zeta protein	317	0.7	0.44
23 kDa Highly Basic Protein	1689	2.0	2.3
α-Tubulin	307	0.57	1.4
β-Actin	236	1.2	1.2
Glyceraldehyde 3-phosphate dehydrogenase	612	0.44	1.1
HLA class I histocompatibility antigen C-4 alpha chain	487	0.94	1.0
Hypoxanthine-guanine phosphoribosyltransferase	59	0.9	3.7
Ribosomal Protein S9	978	1.2	2.1
Ubiquitin	2064	0.8	0.73

[a] Induction ratio from phosphorimage densitometeric measurements of listed gene transcript normalized to the sum total of the detected transcript intensity/pixel density.
[b] Control intensity (grayscale pixel density) adjusted from background. Background was set at the median intensity of the blank space between the six array panels. The subtracted background intensity ranged from 19 to 43.

Table 23.2 HEK Inflammation-Associated Transcripts at 16 Hr Following Sulfur Mustard

Gene Transcript	Gene Ratio[a]		
	Control Intensity[b]	25 µM SM	200 µM SM
CD40	86	4.9	0.3
Interleukin 1 α	67	0.1	1.4
Interleukin 1 β	101	0.6	3.5
Interleukin 2 receptor α subunit	148	0.3	0.4
Interleukin 6	494	0.7	0.6
Interleukin 7 receptor α subunit	131	0.4	0.7
Interleukin 8	16	—[c]	20
Interleukin 13	349	3.0	0.7
Interleukin 15	215	—	0.03
Macrophage inflammatory protein 2α	11	—	13
S19 ribosomal protein	886	0.9	2.1
Tumor necrosis factor α	50	—	1.4

[a] Induction ratio from phosphorimage densitometeric measurements of listed gene transcript normalized to the sum total of the detected transcript density.
[b] Control intensity (grayscale pixel density) adjusted from background. Background was set at the median intensity of the blank space between the six array panels. The subtracted background intensity ranged from 19 to 43.
[c] Transcript not detected above background.

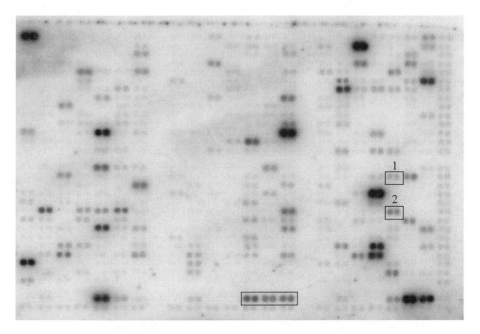

Figure 23.1 Atlas cDNA array nylon blot image. HEK were exposed to 200 μM sulfur mustard for 16 h and mRNA isolated and ^{32}P labeled as cDNA. The array contains double-dot blots of cDNA from 588 transcriptionally regulated genes and 9 housekeeping genes at the bottom of the array (see 3 housekeeping genes in rectangular box). Boxes 1 and 2 show expression of macrophage inflammatory protein 2α and interleukin 8, respectively. These inflammatory transcripts were at very low expression levels in control HEK.

Subtraction Library Construction

mRNA (1 μg) was reverse transcribed using Superscript MMLV (Life Technologies, Gaithersburg, MD) to generate cDNA. The cDNA from one SM concentration and its paired control were used in procedures similar to those described by Diatchenko et al. (1996), which were according to the Clontech PCR-Select cDNA subtraction kit procedures. The prepared subtraction library consisted of the transcripts upregulated by SM.

Subtraction Library Sequence and Analysis

The libraries were cloned into the advantage PCR cloning vector (Clontech) by T/A cloning using the PCR products from the subtraction library. Individual bacterial colonies were cultured overnight and plasmid DNA isolated with a Qiagen plasmid DNA miniprep column. DNA base sequence was determined by cycle sequencing using the Prizm™ reaction kit (PE-Applied Biosystems, Foster City, CA) and reaction analyzed using a DNA sequencer (Applied Biosystems, model 373A). Sequence identification was performed by comparing the cDNA insert sequence data, representing the sense or antisense strand of the isolated mRNA transcript, with all known sequences in the nonrepeating (NR) and the expression sequence tag (EST) databases at the National Center for Biotechnology Information (NCBI) using the base alignment program BLAST 2.06 available on the NCBI Internet web site (http://www.ncbi.nlm.nih.gov). Approximately 100 bacterial colonies from each library were selected for plasmid cDNA insert sequence identification.

RESULTS

One same-lot set of three Atlas™ 588 gene arrays was probed with radiolabeled HEK cDNA derived from HEK isolate 4075. Table 23.1 lists the changes occurring in the housekeeping gene sets of the Atlas™ cDNA array. We initially sought to determine the best housekeeping gene for transcript normalization. However, SM appears to change the expression of many of the levels of these normal transcripts used as housekeeping genes (Table 23.1). Therefore, until more rigorous transcript quantitation experiments are performed through time and SM dose, normalization of gene expression using housekeeping genes was abandoned. For these studies, the global normalization of genes was considered the most accurate measure of gene change.

The Atlas™ cDNA array data were analyzed for inflammatory gene transcript changes. Table 23.2 lists the inflammatory transcripts expressed in HEK. Primary cytokines found on the array at increased levels after 200 μM SM exposure were interleukin 1β (IL-1β), tumor necrosis factor α (TNF-α), and interleukin 1α (IL-1α) (Table 23.2). The largest inductions relative to control levels on the cDNA array were the secondary inflammatory transcripts interleukin 8 (IL-8) and macrophage inflammatory protein 2α (MIP-2α). However, the induction numbers for IL-8 and MIP-2α might not be an accurate calculation of their transcript levels since the control transcript expression levels were very low. Another secondary inflammatory transcript changed was the S19 ribosomal protein with a modest increase at 200 μM SM exposure. Other proinflammatory transcripts such as the interleukin 6 transcript did not change from control expression or interleukin-15 transcript expression that became virtually undetectable after SM exposure. The interleukin receptor subunits IL-2Rα and IL-7Rα were detected in HEK but did not change from control levels at either SM concentration. At 16 hr following the 25 μM SM exposure, transcripts for IL-8 and MIP-2α were not detected in HEK. Also, the primary cytokine TNF-α was not detected, and IL-1α was tenfold lower than control at 25 μM SM exposure. IL-1β did not change from control. Many inflammatory cytokine and cytokine receptor transcripts on the cDNA array blot were not expressed by HEK (data not shown).

Inflammation-associated transcripts isolated by subtraction library differed from those catalogued from the cDNA array except for IL-8. IL-8 was the predominant upregulated transcript, representing over 25% of the isolated transcripts in the 16-hr library produced following 200 μM SM exposure. IL-8 was also isolated in an 8-hr 200 μM SM library, but the transcript was not found in either 8- or 16-hr subtraction libraries generated after 25 μM SM exposure. Another inflammation-associated transcript in the upregulated library isolated at 16 hr after 200 μM SM was nuclear factor of activated T-cells (NF-AT). The 8-hr upregulated 200 μM SM subtraction library also contained annexin I. Upregulated transcripts in libraries produced at the 25 μM SM exposure were tissue factor at 16 hr and interleukin 1α and tissue factor at 8 hr.

DISCUSSION AND CONCLUSIONS

The investigation of SM gene changes using Atlas™ cDNA arrays leads to an initial concern about normalizing data to a specific baseline gene. In past studies, we have normalized our data with the commonly used housekeeping gene glyceraldehyde 3-phosphate dehydrogenase (Schlager et al., 1998). However, this gene was subsequently isolated in series subtraction libraries generated from HEK exposure to SM, which suggests the transcript was changing with SM exposure. Also isolated in HEK subtraction libraries following SM were the housekeeping gene transcripts for α-tubulin, β-actin, 23 kDa highly basic protein, and ribosomal protein S9. For this reason, these transcripts were eliminated from consideration as normalization genes. HLA class I histocompatibility antigen C-4 alpha chain [MHC], ubiquitin, 14-3-3 zeta protein (listed as phospholipase A2) and hypoxanthine-guanine phosphoribosyltransferase were not found in any library. However, the 14-3-3 zeta protein appears to change with SM exposure (Table 23.1) based on global normalization. Ubiquitin was also not considered further due to two concerns. The first was due to its constitutively high transcript expression level that made it difficult to use due to overexposure problems during extended exposure experiments. The second was that multiple proteosome transcripts, which involve digestion of ubiquitinated proteins, were isolated in upregulated subtraction libraries from SM-exposed HEK. This raised concerns about potential changes in ubiquitin protein levels as well as its transcript over time. Hypoxanthine-guanine phosphoribosyltransferase did not produce sufficient expression intensity over background with the short time exposures for the phosphoimage data to be useful for calculations in this study. Finally, the HLA class I histocompatibility antigen C-4 alpha chain [MHC] transcript did appear to be the best single housekeeping gene candidate based on these limited data. However, further quantitative studies using this MHC transcript will be needed to determine its utility for SM exposure concentration and time postexposure data to show whether it is better for transcript normalization compared with use of the total sum density of expressed transcripts.

In this preliminary set of experiments, inflammation-associated transcripts were detected using both techniques. On the cDNA array, the predominant inflammatory transcripts expressed at 16 hr after 200 μM SM were IL-8 and MIP-2α. Our lab has reported increases in HEK IL-8 transcript by SM previously (Schlager, 1998), and recently other investigators reported similar findings (Lardot et al., 1999). Keratinocytes can readily induce IL-8 through diverse noxious stimuli. Subclasses of compounds found to increase HEK IL-8 protein include not only proinflammatory cytokines, but also endotoxins, tumor promoters, cell cycle modulators, and compounds that enhance reactive oxygen species (Wilmer and Luster, 1995). Generally, these transcripts represent a secondary transcript response produced by receptor-specific stimulation through binding of primary cytokines such as by TNF-α on TNF receptor following damage elicitation. Therefore, sulfur mustard could elicit the expression of IL-8 through multiple influences producing an additive stimulus on HEK including increasing the primary cytokine, influencing the cell cycle, changing cellular oxidation state, or directly alkylating or crosslinking specific receptors to produce activated receptors that may initiate a secondary cytokine response.

HEK produce a strong IL-8 expression following SM only at a vesicating concentration, which suggests IL-8 plays an important role in the tissue proinflammatory event(s) contributing to skin pathology. From these limited data, IL-8 also appears to be the most induced transcript, which suggests it could be used as a sensitive biomarker in controlled SM experiments for determining treatment and pretreatment regimens. For *in vivo* screening purposes, the best models would be those with a strong IL-8 response, such as rabbit skin, which has been shown to express IL-8 after SM exposure (Tsuruta et al., 1996), or swine as the skin model, which would also be capable of eliciting an IL-8 response. However, another C-X-C cytokine such as mouse MIP-2 would be required for monitoring in rodents, since MIP-2 is the closest homolog of human IL-8 (Lee et al., 1995).

MIP-2α was the second most amplified inflammatory protein transcript elicited by SM exposure. MIP-2α is a C-X-C chemokine similar to IL-8 known to stimulate migration of human blood monocytes (Roth et al., 1995; Uguccioni et al., 1996), as well as activated memory-type T cells and naive-type T lymphocytes through the blood vessel endothelium (Roth et al., 1995). The mouse macrophage MIP-2 expression can be induced by vanadium, and this induction has been influenced by addition of N-acetylcysteine, which suggests that, like IL-8, oxidative damage could also elicit MIP-2α (Chong et al., 2000). No specific literature reference was found associating MIP-2α with either HEKs or human skin epidermis expression. However, the expression of MIP-2α and IL-8 transcript shows that HEKs are actively recruiting inflammatory cells.

Another inflammation-associated secondary chemokine transcript upregulated at high SM concentration was the S19 ribosomal protein. S19 ribosomal protein forms dimers that were initially isolated in the chronic inflammatory disease rheumatoid arthritis (Yamamoto et al., 1996; Horino et al., 1998) and has been found to produce a monocyte predominate infiltrate (Yamamoto, 2000). How this protein is subsequently expressed in HEK and whether S19 proinflammatory dimers are formed following SM requires further study.

The cDNA array data for 25 μM SM concentration show that this exposure differed dramatically from the 200 μM SM in proinflammatory gene transcription with no overlap in inflammatory mediator induction. The low-dose SM exposure stimulated an increase in two other transcripts, the antiinflammatory transcript IL-13 protein and the proapoptotic and inflammatory nerve growth factor/CD40 ligand receptor. IL-13 receptor stimulation has been shown to block the effects of primary cytokines such as that seen following ultraviolet light B exposure (Saade et al., 2000). No IL-13 receptor transcript was detected in HEK in this study, which suggests that IL-13 expression may protect against stimulation of proinflammatory cytokines from other cells. IL-13 has been found to increase collagen deposition by fibroblasts and inhibit IL-1β-induced matrix metalloproteinase MMP-1 and

MMP-3, and enhance the tissue inhibitor of metalloproteinase (Oriente et al., 2000). This antiinflammatory protein may aid in the modulation of skin proinflammatory transcript induction at subvesicating SM exposure. Also, CD40 tumor necrosis-like receptor was upregulated at low concentration but not found at high concentration. CD40 ligation on keratinocytes can enhance CD54 expression and secretion of IL-8 (Van Kooten and Banchereau, 1997). Increased IL-8 expression did not occur in these cells at this concentration of SM. These findings require further investigation to determine the receptor function and whether it has involvement in proinflammation or a role in creating a proapoptotic state for the cell.

Using the subtraction library procedure, the inflammation-associated transcripts isolated differed considerably from those cataloged from the cDNA array except for the predominant transcript IL-8. IL-8 represented 25% of the library generated at 16 hr following high SM concentration exposure to HEK. Similar to cDNA array data, IL-8 was not detected in the low dose subtraction libraries. Other inflammation-associated transcripts were isolated as single colony observations in both upregulated libraries at 8- and 16-hr studies. Most transcripts were not present on the cDNA array. Further analysis using transcript and protein quantitation methods is required to ensure that these transcripts significantly are changed and to make certain the proteins from these transcripts subsequently participate in the inflammatory protein profile produced by SM.

In this study, the HEK cultured in defined keratinocyte growth medium expressed enhanced levels of three primary cytokines following exposure to high SM concentration, TNF-α, IL-1β, and IL-1α. Each of these transcripts produces a protein cytokine that either singly or in combination can produce a variety of responses depending on the time and level of expression to subsequently induce IL-8. Determining how these primary cytokines are temporally expressed, especially a short time following SM exposure, will be of significant interest, since each cytokine can increase one another as well as the major secondary cytokines found in this study (Boxman et al., 1996).

In conclusion, IL-8 transcript is strongly expressed from SM-exposed HEK and could serve as a biomarker for screening of therapeutic prevention of SM inflammation in human cells and tissues and in animal models that elicit IL-8 (rabbit or pig). Although normal cultured HEK can express a multitude of specific proinflammatory and antiinflammatory transcripts (Schröder, 1995), these data show that HEKs, which are known to be the center of SM tissue damage by histopathology, elicit a specific set of transcripts that would mediate proinflammatory events. The proteins produced from transcript expression would participate in the exacerbation of a skin-blistering event. Using cDNA arrays and subtraction library production as a broad endpoint approach in a simple cell system permits the determination of how an individual human cell type may participate in this complex tissue response. Further investigation using transcript and protein quantitation methods with more complex human and animal skin models is required to understand the participation of these proinflammatory proteins produced from these transcripts in human SM pathology. These present data will be used as better selection criteria for appropriate *in vitro* and *in vivo* models to test treatments and therapy and to evaluate their expression modulation following drug treatment of the SM lesion formation and subsequent healing.

REFERENCES

Boxman, I.L., Ruwhof, C., Boerman, O.C., Lowik, C.W., and Ponec, M. (1996) Role of fibroblasts in the regulation of proinflammatory interleukin IL-1, IL-6 and IL-8 levels induced by keratinocyte-derived IL-1, *Arch. Dermatol. Res.,* 288, 391–398.

Chong, I.W., Lin, S.R., Hwang, J.J., Huang, M.S., Wang, T.H., Tsai, M.S., Hou, J.J., and Paulauskis, J.D. (2000) Expression and regulation of macrophage inflammatory protein-2 gene by vanadium in mouse macrophages, *Inflammation,* 24, 127–139.

Diatchenko, L., Lau, Y.-F.C., Campbell, A.P., Chenchik, A., Moqadam, F., Huang, B., Lukyanov, S., Lukyanov, K., Gurskaya, N., Sverdlov, E.D., and Siebert, P.D. (1996) Suppression subtraction hybridization: a method for generating differentially regulated or tissue-specific cDNA probes and libraries, *Proc. Natl. Acad. Sci. U.S.A.,* 93, 6025–6030.

Farrell, R.E., Jr. (1993) *RNA Methodologies: A Guide for Isolation and Characterization,* Academic Press, San Diego.

Hart, B.W. and Schlager, J.J. (1997) Okadaic acid and calyculin A reverse sulfur mustard-induced G2-M cell-cycle block in human keratinocytes, *J. Am. College Toxicol.,* 15, S36–S42.

Horino, K., Nishiura, H., Ohsako, T., Shibuya, Y., Hiraoka, T., Kitamura, N., and Yamamoto, A. (1998) A monocyte chemotactic factor, S19 ribosomal protein dimer, in phagocytic clearance of apoptotic cells, *Lab. Invest.,* 78, 603–617.

Lardot, C., Dubois, V., and Lison, D. (1999) Sulfur mustard upregulates the expression of interleukin-8 in cultured human keratinocytes, *Toxicol. Lett.,* 110, 29–33.

Lee, J., Cacalano, G., Camerato, T., Toy, K., Moore, M.W., and Wood, W.I. (1995) Chemokine binding and activities mediated by the mouse IL-8 receptor, *J. Immunol.,* 15, 2158–2164.

Oriente, A., Fedarko, N.S., Pacocha, S.E., Huang, S.K., Lichtenstein, L.M., and Essayan, D.M. (2000) Interleukin-13 modulates collagen homeotatis in human skin and keloid fibroblasts, *J. Pharmacol. Exp. Ther.,* 292, 988–994.

Papirmeister, B., Feister, A.J., Robinson, S.I., and Ford, R.D. (1991) *Medical Defense against Mustard Gas: Toxic Mechanisms and Pharmacological Implications,* CRC Press, Boca Raton, FL, pp. 43–78.

Petrali, J.P. and Ogesby-Megee, S. (1997) Toxicity of mustard gas skin lesions, *Microsc. Res. Tech.,* 37, 221–228.

Roth, S.J., Carr, M.W., and Springer, T.A. (1995) C-C chemokines, but not the C-X-C chemokines interleukin-8 and interferon-gamma inducible protein-10, stimulate transendothelial chemotaxis of T lymphocytes, *Eur. J. Immunol.,* 25, 3482–3488.

Saade, N.E., Nasr, I.W., Masaad, C.A., Safieh-Garabedian, B., Jabbar, S.J., and Kaanan, S.A. (2000) Modulation of ultraviolet-induced hyperalgesia and cytokine upregulation by interleukin 10 and 13, *Br. J. Pharmacol.,* 131, 1317–1324.

Schlager, J.J. (1998) Keratinocyte gene transcription changes following sulfur mustard exposure, *Proc. U.S. Army 1998 Med. Def. Bioscience Rev.,* U S. Army Medical Research Institute of Chemical Defense, Aberdeen Proving Ground, MD.

Schröder, J.-M. (1995) Cytokine networks in the skin, *J. Invest. Dermatol.,* 105, 20S–24S.

Smith, W.J., Saunders, K.M., Ruddle, S.E., and Gross, C.L. (1993) Cytometric analysis of DNA changes induced by sulfur mustard, *J. Toxicol. Cutaneous Ocular Toxicol.,* 12, 337–343.

Tsuruta, J., Sugisaki, K., Dannenberg, A.M., Jr., Yoshimura, T., Abe, Y., and Mounts, P. (1996) The cytokines NAP-1 (IL-8), MCP-1, IL-1 beta, and GRO in rabbit inflammatory skin lesions produced by the chemical irritant sulfur mustard, *Inflammation,* 20, 293–318.

Uguccioni, M., D'Apuzzo, M., Loetscher, M., Dewald, B., and Baggiolini, M. (1996) Actions of the chemotactic cytokines MCP-1, MCP-2, MCP-3, RANTES, MIP-1 alpha and MIP-1 beta on human monocytes, *Eur. J. Immunol.*, 25, 64–68.

Van Kooten, C. and Banchereau, J. (1997) Functions of CD40 on B cells, dendritic cells and other cells, *Curr. Op. Immunol.*, 9, 330–337.

Wilmer, J.L. and Luster, M.I. (1995) Chemical induction of interleukin-8, a proinflammatory chemokine, in human epidermal keratinocyte cultures and its relation to cytogenetic toxicity, *Cell Biol. Toxicol.*, 11, 37–50.

Yamamoto, T. (2000) Molecular mechanisms of monocyte predominate infiltration in chronic inflammation: mediation by monocyte chemotactic factor, S19 ribosomal protein dimmer, *Pathol. Int.*, 50, 863–871.

Yamamoto, T., Nishiura, H., and Nishida, H. (1996) Molecular mechanisms to form leukocyte infiltration patterns distinct between synovial tissue and fluid of rheumatoid arthritis, *Semin. Thromb. Hemost.*, 22, 507–511.

CHAPTER 24

Evaluation of Cytotoxicity Assays of Human Epidermal Keratinocytes Exposed *In Vitro* to Sulfur Mustard

Susan A. Kelly, Juanita J. Guzman, Clark L. Gross, and William J. Smith

CONTENTS

INTRODUCTION

Sulfur mustard (2,2′-dichlorodiethyl sulfide, HD) is a vesicating chemical warfare agent that produces injury to the skin, eyes, and lungs. It has been a military threat since World War I. To develop therapeutic regimens, PBL and HEKs have been used as models to study the cytotoxic effects of HD. Previous studies have demonstrated that cell viability decreases when cells are exposed to HD (Smith et al., 1990, 1991). However, there have been problems with dye uptake as a measure of cytotoxicy in HEKs (Smith et al., 1996). This dye uptake problem may be the result of the trypsinization process required for isolation of the HEKs. The assays we screened allowed the cells to remain in 24-well plates for the entire procedure.

EXPERIMENT

Reagents

Keratinocyte growth media (KGM) and HEKs were purchased from Clonetics Corporation, San Diego, CA. Calcein AM was purchased from Molecular Probes, Eugene, OR. Alamar blue was purchased from AccuMed International, Inc., Chicago, IL. Neutral red, propidium iodide, and other laboratory chemicals were purchased from Sigma Chemical Co., St. Louis, MO. Sulfur mustard (HD, CAS registry 505-60-2, 98% pure) was obtained from The U.S. Army Edgewood Research, Development and Engineering Center, Aberdeen Proving Ground, MD.

Keratinocyte Growth

Normal human epidermal keratinocytes were purchased as second passage cells from Clonetics. The cells were grown and subcultured and then dispensed into tissue culture plates at the appropriate density for experimentation.

Agent Exposure

HD (98% pure obtained from the Edgewood Chemical Biological Center, Aberdeen Proving Ground, MD) was diluted with KGM (Keratinocyte growth media) and added to the cell culture plates to yield a final concentration from 50 B 300 μM. After 1 hr at room temperature in a chemical surety hood, the tissue culture plates were transferred to a 37°C incubator for the duration of the postexposure incubation period.

Calcein AM

At 24 hr postexposure, the media were removed from each well. In the dark, 1 ml of calcein-AM (10 μM) was added to each well. The trays were incubated for 1 hr at 37°C. The calcein-AM was then removed from each well, and 300 μl of RPMI 1640 (without phenol red) was added. The plates were read on a Cytofluor multiwell plate reader with the excitation set at 485 nm and emission read at 530 nm.

Alamar Blue

At 24 hr postexposure, the media were removed and each well was rinsed three times with RPMI 1640 (without phenol red). After the third rinse, 500 μl of alamar blue (5% v/v) were added to each well, in the dark. The plate was then incubated at

37°C for 90 min. At the end of the incubation time, the cell culture plate was read on a Cytofluor multiwell plate reader with the excitation set at 530 nm and emission read at 590 nm.

Neutral Red

At 24 hr postexposure, in the dark, 1 ml of neutral red (500 µg/ml) was added to each well. The plate was then incubated for 1 hr at 37°C. The neutral red was removed, and 1 ml of a 50% ethanol/1% acetic acid solution was added to each well. The plate was incubated for 30 min at 37°C. Two hundred microliters of each sample was transferred to a clean 96-well plate. The 96-well plate was placed in the microplate scanning spectrophotometer, and the absorbance at 550 nm was determined.

MTS

A colorimetric assay of cell viability from Promega (Madison, WI) that employs a methoxy tetrazolium salt (MTS) in the presence of an electron coupling agent phenazine methosulfate (PMS) was evaluated. At 24 hr postexposure, 200 µl of MTS/PMS solution was added to each well in the dark. The tray was incubated at 37°C for 2 hr. Two hundred microliters of each sample were transferred to a clean 96-well plate. The 96-well plate was placed in the microplate scanning spectrophotometer, and the absorbance at 500 nm was determined.

Propidium Iodide

At 24 hr postexposure to HD, 200 µL of each sample was transferred to a 12 × 75-mm test tube. Two hundred microliters of KGM was added to each tube. Fifty microliters of propidium iodide (0.3 mg/ml) was added to each tube and incubated at room temperature for approximately 3 to 5 min. The tubes were then placed in the flow cytometer, and viabilities were determined with excitation at 488 nm and emission between 580 and 650 nm.

RESULTS

HEKs were exposed to 50, 100, and 300 µM concentrations of HD and then incubated for 24 hr at 37°C. Viabilities were determined using calcein AM (measures membrane integrity), alamar blue (indicator of mitochondrial metabolism), neutral red (indicator of lysosomal activity), and MTS (indicator of mitochondrial dehydrogenase activity) as described in the experimental section. As shown in Figure 24.1, calcein AM, alamar blue, and PI demonstrated about a 40% loss in viability when HEKs are exposed to 300 µM HD. There was very little loss in viability at 50 and 100 µM HD levels. Neutral red and MTS only show about a 10% decrease in viability of HEKs exposed to 300 µM HD. These can be compared to our historic data for viable cell number, which shows almost a 70% loss in viability at 300 µM HD.

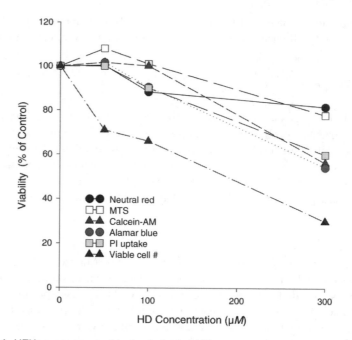

Figure 24.1 HEKs were exposed to the indicated HD concentrations and then incubated for 24 hr at 37°C. Viabilities were determined by using these dyes as described in the Experimental section.

DISCUSSION

Both chromogenic and fluorometric dyes can be used to assess viability in HEKs exposed *in vitro* to HD. Six different measures of cell viability have been analyzed. Viable cell number appears to be the most sensitive indicator of HD cytotoxicity. The fluorescent dyes, calcein AM (an indicator of membrane integrity), alamar blue (an indicator of mitochondrial metabolism), and PI uptake appear to be the next most sensitive assays for analysis of viability in HEKs. MTS and neutral red appeared to be equal in sensitivity, but not good indicators of HEK cell viability. Calcein AM and alamar blue appear to be reliable indicators of the viability status of HD-exposed HEKs assessed *in situ* in microplates. They may not be as sensitive a measurement as the viable cell number using trypsinized HEKs, but it is not known at this time whether the trypsinization step leads to artifactual results.

REFERENCES

Gross, C.L., Corun, C.M., Kelly, S.A., and Smith, W.J. (1998) A Rapid Assay for Cytoxicity in Sulfur Mustard Exposed Isolated Human Peripheral Blood Lymphocytes, paper presented at the Proceedings of the 1998 Medical Defense Bioscience Review.

Smith, W.J., Blank, J.A., Starner, R.A., Menton, R.G., and Harris, J. (1996) Effect of Sulfur Mustard Exposure on Human Epidermal Keratinocyte Viability and Protein Content, paper presented at the Proceedings of the 1996 Medical Defense Bioscience Review (DTIC accession AD A321841).

Smith, W.J., Gross, C.L., Chan, P., and Meier, H.L. (1990) The use of human epidermal keratinocytes in culture as a model for studying the biochemical mechanisms of sulfur mustard toxicity, *Cell Biol. Toxicol.*, 6, 285–291.

Smith, W.J., Sanders, K.M., Gales, Y.A., and Gross, C.L. (1991) Flow cytometric analysis of toxicity by vesicating agents in human cells *in vitro*, *J. Toxicol. Cutaneous Ocular Toxicol.*, 10, 33–42.

CHAPTER **25**

Comparison of Spectrophotometric and Fluorometric Assays of Proteolysis in Cultured Human Cells Exposed to Sulfur Mustard

Susan A. Kelly, Charlene M. Corun, Marian R. Nelson, Clark L. Gross, and William J. Smith

CONTENTS

INTRODUCTION

Sulfur mustard (2,2'-dichlorodiethyl sulfide, HD) is a potent vesicating agent whose mechanism of blister formation is poorly understood. Microscopic examination of the lesion intimates the involvement of proteolysis in the cascade of events leading to the epidermal–dermal separation and consequent formation of the blister (Papirmeister et al., 1985). HD exposure of isolated human blood lymphocytes (PBLs, Meier and Johnson, 1992), human epidermal keratinocytes (HEKs, Smith et al., 1990), living skin equivalent cultures (Cowan et al., 1993), and hairless guinea pig skin (Cowan et al., 1994) has demonstrated increased serine protease activity in these model systems. These results have led to the design of medical countermeasures against the vesicating activity of sulfur mustard, and many candidate antivesicant compounds have been synthesized that require screening for efficacy. The screening process demands the development of both sensitive and reproducible *in vitro* assays that can be used to quantitate the biomarkers formed as the result of HD exposure in target tissues. We have investigated the use of commercial protease substrates with either chromogenic or fluorogenic properties to measure the biomarker, proteolytic activity, in both PBLs and HEKs that have been exposed to HD. The measurement of proteolytic activity was quantitated by both spectrophotometric and fluorometric methods. Suitability of these assays for the screening of potential medical countermeasure efficacy will be assessed.

MATERIALS AND METHODS

Reagents

RPMI 1640 tissue culture media, gentamycin, and other laboratory chemicals were obtained from Sigma Chemical Co., St. Louis, MO. Percoll was obtained from Pharmacia, Piscataway, NJ. Chromozym® substrates were obtained from Boehringer-Mannheim, Indianapolis, IN. CellProbe® enzyme substrates were obtained from Coulter Corporation, Miami, FL. Keratinocyte growth media (KGM) and HEKs were purchased from Clonetics Corporation, San Diego, CA. Sulfur mustard (HD, CAS registry 505-60-2, 98% pure) was obtained from the Edgewood Chemical Biological Center, Aberdeen Proving Ground, MD.

Lymphocyte Isolation

Human PBLs were obtained from whole blood by venipuncture from human volunteers under an approved human use protocol. The lymphocytes were isolated by Percoll (density = 1.08) centrifugation (Meier and Johnson, 1992), and the mononuclear layer was collected, washed, and diluted in RPMI containing gentamycin (50 µg/ml) to a final concentration of 2×10^7 cells/ml. Cells were then dispensed into tissue culture plates at the appropriate density for experimentation.

Keratinocyte Growth

Normal human epidermal keratinocytes were purchased as second passage cells from Clonetics. The cells were grown, subcultured, and then dispensed into tissue culture plates at the appropriate density for experimentation (Smith et al., 1991).

HD Exposure

HD was diluted into either KGM (for keratinocytes) or RPMI (for lymphocytes) and added to the appropriate cell culture plates in a chemical surety hood to yield final HD concentrations ranging from 50 to 300 μM. After 1 hr at room temperature to allow hydrolysis of agent, the tissue culture plates were transferred to a 37°C incubator under a humidified 5% CO_2 atmosphere for the duration of the postexposure incubation period.

Chromozym® Assay (24 hr Postexposure to HD)

Keratinocytes

Twenty microliters of the appropriate Chromozym substrate was added to each well of the 24-well plate. The plates were incubated for 1 hr at 37°C. Fifty microliters of supernate was removed from each sample and placed into a 96-well plate. The 24-well plate was returned to the incubator. The 96-well plate was placed in the microplate scanning spectrophotometer and the absorbance at 405 nm was determined. The last two steps were repeated again at 4 hr.

Lymphocytes

Supernate, 100 µl, was removed and discarded from each well. An aliquot of 100 µl of 2.5×10^{-3} M Chromozym® TH was added to each well for a final volume of 150 µl. The plate was incubated at 37°C for 1 hr. An aliquot of 100 µl of supernate was removed and added to a clean 96-well plate. The 96-well plate was placed in the microplate scanning spectrophotometer, and the absorbance at 405 nm was determined.

Intracellular Protease Activity

At 20 hr postexposure to HD, 25 µl of each CellProbe enzyme substrate was added to the appropriate wells of the 24-well plate. The plates were then incubated for 4 hr at 37°C. Fluorescence was then measured using the CytoFluor multiwell plate reader with excitation set at 485 nm and emission read at 530 nm.

RESULTS

The compounds used in this investigation are found in Figure 25.1.

Chromozym® Substrates
Chromozym® TH   Tosyl-glycyl-prolyl-arginine-4-nitranilide acetate
Chromozym® t-PA   N-Methylsulfonyl-D-Phe-Gly-Arg-4-nitranilide acetate
Chromozym® TRY   Carbobenzoxy- valyl-glycyl-arginine-4-nitrilanilide acetate
Chromozym® U   Benzoyl-β-alanyl-glycyl-arginine-4-nitranilide acetate

CellProbe® Enzyme Substrates:
Nonfluorescent   (aa)x -Fl   Fluorescent Dye +
Substrate-Dye complex   ⇒⇒⇒   Nonfluorescent
                                                Substrate leaving group

Enzyme	Substrate
AAPV- Elastase (AAPV)	Dl-Alanyl-Alanyl-Prolyl-Rho 110
D-aminopeptidase A (DAA)	Asp-Asp-Rho 110
K-Aminopeptidase B (KAB)	Lysine-Lysine-Rho 110
G-Aminopeptidase (GA)	Gly-Gly-Rho 100
L- Aminopeptidase (LA)	Leu-Leu-Rho
A- Aminopeptidase M (AAM)	Alanine-Alanine-Rho 110
R- Aminopeptidase B (RAB)	Arginine-Arginine-Rho 110

Figure 25.1 Substrate descriptions.

Chromozym® Assay

Protease activity of PBL was measured in two donors as a function of cell number, and 2×10^6 cells/well exhibited a better response than 1×10^6 cells/well (Figure 25.2). When the concentration was increased to 3×10^6 cells/well, the response was no better than 2×10^6 cells/well.

The response was also found to be donor dependent. Out of the 11 donors that were screened, 5 exhibited a reproducible, positive response and had consistent responses from study to study. The PBLs from these 5 donors were then exposed to HD and incubated for 24 hr, and the protease activity was measured by using the Chromozym® TH substrate as described in the Materials and Methods section. There was a significant reproducible increase in protease activity as shown in Figure 25.3.

HEK that had been exposed to HD and incubated for 24 hr showed a significant increase in urokinase and tissue plasminogen activator-like activity at 300 μM HD (Figure 25.4). There was little change in the trypsin and thrombin levels. As consistent with previous reportings, keratinocytes only show response in 50% of the studies conducted, but the reason for this variation is currently unknown.

CellProbe® Assay

Protease activity in HEK after HD exposure was measured fluorometrically as described in the Materials and Methods section. Substrates K aminopeptidase B and G aminopeptidase were hydrolyzed significantly above the control values, while elastase AAPV and D aminopeptidase showed a decrease in enzyme activity (Figure 25.5). Substrates A Aminopeptidase and R Aminopeptidase B exhibited a small increase in activity, while substrate L Aminopeptidase showed no response.

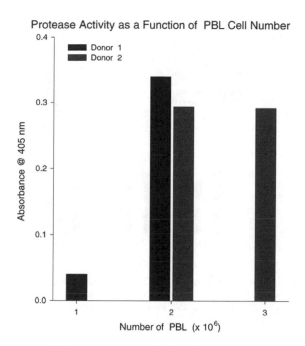

Figure 25.2 Protease activity was measured in two donors as a function of cell number. Increasing the cell concentration above 2 × 10⁶/well did not increase protease activity and this concentration was used in all subsequent studies.

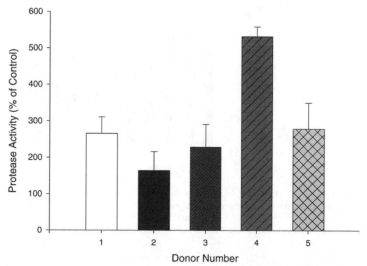

Figure 25.3 PBL from five different donors were exposed to 250 μ*M* HD and then incubated for 24 hr. Protease activity using the Chromozym® TH substrate was measured as described in Material and Methods. Significant protease activity occurred reproducibly. All assays were run in triplicate and all donors were evaluated multiple times on different days.

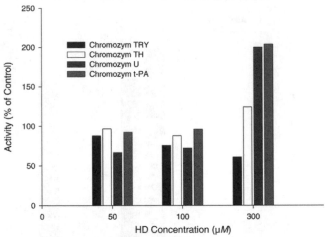

Figure 25.4 HEK were exposed to indicated HD concentrations and incubated for 20 hr. Chromogenic protease assays were performed as described in the Materials and Methods. The protease activity was only evident at the highest concentration of HD, and only the Chromozym® U and Chromozym® t-PA substrates were significantly hydrolyzed.

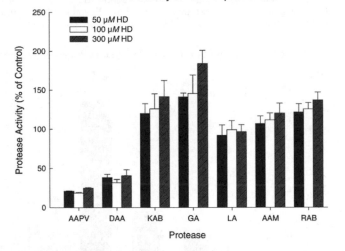

Figure 25.5 HEK were exposed to HD at the indicated concentrations, and protease activity was measured fluorometrically 24 hr later as described in the Material and Methods section. KAB and GA substrates were significantly hydrolyzed above the control values while elastase (AAPV) and DAA were decreased.

SUMMARY

Protease profiles were different in the two *in vitro* models tested here. PBLs showed a significant increase in proteolysis using the serine protease substrates

Chromozym® TH and Chromozym® TRY. Reproducible protease activity was found in 5 out of the 11 donors tested. We have previously reported that PBLs show a general decline in all aminopeptidase activity tested when using fluorescent substrates (Smith et al., 1998). Protease profiles were more complicated when HEKs were assessed. No changes in aminopeptidase activities were detected after exposure to HD when HEKs were trypsinized and analyzed by flow cytometry. However, HEKs assayed *in situ* in microplates showed an increase in K aminopeptidase B and G aminopeptidase and a decrease in elastase and D aminopeptidase A, but L aminopeptidase was unchanged. The reason for this variability is unknown, but may be due to culturing and handling procedures. Before HEK can be used as an *in vitro* method to screen compounds, a considerable amount of research must be done to determine the cause of these variabilities.

REFERENCES

Cowan, F.M., Bongiovanni, R., Broomfield, C.A., Shultz, S.M., and Smith, W.J. (1994) Sulfur mustard increases elastase-like activities in homogenates of hairless guinea pig skin, *J. Toxicol. Cutaneous Ocular Toxicol.,* 13, 221–229.

Cowan, F.M., Yourick, J.J., Hurst, C.G., Broomfield, C.A., and Smith, W.J. (1993) Sulfur mustard increased-proteolysis following *in vitro* and *in vivo* exposures, *Cell Biol. Toxicol.,* 9, 253–261.

Meier, H.L. and Johnson, J.B. (1992) The determination and prevention of cytotoxic effects induced in lymphocytes by the alkylating agent 2,2'dichlorodiethyl sulfide (sulfur mustard, HD), *Toxicol. Appl. Pharmacol.,* 113, 234–239.

Papirmeister, B., Gross, C.L., Meier, H.L., Petrali, J.P., and Johnson, J.B. (1985) Molecular basis for mustard-induced vesication, *Fundam. Appl. Toxicol.,* 5, 134–149.

Smith, W.J., Gross, C.L., Chan, P., and Meier, H.L. (1990) The use of human epidermal keratinocytes in culture as a model for studying the biochemical mechanisms of sulfur mustard toxicity, *Cell Biol. Toxicol.,* 6, 285–291.

Smith, W.J., Kelly, S.A., Clark, O.E., III, DeJoseph, M.E., and Gross, C.L. (1998) Fluorometric analysis of intracellular changes induced by sulfur mustard in cultured human epidermal keratinocytes, *Int. Soc. Anal. Cytol.* (Colorado), 1998.

Smith, W.J., Sanders, K.M., Gales, Y.A., and Gross, C.L. (1991) Flow cytometric analysis of toxicity by vesicating agents in human cells *in vitro, J. Toxicol. Cutaneous Ocular Toxicol.,* 10, 33–42.

CHAPTER **26**

Effects of Low Dose Sulfur Mustard on Growth and DNA Damage in Human Cells in Culture

William J. Smith, Bethany S. Toliver, Offie E. Clark III, Janet Moser, Eric W. Nealley, Juanita J. Guzman, and Clark L. Gross

CONTENTS

INTRODUCTION

Sulfur mustard (2,2'-dichloroethyl sulfide, Army designation HD) is a potent cytotoxic chemical agent with vesicating (blistering) properties upon contact with human skin. Development of medical countermeasures to protect individuals from injury following attack by this chemical warfare weapon requires an understanding of the mechanisms by which the pathology is generated. DNA is believed to be a major macromolecular target of HD in the epidermis. Using human epidermal keratinocytes (HEKs) and human peripheral blood lymphocytes (PBLs) in culture, we evaluated the effects of HD on DNA as assessed by the comet single cell electrophoresis assay. In addition, we evaluated survival and growth of HEKs through the measurement of viable cell number, metabolic fluorescence of alamar blue, and membrane integrity assessment by calcein-AM at various times after exposure to low doses (0.01 to 5.0 μM) of HD. At 5 μM HD, growth of HEKs is retarded for 72 hr but then returns to control levels. Below 5 μM, no inhibition of growth is detected. At 5 μM HD, cross-links formed in PBL DNA inhibit the expression of H_2O_2-induced single strand breaks in the comet assay. Below 5 μM, inhibition of single strand breaks is not observed. Most research with mustard toxicity is conducted at significantly higher dose ranges, >100 μM; such concentrations are believed to be equivalent to the vesicating doses on skin. At those high doses, it is difficult to assess the genotoxicity or growth potential of HEKs exposed to HD *in vitro*. These studies suggest that cells can be exposed to a concentration of HD (1 to 5 μM) that should generate significant DNA damage and still survive the insult. Understanding the biochemical effects at this lower level of exposure may lead to medical countermeasures against the higher, injurious levels of HD damage seen in battlefield conditions.

PURPOSE

- Develop concentration response range for HD-induced inhibition of comet assay detection of single strand breaks by H_2O_2 (Moser et al., 1999).
- Determine whether HEKs behave similarly to PBLs in the comet assay.
- Determine whether monofunctional alkylating agents, i.e., chloroethyl ethyl sulfide (CEES), behave like bifunctional alkylators, i.e., HD, in the comet assay.
- Determine the highest HD concentration that will allow full HEK growth recovery.

MATERIALS AND METHODS

PBL Isolation

Human PBLs were collected from volunteers using an approved human use protocol and then isolated by buoyant density centrifugation.

PBL Exposure

HD or its single-arm mustard analog, chloroethyl ethyl sulfide (CEES) was diluted in RPMI medium and added to the tubes, yielding final concentrations of 0.1 to 50 μM. The tubes were left in the chemical hood at room temperature for 1 hr, then placed in a 37°C, 5% CO_2 incubator for the remainder of the 4-hr time period. Immediately following this end-point, half of the cells from each tube were exposed to 0.001% H_2O_2 for 5 min and the other half of the cells served as agent-exposed controls.

HEK Cultures

Primary cultures of human epidermal keratinocytes (HEKs) were obtained from Clonetics Div, Cambrex (Walkersville, MD). Secondary cultures were set up in 150-cm^2 tissue-culture flasks using keratinocyte growth medium (KGM, Cambrex) and then subcultured as tertiary cultures into tissue culture flasks or multiwell plates. All cultures were maintained in an incubator at 37°C and 5% CO_2.

HEK Exposure

HD or CEES was diluted in KGM and added to the culture vessels, yielding final concentrations of 0.05 to 1000 μM. The vessels were left in the chemical hood at room temperature for 1 hr, then placed in a 37°C, 5% CO_2 incubator for the remainder of the incubation period. Immediately following the incubation period, the HEKs were either harvested by trypsinization for the comet and growth curve assays or left in the wells for the alamar blue and calcein viability assays. For the comet studies, half of the cells from each concentration were exposed to 0.002% H_2O_2 for 5 min and the other half of the cells served as agent-exposed controls.

Comet Assay

Both cell types underwent a slightly modified version of Singh's comet assay protocol (Singh et al., 1988). DNA damage was analyzed using Komet 3.1 imaging software (Kinetic Imaging, Cheshire, U.K.), and the results were expressed as "comet moment," i.e., percentage DNA in tail × tail length. Unexposed cells served as negative controls; cells exposed solely to H_2O_2 were the positive controls.

Viability Assays

At 24, 48, 72, or 96 hr after HD exposure, the media were removed and the wells were washed three times with RPMI. Either alamar blue (5% v/v) or calcein-AM (10 $\mu g/mL$) was added to each well and the plates were returned to the incubator for 1 to 1.5 hr. The plates were then read on a Cytofluor multiwell plate reader (Ex: 530/Em: 590 for alamar blue; Ex: 485/Em: 530 for calcein).

Growth Curve Assay

The cell suspension was removed from each well and washed in phosphate buffered saline. Cell numbers were determined using a Coulter model ZM cell counter. Cell viability was determined by propidium iodide (PI) analysis on a FACSort flow cytometer (Becton Dickinson, San Jose, CA). Viable cell number was calculated as the product of cell number and percent PI positive.

RESULTS

At concentrations greater than 5 μM HD in human PBLs, the expression of hydrogen peroxide DNA fragmentation in the comet assay is blocked (Figure

26.1). A similar pattern is observed in HEKs (Figure 26.2). When cells are exposed to the single arm mustard CEES, no blockage of DNA fragmentation detection is observed in either PBLs (Figure 26.3) or HEKs (Figure 26.4). When the comet

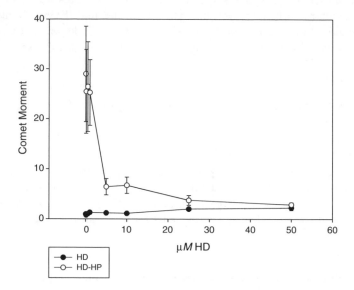

Figure 26.1 PBLs were exposed to buffer or to buffer plus HD. Four hours following exposure, cells were harvested and treated with 0.001% H_2O_2 or buffer. HD concentrations of 5 μM or greater inhibited expression of SSB in the comet assay. Points represent mean ±SEM from two experiments.

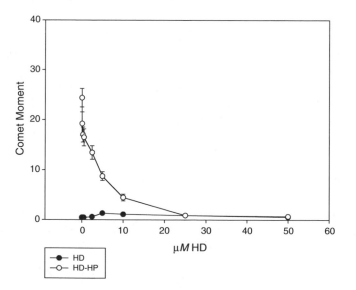

Figure 26.2 HEKs were exposed to buffer or to buffer plus HD. Four hours following exposure, cells were harvested and treated with 0.002% H_2O_2 or buffer. Results are similar to those seen with PBLs. Points represent mean ±SEM from two experiments.

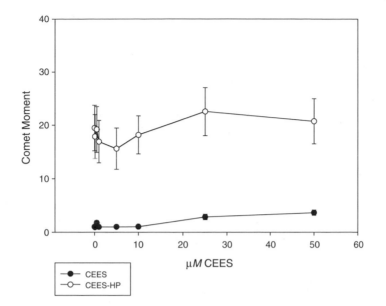

Figure 26.3 PBLs were exposed to buffer or to buffer plus CEES. Four hours following exposure, cells were harvested and treated with 0.001% H_2O_2 or buffer. CEES did not inhibit expression of H_2O_2-induced SSB. Points represent mean ±SEM from two experiments.

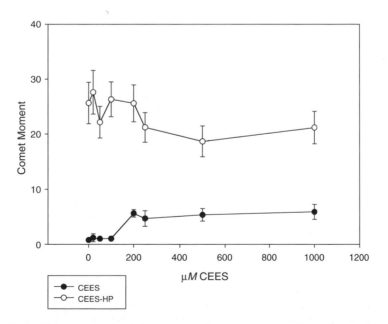

Figure 26.4 HEKs were exposed to buffer or to buffer plus CEES. Four hours following exposure, cells were harvested and treated with 0.002% H_2O_2 or buffer. Results are similar to those seen with PBLs. Points represent mean ±SEM from two experiments.

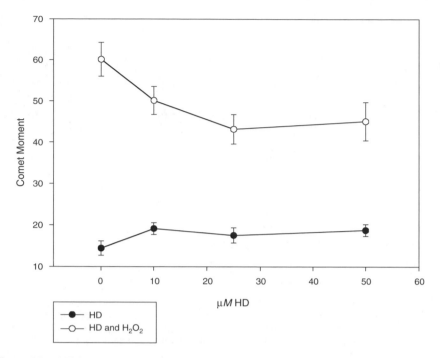

Figure 26.5 HEKs were exposed to buffer or to buffer plus HD. Eighteen hours following exposure, cells were harvested and treated with 0.002% H_2O_2 or buffer. Points represent mean ±SEM from two experiments.

assay was run at 18 hr after HD exposure, the inhibition of H_2O_2-induced fragmentation was markedly reduced (Figure 26.5). By 24 hr after exposure, the inhibition was no longer evident and an additive effect of HD on the detected fragmentation is apparent (Figure 26.6). At concentrations of HD equal to or less than 5 μM, only limited disruption of cell viability (data not shown) or growth was observed (Figure 26.7).

CONCLUSIONS

- The detection of H_2O_2-induced single strand DNA breaks (SSBs) in the comet assay is masked by the bifunctional alkylator sulfur mustard (HD) presumably through cross-link formation.
- The masking function of HD in the comet assay diminishes below 5 μM.
- Keratinocytes behave similarly to PBLs in the comet assay.
- The monofunctional alkylator CEES does not exhibit masking of H_2O_2-induced SSB either in PBLs or HEKs.
- By 24 hr, the inhibitory effects of the presumed crosslinks is no longer evident.
- HEKs can establish a normal growth rate after exposure to 5 μM HD after a lag period of 72 hr.
- Concentrations of HD below 5 μM, while partially masking SSB formation in the comet assay, do not inhibit HEK growth or viability.

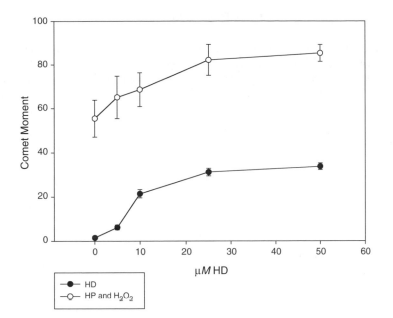

Figure 26.6 HEKs were exposed to buffer or to buffer plus HD. Twenty-four hours following exposure, cells were harvested and treated with 0.002% H_2O_2 or buffer. Points represent mean ±SEM from two experiments.

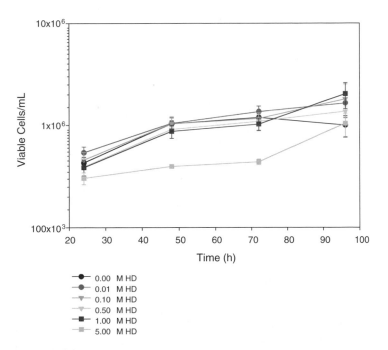

Figure 26.7 Growth curves for HEKs following exposure to HD in culture. Lowest line is for 5 μM concentration.

REFERENCES

Moser, J. et al. (1999) Crosslinking interferes with assessing sulfur mustard-induced DNA damage in human lymphocytes using the comet assay, *Toxicol. Sci.*, 48, 122.

Singh, N.P. et al. (1988) A simple technique for quantitation of low levels of DNA damage in individual cells, *Exp. Cell Res.*, 175, 184–191.

CHAPTER 27

Imaging Sulfur Mustard Lesions in Basal Cells and Human Epidermal Tissues by Confocal and Multiphoton Laser Scanning Microscopy

Robert J. Werrlein and Janna S. Madren-Whalley

CONTENTS

INTRODUCTION

Sulfur mustard [HD, di(2 chloroethyl) sulfide] is a blistering agent that has been used by warring nations for more than 80 years. There is still no completely effective treatment for its vesicating lesions, and that presents a fundamental question. How is skin altered by sulfur mustard so that structural bonds between basal cells and basement membrane are selectively disrupted? We have postulated that, like blistering diseases of the skin, HD may potentiate dermal–epidermal separations by altering molecules of the basal cell's adhesion complex (Werrlein and Madren-Whalley, 2000). Accordingly, we are using confocal and multiphoton laser scanning techniques in an attempt to determine whether there are detectable postexposure changes in the interactive attachment molecules. The adhesion complex model in Figure 27.1 shows a dermal–epidermal separation typical of an HD blister, including the cleavage plane that displaces hemidesmosomes toward the roof of the blister and basement

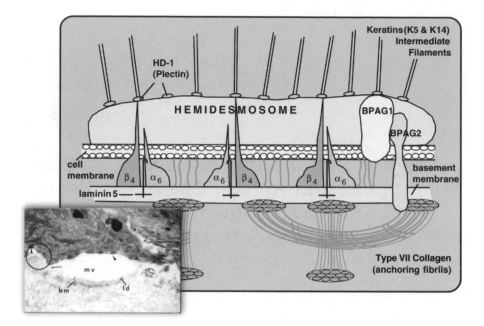

Figure 27.1 Basal cell adhesion complex. A microvesicle (lower left panel) showing details of the dermal–epidermal separations characteristic of a sulfur mustard blister. Hemidesmosomes (arrowhead), at the roof of the blister, are well displaced from the basement membrane (bm) and lamina densa (ld). An expanded model of the intact adhesion complex (circumscribed area) includes the intracellular keratin filaments K5 and K14 and their facilitated attachments to the transmembrane $\alpha_6\beta_4$ integrin receptors. The exodomains of $\alpha_6\beta_4$ are shown linked by laminin 5 to the basement membrane zone.

membrane to the floor of the blister. Postexposure images obtained from the following studies of keratinocyte cultures and epidermal tissues indicate a substantial involvement of the attachment molecules. We are using noninvasive, laser-scanning techniques to determine the onset of these structural and functional changes and to enhance our capacity to develop more effective therapies.

MATERIALS AND METHODS

Human epidermis and keratinocyte (HEK) cultures were prepared as previously described (Werrlein et al., 1999) by gentle proteolytic treatment of surgical explants obtained from the Cooperative Human Tissue Network (Ohio State University, Columbus, OH). HEKs were grown on glass coverslips in keratinocyte growth medium (KGM; Clonetics/Cambrex, Walkersville, MD) at 37°C in a humidified, 5% CO_2 and air incubator and were approximately 70% confluent when subjected to exposure.

Exposure to sulfur mustard was similar for epidermis and HEK cultures. Freshly isolated epidermal tissues were maintained in KGM at 6°C and warmed to room temperature immediately prior to exposure. HEKs were maintained in exponential growth and were subjected to medium renewal with KGM 2 hr prior to exposure.

At exposure, the supernatant media were replaced with 37°C KGM containing 400 μM HD, or KGM only for sham-treated controls. After 5 min, cells and tissues were washed 3× with fresh KGM and returned to the CO_2 incubator.

Fixing and staining of HEK and epidermal tissues at 1 and 2 hr postexposure began with 4% paraformaldehyde at room temperature (10 min for HEK, and 30 min for epidermis). For keratins K5 and K14, HEKs were postfixed with 100% acetone for 3 min at −20°C, then incubated 1 hr at room temp with a 1:50 dilution (in phosphate buffered saline [PBS]) of primary antibody, either mouse antihuman K5 and 8 (clone RCK102; Accurate Chemical and Scientific Co., Westbury, NY) or K14 (clone CKB1; Sigma Chemical Co., St. Louis, MO). For $\alpha_6\beta_4$ integrins, primary antibodies were a 1:50 dilution of mouse antihuman α_6 (clone 4F10; Harlan, Sera-Lab LTD, Loughborough, England) and a 1:100 dilution of mouse antihuman β_4 (clone 3E1; Gibco BRL, Gaithersburg, MD). After a thorough washing with PBS, cells and tissues were incubated 1 hr at room temp with a 1:50 dilution of fluorescein isothiocyanate (FITC)-conjugated goat antimouse IgG (H&L [heavy and light chain]) from Accurate Chemical and Scientific Co. Mouse antihuman keratin 8 (clone M20; Sigma Chemical Co.) was used in replicate HEK cultures to confirm the absence of K8 expression.

Confocal imaging and multiphoton imaging were performed with a Meridian ACAS-570, and an MRC-1024 multiphoton laser scanning microscope (Bio-Rad, Hemel Hempstead, U.K.). Excitation was by a 488 laser line from a 5-Watt argon laser for confocal studies and by a Mira 900 Ti:sapphire pulsed laser (Coherent Laser Group, Santa Clara, CA) at 780 nm for multiphoton studies.

Analyses of confocal images were performed with Meridian quantitative software and Microsoft Excel. Average results for control and HD-exposed populations are presented as the mean ± SEM. Student's t-test was used for statistical comparisons with probabilities of $p < 0.01$ being regarded as statistically significant.

RESULTS

Multiphoton images of keratin 5 in control cultures of HEKs revealed an elaborate cytoskeletal network of intermediate filaments (Figure 27.2A) that was well distributed throughout the cell cytoplasm. Analysis of confocal images from K5 controls and HD-exposed populations (Figures 27.2B,C) showed a statistically significant ($p < 0.01$) 29.2% decrease in image intensity at $T = 1$ hr postexposure. Exposure to HD disrupted but did not affect dissolution of the keratin filaments, nor did it cause a progressive decrease in K5 expression.

Multiphoton images of keratin 14 in control cultures of HEK were very similar to those of keratin 5 (Figure 27.3A). At $T = 1$ hr after exposure to sulfur mustard, there was an obvious disruption of these type I filaments (Figure 27.3B), resulting in their withdrawal from the plasma-membrane margins and in the appearance of punctate, K14 nodules.

Exposure to sulfur mustard caused a statistically significant ($p < 0.01$) 30.14% decrease in the image intensity of K14 at 1 hr postexposure (Figures 27.4A,B), which was similar to the decrease in keratin 5. Unlike K5, however, images obtained

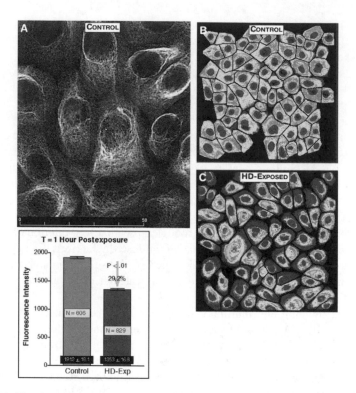

Figure 27.2 Keratin 5 images from control cultures of HEK recorded by multiphoton imaging (A), showed the elaborate cytoskeletal matrix and distribution of these filaments within the cell cytoplasm. Image intensity and K5 concentration were greatest around the nucleus of each cell, and a lacy network of delicate filaments projected out toward the cell extremities. Analysis of confocal images from K5 controls (B) and HD-exposed populations (C) showed a statistically significant ($p < 0.01$) 29.2% decrease in intensity at 1 hr postexposure to sulfur mustard.

with K14 antibody (clone CKB1) indicated a progressive and nearly complete loss of K14 expression at 2 hr postexposure (Figures 27.4C,D).

Multiphoton images of α_6 integrin in the stratum basale of human epidermis provided two-dimensional, three-dimensional, and stereo image details of the *in situ* organization of these heterodimeric, $\alpha_6\beta_4$ receptor subunits. Serial slices (Figures 27.5A,B) provided the outline of organized α_6 in successive cross sections through the skin's epidermal rete pegs and ridges. By three-dimensional reconstruction (Figure 27.5C) and stereo projection of these image slices (Figure 27.5D), we were able to show the topographic complexity of the ventral epidermis and, from it, the extensive distribution and shape of organized α_6-integrin subunits. Optical slices through the intact human epidermis also produced images of β_4 integrin that were distributed and organized on the basal cell surface in small, circular shapes similar to those of α_6 integrin (Figure 27.6).

Exposure of epidermal tissues to HD was associated with disruption and unraveling of the $\alpha_6\beta_4$ integrin circlets and concomitant movement of these receptor subunits toward the basolateral margins of the constituent basal cells (Figure 27.7A).

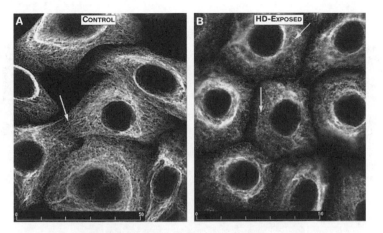

Figure 27.3 Multiphoton keratin 14 images from control HEK cultures (A) showed elaborate cytoskeletal distribution comparable to that of keratin 5. Image intensity and K14 concentration were greatest around the nucleus. Lacy networks of filaments projected out to the cell extremities where they interfaced closely with those of adjacent cells (arrow). At 1 hr postexposure to sulfur mustard, K14 images (B) indicated a disruption of organization, resulting in withdrawal of filaments from the plasma membrane margins, appearance of punctate nodules (arrows), and a substantial loss of cytoskeletal definition.

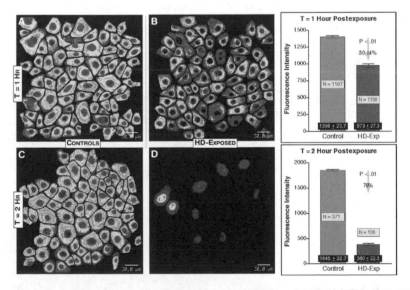

Figure 27.4 Analysis of K14 confocal images from replicate cultures of HEK sham-treated controls (A and C) and HD-exposed populations (B and D) showed a statistically significant (p < 0.01) 30.14% decrease in image intensity (K14 expression) at 1 hr postexposure and a nearly complete loss of expression (79% decrease in image intensity) at 2 hr.

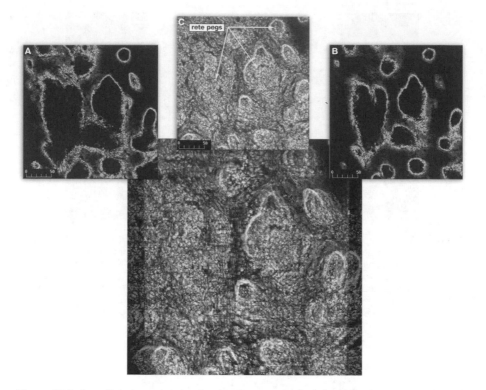

Figure 27.5 A multiphoton montage showing the organization of α_6 integrins on an explant of human epidermis. Serial slices (A and B) illustrate the receptor outline on successive cross sections through the epidermal rete pegs. The three-dimensional reconstruction (C) and the stereo image (D) are from the same Z-series of serial slices. Together, they show the topographic complexity of ventral epidermis plus the circular shape and extensive distribution of $\alpha_6\beta_4$-integrin receptors.

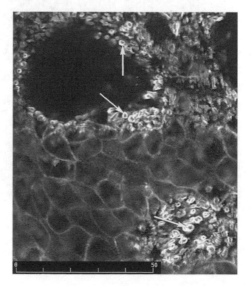

Figure 27.6 A multiphoton image (slice) of human epidermis showing in cross section the distribution and circular shape of β_4 integrins (arrows) on the basal cell surface.

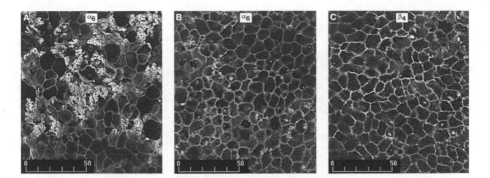

Figure 27.7 Multiphoton images of $\alpha_6\beta_4$ receptors in human epidermis exposed to sulfur mustard indicated unraveling and loss of circular shape at 1 hr postexposure (A) and an almost total loss of $\alpha_6\beta_4$ expression at the basal cell surface by 2 hr postexposure (B, C). At 2 hr postexposure, only a basolateral pattern of residual fluorescence remained to outline the constituent basal cells. Loss of α_6 and β_4 integrin also occurred spontaneously in epidermal tissues following dermal–epidermal separation; therefore, the effects may not be strictly related to sulfur mustard exposure.

By 2 hr postexposure, there was an almost total loss of α_6 and β_4 integrin expression (Figures 27.7B,C).

These integrin events cannot be strictly related to sulfur mustard exposure because the loss of α_6 and β_4 integrin organization also occurred spontaneously following dermal–epidermal separation. However, the basolateral pattern of integrin fluorescence in the exposed epidermis at $T = 2$ hr was strikingly similar to the pattern produced in basal-cell cultures (Figure 27.8), where dermal–epidermal separation is not a factor.

Analysis of the α_6 and β_4 integrins in replicate cultures of control and HD-exposed keratinocytes showed a statistically significant ($p < 0.01$) postexposure decrease in image intensity of 27.3% and 26.3%, respectively (Figure 27.8). In each case, the decrease in α_6 and β_4 integrin was characterized by a loss of fluorescence from the surface of the attached keratinocytes and resulted in a residual, basolateral pattern of fluorescence.

DISCUSSION

Images of molecules from the adhesion complex of HEKs were produced by confocal and multiphoton laser scanning microscopy before and after exposure to vesicating doses of sulfur mustard. The combined qualitative and quantitative results indicate that in culture, the basal-cell keratins K5 and K14 are early targets of HD alkylation. Analyses of the confocal images (Figures 27.2 and 27.4) suggest that the initial decrease in epitope expression for K5 (29.2%) and K14 (30.14%) at 1 hr postexposure was the result of alkylation *per se*. However, the progressive decrease of K14 expression during the postexposure absence of sulfur mustard was inconsistent with further alkylation. Multiphoton images (Figure 27.3) indicate that

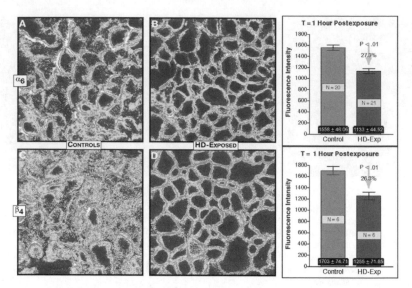

Figure 27.8 Analysis of confocal images from HEK in replicate control and HD-exposed cultures indicated a statistically significant ($p < 0.01$) decrease of 27.3% and 26.3% in image intensity of α_6 and β_4 integrins, respectively, at 1 hr postexposure. The decrease was characterized by a loss of fluorescence from the surface of attached basal cells, resulting in a honeycomb pattern of residual, basolateral fluorescence. Postexposure image patterns from cultures were very similar to those recorded from intact epidermal tissues (see Figures 27.7B,C).

exposure to HD destabilized the cytoskeleton, causing retraction of K14 filaments from the plasma membrane margins, formation of punctate K14 nodules, obvious disruption, and almost certainly an associated loss of K14 continuity with the basal cell's $\alpha_6\beta_4$-integrin receptors. Postexposure collapse of the K14 cytoskeleton has recently been demonstrated using multiphoton microscopy and mouse antihuman keratin 14 clone LL002 (Werrlein and Madren-Whalley, 2002). Disruption of K14 in the mutagenic studies of Fuchs (1995, 1996, 1997) and co-workers (Uttam et al., 1996) has been associated with epidermolysis bullosa simplex (EBS, a family of blistering skin diseases); however, EBS blisters occur above the hemidesmosomes and are not characteristic of the dermal–epidermal separations induced by sulfur mustard (Papirmeister et al., 1991; Zhang et al., 1995). Progressive disruption of alkylated K14 might be due to destabilization of its highly conserved carboxyl and/or amino terminal ends or to interaction with proteases, which are generally resistant to sulfur mustard (Dixon and Needham, 1946). Multiphoton, three-dimensional images of the human epidermis showed elaborate organization of $\alpha_6\beta_4$ integrins into circular receptors on the basal cell's ventral surface (Figure 27.6). The structure and functional role of these receptors and ultimately stabilization of the dermal–epidermal junction are well served by the rete pegs (Figure 27.5), which increase the epidermal surface area of the stratum basale and, accordingly, the number of anchoring sites for $\alpha_6\beta_4$-laminin 5 attachments. Disruption of the $\alpha_6\beta_4$-integrin's epidermal organization was observed following exposure to sulfur mustard (Figures 27.6 and 27.7). However, disruption of $\alpha_6\beta_4$-integrin organization also occurred spontaneously following dermal–epidermal separation and could not be strictly related to HD exposure. Nevertheless, HD induced similar disruption in HEK cultures where dermal–epidermal separation was not a factor. The latter was characterized by postexposure loss of fluorescence from the HEK surface, resulting in a residual, basolateral pattern of fluorescence that outlined the constituent cells. Within the context of the adhesion complex (Figure 27.1), disruption and loss of $\alpha_6\beta_4$-integrin could be expected to reduce the number of docking sites for the G domain of laminin 5 and to destabilize the dermal–epidermal junction. Based on these and related results (Werrlein and Madren-Whalley, 2002), we are persuaded that HD-induced disruption of adhesion-complex molecules precedes and potentiates vesication. Our images indicate that the molecular lesions affected by sulfur mustard would interfere with homeostatic maintenance and repair of the adhesion complex by corrupting inside-out and outside-in communication between basal cells and the basement membrane. That postulate is consistent with results from our current studies and with evolving concepts linking $\alpha_6\beta_4$ integrin, keratin filaments, hemidesmosomes, and receptor-ligand attachments to signal transduction (Quaranta and Jones, 1991; Spinardi et al., 1993; Mainiero et al., 1995; Baker et al., 1996; Borradori and Sonnenberg, 1999; van der Flier and Sonnenberg, 2001; Kaltschmidt and Arias, 2002). Understanding how those molecules affect maintenance and repair of the adhesion complex will help to explain the clinical latent period between HD exposure and vesication and should provide a mechanistic basis for developing more effective HD treatments.

REFERENCES

Baker, S.E., Hopkinson, S.B., Fitchmun, M., Andreason, G.L., Frasier, F., Plopper, G., Quaranta, V., and Jones, J.C.R. (1996) Laminin-5 and hemidesmosomes: role of the α3 chain subunit in hemidesmosome stability and assembly, *J. Cell Sci.*, 109, 2509–2520.

Borradori, L. and Sonnenberg, A. (1999) Structure and function of hemidesmosomes: more than simple adhesion complexes, *J. Invest. Dermatol.*, 112, 411–418.

Dixon, M. and Needham, D.M. (1946) Biochemical research on chemical warfare agents, *Nature,* 158, 432–438.

Fuchs, E. (1995) Keratins and the skin, *Annu. Rev. Cell Dev. Biol.*, 11, 123–153.

Fuchs, E. (1996) The cytoskeleton and disease: genetic disorders of intermediate filaments, *Annu. Rev. Genet.*, 30, 197–231.

Fuchs, E. (1997) Of mice and men: genetic disorders of the cytoskeleton, Keith Porter Lecture, *Mol. Biol. Cell,* 8, 189–203.

Kaltschmidt, J.A. and Arias, A.M. (2002) A new dawn for an old connection: development meets the cell, *Trends Cell Biol.,* 12, 316–320.

Mainiero, F., Pepe, A., Wary, K.K., Spinardi, L., Mohammadi, M., Schlessinger, J., and Giancotti, F.G. (1995) Signal transduction by the α6β4 integrin: distinct β4 subunit sites mediate recruitment of Shc/Grb2 and association with the cytoskeleton of hemidesmosomes, *EMBO J.,* 14, 4470–4481.

Papirmeister, B., Feister, A.J., Robinson, S.I., and Ford, R.D. (1991) *Medical Defense against Mustard Gas: Toxic Mechanisms and Pharmacological Implications,* CRC Press, Boca Raton, FL.

Quaranta, V. and Jones, J.C.R. (1991) The internal affairs of an integrin, *Trends Cell Biol.*, 1, 2–4.

Spinardi, L., Ren, Y.L., Sanders, R., and Giancotti, F.G. (1993) The β4 subunit cytoplasmic domain mediates the interaction of α6β4 integrin with the cytoskeleton of hemides-mosomes, *Mol. Biol. Cell,* 4, 871–884.

Uttam, J., Hutton, E., Coulombe, P.A., Anton-Lamprecht, I., Yu, Q., Gedde-Dahl, T., Jr., Fine, J., and Fuchs, E. (1996) The genetic basis of epidermolysis bullosa simplex with mottled pigmentation, *Proc. Natl. Acad. Sci. U.S.A.,* 93, 9079–9084.

Van der Flier, A. and Sonnenberg, A. (2001) Function and interactions of integrins, *Cell Tissue Res.*, 305, 285–298.

Werrlein, R.J., Hamilton, T.A., and Madren-Whalley, J.S. (1999) Development of human keratinocyte colonies for confocal microscopy and for study of calcium effects on growth differentiation and sulfur mustard lesions, *a model,* in *Toxicity Assessment Alternatives: Methods, Issues, Opportunities,* Salem, H. and Katz, S.A. Eds., Humana Press, Totowa, NJ, pp. 165–174 .

Werrlein, R.J. and Madren-Whalley, J.S. (2000) Effects of sulfur mustard on the basal cell adhesion complex, *J. Appl. Toxicol.*, 20, S115–S123.

Werrlein, R.J. and Madren-Whalley, J.S. (2002) Imaging sulfur mustard lesions in human epidermal tissues and keratinocytes by confocal and multi-photon microscopy, in *Proceedings of SPIE,* 4620, 231–241.

Zhang, Z., Peters, B.P., and Monteiro-Riviere, N.A. (1995) Assessment of sulfur mustard interaction with basement membrane components, *Cell Biol. Toxicol.*, 11, 89–101.

CHAPTER 28

Suppression of Sulfur Mustard-Increased IL-8 in Human Keratinocyte Cell Cultures by Serine Protease Inhibitors: Implications for Toxicity and Medical Countermeasures*

Fred M. Cowan, Clarence A. Broomfield, and William J. Smith

CONTENTS

INTRODUCTION

Sulfur mustard (2,2'-dichlorodiethyl sulfide, HD) has been known as a chemical warfare blistering agent for nearly a century. Although, HD pathology is fairly well understood and the basic histopathology and toxicology of HD exposure have been reviewed, the toxicological mechanisms of HD remain obscure and no antidote exists (Papirmeister et al., 1991, 1995; Cowan and Broomfield, 1993). HD has radiomimetic, mutagenic, and cytotoxic properties and predominantly targets the epithelial

* The opinions or assertions contained herein are the private views of the authors and are not to be construed as official or as reflecting the views of the Department of the Army or the Department of Defense.

tissues of skin, eye, and respiratory tract, yielding site specific symptoms, e.g., vesication, conjunctivitis, bronchopneumonia (Papirmeister et al., 1991, 1995). The degree of HD pathology (Papirmeister et al., 1991, 1995) is dose dependent, causing irritation, edema, necrosis, ulceration, and systemic symptoms only at relatively high exposures. The basic histopathology of HD-induced cutaneous lesions includes degeneration of epidermal cells, especially in the basal layer, followed by vesication (Papirmeister et al., 1991, 1995). The accompanying dermal-epidermal separation is similar to that caused by proteolysis and certain bullous diseases, and this has fostered the hypotheses that HD vesication involves proteolytic and/or inflammatory responses (Papirmeister et al., 1991, 1995; Cowan and Broomfield, 1993). HD-increased proteases and the expression of inflammatory enzymes, gene products, mediators, and receptors in tissue or cell cultures and inflammatory enzymes and cytokines in the skin of HD-exposed animals are well documented in the literature (Higuchi et al., 1988; Papirmeister et al., 1991, 1995; Cowan et al., 1993, 1994, 1996, 1997, in press; Cowan and Broomfield, 1993; Arroyo et al., 1995; Sabourin and Casillas, 1998).

IL-8 is a potent neutrophil chemotactic cytokine that is increased in skin exposed to HD (Tsuruta et al., 1996) and HEK cell cultures following exposure to ultraviolet light (Takematsu et al., 1990) or HD (Arroyo et al., 1999). Most of the drugs with efficacy for HD toxicity are anti-inflammatory compounds (Table 28.1) (Casillas et al., 1996, 2000), and HD-increased IL-8 has been proposed as a marker for HD-induced inflammation (Arroyo et al., 1999). However, no *in vitro* assay is in current use for screening of potential anti-inflammatory HD antidotes. Since IL-8 is at the apex of many inflammatory cascades, HD-increased IL-8 in HEK cell culture might provide a suitable *in vitro* assay system and reduce the need for animal use for screening of anti-inflammatory HD antidotes. In addition to HD toxicity, protease inhibitors are being considered for treatment of numerous pathological conditions and can suppress protease-induced IL-8 in HEKs (Siefe, 1997; Wakita et al., 1997). In this study the serine protease inhibitor TLCK, as well as the protease inhibitors that reduce HD toxicity such as compound 1579 (Table 28.1), suppresses HD-increased IL-8 in HEK cell cultures.

METHODS

Reagents

Sulfur mustard (HD, 2,2′-dichlorodiethyl sulfide) with a purity of >98% was obtained from the U.S. Army Edgewood Chemical Biological Center, Aberdeen Proving Ground, MD. Human epidermal keratinocytes (HEKs) and keratinocyte growth serum free media (KGM) were purchased from Cambrex, Walkersville, MD. *N*-Tosyl-ʟ-lysine chloromethyl ketone (TLCK) was obtained from Sigma, St. Louis, MO. Ethyl *p*-guanidino benzoate hydrochloride (compound 1579) was obtained from in-house antivesicant screening program (U.S. Army Medical Research Institute of Chemical Defense, Aberdeen Proving Ground, MD).

Table 28.1 Candidate Antivesicant Drug Screening: Statistically Positive Reduction of at Least 50% in Edema or Histopathology in the Mouse Ear or Hairless Mouse

	Edema	Histopathology
Anti-Inflammatory Drugs		
Fluphenazine dihydrochloride		50
Indomethacin	63	96
Olvanil	53	91
Hydrocortisone	65	71
Olvanil (saturated)		53
Retro olvanil	62	84
Olvanil (urea analog)		81
Octyl homovanillamide	65	100
Dexamethasone		72
Scavenger Drugs		
2-Mercaptopyridine-1-oxide		65
6-Methyl-2-Mercaptopyridine-1-oxide		56
4-Methyl-2-Mercaptopyridine-1-oxide	57	94
Dimercaprol	43	92
Protease Inhibitor		
1-(4-aminophenyl)-3-(4-chlorophenyl)urea HCl		54
N-(OP)-L-Ala-L-Ala-benzy ester hydrate		63
1(G-T)-4-(4-methyl phenylsemithiocarbazide)		50
PADPRP Inhibitor		
3-(4'-Bromophenyl)ureidobenzamide		74
Benzoylene urea		54
Other		
Hydrogen peroxide gel, 3%		58

Data generated by the U.S. Army Medical Research Institute of Chemical Defense Anti-vesicant Drug Screen.

Sulfur Mustard Exposure

HEKs in 24-well tissue culture plates were incubated at 37°C in a 5% CO_2 incubator using standard procedures provided by Clonetics. Subculturing was done using Clonetics trypsin-EDTA. HEKs at 100% confluence were exposed to 200 μM HD per well. The plates were maintained at room temperature in a fume hood for 1 hr to allow venting of volatile agent and then transferred to a 5% CO_2 incubator at 37°C for a total incubation time of 8 to 24 hr.

Protease Inhibitors

The serine protease inhibitors N-tosyl-L-lysine chloromethyl ketone (TLCK) and ethyl p-guanidino benzoate hydrochloride (1579) were added to HEK cell cultures 1 hr after HD exposure at concentrations from 1000 to 31.25 μM.

DATA ANALYSIS

Data from single experiments are representative of triplicate experiments. Statistical significance was determined using Student's *t*-test, and data are presented with standard deviations.

RESULTS

Exposure of HEKs to 200 μ*M* HD demonstrated an increase in IL-8 in culture media 24 hr after HD exposure, as previously reported by Arroyo et al. (1999) and confirmed by Lardot et al. (1999). Levels of IL-8 were generally less than 30 pg/ml in control HEK tissue culture media and above 1500 pg/ml in HEK media 24 hr after HD exposure. A dose-dependent suppression of the HD-enhanced IL-8 in HEK cell cultures was achieved by adding the serine protease inhibitors TLCK and compound 1579 (1000, 500, 250, 125, 62.5, and 31.25 μ*M*) (Figures 28.1 and 28.2). Solubility of some of the protease inhibitors that reduced HD vesication in tissue culture media proved difficult and made testing of these compounds in this assay system difficult. However, *N*-(OP)-L-Ala-L-Ala-benzy ester hydrate (compound 2780) dissolved in ETOH and, added to the assay at a final concentration of 5% ETOH in HEK cell cultures, inhibited HD-increased IL-8. Protease inhibitor-treated HD-exposed HEK cell cultures often appeared morphologically more like negative control HEK monolayers with classic cobblestone appearance than positive control HD-exposed HEK cell cultures that lose cell-to-cell contact and can be round in appearance.

DISCUSSION

The use of serine protease inhibitors to suppress HD-increased IL-8 in HEK cell cultures demonstrates that proteolysis participates in HD-increased IL-8

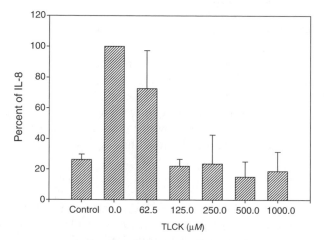

Figure 28.1 Percent IL-8 of HD-exposed HEK following treatment with TLCK.

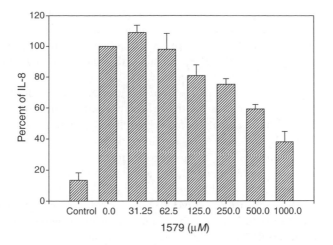

Figure 28.2 Percent IL-8 of HD-exposed HEK following treatment with 1579.

production *in vitro*. This may reflect the efficacy of these compounds for HD vesication in the mouse ear. Predicting the interplay between the toxicological mechanisms of HD and pharmacological actions of antivesicant drugs may prove key to the development of the best medical countermeasures for HD toxicity. Our institute, in conjunction with Battelle, has screened nearly 400 compounds in the mouse ear model for HD cutaneous injury (Table 28.1) (Casillas et al., 2000). Twenty-one compounds reduced HD histopathology greater than 50% (Table 28.1). Of these drugs, five are scavengers and one other drug, hydrogen peroxide, most likely neutralizes HD molecules, effectively reducing the dose. Of the remaining drugs, four are protease inhibitors, one is a poly(ADP-ribose) polymerase (PADPRP) inhibitor, and ten are anti-inflammatory drugs. The anti-inflammatory drugs include two corticoid steroids, five capsaicin analogues, two cyclooxygenase (COX) inhibitors, and a calmodulin inhibitor.

The diverse chemistry and actions of these classes of drugs create some ambiguity as to their mechanism(s) of efficacy against HD toxicity. However, some commonality of action exists between many of these drugs. Serine protease inhibitors, corticosteroids, capsaicin analogues, and PADPRP inhibitors (Hassa and Hottiger, 1999; Oliver et al., 1999) can all suppress activation of the transcription factor NF-κB (reviewed, Cowan et al., 2000). Such inhibition of transcription could affect the expression of numerous molecules that include many proinflammatory mediators such as IL-8. In addition to protease inhibitors described in this study, all other classes of compounds that work against HD vesication in rodents so far tested, e.g., COX inhibitor indomethacin, calmodulin antagonist fluphenazine, and the PADPRP inhibitor 3-(4′-bromophenyl)ureidobenzamide, also suppress HD-increased IL-8 in HEK cell cultures (Cowan et al., unpublished observations). However, inhibition of transcription does not totally explain the efficacy of the diverse classes of drugs that affect HD toxicity. HD vesication in rodent models is reduced by dexamethasone (Casillas et al., 2000) but not by the closely related corticosteroid betamethasone (Casillas et al., Cowan et al., unpublished observations). Both drugs have about equal genomic effects on transcription; however, dexamethasone has better nongenomic action and is a potent inhibitor of concanavalin A-stimulated respiration, while betamethasone has little effect on this toxicity (Buttgereit et al., 1999). Thus, HD vesication may involve both genomic and oxidative pathways.

One potential inflammatory pathway of keratinocytes that could account for the mechanistic actions for most of the drugs that reduce HD toxicity involves oxidative or other stimuli causing increased synthesis of platelet activating factor (PAF), COX-2, and IL-8 (24). PAF is a dual proinflammatory and neuromessenger phospholipid molecule that is involved in many normal physiological processes, is implicated in lethal anaphylaxis, and is implicated as a causative factor in neuronal degeneration and bullous disease blisters (Tanniere-Zeller et al., 1989; Bazan and Allan, 1996; Travers et al., 1998). PAF can further cause neutrophil infiltration and increase the synthesis of proteases such as t-PA and gelatinase that are implicated in bullous phemphigoid and HD toxicity (Emeis and Kluft, 1985; Harvath, 1991; Liu et al., 1997; Millard et al., 1997; Calvet et al.,1999; Shan et al., 1999). Bazan & Tao (1997) suggest that PAF antagonists could suppress synthesis of proteases and reduce degradation of the epithelial extracellular matrix.

Antivesicant candidate drugs that are more likely to have a single site of action have shown lesser efficacy for HD pathology than drugs with more potential for multiple sites of actions that include PAF activity. The COX inhibitor indomethacin, which gave 100% inhibition of HD vesication in the mouse ear, can, at higher concentrations, also antagonize enzymes that mediate the synthesis of PAF (Hurst and Bazan, 1997). Furthermore, indomethacin could suppress HD-increased IL-8 in HEK cell cultures only at concentrations far in excess of that expected to inhibit COX and consistent with inhibition of PAF synthesis (Cowan et al., unpublished observation). The corticoid steroid dexamethasone and the capsaicin analogue homovanillamide are very effective against HD toxicity, whereas the specific calmodulin antagonist fluphenazine inhibited HD histopathology by only 50% (Table 28.1). Dexamethasone can influence both genomic and oxidative pathways (Bazan and Allan, 1996), and homovanillamide is a capsaicin receptor antagonist that, like fluphenazine, is also a potent calmodulin antagonist (Savitha et al., 1990). Both dexamethasone and homovanillamide can further inhibit PAF-mediated activity (Brand et al., 1990; Han et al., 1999).

The experimental record strongly indicates that proteolysis produced by metabolic disruption of skin cells and/or inflammation may contribute to HD pathology. Protease inhibitors and most of the other drugs that have shown efficacy for HD pathology can target a combination of oxidative, genomic, enzyme, or proteolytic pathways that influence the synthesis or action of proteases, cytokines, and other mediators of inflammatory cascades. Research on compounds such as protease inhibitors that inhibit HD-increased IL-8 in HEK cell cultures may enhance our understanding of the toxicity of HD and the efficacy of prophylactic and therapeutic compounds. This approach could further predict and lead to new medical countermeasures for HD toxicity.

REFERENCES

Arroyo, C.M., von Tersch, R.L., and Broomfield, C.A. (1995) Activation of alpha-human tumour necrosis factor (TNF-α) by human monocytes (TNP-1) exposed to 2-chloro-ethyl ethyl sulphide (H-MG), *Hum. Exp. Toxicol.,* 14, 547–553.

Arroyo, C.M., Schafer, R.J., Kurt, E.M., Broomfield, C.A., and Carmicheal, A.J. (1999) Response of normal human keratinocytes to sulfur mustard (HD): cytokine release using a non-enzymatic detachment procedure, *Hum. Exp. Toxicol.,* 18, 1.

Bazan, N.G. and Allan, G. (1996) Platelet-activating factor in the modulation of excitatory amino acid neurotransmitter release and of gene expression, *J. Lipid Mediat. Cell Signal,* 14, 321–330.

Bazan, H.E. and Tao, Y. (1997) PAF antagonists as possible inhibitors of corneal epithelial defects and ulceration, *J. Ocul. Pharmacol. Ther.,* 13, 277–285.

Brand, L.M., Skare, K.L., Loomans, M.E., Reller, H.H., Schwen, R.J., Lade, D.A., Bohne, R.L., Maddin, C.S., Moorehead, D.P., and Fanelli, R. (1990) Anti-inflammatory pharmacology and mechanism of the orally active capsaicin analogs, NE-19550 and NE-28345, *Agents Actions,* 31, 329–340.

Buttgereit, F., Brand, M.D., and Burmester, G.R. (1999) Equivalent doses and relative drug potencies for non-genomic glucocorticoid effects: a novel glucocorticoid hierarchy, *Biochem. Pharmacol.,* 58, 363–368.

Calvet, J.-J. et. al. (1999) Matrix metalloproteinase gelatinases in sulfur mustard-induced acute airway injury in guinea pigs, *Am. J. Physiol.,* 276, L754–L762.

Casillas, R.P., Smith, K.J., Lee, R.B., Castrejon, L.R., and Stemler, F.W. (1996) Effect of topically applied drugs against HD-induced cutaneous injury in the mouse ear edema model, paper presented at the proceedings of the 1996 Medical Defense Bioscience Review. U.S. Army Medical Research Institute of Chemical Defense, AD A321841, 2, 801–809.

Casillas, R.P., Babin, M.C., Ricketts, K.M., Castrejon, L.R., Baker, L.M., Mann, J., Jr., Shumaker, S.M., Truxall, J.A., Blank, J.A., and Kiser, R.C. (2000) *In vivo* therapeutic prophylactic protection against cutaneous sulfur mustard injury using the mouse ear veicant model (MEVM), paper presented at the proceedings of the 2000 Medical Defense Bioscience Review. U.S. Army Medical Research Institute of Chemical Defense.

Cowan, F.M. and Broomfield, C.A. (1993) Putative roles of inflammation in the dermatopa-thology of sulfur mustard, *Cell Biol. Toxicol.,* 9, 201–213.

Cowan, F.M., Broomfield, C.A., and Smith, W.J. (1997) Sulfur mustard exposure enhances Fc receptor expression on human epidermal keratinocytes in cell culture: implications for toxicity and medical countermeasures, *Cell Biol. Toxicol.,* 14, 1–6.

Cowan, F.M., Broomfield, C.A., and Smith, W.J. (in press) Exposure of human epidermal keratinocytes cell cultures to sulfur mustard promotes binding of complement C1q: implications for toxicity and medical countermeasures, *J. Appl. Toxicol.*

Cowan, F.M., Yourick, J.J., Hurst, C.G., Broomfield, C.A., and Smith, W.J. (1993) Sulfur mustard-increased proteolysis following *in vitro* and *in vivo* exposures, *Cell Biol. Toxicol.,* 9, 253–261.

Cowan, F.M., Bongiovanni, R., Broomfield, C.A., Yourick, J.J., and Smith, W.J. (1994) Sulfur mustard increases elastase-like activities in homogenates of hairless guinea pig skin, *J. Toxicol. Cutaneous Ocular Toxicol.,* 13, 221–229.

Cowan, F.M., Anderson, D.R., Broomfield, C.A., Byers, S., and Smith, W.J. (1996) Bio-chemical alterations in rat lung lavage fluid following acute sulfur mustard inhalation. II. increases in proteolytic activity, *Inhalation Toxicol.,* 9, 53–61.

Cowan, F.M. et al. (2000) Putative Role of Proteases and Other Inflammatory-Neuronal Molecules in the Toxicity of Nerve and Blister Chemical Warfare Agents, paper presented at the proceedings of the 2000 Medical Defense Bioscience Review. U.S. Army Medical Research Institute of Chemical Defense.

Emeis, J.J. and Kluft, C. (1985) PAF-acether-induced release of tissue-type plasminogen activator from vessel walls, *Blood*, 66, 86–91.

Han, S.J., Choi, J.H., Ko, H.M., Yang, H.W., Choi, I.W., Lee, H.K., Lee, O.H., and Im, S.Y. (1999) Glucocorticoids prevent NF-kappaB activation by inhibiting the early release of platelet-activating factor in response to lipopolysaccharide, *Eur. J. Immunol.*, 29, 1334–1341.

Harvath, L. (1991) Neutrophil chemotactic factors, EXS 59, 35–52.

Hassa, P.O. and Hottiger, M.O. (1999) A role of poly (ADP-ribose) polymerase in NF-kappaB transcriptional activation, *Biol. Chem.*, 380, 953–959.

Higuchi, K., Kajiki, A., Nakamura, M., Harada, S., Pula, P.J., Scott, A.L., and Dannenburg, A.M. (1988) Protease released in organ culture by acute inflammatory lesions produced *in vivo* in rabbit skin by sulfur mustard: hydrolysis of synthetic peptide substrates for trypsin-like and chymotrypsin-like enzymes, *Inflammation*, 12, 311–334.

Hurst, J.S. and Bazan, H.E. (1997) The sensitivity of bovine corneal epithelial lyso-PAF acetyltransferase to cyclooxygenase and lipoxygenase inhibitors is independent of arachidonate metabolites, *J. Ocul. Pharmacol. Ther.*, 13, 415–426.

Lardot, C., Dubois, V., and Lison, D. (1999) Sulfur mustard upregulates the expression of interleukin-8 in cultured human keratinocytes, *Toxicol. Lett.*, 29, 29–33.

Liu, Z. et al. (1997) A major role for neutrophils in experimental bullous phemphigoid, *J. Clin. Invest.*, 100, 1256–1263.

Millard, C.B., Bongiovanni, R., and Broomfield, C.A. (1997) Cutaneous exposure to bis-(2-chloroethyl)sulfide results in neutrophil infiltration and increased solubility of 180,000 Mr subepidermal collagens, *Biochem. Pharmacol.*, 53, 1405–1412.

Oliver, F.J., Menissier-de Murcia, J., Nacci, C., Decker, P., Andriantsitohaina, R., Muller, S., de la Rubia, G., Stoclet, J.C., and de Murcia, G. (1999) Resistance to endotoxic shock as a consequence of defective NF-kappaB activation in poly (ADP-ribose) polymerase-1 deficient mice, *Embo. J.*, 18, 4446–4454.

Papirmeister, B., Feister, A.J., Robinson, S.I., and Ford, R.D. (1991) *Medical Defense against Mustard Gas: Toxic Mechanisms and Pharmacological Implications*, CRC Press, Boston.

Papirmeister, B., Gross, C.L., Meier, H.L., Petrali, J.P., and Johnson, J.B. (1995) Molecular basis for mustard-induced vesication, *Fund. Appl. Toxicol.*, 5, S134–S149.

Pei, Y., Barber, L.A., Murphy, R.C., Johnson, C.A., Kelley, S.W., Dy, L.C., Fertel, R.H., Nguyen, T.M., Williams, D.A., and Travers, J.B. (1998) Activation of the epidermal platelet-activating factor receptor results in cytokine and cyclooxygenase-2 biosynthesis, *J. Immunol.*, 161, 1954–1961.

Sabourin, C.L.K. and Casillas, R.P. (1998) Inflammatory gene expression in mouse skin following sulfur mustard exposure, *Toxicol. Sci.*, 42, 393.

Savitha, G., Panchanathan, S., and Salimath, B.P. (1990) Capsaicin inhibits calmodulin-mediated oxidative burst in rat macrophages, *Cell Signal*, 2, 577–585.

Shan, L. et al. Platelet-activating factor increases the expression of metalloproteinase-9 in human bronchial epithelial cells, *Eur. J. Pharmacol.*, 374, 147–56.

Siefe, C. (1997) Blunting nature's Swiss army knife, *Science*, 277, 1602–1603.

Takematsu, H., Isono, N., Kato, T., and Tagami, H. (1990) Normal human epidermal keratinocyte-derived neutrophil chemotactic factor, *Tohoku J. Exp. Med.*, 162, 1–13.

Tanniere-Zeller, M., Rochette, L., and Bralet, J. (1989) PAF-acether-induced mortality in
    mice: protection by benzodiazepines, *Drugs Exp. Clin. Res.,* 15, 553–558.
Travers, J.B., Murphy, R.C., Johnson, C.A., Pei, Y., Morin, S.M., Clay, K.L., Barber, L.A.,
    Hood, A.F., Morelli, J.G., and Williams, D.A. (1998) Identification and pharmaco-
    logical characterization of platelet activating factor and related 1-palmitoyl species
    in human inflammatory blistering diseases, *Prostaglandins Other Lipid Mediat.,* 56,
    305–324.
Tsuruta, J., Sugisaki, K., Dannenberg, A.M., Jr., Yoshimura, T., Abe, Y., and Mounts, P. (1996)
    The cytokines NAP-1 (IL-8), MCP-1, IL-1 beta, and GRO in rabbit inflammatory
    skin lesions produced by the chemical irritant sulfur mustard, *Inflammation,* 20,
    293–318.
Wakita, H., Furukawa, F., and Takigawa, M. (1997) Thrombin and trypsin induce granulocyte-
    macrophage colony-stimulating factor and interleukin-6 gene expression in cultured
    normal human keratinocytes, *Proc. Assoc. Am. Physicians,* 109, 190–207.

CHAPTER 29

Development of Medical Countermeasures to Sulfur Mustard Vesication

William J. Smith, Michael C. Babin, Robyn C. Kiser, and Robert P. Casillas

CONTENTS

INTRODUCTION

Although many of the toxic manifestations that follow sulfur mustard (2,2′-dichloroethyl sulfide, Army designation HD) exposure have been defined, the actual mechanisms of pathology remain elusive. Much of the research in this area has been conducted in the Pharmacology and Drug Assessment Divisions of the U.S. Army Medical Research Institute of Chemical Defense (USAMRICD), the laboratories of our NATO allies, and laboratories funded through the Medical Research and Material Command (USAMRMC) extramural contract program. Based on the technological database developed through this program, we have been able to generate a unifying hypothesis for cellular and tissue events that explains the formation of cutaneous blisters following exposure to HD. Studies of individual toxic events, such as alkylation of cellular macromolecules, formation of DNA strand breaks, activation of poly(ADP-ribose) polymerase (PARP or PADPRP), disruption of calcium regulation, proteolytic activation, and tissue inflammation, have together led to the formulation of six strategies for therapeutic intervention (Smith et al., 1996, 1999). The proposed pharmaceutical strategies are intracellular scavengers, DNA cell cycle modulators, PARP inhibitors, calcium modulators, protease inhibitors, and antiinflammatory compounds.

These compound classes are currently being evaluated as medical countermeasures against HD dermatotoxicity. We have validated four *in vitro* testing modules for compound screening: solubility, direct toxicity, protection against HD-induced cytotoxicity, and protection against HD-induced depletion of cellular nicotinamide adenine dinucleotide (NAD+) levels. Two additional *in vitro* modules, preservation of cellular adenosine triphosphate (ATP) levels and inhibition of proteolysis, are in the final stages of validation. For *in vivo* screening, we have used the mouse ear vesicant model (MEVM) with associated histopathological evaluation (Casillas et al., 1997) and cutaneous vapor exposure in hairless guinea pigs (Yourick et al., 1991). For systemic drug therapy, we are validating a hairless mouse cutaneous vapor exposure model.

EXPERIMENTAL DESIGN

Decision Tree Network (DTN)

A DTN has been devised to outline the selection process used to evaluate candidate pretreatment or treatment compounds. This DTN consists of pathways through *in vitro* and *in vivo* compound screening modules based on known characteristics of the compounds being evaluated.

In Vitro Screening Modules

As compounds are placed in the drug assessment compound tracking system, they are assigned to specific functional categories. Based on their categorization, they are evaluated through a series of assays such as aqueous solubility, direct cytotoxicity in human lymphocytes (PBL), protection of PBL against the cytotoxicity of HD, depletion of metabolic factors (NAD+ or ATP), and inhibition of HD-induced proteolysis. Results from these assays are used to prioritize movement of candidate compounds into the *in vivo* screening modules.

In Vivo Screening Modules

Compounds passing the *in vitro* modules or compounds from classes not applicable to *in vitro* screening (i.e., anti-inflammatory compounds) are tested in the MEVM for edema and histopathologic (i.e., epidermal–dermal separation and epidermal necrosis) evaluation. Other *in vivo* assays available for additional testing as required include cutaneous HD vapor exposure in the hairless guinea pig or the domestic swine and cutaneous HD vapor and liquid exposures in the hairless mouse. These modules usually employ topical treatment with candidate compounds, but new modules are being designed for systemic treatment regimes.

RESULTS AND DISCUSSION

Basic Research

After its introduction onto the battlefield in World War I and through the 1940s, most of the research efforts directed toward HD focused on defining the histopathological sequelae of exposure in humans. Attempts were also made to establish relevant animal model systems. Beginning in the 1950s, research turned more toward the biochemical effects of HD, and empirical studies were conducted with the aim of identifying therapeutic modalities. While the biochemical studies led to significant inroads for our understanding of the toxic mechanisms, the therapeutic approaches were futile. In the 1960s and 1970s, HD research focused mostly on DNA damage and repair, cytotoxic mechanisms, and mutagenesis.

Around 1990, the U.S. Army decided to focus its efforts for developing medical intervention strategies for HD injury through the formulation of an Army Science and Technology Objective (STO) titled *Medical Countermeasures against Vesicant Agents*. This STO presented three technical milestones: by 1996, define technological and pathophysiological databases and establish pharmacological intervention strategies for the HD injury; by 1997, show efficacy of a candidate medical countermeasure in an animal model; and by 2000, prepare a milestone 0 drug development decision.

The first technical milestone for 1996 was met through the research efforts of the USAMRICD, the extramural contract program of the USAMRMC, and the medical research programs of our allied nations. From this research, we were able to construct a schema of the major events of the pathological processes documented in cells and tissues exposed to HD (Figure 29.1). This schema was presented at numerous Department of Defense and professional scientific forums, including the 20th Army Science Conference (Smith et al., 1996). The research findings of this program served as the core of a NATO sponsored monograph on HD research (Smith and Mol, 1997).

The second part of the 1996 milestone, i.e., define strategies for pharmacological protection against the vesicant injury, was met by using the information developed for the pathology schema. We identified six specific areas of the pathologic mechanism that could serve as points of pharmacological intervention into the HD injury. These were presented along with the pathology schema at numerous meetings and are presented in Table 29.1 along with prototypic compounds, in each area, that have been shown to be efficacious against HD toxicity in various model systems.

The 1997 technical milestone called for the demonstration of efficacy by a candidate countermeasure in an animal model. This was first met by research in hairless guinea pigs by Yourick et al. (1991) and subsequently confirmed in the MEVM (Casillas et al., 1997; Smith et al., 1998).

Proposed Mechanism of HD Action

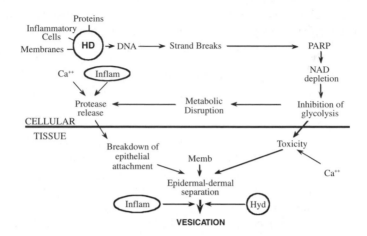

Figure 29.1 The cellular and tissue alterations induced by HD that are proposed to result in blister formation. HD can have many direct effects such as alkylation of proteins and membrane components (Memb), as well as activation of inflammatory cells. One of the main macromolecular targets is DNA, with subsequent activation of poly(ADP-ribose) polymerase (PARP). Activation of PARP can initiate a series of metabolic changes culminating in protease activation. Within the tissue, the penultimate event is the epidermal–dermal separation that occurs in the lamina lucida of the basement membrane zone. Accompanied by a major inflammatory response and changes in the tissue hydrodynamics (Hyd), fluid fills the cavity formed at this cleavage plane and presents as a blister.

Table 29.1 Strategies for Pharmacologic Intervention of the HD Lesion

Biochemical Event	Pharmacologic Strategy	Example
DNA alkylation	Intracellular scavengers	N-acetyl cysteine
DNA strand breaks	Cell cycle inhibitors	Mimosine
PARP activation	PARP inhibitors	Niacinamide
Disruption of calcium	Calcium modulators	BAPTA[a]
Proteolytic activation	Protease inhibitors	AEBSF[a]
Inflammation	Antiinflammatories	Indomethacin; Olvanil

[a] BAPTA is a calcium chelator; AEBSF is a sulfonyl fluoride compound.

Candidate Compound Screening

In fiscal year 1997, the program was converted from an Army STO to a defense technology objective (DTO), CB.22, and while the technical milestones remained intact, a new metric was imposed on the drug development effort. Rather than identifying compounds that just significantly reduced our pathological endpoints, we were required to attain at least 50% reduction of indicators of morbidity.

Over 500 candidate prophylactic or therapeutic compounds have been evaluated through the antivesicant DTN. Sixty-two compounds have demonstrated an ability to provide significant modulation of edema and/or histopathology caused by HD *in vivo*. Of these 62 compounds, 19 have demonstrated at least 50% protection against

Table 29.2 Candidate Countermeasures with Greater Than 50% Efficacy in Mouse Ear Model

	Percentage Reduction in Pathology
Anti-Inflammatory Drugs	
Fluphenazine dihydrochloride	50
Indomethacin	96
Olvanil	91
Olvanil (saturated)	53
Retro olvanil	84
Olvanil (urea analog)	81
Octyl homovanillamide	100
Scavenger Drugs	
2-Mercaptopyridine-1-oxide	66
6-Methyl-2-mercaptopyridine-1-oxide	56
4-Methyl-2-mercaptopyridine-1-oxide	94
Dimercaprol	78
Na 3-sulfonatopropyl glutathionyl disulfide	64
Hydrogen peroxide gel, 3%	58
Protease Inhibitors	
1-(4-aminophenyl)-3-(4-chlorophenyl) urea	54
N-(OP)-L-Ala-L-Ala-benzy ester hydrate	62
Ethyl p-guanidino benzoate hydrochloride	62
PARP Inhibitors	
3-(4'-Bromophenyl)ureidobenzamide	74
Benzoylene urea	54
4-Amino-1-naphthol hydrochloride tech	80
Total number of positive compounds = 19	

the pathological indicators of mustard injury (Table 29.2). All of these 19 successful candidates fall into four of our six original proposed strategies: antiinflammatories (Smith and Mol, 1997), antiproteases (Smith et al., 1996), scavengers (Yourick et al., 1991), or PARP inhibitors (Smith et al., 1996).

With these compounds as proof of concept, we received approval for transition to concept development in November 2000. A new DTO (CB.30) has been approved, and work has been initiated to drive the drug development process through concept exploration toward a transition to advanced development in the fiscal year 2003/2004 time period.

Future

Having established proof of concept for the potential development of a medical countermeasure against vesicant agents, we will move the 19 most successful candidate compounds from basic research into the concept exploration phase of the drug development process. Through a downselection process currently under way, we will present to the U.S. Army Medical Materiel Development Activity the optimal candidate, route of administration, and timing of dosage for transition to advanced drug development within 3 years.

CONCLUSIONS

This research has been directed at meeting the medical chemical defense DTO *Medical Countermeasures against Vesicant Agents*. Based on results to date, we have met every milestone of the DTO, i.e., "to develop a technological database and define therapeutic strategies that protect against the vesicant injury," and "demonstrate efficacy in an animal model." Having identified at least 19 compounds that are capable of protecting against the *in vivo* pathology of HD, we now have the means to move from the research phase of pharmaceutical investigation into the concept exploration phase of drug development. This work, the combined efforts of army, academic, industrial, and contracted research laboratories has set the stage for development of a fielded medical countermeasure against HD. For the first time since HD's introduction onto the battlefield more than 80 years ago, we have the true potential to protect our war fighters against this insidious weapon through pharmacological therapy.

REFERENCES

Casillas, R.P., Mitcheltree, L.W., and Stemler, F.W. (1997) The mouse ear model of cutaneous sulfur mustard injury, *Toxicol. Methods*, 7, 381–397.
Papirmeister, B., Feister, A.J., Robinson, S.I., and Ford, R.D. (1991) *Medical Defense against Mustard Gas: Toxic Mechanisms and Pharmacological Implications*, CRC Press, Boca Raton, FL.
Smith, W.J. and Dunn, M.A. (1991) Medical defense against blistering chemical warfare agents, *Arch. Dermatol.*, 127, 1207–1213.
Smith, W.J. and Mol, M.A.E. (1997) Progress and Future Direction of Research into the Toxicity and Treatment of Sulfur Mustard Exposure, NATO Technical Report AC/243 (Panel 8) TR/19.
Smith, W.J., Martens, M.E., Gross, C.L., Clark, O.E., Cowan, F.C., and Yourick, J.J. (1996) Therapeutic Approaches to Cutaneous Injury by Sulfur Mustard, paper presented at the proceedings of the 20th Army Science Conference, Vol. 2, pp. 699–703.
Smith, W.J., Casillas, R.P., Gross, C.L., and Koplovitz, I. (1998) Therapeutic Approaches to Dermatotoxicity by Sulfur Mustard, paper presented at the *U.S. Army MRMC Bioscience Review*.
Smith, W.J. et al. (1999) The Use of *In Vitro* Systems to Define Therapeutic Approaches to Cutaneous Injury by Sulfur Mustard, in *Toxicity Assessment Alternatives: Methods, Issues, Opportunities*, Salem, H. and Katz, S., Eds., Humana Press, Totowa, NJ, pp. 205–212.
Yourick, J.J., Clark, C.R., and Mitcheltree, L. (1991) Niacinamide pretreatment reduces microvesicle formation in hairless guinea pigs cutaneously exposed to sulfur mustard, *Fundam. Appl. Toxicol.*, 17, 533–542.

PART V

Neurotoxicology: Molecular Biomarkers, Transgenics, and Imaging Technologies

WILLIAM J. SLIKKER, JR. AND THOMAS J. SOBOTKA

SUMMARY

Understanding the linkage between the environment and the genome represents a major challenge to the toxicologist. Within the nervous system, the multitude of cell types and regional functionalities increases the difficulty of understanding signal transduction by an order of magnitude over less complex organ systems. New tools, including genomics, proteomics, transgenics, knockouts, and imaging techniques, are needed to unravel the complexity of the nervous system. The development and understanding of markers for generic responses by the nervous system to toxic agents offers one avenue to screen for neurotoxic effects of broad classes of chemicals or chemical mixtures. The identification of sensitive, early molecular biomarkers of neurotoxicity—including members of the family of cell adhesion molecules known as integrins that regulate cell migration, attachment to the extracellular matrix, and contacts with other cells—provides mechanistic data linking exposure with adverse effects and/or susceptibility. Gene-expression patterns (assessed by gene-array technologies, filter or microarray), proteomics (assessed by analytical mass spectrometry), and toxicant-induced cell-signaling (assessed by phospho-state-specific antibodies linked to gene transcription) offer the potential for detection and characterization of novel markers of neural injury associated with the above-mentioned neurotoxic responses. Developing a database of novel neural injury markers using these techniques can provide molecular and cellular bases for interpretation and validation of data obtained with emerging noninvasive imaging technologies. While techniques such as positron emission tomography (PET) and single photon emission computed tomography (SPECT) provide important information on the localization of pharmacological agents and their pharmacodynamics and pharmacokinetics, new applications of magnetic resonance imaging (MRI) and PET provide the ability to noninvasively detect gene expression in higher organisms. The development of *in vitro* imaging techniques that employ trophic factor stimulated and differentiated rat pheochromocytoma (PC12) cells in culture can recapitulate early and later events in the processes common to neuronal differentiation. These new approaches employ quantitative morphological methods to evaluate both pharmacological and toxicological effects. In so doing, rapid, cost-effective, imaging-based approaches to neurotoxicity assessment can be implemented with an associated reduction in animal usage.

GENOMICS/PROTEOMICS

As neurotoxicologists, we stand on the threshold of unleashing powerful techniques to solve the conundrum of neurotoxicity and neurodegenerative diseases. The tools available include genomics and proteomics, the ability to simultaneously examine the expression of hundreds of genes and their resultant protein products. Although few studies have been completed to date, there are clear examples where complex molecular relationships have been defined that underlie the altered biology (Geschwind, 2000; Mirnics et al., 2000). This microarray analysis approach has been used to suggest that schizophrenic subjects show a common abnormality in presynaptic function (Mirnics et al., 2000).

The application of genomics in solving important problems concerning nervous system function is not without difficulties. Reservations have been raised because of the relatively small changes (often less than twofold) in the expression of genes in the phenotypically diverse nervous system (Collinge and Curtis, 1991; Akbarian et al., 1995; Woo et al., 1998). Application of these approaches to human subjects has been further complicated by confounders such as concurrent or previous drug use, time lapse from exposure until tissue collection, and lifestyle influences on human clinical populations (Mirnics et al., 2001). Most of these problems can be solved, however, by the careful selection of matched controls and affected subjects, comparison of carefully collected and well-characterized tissue specimens, and the use of proper quality controls. Many of these considerations, including proper selection of microarrays and careful interpretation of data and verification strategies, have been recently reviewed (Mirnics et al., 2001).

The application of genomics to animal models provides a powerful tool to describe neurotoxicant-induced alterations in gene expression. Microarray technology can be useful in the screening mode to uncover previously unknown expression changes or to direct further investigation. Perhaps the most fruitful application of microarrays, however, is accomplished when their use is applied to hypothesis-driven studies where several well-understood biomarkers are available and a mode of action, if not mechanism of action, has been described. This focused use of genomics allows the testing of critical hypotheses and winnowing in or out a limited number of possible mechanisms. Researchers must have a firm understanding of the endpoints affected, the dose-response characteristics, and possible mechanism(s) of action before the judicious but highly effective application of genomic approaches is made.

In addition to genomics, the associated techniques of proteomics (protein analysis) and metabonomics (metabolite analysis) are also valuable for addressing neurotoxicological problems (Dove, 1999). Defining the quantity or relative change of critical proteins may prove to be more informative than defining the relative abundance or change of messenger RNA. After all, gene expression can be regulated at the level of translocation, and various other controlling mechanisms can occur, including half-life variation, posttranslational modification, and compartmentalization in protein complexes (Dove, 1999). Therefore, functional genomics, including protein and downstream metabolite profiles, may be considered the wave of the future.

IMAGING

The structural information provided by magnetic resonance imaging (MRI) has been appreciated in the clinical setting since the middle 1980s. More recently, application of MRI to animal studies is proving both practical and efficient. Based on T_2-weighted MRI, Palmer et al. (2001) were able to determine the degrees of hypoxia-induced insult and the protection against such insults by neuroprotective agents.

The ability to determine noninvasively the regional distribution of chemicals within the nervous system is a relatively new capability with great potential. For example, the brain levels of fluoxetine, a well-known antidepressant, were determined in humans by applying magnetic resonance spectroscopy (Karson et al., 1992). Although currently limited to agents containing "visible" atoms including fluorine and lithium, the ability to obtain real time, repeated, and noninvasive measurements of drugs in the nervous system is possible (Komoroski et al., 1990).

In addition, positron emission tomography (PET), which allows for the real time description of ligand-receptor localization, is becoming available for animal use. The abundance of dopamine receptors and, thus, dopamine neurons in the basal ganglia can be determined over a protracted time course of treatment in the same animal. New "table top" microPET instruments, as described by Cherry et al. (1997), will revolutionize the application of these powerful noninvasive tools in animal models.

Finally, by combining imaging techniques and "*omics*" methodology ("imaginomics"), the promise of the noninvasive assessment of gene expression becomes feasible. As the resolution of the imaging technologies improve and the cost of equipment and genetic assessment tools is reduced, these procedures will be more widely and routinely used. The advantages of noninvasive data collection over time include the ability to use longitudinal study designs and to reduce the overall number of animals necessary for selected safety assessment and drug efficacy studies.

SECTION OUTLINE

The selection of presentations for this section was intended to offer a more focused discussion of representative new technologies, including molecular biomarkers, transgenic models, and imaging, and to discuss some of the progress in applying these tools to the study of neurotoxicity. Jean L. Cadet's contribution to the section, Chapter 30, is a discussion of methamphetamine-induced neurotoxicity titled Molecular Neurotoxicology of 6-Hydroxydopamine and Methamphetamine: Lessons Derived from Transgenic Models. Laurie Roszell, B. C. Kramer, and Glen Leach wrote Chapter 31, A Microassay Method Using a Neuroblastomsa Cell Line to Examine Neurotoxicity of Organophosphate Mixtures. The contribution by Joyce Royland, Chapter 32, is titled Development of Integrin Expression as a Molecular Biomarker for Early, Sensitive Detection of Neurotoxicity. In the final chapter of the section, Chapter 33, Dong and his colleagues present Two Photon Fluorescence Microscopy: A Review of Recent Advances in Deep Tissue Imaging.

REFERENCES

Akbarian, S. et al. (1995) Gene expression for glutamic acid decarboxylase is reduced without loss of neurons in prefrontal cortex of schizophrenics, *Arch. Gen. Psychiatry,* 52, 258–266.

Cherry, S.R. et al. (1997) MicroPET: a high resolution PET scanner for imaging small animals, *IEEE Trans. Nucl. Sci.,* 44, 1161–1166.

Collinge, J. and Curtis, D. (1991) Decreased hippocampal expression of a glutamate receptor gene in schizophrenia, *Brit. J. Psychiatry,* 159, 857–859.

Dove, A. (1999) Proteonics: translating genomics into products, *Nature Biotech.,* 17, 233–236.

Geschwind, D.H. (2000) Mice, microarrays, and the genetic diversity of the brain, *Proc. Natl. Acad. Sci. U.S.A.,* 97, 10676–10678.

Karson, C.N. et al. (1992) Fluoxetine and trifluoperazine in human brain: a 19F-nuclear magnetic resonance spectroscopy study, *Psychiatry Res.,* 45, 95–104.

Komoroski, R.A. et al. (1990) *In vivo* NMR spectroscopy of lithium-7 in humans, *Magn. Reson. Med.,* 15, 347–356.

Mirnics, K., Lewis, D.A., and Levitt, P. (2001) DNA microarrays and human brain disorders, in *Methods in Neurogenetics,* CRC Press, Boca Raton, FL, pp. 1–48.

Mirnics, K. et al. (2000) Molecular characterization of schizophrenia viewed by microarray analysis of gene expression in prefrontal cortex, *Neuron,* 28, 53–67.

Palmer, G.C. et al. (2001) T_2-weighted MRI correlate with long-term histopathology, neurology scores, and skilled motor behavior in a rat stroke model, *Neuroprotective Agents,* New York Academy of Sciences, Vol. 939.

Woo, T.U. et al. (1998) A subclass of prefrontal gamma-aminobutyric acid axon terminals are selectively altered in schizophrenia, *Proc. Natl. Acad. Sci. U.S.A.,* 95, 5341–5346.

CHAPTER 30

Molecular Neurotoxicology of 6-Hydroxydopamine and Methamphetamine: Lessons Derived from Transgenic Models

Jean Lud Cadet

CONTENTS

INTRODUCTION

Parkinson's disease (PD) is an idiopathic neurodegenerative disease whose signs include tremor, hypokinesia, and muscular rigidity (Bernheimer et al., 1973; Marsden, 1990). Secondary Parkinsonism has been reported after exposure to various neurotoxic agents (Ikeda et al., 1978). These signs and symptoms are secondary to the degeneration of pigmented nuclei observed in the brainstem of these patients (Fahn et al., 1971; Bernheimer et al., 1973; Agid et al., 1987). Specifically, the *pars compacta* of the *substantia nigra* (SNpc) is characterized by severe loss of dopamine (DA)-containing neurons of PD patients (Ikeda et al., 1978).

Recent observations have suggested a role for free radicals in the causation of PD (Fahn and Cohen, 1992). For example, lipid peroxidation products are significantly elevated in the brains of these patients (Dexter et al., 1989, 1992, 1994), and abnormal iron metabolism has been demonstrated in the basal ganglia of PD subjects (Dexter et al., 1987, 1989; Sofic et al., 1988; Reiderer et al., 1989; Hirsch et al., 1991; Jellinger et al., 1993; Reichmann et al., 1995). There are also decreased brain ferritin levels (Dexter et al., 1992) and increased ferritin-like immunoreactivity in the proliferating microglia located adjacent to degenerating nigral neurons (Jellinger et al., 1993). The levels of free radical scavengers are reported to be abnormal in PD patients (Ambani et al., 1975; Martilla et al., 1988; Saggu et al., 1989; Adams et al., 1991). There are increases in mitochondrial Mn-superoxide dismutase (SOD) (Saggu et al., 1989) and in CuZn-SOD (Martilla et al., 1988).

A few neurotoxin-based models have been used to attempt to decipher the mechanisms involved in causing PD. These include, among others, 6-hydroxy-dopamine (6-OHDA) (Asanuma et al., 1998) and methamphetamine (Cadet et al., 1994). The purpose of this chapter is to provide a brief overview of the recent use of transgenic and knockout mice to test the idea that free-radical mediated or triggered events may be responsible for the destruction of DA terminals and cell bodies.

SIX-OHDA-INDUCED NEURODEGENERATION

Six-OHDA is a neurotoxin that destroys catecholaminergic neurons selectively (Cadet and Brannock, 1998). Its injection into the SNpc and in the striatum results in loss of nigral DA cell bodies and striatal DA depletion (Berger et al., 1990; Cadet et al., 1991; Cadet and Zhu, 1992).

The toxicity of 6-OHDA is thought to be related to the production of oxygen-based radicals (Cohen and Heikkila, 1974; Cohen et al., 1976; Cohen, 1987; Perumal et al., 1989). Specifically, the production of superoxide radicals, H_2O_2, and of hydroxyl radicals appears to be involved (Cohen and Heikkila, 1974; Cohen et al., 1976). We tested the possible protective effects of the overexpression of CuZn-superoxide dismutase (SOD) activity (an enzyme that breaks down superoxide radicals) on dopaminergic neuronal damage caused by 6-OHDA (Asanuma et al., 1998) by measuring the effects of 6-OHDA on striatal and nigral dopamine trans-porters and nigral tyrosine hydroxylase-immunoreactive neurons in the transgenic mice. Intracerebal injection of 6-OHDA caused marked decreases in striatal and nigral dopamine transporters in the mouse striatum, as well as decreased cell number and size of tyrosine hydroxylase-immunoreactive dopamine neurons in the SNpc of the wild-type mice. In contrast, SOD transgenic mice were significantly protected against these neurotoxic effects. These results provide evidence for a role of the superoxide anion in the toxic effects of this drug.

The protooncogene Bcl-2 rescues cells from a wide variety of insults including free radicals (Chakraborti et al., 1999). Recently, it was shown that the toxicity of 6-OHDA can be attenuated in transgenic mice overexpressing bcl-2 (Offen et al., 1998). Specifically, 6-OHDA caused cell death of essentially all neurons obtained from normal mice. However, cultures generated from heterozygous and homozygous NSE-nbcl-2 transgenic mice were almost completely protected, as with homozygous mice.

METHAMPHETAMINE-INDUCED NEURODEGENERATION

Methamphetamine (meth) is an illicit drug of abuse that causes degeneration of DA systems (Cadet et al., 1994; Cadet and Brannock, 1998). A number of investigators have hinted to a role for oxygen-based free radicals in the actions of this drug (Wagner et al., 1980; DeVito and Wagner, 1989; Cubells et al., 1994; Giovanni et al., 1995; Hirata et al., 1996, 1998). We have tested the role of superoxide radicals in meth neurotoxicity (Cadet et al., 1994; Hirata et al., 1996) used transgenic (Tg) mice that express the human CuZnSOD gene (Epstein et al., 1987). These mice have much higher CuZn-SOD activity than wild-type animals from similar backgrounds (Jayanthi et al., 1998). The toxic effects of meth were significantly attenuated in a gene dosage fashion, with homozygous SOD-Tg mice showing greater protection (Hirata et al., 1996). Subsequent studies have suggested that the administration of meth is associated with a toxic cascade that involves the production of superoxides, hydrogen peroxide, and hydroxyl radicals (Jayanthi et al., 1998) as well as quinone production (LaVoie and Hastings, 1999).

The role of glutamate in meth neurotoxicity has been investigated using glutamate antagonists against the toxic effects of the drug (Sonsalla et al., 1989; Weihmuller et al., 1992; O'Dell et al., 1994; Stephans and Yamamoto, 1994). Other studies using lesions of intrinsic striatal cells that contain glutamate receptors have also supported a role of glutamate in this model (O'Dell et al., 1994). Because glutamate appears to cause some of its neurotoxic effects via the production of NO (Dawson et al., 1993) the involvement of NO was tested and shown to participate in meth neurotoxicity (Itzhak and Ali, 1996; Sheng et al., 1996; Ali and Itzhak, 1998). The role of NO in the toxic effects of meth was further supported by the report that meth can cause overexpression of nNOS in the mouse brain (Deng and Cadet, 1999).

The involvement of p53 in meth has also been assessed using p53 knockout mice. We had suggested that if the p53 protein is an important determinant of meth-induced neurotoxicity, animals lacking the gene for the p53 protein would be protected against meth neurotoxicity. This contention was proved by the demonstration that the p53-knockout phenotype attenuated the long-term neurotoxic effects of meth on striatal dopaminergic terminals and on midbrain DA cell bodies (Hirata and Cadet, 1997). We also showed that meth could cause accumulation of p53. It is also of interest to relate the observed protection against meth-induced toxicity in the p53-knockout mice to recent reports that these mice show decreases in Bax protein but no changes in bcl-2 in their brains (Miyashita et al., 1994). Because Bax is a known inhibitor of the antioxidant effects of bcl-2 and a promoter of apoptosis (Oltvai et al., 1993), it is possible that the protective effects observed in the knockout mice might be due to the relative greater abundance of bcl-2 in these animals (Miyashita et al., 1994). This reasoning is consistent with our recent demonstration that bcl-2 can protect against the apoptotic effects of meth *in vitro* (Cadet et al., 1997).

CONCLUSIONS

The purpose of this review was to document the possible involvement of complex mechanisms in the neurotoxicity of drugs that affect monoaminergic systems.

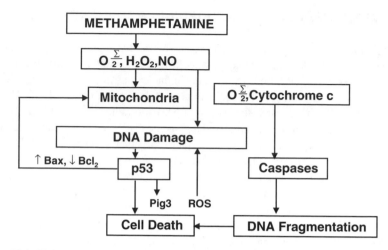

Figure 30.1 Molecular neurotoxicology of methamphetamine.

Because free radicals can trigger cell death by stimulating complex interactions between apparently parallel as well as sequential molecular events (see Figure 30.1 for working model of the neurotoxicity of meth), it is to be expected that the elucidation of DA cell death will necessitate a thorough molecular understanding and dissection of cell death pathways. This will include the use of the recently developed microarray technology.

REFERENCES

Adams, J.D., Klaidman, L.K., Odunze, I.N., Shen, H.C., and Miller, C.A. (1991) Alzheimer's and Parkinson's disease: brain levels of glutathione, glutathione disulfide, and vitamin E, *Mol. Chem. Neuropathol.*, 14, 213–226.

Agid, Y., Javoy-Agid, F., and Ruberg, M. (1987) Biochemistry of neurotransmitters in Parkinson's disease, in *Movement Disorders 2,* Marsden, C.D. and Fahn S., Eds., Butterworths, London, pp. 166–230.

Ali, S.F. and Itzhak Y. (1998) Effects of 7-nitroindazole, an NOS inhibitor, on methamphetamine-induced dopaminergic and serotonergic neurotoxicity in mice, *Ann. NY Acad Sci.*, 844, 122–130.

Ambani, L.M., Van Woert, M.H., and Murphy, S. (1975) Brain peroxidase and catalase in Parkinson's disease, *Arch. Neurol.*, 32, 114–118.

Asanuma, M., Hirata, H., and Cadet, J.L. (1998) Attenuation of 6-hydroxydopamine-induced dopaminergic nigrostriatal lesions in superoxide dismutase transgenic mice, *Neuroscience*, 85, 907–917.

Berger, K., Przedborski, S., and Cadet, J.L. (1990) Retrograde degeneration of nigrostriatal neurons induced by intrastriatal 6-hydroxydopamine injection in rats, *Bran Res. Bull.*, 26, 301–307.

Bernheimer, R.S., Birkmayer, W., Hornykiewicz, O., Jellinger, K., and Seitelberger, F. (1973) Brain dopamine and the syndromes of Parkinson and Huntington: clinical, morphological and neurochemical correlations, *J. Neurol. Sci.*, 20, 415–455.

Cadet, J.L. and Brannock, C. (1998) Free radicals and the pathobilogy of the brain dopamine systems, *Neurochemistry*, 32, 117–131.

Cadet, J.L., Ordonez, S.V., and Ordonez, J.V. (1997) Methamphetamine induces apoptosis in immortalized neural cells: protection by the proto-ocogene, bcl-2, *Synapse* 25, 176–184.

Cadet, J.L. and Zhu, S.M. (1992) The instrastriatal 6-hydroxydopamine model of hemiparkinsonism: quantitative receptor autoradiographic evidence of correlation between circling behavior and presynaptic nigrostriatal markers in the rat, *Brain Res.*, 595, 316–326.

Cadet, J.L., Last, R., Kostic, V., Przedborski, S., and Jackson-Lewis, V. (1991) Long-term behavioral and biochemical effects of intrastriatal injections of 6-hydroxydopamine, *Brain Res. Bull.*, 26, 707–713.

Cadet, J.L., Sheng, P., Ali, S., Rothman, R., Carlson, E., and Epstein, C. (1994) Attenuation of methamphetamine-induced neurotoxicity in copper/zinc superoxide dismutase transgenic mice, *J. Neurochem.*, 62, 380–383.

Chakraborti, Y., Das, S., Mondal, M., Roychoudbury, S., and Chakraborti, S. (1999) Oxidant, mitochondria and calcium: an overview, *Cell Signal*, 11, 77–85.

Cohen, G. (1987) Monoamine oxidase, hydrogen peroxide, and Parkinson's disease, *Adv. Neurol.*, 45, 119–125.

Cohen, G. and Heikkila, R.E. (1974) The generation of hydrogen peroxide, superoxide radical and hydroxyl radical by hydroxydopamine, dialuric acid, and related cytotoxic agents, *J. Biol. Chem.*, 249, 2447–2452.

Cohen, G., Heikkila, R.E., Allis, B., Cabbat, D., Bembiec, D., MacNamee, D., Mytlineou, C., and Winston, B. (1976) Destruction of sympathetic nerve terminals by 6-hydroxydopamine: Protection by 1-phenyl-3-(2-thiazolyl)-2-thiourea, diethyldithiocarbamate, methimazole, cysteamine, ethanol, and n-butanol, *J. Pharmacol. Exp. Ther.*, 199, 336–352.

Cubells, J.F., Rayport, S., Rajndron, G., and Sulzer, D. (1994) Methamphetamine neurotoxicity involves vacuolation of endoxytic organelles and dopamine-dependent intracellular oxidative stress, *J. Neurosci.*, 14, 2260–2271.

Dawson, V.L., Dawson, T.M., Bartley, D.A., Uhl, G.R., and Snyder, S.M. (1993) Mechanisms of nitric oxide-mediated neurotoxicity in primary brain cultures, *J. Neurosci.*, 13, 2651–2661.

Deng, X. and Cadet, J.L. (1999) Methamphetamine administration causes overexpression of nNOS in the mouse striatum, *Brain Res.*, 851, 254–257.

DeVito, M.J. and Wagner, G.C. (1989) Methamphetamine-induced neuronal damage: a possible role for free radicals, *Neuropharmacology*, 28, 1145–1150.

Dexter, D.T., Wells, F.R., Agid, F., Agid, Y., Lees, A., Jenner, P., and Marsden, C.D. (1987) Increased nigral iron content in post-mortem Parkinsonism brain, *Lancet*, 11, 219–220.

Dexter, D.T., Carter, C.J., Wells, F.R., Javoy-Agid, F., Agid, Y., Lees, A., Jenner, P., Marsden, C.D. (1989) Basal lipid peroxidation in substantia nigra is increased in Parkinson's disease, *J. Neurochem.*, 52, 381–389.

Dexter, D.T., Jenner, P., Schapira, A.H.V., and Marsden, C.D. (1992) Alterations in levels of iron, ferritin, and other trace metals in neurodegenerative diseases affecting the basal ganglia, *Ann. Neurol.*, 32, 94–100.

Dexter, D.T., Sian, J., Rose, S., Hindmarsh, J.G., Mann, V.M., Cooper, J.M., Wells, F.R., Daniel, S.E., Lees, A., Schapira, A.H.V., Jenner, P., and Marsden, C.D. (1994) Indices of oxidative stress and mitochondrial function in individuals with incidental Lewy body disease, *Ann. Neurol.*, 35, 38–44.

Epstein, C.J., Avraham, K.B., Lovett, M., Smith, S., Elroy-Stein, O., Rotman, G., Bry, C., and Groner, Y. (1987) Transgenic mice with increased CuZn-superoxide dismutase activity: animal model of dosage effects in Down's Syndrome, *Proc. Natl. Acad. Sci. U.S.A.*, 84, 8044–8048.

Fahn S. and Cohen, G. (1992) The oxidant stress hypothesis in Parkinson's disease: evidence supporting it, *Ann. Neurol.*, 32, 804–812.

Fahn, S., Libsch, L.R., and Cutler, R.W. (1971) Monoamines in the human neostriatum: topographic distribution in normals and in Parkinson's disease and their role in akinesia, rigidity, chorea, and tremor, *J. Neurol. Sci.*, 14, 427–455.

Giovanni, A., Liang, L.P., Hastings, T.G., and Zigmond, M.J. (1995) Estimating hydroxyl radical content in rat brain using systemic and intraventricular salicylate: Impact of methamphetamine, *J. Neurochem.*, 64, 1819–1825.

Hirata, H., Asanuma, M., and Cadet, J.L. (1998) Melatonin attenuates methamphetamine-induced toxic effects on dopamine and serotonin terminals in mouse brain, *Synapse*, 30, 150–155.

Hirata, H. and Cadet, J.L. (1997) p53-knockout mice are protected against the long-term effects of methamphetamine on dopaminergic terminals and cell bodies, *J. Neurochem.*, 69, 780–790.

Hirata, H.H., Ladenheim, B., Carlson, E., Epstein, C., and Cadet, J.L. (1996) Autoradiographic evidence for methamphetamine-induced striatal dopaminergic loss in mouse brain: attenuation in CuZn-superoxide dismutase transgenic mice, *Brain Res.*, 714, 95–103.

Hirsch, E.C., Brandel, J.P., Galle, P., and Javoy-Agid, Y. (1991) Iron and aluminum increases in the substantia nigra of patients with Parkinson's disease: an x-ray microanalysis, *J. Neurochem.* 56, 446–451.

Itzhak, Y. and Ali, S.F. (1996) The neuronal nitric oxide synthase inhibitor, 7-nitoindazole, protects against methamphetamine-induced neurtoxicity *in vivo*, *J. Neurochem.*, 67, 1770–1773.

Ikeda, R., Ikeda, S., Yoshimura, T., Kato, K., and Namba, M. (1978) Resistance of neuronal nitric oxide synthase-deficient mice to methamphetamine-induced dopaminergic neurotoxicity, *J. Pharmacol. Exp. Ther.*, 284, 1040–1047.

Jayanthi, S., Ladenheim, B., and Cadet, J.L. (1998) Methamphetamine-induced changes in antioxidant enzymes and lipid peroxidation in copper/zinc-superoxide dismutase transgenic mice, *Ann. NY Sci.*, 844, 92–102.

Jellinger, K.A., Kienzl, E., Rumpelmaier, G., Parelus, W., Reiderer, P., Stachelberger, H., Youdin, M.B.H., and Ben-Shachar, D. (1993) Iron and ferritin in substantia nigra in Parkinson's Disease, *Adv. Neurol.*, 60, 267–272.

LaVoie, M.J. and Hastings, T.G. (1999) Dopamine quinone formation and protein modification associated with the striatal neurotoxicity of methamphetamine: evidence against a role for extracellular dopamine, *J. Neurosci.*, 19, 1484–1491.

Marsden, C.D. (1990) Parkinson's disease, *Lancet*, 335, 948–952.

Martilla, R.J., Lorentz, H., and Rinne, U.K. (1988) Oxygen toxicity protecting enzymes in Parkinson's disease. Increase of superoxide dismutase-like activity in the substantia nigra and the basal nucleus, *J. Neurol. Sci.*, 86, 321–331.

Miyashita, T., Krajewski, S., Krajewski, M., Wang, H.G., Lin, H.K., Liebermann, D.A., Hoffman, B., and Reed, J.C. (1994) Tumor suppressor p53 is a regulator of bcl-2 and bax gene expression *in vitro* and *in vivo*, *Onogene*, 9, 1799–1805.

O'Dell, S.J., Weihmuller, F.B., McPherson, R.J., and Marshall, J.F. (1994) Excitotoxic striatal lesions protect against subsequent methamphetamine-induced dopamine depletions, *J. Pharmacol. Exp. Ther.*, 269, 319–325.

Offen, D., Beart, P.M., Cheung, N.S., Pascoe, C.J., Hochman, A., Gorodin, S., Melamed, E., Bernard, R., and Bernard, O. (1998) Transgenic mice expressing human Bcl-2 in their neurons are resistant to 6-hydroxydopamine and 1-methyl-4-phenyl-1,2,3,6-tetrahydropyridine neurotoxicity, *Proc. Natl. Acad. Sci. U.S.A.*, 95, 5789–5794.

Oltvai, Z.N., Milliman, C.L., and Korsmeyer, S.J. (1993) Bcl-2 heterodimerizes *in vivo* with a conserved homolog, Bax, that accelerates programmed cell death, *Cell*, 74, 609–619.

Perumal, A.S., Tordzro, W.K., Katz, M., Jackson-Lewis, V., Cooper, T.B., Fahn, S., and Cadet, J.L. (1989) Regional effects of 6-hydroxydopamine (6-OHDA) on free radical scavengers in rat brain, *Brain Res.*, 504, 139–141.

Reichmann, H., Joanetsky, B., and Reiderer, P. (1995) Iron-dependent enzymes in Parkinson's disease, *J. Neural. Transm.*, 46, 157–164.

Reiderer, P., Sofic, E., Rausch, W.D., Schmidt, B., Reynolds, G.P., Jellinger, K., and Youdim, M.B.H. (1989) Transition metals, ferritin, glutathione, and ascorbic acid in Parkinsonian brains, *J. Neurochem.*, 52, 515–520.

Saggu, H., Cooksey, J., Dexter, D., Wells, F.R., Lees, A., Jenner, P., and Marsden, C.D. (1989) A selective increase in particulate superoxide dismutase activity in Parkinsonian substantia nigra, *J. Neurochem.*, 53, 692–697.

Sheng, P., Cerruti, C., Ali, S., and Cadet, J.L. (1996) Nitric oxide is a mediator of methamphetamine (METH)-induced neurotoxicity: *In vitro* evidence from primary cultures of mesencephalic cells, *Ann. NY Acad. Sci.*, 801, 174–186.

Sofic, E., Reiderer, P., Heinsen, H., Beckmann, H., Reynolds, G.P., Hebenstreit, G., and Youdim, M.B. (1988) Increases iron (III) and total iron content in post-mortem substantia nigra of Parkinsonian brain, *J. Neural Transmittal*, 74, 199–205.

Sonsalla, P.K., Nicklas, W.J., and Heikkila, R.E. (1989) Role for excitatory amino acids in methamphetamine-induced dopaminergic toxicity, *Science*, 243, 398–400.

Stephans, S.E. and Yamamoto, B.Y. (1994) Methamphetamine-induced neurotoxicity: roles for glutamate and dopamine efflux, *Synapse*, 17, 203–209.

Wagner, G.C., Ricaurte, G.A., Seiden, L.S., Schuster, C.R., Miller, R.J., and Westley, J. (1980) Long-lasting depletions of striatal dopamine and loss of dopamine uptake sites following repeated administration of methamphetamine, *Brain Res.*, 181, 151–160.

Weihmuller, F.B., O'Dell, S.J., and Marshall, J.F. (1992) MK-801 protection against methamphetamine-induced striatal dopamine terminal injury is associated with attenuated dopamine overflow, *Synapse*, 11, 155–163.

CHAPTER 31

A Microassay Method Using a Neuroblastoma Cell Line to Examine Neurotoxicity of Organophosphate Mixtures

Laurie E. Roszell, Benjamin C. Kramer, and Glen J. Leach

CONTENTS

INTRODUCTION

The inhibition of acetylcholinesterase (AChE) by organophosphates (OPs) results in an accumulation of acetylcholine and sustained cholinergic stimulation. Current federal testing regulations for OP insecticides require studies on the dose-dependent inhibition of AChE activity in experimental animals. Difficulties with this approach include the time and cost constraints of using animals, as well as the uncertainty of extrapolating animal data to human risk. Immortal cell lines have been demonstrated to exhibit many of the same activities as their *in vivo* counterparts, including the production of various enzymes. One such cell line is SH-SY5Y, a neuroblastoma derived from human tissue. These cells produce AChE as well as neurotoxic esterase (NTE); inhibition of NTE results in a delayed neuropathy known as organophosphate-induced delayed neurotoxicity. It has been recently demonstrated that SH-SY5Y neuroblastomas can be used to assess AChE activity (Veronesi and Ehrich, 1993). The OP-induced inhibition of AChE activity in these cells was demonstrated to be similar to that seen in animal models (Ehrich et al., 1997).

The goal of these experiments was to adapt the method of Ehrich et al. (1997) to a 96-well plate format, in order to provide a screening assay in which more samples could be run with fewer cells and in less time. This modified method was then tested by assessing the inhibition of AChE activity in the presence of two OPs, paraoxon and dichlorvos, individually and in various dose combinations.

MATERIALS AND METHODS

All chemicals were obtained from Sigma Chemicals (St. Louis, MO) unless otherwise specified. The SH-SY5Y neuroblastoma cell line was purchased from American Type Culture Collection (Manassas, VA).

SH-SY5Y neuroblastomas were cultured in a humidified atmosphere at 37°C and 5% CO_2. The culture media was Ham's F-12 media supplemented with 15% fetal bovine serum and penicillin/streptomycin (5,000 IU/ml, 5,000 µg/ml).

To determine the optimal number of cells for use in the 96-well plate format, the neuroblastomas were harvested, resuspended in culture media, and added to triplicate wells of a 96-well plate at concentrations ranging from 8×10^3 to 1×10^6 cells/well. Plates with cells were then allowed to incubate for 18 to 24 hr. At the end of this period, the plates were centrifuged for 3 min at $100 \times g$ and the media removed from the wells and replaced with 100 µL of phosphate buffered saline (PBS). AChE activity was measured by adding 100 µL of AChE reagent (Sigma Diagnostics Cholinesterase (PTC) procedure 422) to each well and measuring the absorbance at 405 nm every 15 min for 1 hr. Triplicate wells were prepared for each cell concentration. Matched controls for each sample had 100 µL PBS added rather than AChE reagent. A substrate control contained 100 µL each PBS and AChE reagent in the absence of cells.

Dichlorvos (Chem Service, Inc., West Chester, PA) and paraoxon were initially made as 0.1 M stocks in absolute ethanol; subsequent dilutions were in PBS. For all experiments with OPs, a dosing plate was prepared containing the appropriate dilutions of individual or mixtures of OPs. For experiments in which neuroblastomas were exposed to individual OPs, dichlorvos was diluted to concentrations ranging from 10 to 10^{-2} µM and paraoxon was diluted to concentrations ranging from 10^{-1} to 10^{-7} µM. For experiments in which combinations of OPs were used, dichlorvos or paraoxon were diluted in PBS at concentrations of 2.0, 2×10^{-1}, or 2×10^{-2} µM and 2×10^{-3}, 2×10^{-4}, and 2×10^{-5} µM, respectively. Equal amounts of the appropriate dilution of each compound were added to the dosing plate to achieve final concentrations of 10^{-3}, 10^{-4}, and 10^{-5} µM paraoxon and 1.0, 10^{-1}, and 10^{-2} µM dichlorvos. All combinations of these OPs, nine total, were tested. These concentrations were found to be nonlethal as determined by a cytotoxicity assay using the reduction of MTT as an indicator of cellular viability.

For the experiments assessing AChE activity following exposure to paraoxon and dichlorvos, cells were transferred to 96-well plates at a concentration of 100,000 cells/well one day prior to running the assay. On the day of the assay (18 to 24 hr after cells were plated), media in all wells was replaced with 100 µL of individual or combined organophosphates from the dosing plate. The cells were incubated for

1 hr in a humidified atmosphere at 37°C, 5% CO_2, and ambient oxygen. After this time, AChE activity was measured as described above. Triplicate wells were prepared for each individual or combined concentration. Matched controls for each sample had 100 μL PBS added rather than AChE reagent. A substrate control contained 100 μL each PBS and AChE reagent in the absence of cells.

Data were analyzed for significance by performing a Kruskal-Wallis one-way analysis of variance on ranks, followed by multiple comparisons of OP-treatments vs. the control group using Dunn's method.

RESULTS

The results of the experiments to determine optimal cell number and reaction time are shown in Figure 31.1. After 60 min, all concentrations of cells showed similar AChE activity. Differences were seen in the time required for AChE activity to plateau, with wells containing 31,000 or more cells reaching a plateau at about 45 min. Based on these results, a concentration of 100,000 cells/well and a reaction time of 60 min were selected for experiments with the OPs.

Exposure to both paraoxon and dichlorvos resulted in a dose-dependent inhibition of AChE activity (Figure 31.2). Paraoxon was more potent than dichlorvos. AChE activity was significantly inhibited ($p < 0.05$) at paraoxon concentrations greater than 1×10^{-4} μM. The highest concentration of paraoxon, 10^{-1} μM, resulted in nearly 100% inhibition of AChE activity. Dichlorvos significantly inhibited AChE activity at concentrations above 5×10^{-1} μM. The highest concentration of dichlorvos, 1 μM, resulted in an inhibition of approximately 50%. Concentrations above this resulted in decreased cellular viability (data not shown). The apparent EC50 for paraoxon was 1.75×10^{-3} μM, while the apparent EC50 for dichlorvos was 5.26 μM. These values are in agreement with those of Ehrich et al. (1997) in which similar experiments were performed with terminally differentiated SH-SY5Y neuroblastomas.

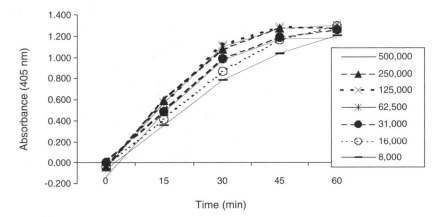

Figure 31.1 Determination of optimal cell number per well and reaction time for AChE activity.

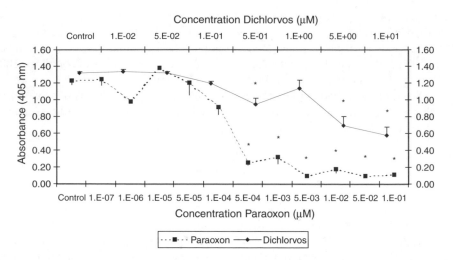

Figure 31.2 Effect of dichlorvos or paraoxon on AChE activity of SH-SY5Y neuroblastomas. $^*p < 0.05$.

Based on the above experiments, three concentrations of each OP were chosen to assess the effects of a mixture: 10^{-3}, 10^{-4}, and 10^{-5} μM paraoxon and 1.0, 10^{-1}, and 10^{-2} μM dichlorvos. These concentrations were chosen to include both inhibitory and noninhibitory concentrations of the individual compounds.

Figure 31.3 shows the effect of the single and combined compounds on AChE activity as demonstrated by the change in absorbance at 405 nm. The actual values for these mixtures are shown in Table 31.1. Additionally, Table 31.1 shows the values expressed as percent inhibition (as compared to the control values) and the predicted and actual inhibition by the mixtures. In general, combinations of these OPs appeared

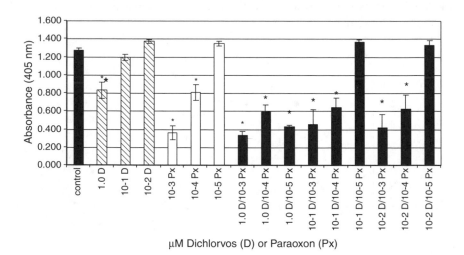

Figure 31.3 Effect of dichlorvos (D) or paraoxon (Px) alone or in combination on AChE activity of SH-SY5Y neuroblastomas. $^*p < 0.05$.

Table 31.1 Effect of Paraoxon (Px) or Dichlorvos (D) on AChE Activity of SH-SY5Y Neuroblastomas, Significance Level 0.05

OP concentration (μM)	Absorbance at 405 nm ± SEM	Measured inhibition (%)	Predicted inhibition (%)	Significant vs. control?
control	1.269 ± 0.031			
10^{-2} D	1.373 ± 0.091	−8		
10^{-1} D	1.198 ± 0.033	6		
1.0 D	0.831 ± 0.023	34		x
10^{-5} Px	1.352 ± 0.081	−7		
10^{-4} Px	0.811 ± 0.086	36		x
10^{-3} Px	0.362 ± 0.024	72		x
10^{-2} D/10^{-5} Px	1.332 ± 0.042	−5	−15	
10^{-2} D/10^{-4} Px	0.630 ± 0.077	50	28	x
10^{-2} D/10^{-3} Px	0.418 ± 0.017	67	63	x
10^{-1} D/10^{-5} Px	1.370 ± 0.167	−8	−1	
10^{-1} D/10^{-4} Px	0.647 ± 0.104	49	42	x
10^{-1} D/10^{-3} Px	0.453 ± 0.027	64	77	x
1.0 D/10^{-5} Px	0.432 ± 0.151	66	28	x
1.0 D/10^{-4} Px	0.590 ± 0.156	54	71	x
1.0 D/10^{-3} Px	0.339 ± 0.052	73	106	x

to inhibit AChE activity in an additive manner. As with the individual compounds, inhibition was dose-dependent. In each mixture that was significantly different from the control, at least one of the individual components also significantly inhibited AChE activity.

DISCUSSION

Currently, *in vivo* models are recommended by the U.S. EPA to assess the anticholinergic properties of OPs. Difficulties with this approach include the time and cost constraints of using animals, interlaboratory variability, and the uncertainty associated with extrapolating animal data to human risk. It has been previously demonstrated that SH-SY5Y neuroblastomas can be used to assess AChE activity (Veronesi and Ehrich, 1993) and its inhibition by OPs (Ehrich et al. 1997; Barber et al., 1999). Our results with paraoxon and dichlorvos alone are in agreement with those of Ehrich et al. (1997), as well as with studies performed in brain homogenates from hens (Lotti and Johnson, 1978), further validating the use of these cells.

In the absence of mixture-specific data, current guidance on mixtures recommends that effects of individual components be assumed to interact in an additive manner. This assumption was supported by the current work, in which the mixtures of dichlorvos and paraoxon appeared to be additive in their inhibition of AChE activity. A more accurate method to determine interaction types is through the use of isobolographic analysis. This method, by providing graphical representation of chemical interactions in two dimensions, allows differences in mixtures to be clearly perceived (Gessner, 1995). Therefore, further experiments are required to verify that the apparent interactions are indeed additive.

In contrast to the results reported herein, there have been other research efforts demonstrating that mixtures of pesticides do not always act in an additive manner. In a series of experiments with pesticides including dimethoate, azinphos-methyl, diazinon, pirimiphos methyl, and benomyl, Marinovich et al. (1996) found that the inhibition of AChE by a mixture was equal to the inhibition induced by the most potent component. The differences in the current work and that of Marinovich et al. demonstrate that assuming additive interactions is not always appropriate for OPs and emphasize the need to screen environmentally relevant mixtures of OPs for possible interactions. The work described here demonstrates that the 96-well plate format can be an effective first step in screening OP mixtures.

REFERENCES

Barber, D., Correll, L., and Ehrich, M. (1999) Comparison of two *in vitro* activation systems for protoxicant Organophosphorus esterase inhibitors, *Toxicol. Sci.,* 47, 16–22.

Ehrich, M., Correll, L., and Veronesi, B. (1997) Acetylcholinesterase and neuropathy target esterase inhibitions in neuroblastoma cells to distinguish organophosphorus compounds causing acute and delayed neurotoxicity, *Fundam. Appl. Toxicol.,* 38, 55–63.

Gessner, P.K. (1995) Isobolographic analysis of interactions: an update on applications and utility, *Toxicology,* 105, 161–179.

Lotti, M. and Johnson, M.K. (1978) Neurotoxicity of organophosphorus pesticides: Predictions can be based on *in vitro* studies with hen and human enzymes *Arch. Toxicol.,* 41, 215–221.

Marinovich, M., Ghilardi, G., and Galli, C.L. (1996) Effect of pesticide mixtures on *in vitro* nervouscells: comparison with single pesticides, *Toxicol.,* 108, 206–210.

Veronesi, B. and Ehrich, M. (1993) Using neuroblastoma cell lines to examine organophosphate neurotoxicity, *In Vitro Toxicol.,* 6, 57–65.

CHAPTER 32

Development of Integrin Expression as a Molecular Biomarker for Early, Sensitive Detection of Neurotoxicity

Joyce E. Royland

CONTENTS

INTRODUCTION

The Environmental Protection Agency (EPA) has a long-term interest in neurotoxicity testing as one endpoint in the development of toxicity reference doses. As early as 1982, the Office of Pesticide Programs began publishing neurotoxicity testing guidelines for pesticides and other toxic substances. The goal of these documents was to provide a framework of experimental protocols that when used would provide a consistent data set for risk analysis. Recently the Guidelines for Neurotoxicity Risk Assessment (U.S. EPA, 1998) were formulated to facilitate interpretation of neurotoxicity data in a risk assessment context. A multifaceted approach for the evaluation of risk to humans, the guidelines include four main topics for consideration: hazard characterization, quantitative dose response assessment, exposure assessment, and risk characterization. As a number of unknowns can exist in each of these areas, assumptions must be made when determining risk. For example, in dose response assessments, extrapolation from animal data to humans is a primary concern. In this instance, the study of proteins in major physiological processes, which often share considerable amino acid homology across species, might be one approach to reduce uncertainty. The identification of such protein molecular bio-markers that serve as predictors of neurotoxic insult and are independent of species differences or are well characterized in several species would help to address issues of this kind.

The new guidelines further the concept that behavioral, neurophysiological, neurochemical, and neuroanatomical manifestations should be combined with mechanistic and pharmacokinetic data to reduce uncertainty in risk assessments. In the past, toxicity often has been evaluated based on acute and/or high dose exposure data. It is now apparent that the consequences of multiple low dose or chronic exposures and exposure to mixtures also must be considered. To improve our ability to identify potential neurotoxicants and to evaluate known neurotoxicants at low exposures, it is necessary to be able to identify conditions that precede overt toxicity and to recognize more subtle adverse effects if hazard characterization is to include outcomes such as subtle changes in cognition and learning or long-term effects after early insult. The focus of biomarker research is to provide the means by which the ability to identify neurotoxicity can be improved.

Biomarker research is divided into three categories: *biomarkers of exposure, biomarkers of effect,* and *biomarkers of susceptibility. Biomarkers of exposure* can include exogenous compounds, their metabolites, or the products of the interaction between the compound and target molecules. *Biomarkers of effect* are measurable changes in endogenous compounds that can be tied to a toxic effect or disease. *Biomarkers of susceptibility* are indicators of inherent or acquired properties that affect organisms' response to compounds. Biomarkers that can be measured in easily available samples such as blood or urine are preferred in many toxicological studies. However, changes may occur in tissues that affect function, yet are not reflected in body fluids. This is particularly true in neurotoxicity studies where the blood–brain barrier can prevent release of proteins or compounds to the peripheral circulation and where small changes in structure can have profound consequences (e.g., dendritic spine formation in learning and memory). Our research focuses on the use of cell adhesion molecules as biomarkers of effect, but they also have the potential to be useful as biomarkers of susceptibility.

The development of the nervous system requires a precise sequence of events proceeding from cell migration and differentiation, through growth cone formation and axonal elongation to neurite extension and target recognition. Each of these processes requires specific cell-to-cell and/or cell-to-extracellular matrix interactions that result in initiation of signaling cascade events, morphometric or cytoskeletal changes, or regulation of gene expression. Cell-to-cell and cell-to-extracellular matrix interactions are mediated by a number of different cell adhesion molecules (CAMs) derived from relatively few protein families. In most cases, CAMs are transmembrane proteins that require divalent cations for activity. The different families of CAMs mediate varying levels of cell adhesion and serve specific physiological needs.

Integrins are the cell adhesion molecules of primary importance in neural interactions. As such they are likely candidates to be molecular biomarkers for

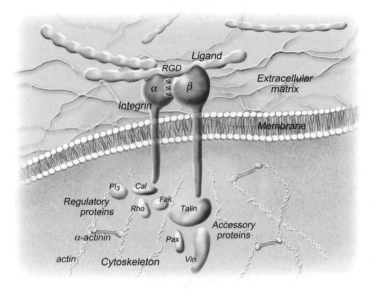

Figure 32.1 Integrin heterodimers transduce signals both into and out of the cell via interactions with extracellular ligands and cytoplasmic accessory or regulatory proteins, the cytoskeleton, and signal transduction proteins. Abbreviations: arginine-glycine-aspartic acid peptide (RGD), calreticulin (Cal), focal adhesion kinase (Fak), paxillin (Pax), phosphatidylinositol-3 kinase (PI3), vinculin (Vin).

neurotoxic effects. Composed of transmembrane heterodimers of noncovalently bound α and β subunits, integrins link the cytoskeleton with the extracellular environment via cell-to-cell or cell-to-extracellular matrix (ECM) interactions (Figure 32.1). Each subunit is composed of a large extracellular domain with a globular head and a small cytoplasmic tail. The head of the α subunit contains 2 to 3 divalent cation binding sites that must be filled for ligand binding to occur and in some cases for subunit association (Kirchhofer et al., 1991). The cytoplasmic tail of the β subunit interacts with the cytoskeleton through a number of accessory proteins (e.g., vinculin, talin, paxillin) that activate a number of downstream signal transduction pathways. Analysis of the beta1 family of integrins has shown ligand affinity and specificity to be determined largely by the alpha subunit (Fernandez et al., 1998).

The extracellular portions of the α and β subunits serve as a receptor for recognition sites on extracellular ligands or other cell surfaces. The extracellular ligands are most often large glycoproteins (e.g., collagens, fibronectin, laminins) that assemble into the three-dimensional arrays of the extracellular matrix. The most common recognition site found to date is the Arg-Gly-Asp (arginine-glycine-asparagine, RGD) sequence found in collagen, fibronectin, and a number of other ECM ligands, but other recognition sequences have been identified (for review, see Hynes, 1992). Interaction of the extracellular ligand with the integrin receptors initiates outside-in signaling via signal transduction pathways. The accessory proteins serve to connect the cytoplasmic domains of the integrin subunits with the cytoskeleton and intracellular regulatory proteins (e.g., calreticulin, PI3) for inside-out signaling.

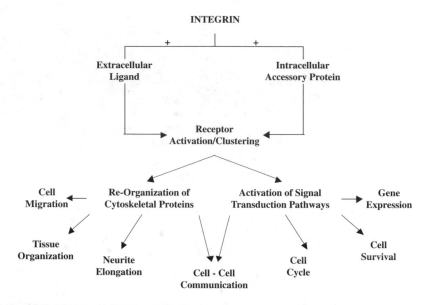

Figure 32.2 Integrin-mediated cell functions.

Integrin outside-in activation results in a number of cellular responses including phosphoinositide metabolism (McNamee et al., 1993); activation of Rho family GTPases leading to changes in cytoskeleton structure (Defilippi et al., 1997b); and activation of protein tyrosine kinases (focal adhesion kinase [FAK], nitrogen-activated protein kinase [MAP]) and phosphatases (Src) (Schlaepfer et al., 1998), which in turn induce nuclear signaling pathways leading to gene expression (Brizzi et al., 1999) and translation (Pabla et al., 1999). As is often the case, members of one transduction pathway can modify the activity of one or more of the others, either enhancing or repressing their function (for review, see Defilippi et al., 1997a). Activation of these signaling pathways leads to changes in cell cycle, cell survival, and gene expression in addition to the better known integrin functions in cell adhesion and migration (Figure 32.2).

Integrin activation state also can be mediated by intracellular events. Known as inside-out signaling, proteins binding to the cytoplasmic tails of integrin subunits can cause conformational changes in the subunit extracellular head that regulate receptor-mediated adhesion to the extracellular ligands (affinity modulation) or mediate lateral movement within the plasma membrane during receptor clustering (avidity modulation) (Hughes and Pfaff, 1998). Integrin-mediated cell adhesion often is required for cell survival.

Integrin activation even in the absence of cell adhesion has been shown to protect against apoptosis. SK-N-BE cells, a neuroblastoma cell line, become apoptotic and die under nonadherent conditions. Stimulation of suspended SK-N-BE cells by soluble collagen I induces clustering of $\alpha 1$, $\alpha 3$, αV, $\beta 1$, and $\beta 3$ integrins; increases expression of the antiapoptotic bcl-2 gene; and protects against apoptosis in a *de novo* protein synthesis-dependent manner (Bozzo et al., 1997). However, not all cell types can be rescued by this method. Endothelial cells have been shown to require attachment and cytoskeletal rearrangements to prevent cell death (Re et al., 1994).

It has been hypothesized that synaptic plasticity in the form of structural changes occurring in the postsynaptic dendritic spines during long-term potentiation (LTP) are an integral part of learning and memory. Integrin-mediated changes in cytoskeleton could play a role in spine formation and stabilization (Lee et al., 1980). Staubli et al. (1990, 1998) found that inhibition of integrin-ligand binding had no effect on LTP induction or degree of potentiation but did decrease LTP retention time. In addition, immunohistochemical studies have identified the α8 integrin subunit (Einheber et al., 1996) and the αVβ8 heterodimer (Nishimura et al., 1998) within the spines and postsynaptic densities of dendrites, providing further evidence for a role of integrins in the formation, maintenance, or plasticity of synapses.

Not only are integrins involved in a number of critical physiological functions, their expression varies with cell type and state of differentiation. For example, in the developing brain, neurite outgrowth is mediated by the α1 integrin subunit, whereas glial cell process extension involves the αV integrin subunit (Tarone et al., 2000). Additional specificity may be determined by the ability of cells to regulate the binding affinity of the integrin receptor (e.g., by inside-out modifications). Thus in platelets, α2β1 is specific for collagen (Staaz et al., 1989), but in other cell types it can recognize both collagen and laminin (Kirchhofer et al., 1990). Most cells express more than one integrin receptor, giving them the ability to bind to more than one ligand; consequently, the selectivity of a given cell type for specific ligands is largely due to their pattern of integrin expression (Hynes and Lander, 1992). This definitive cell type and state integrin expression contributes to their potential usefulness as molecular biomarkers.

Integrin heterodimers have been shown to be present at the site of damage in several neurodegenerative diseases. For example, integrin α3, α4, α6, and β1 subunits have been found within neuritic plaques of Alzheimer's disease (Eikelenboom et al., 1994; Van Gool et al., 1994). The major protein of neuritic plaques, β-amyloid (βA), is derived from the amyloid precursor protein (APP) via cleavage by β- and γ-secretases (Selkoe, 1994). Recent *in vitro* studies on the normal function of APP show it is expressed in adhesion patches and colocalizes with integrin α1β1 and α5β1 heterodimers, which suggests APP plays a role in cell adhesion, neurite extension, and synaptic plasticity either directly via integrin interactions or by similar pathways (Sabo et al., 1995; Storey et al., 1996a,b; Yamazaki et al., 1997). Neurons and glia, in contrast to nonneuronal cells, secrete small amounts of APP, which has been reported to become embedded in the extracellular matrix (Klier et al., 1990), where it could mediate cell attachment via an Arg-His-Asp (RHD) sequence that mimics the RGD integrin β1 subunit recognition sequence of fibronectin (Ghiso et al., 1992). Therefore, disruption of normal neuronal cell adhesion functions could contribute to pathology of the disease. In contrast, Matter et al. (1998) demonstrated that the integrin fibronectin receptor, α5β1, is capable of binding the soluble non-fibrillar βA toxic APP breakdown product, facilitating its internalization and degradation by cells and decreasing the extracellular formation of toxic fibrils and consequent cell apoptosis. In this context, integrins appear to play a neuroprotective role, suggesting a careful balance must be maintained between multiple members of a complex interactive system.

Integrin activity also has been implicated in the induction and chronicity of multiple sclerosis (MS) and Guillain-Barré syndrome (GBS), immune-mediated inflammatory diseases of the central and peripheral nervous systems, respectively (Archelos et al., 1999). Integrins modulate critical processes important in disease pathogenesis such as T-cell activation and recruitment, cytokine induction, and ECM synthesis. They mediate entrance of mononuclear cells through the blood-brain and blood-neuronal barriers and antigen presentation for T-cell activation, which is believed to be required for initiation and maintenance of the inflammation leading to demylination and loss of function in MS (Hart and Fabry, 1995). Components of the ECM in conjunction with integrins contribute both to cell damage by co-stimulating T-cell activation and to neuronal recovery by modulating remyelination and axonal outgrowth (Sobel, 1998).

APPROACH

A multitiered approach is being used to determine whether integrins can be used as biomarkers of neurotoxicity (Figure 32.3). Molecular and cellular biological techniques, including Northern Blot and/or RNAse protection assays (mRNA) and Western Blot (protein), will be used to monitor mRNA and protein expression levels. A series of glial and neuronal cell lines (e.g., C6, N2A, PC12) and isolated cell types from tissue culture (e.g., isolated astrocytes, oligodendrocytes, or neurons) will be tested to identify *in vitro* systems for monitoring response to toxicant exposure. Investigation of possible cell-to-cell interactions can be carried out using primary cultures and/or various co-culture techniques (e.g., plating neurons on an astrocyte monolayer or using cell culture plate inserts). So that the efficacy of integrins as markers of neurotoxicity can be assessed, time and dose studies to determine critical windows of exposure and the relative sensitivity of individual integrin subunits will be carried out using known neurotoxicants. Exposure levels that affect integrin expression without causing cell mortality will be chosen to reduce concerns over general whole cell toxicity effects. Changes found in integrin expression levels will be assessed further by cell adhesion assays to determine functional consequences. Morphometric changes and/or possible changes in timing of differentiation (e.g., changes in proliferation or time of expression of markers) will be monitored as additional indicators of cell health and functional changes. Information gained from the above studies will be used to design targeted *in vivo* studies using some of the same compounds. Reproducing changes found in *in vitro* testing in an *in vivo* model is a necessary step in the validation of integrin expression as a biomarker of neurotoxicity. Once validated, both *in vitro* and *in vivo* test systems can be used to gain information on neurotoxicants for which the mechanism is not known or to evaluate new compounds that are suspected to have neurotoxicant activity.

Our initial efforts are directed at identifying profiles of integrin message and protein expression in the PC12 adrenal pheochromocytoma cell line. PC12 cells differentiate into a sympathetic neuronal phenotype following treatment for 7 d with nerve growth factor (NGF) (Greene and Tischler, 1976). NGF exposure stops cell division, induces expression of neuronal specific markers, induces neurite extension,

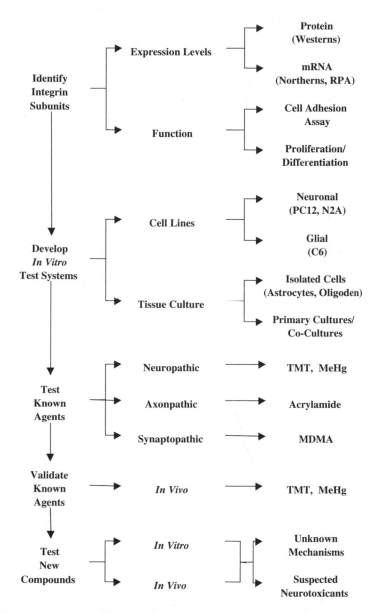

Figure 32.3 Approach to validation of integrin subunit expression levels as molecular biomarkers of neurotoxicity. Abbreviations: trimethyltin (TMT), methylmercury (MeHg), 3,4-methylenedioxymethamphetamine (MDMA), RNAse protection assay (RPA).

and causes cells to become electrically excitable (see review by Fujita et al., 1989). PC12 cells have been used extensively as a model of neurite outgrowth to study cytoskeletal assembly and signal transduction pathways during neurite extension (Keegan and Halegoua, 1993; Marshall, 1995). They also have been shown to be sensitive to the effects of known neurotoxicants including mercuric compounds

(Parran et al., 2001), PCBs (Angus and Contreras, 1994), lead (Crumpton et al., 2001), and the acetylcholine esterase inhibitor, chlorpyrifos (Das and Barone, 1999; Song et al., 1998).

Critical to the current study, PC12 cells have been shown to express a number of integrin receptor subtypes in common with the brain (Pinkstaff et al., 1999). Differentiated PC12 cells have been shown to express integrin $\alpha1\beta1$ and $\alpha3\beta1$ heterodimers in point contacts at the cell/ECM interface similar to dorsal root ganglion cells (Arregui et al., 1994). And the integrin $\alpha5\beta1$ heterodimer has been identified by confocal laser scanning microscopy in the filopodia of PC12 cells, where it is concentrated in the growth cones (Yanagida et al., 1999). Functionally, NGF-treated PC12 cells adhere to collagen I and IV via the integrin $\alpha1\beta1$ heterodimer and to laminin via both $\alpha1\beta1$ and $\alpha3\beta1$ heterodimers by distinct binding sites. Antibodies to the $\alpha1$, $\alpha3$, and $\beta1$ integrin subunits block this cell adhesion and inhibit neurite extension (Tomaselli et al., 1990). Arregui et al. (1994) demonstrated a direct relationship between levels of specific extracellular matrix receptors and cell adhesion levels. And recently in a study on manganese-induced neurite outgrowth in PC12 cells, the $\alpha V\beta1$ integrin complex was identified as the activated adhesion receptor (Lein et al., 2000).

This study concentrates on integrin subunits expressed both in PC12 cells and the brain (e.g., $\alpha1$, $\alpha3$, αV, and $\beta1$). Subunit mRNAs and protein expression levels are determined both in differentiating PC12 cells as a model of early neuronal development and in the NGF primed cells as a model of late development or plasticity. Control levels are compared to integrin expression after time and dose effect experiments using known (methyl mercury), suspected (chlorpyrifos), and potential (dimethyltin) neurotoxicants.

DISCUSSION

Identification of a new molecular biomarker of effect entails defining a number of criteria. The protein must be part of a biochemical pathway or physiological process that is likely to be impacted by toxicant exposure. Integrins participate in a number of critical neural functions both developmentally and in the adult. Their activation can lead to changes in signal transduction pathways and induction of gene expression. In addition, they play an important role in a cell's interaction with its external environment and neighboring cell types. A biomarker should be specific for a cell type or function. Integrin expression profiles display both cell type and function specificity. It is useful if a biomarker has been associated with disease processes. Integrins have been associated with Alzheimer's disease as well as with immune-related diseases of the nervous system (Archelos et al., 1999). And finally, a biomarker must be found to be changed by toxicant exposure in the system for which it is to be used. This last criteria is the primary aim of the current study.

Part of the identification and validation process of a molecular biomarker is to determine whether it is affected by known toxicants. It is also necessary to determine whether the biomarker is specific to a given family of toxicants or has wider application; therefore, it needs to be tested against a number of different compounds with different mechanisms of action. This project includes monitoring the effects of prototypic (e.g., mercury), suspected (e.g., chlorpyrifos), and potential (e.g., butyltin compounds) neurotoxicants on integrin expression (type and localization) in cell lines and in tissue culture systems. Methylmercury is a known developmental neurotoxicant that may have direct or indirect effects on integrin expression and/or function. For instance, levels of expression of growth factors, known modulators of integrin cell surface receptors (Rossino et al., 1990; Santala and Heino, 1991), are affected by exposure to methylmercury. Chlorpyrifos is an acetylcholine esterase (AChE) inhibiting pesticide that has been shown to have neurotoxic effects separate from its AChE inhibiting ability (Das and Barone, 1999). Integrins may participate in that toxicity via receptor crosstalk with muscarinic acetylcholine receptors (Slack, 1998). And the butyltin compounds have been identified by the EPA Office of Water as potential candidates for neurotoxicity and are listed on the contaminate candidate list as high priority compounds for investigation.

Use of an *in vitro* model allows us to dissect out questions on order of cause and effect and on possible sites of action in a relatively quick and non-animal intensive manner. Questions such as whether a given neurotoxicant perturbs integrin function directly with consequences on cell attachment, function, or survival or whether a disruption in cell function/survival is reflected in level of integrin expression (i.e., an indirect effect) can be answered by examining the relative timing of changes in function and integrin expression. By progressing from cell lines to increasingly more specific and complex models, knowledge of possible mechanisms of action of various neurotoxicants can be gained in addition to validation of integrins as potential molecular biomarkers.

For earlier, more sensitive detection of toxicity, changes in the selected molecular biomarker should be reflected in changes in a physiological endpoint. NGF-induced differentiation of PC12 cells has been shown to cause a tenfold increase in integrin $\alpha 1$ subunit expression before measurable neurite outgrowth occurs (Rossino et al., 1990). Since expression of the $\beta 1$ subunit is constitutive, the expression of the different α subunits often controls the amount of the functional heterodimeric receptor (Zhang et al., 1993). Consequently, the induction of $\alpha 1$ subunit expression preceding neurite outgrowth suggests that integrin subunit expression levels can be used as early, sensitive biomarkers of neurotoxicants that affect neuronal differentiation or neurite extension.

For the successful identification and validation of a new biomarker, the tools must be available to investigate the potential candidate(s). Since their discovery a little less than 25 years ago, research into integrin types, distribution, and function has increased exponentially. A preliminary review of research articles listed on Medline shows that since their first mention in 1977 through the year 2001, nearly 21,000 integrin-related papers have been published. Of those papers, approximately 900 deal specifically with integrins and the nervous system. Paralleling the increase in scientific interest in integrins is increasing availability of the tools to study them. For instance, between 2000 and 2002, one major supplier of integrin antibodies added 84 new antibodies to their catalogue—antibodies to different subunit epitopes and with different functional capabilities that expand the researcher's investigative options. Similarly, there have been improvements in available protein extraction protocols (e.g., separation of membrane and cytoplasmic proteins) and increased variety and improved sensitivity in detection methods. Industry has taken note of the high interest in and multiple functions of integrins and has included them in new research technologies. Vendors for genomic-related supplies include members of the integrin family, their regulatory and accessory proteins, and components of the ECM on microarrays targeted to toxicology research. And select integrins have been included on a recently available signal transduction protein array.

We have identified only one study to date on the consequences of toxicant exposure on integrin expression in any neural cell system. In that study, Zhang et al. (1994) found treatment with hydrogen peroxide inhibited both integrin specific PC12 cell attachment to collagen and caused adhered cells to detach. Intracellular ATP also was found to be profoundly decreased. As integrins mediate interactions between the ECM and the cytoskeleton in an energy-dependent manner, it was suggested that loss of intracellular ATP interfered with integrin complexing with cytoskeletal elements. So yet another mechanism has been proposed by which integrins may be impacted by neurotoxicant exposure. Our study is designed to provide new information on this important family of cell adhesion molecules and how changes in their expression levels may have applicability as molecular biomarkers of neurotoxicity.

ACKNOWLEDGMENTS

This document has been reviewed in accordance with the U.S. Environmental Protection Agency policy and approved for publication. Mention of trade names or commercial products does not constitute endorsement or recommendation for use. We thank John Havel for drafting the drawing in Figure 32.1.

REFERENCES

Angus, W.G. and Contreras, M.I. (1994) The effects of Aroclor 1254 on undifferentiated and NGF stimulated PC12 cells, *Neurotoxicology,* 15, 809–817.

Archelos, J.J., Previtali, S.C., and Harung, H.-P. (1999) The role of integrins in immune-mediated diseases of the nervous system, *Trends Neurosci.,* 22, 30–38.

Arregui, C.O., Carbonetto, S., and McKerracher, L. (1994) Characterization of neural cell adhesion sites: point contacts are the sites of interaction between integrins and the cytoskeleton in PC12 cells, *J. Neurosci.,* 14, 6967–6977.

Bozzo, C., Bellomo, G., Silengo, L., Tarone, G., and Altruda, F. (1997) Soluble integrin ligands and growth factors independently rescue neuroblastoma cells from apoptosis under nonadherent conditions, *Exp. Cell Res.,* 237, 326–337.

Brizzi, M.F., Defilippi, P., Rosso, A., Ventmino, M., Garbarino, G., Mayajima, A., Silengo, L., Tarone, G., and Pegoraro, L. (1999) Integrin-mediated adhesion of endothelial cells induces JAK2 and STAT5A activation: role in the control of c-fos gene expression, *Mol. Biol. Cell.,* 103, 3463–3471.

Crumpton, T., Atkins, D.S., Zawia, N.H., and Barone, S., Jr. (2001) Lead exposure in pheo-chromocytoma (PC12) cells alters neural differentiation and SP1 DNA-binding, *Neurotoxicology,* 22, 49–62.

Das, K.P. and Barone, S., Jr. (1999) Neuronal differentiation in PC12 cells is inhibited by chlorpyrifos and its metabolites: is acetylcholinesterase inhibition the site of action?, *Toxicol. Appl. Pharmacol.*, 160, 217–230.

Defilippi, P., Giondi, A., Santoni, A., and Tarone, G. (1997a) *Signal Transduction by Integrins*, Landes Bioscience, Austin, pp. 29–155.

Defilippi, P., Venturino, M., Gulino, D., Duperray, A., Boquet, P., Fiorentini, C., Volpe, G., Palmieri, M., Silengo, L., and Tarone, G. (1997b) Dissection of pathways implicated in integrin-mediated actin cytoskeleton assembly. Involvement of protein kinase C, RHO GTPase, and tyrosine phosphorylation, *J. Biol. Chem.*, 35, 21726–21734.

Eikelenboom, P., Shan, S.S., Kamphorst, W., van der Valk, P., and Rozemuller, J.M. (1994) Cellular and substrate adhesion molecules (integrins) and their ligands in cerebral amyloid plaques in Alzheimer's disease, *Virchows Arch.*, 424, 421–427.

Einheber, S., Schnapp, L.M., Salzer, J.L., Cappiello, Z.B., and Milner, T. (1996) Regional and ultrastructural distribution of the $\alpha 8$ integrin subunit in developing and adult rat brain suggests a role in synaptic function, *J. Comp. Neurol.*, 370, 105–134.

Fernandez, C., Clark, K., Burrows, L., Schofield, N.R., and Humphries, M.J. (1998) Regulation of the extracellular ligand binding activity of integrins, *Frontiers Biosci.*, 3, 5864–700.

Fujita, K., Lazarovici, P., and Guroff, G. (1989) Regulation of the differentiation of PC12 pheochromocytoma cells, *Environ. Health Perspec.*, 80, 127–142.

Ghiso, G., Rostagno, A., Gardella, J.E., Liem, L., Gorevic, P.D., and Frangione, J. (1992) A 109-amino acid C-terminal fragment of Alzheimer's-disease amyloid precursor protein contains a sequence, -RHDS-, that promotes cell adhesion, *Biochem. J.*, 288, 1053–1059.

Greene, L.A. and Tischler, A.S. (1976) Establishment of a noradrenergic clonal line of rat adrenal pheochromocytoma cells which respond to nerve growth factor, *Proc. Natl. Acad. Sci. U.S.A.*, 73, 2424–2428.

Hart, M.N. and Fabry, Z. (1995) CNS antigen presentation, *Trends Neurosci.*, 18, 475–481.

Hughes, P.E. and Pfaff, M. (1998) Integrin affinity modulation, *Trends Cell Biol.*, 8, 359–364.

Hynes, R.O. (1992) Integrins: versatility, modulation, and signaling in cell adhesion, *Cell*, 69, 11–25.

Hynes, R.O. and Lander, A.D. (1992) Contact and adhesive specificities in the associations, migration, and targeting of cells and axons, *Cell*, 68, 303–322.

Keegan, K. and Halegoua, S. (1993) Signal transduction pathways in neuronal differentiation, *Curr. Opin. Neurobiol.*, 3, 14–19.

Kirchhofer, D., Grzesiak, J., and Pierschbacher, M.D. (1991) Calcium as a potential physiological regulator of integrin-mediated cell adhesion, *J. Biol. Chem.*, 266, 4471–4477.

Kirchhofer, D., Languino, L.R., Ruoslahti, E., and Pierschbacher, M.D. (1990) $\alpha 2\beta 1$ integrins from different cell types show different binding specificites, *J. Biol. Chem.*, 265, 615–618.

Klier, F.G., Cole, G., Stallcup, W., and Schubert, D. (1990) Amyloid beta-protein precursor is associated with extracellular matrix, *Brain Res.*, 515, 336–342.

Lee, K., Schottler, F., Oliver, M., and Lynch, C. (1980) Brief bursts of high frequency stimulation produce two types of structural changes in rat hippocampus, *J. Neurophysiol.*, 44, 247–258.

Lein, P., Gallagher, P.J., Amodeo, J., Howie, H., and Roth, J.A. (2000) Manganese induces neurite outgrowth in PC12 cells via upregulation of α_v integrins, *Brain Res.*, 885, 220–230.

Marshall, C.J. (1995) specificity of receptor tyrosine kinase signaling: transient versus sustained extracellular signal-regulated kinase activation, *Cell*, 80, 179–185.

Matter, M.L., Zhang, Z., Nordstedt, C., and Ruoslahti, E. (1998) The α5β1 integrin mediates elimination of amyloid-β peptide and protects against apoptosis, *J. Cell Biol.,* 141, 1019–1030.

McNamee, H.P., Ingberg, D.E., and Schwartz, M.A. (1993) Adhesion to fibronectin stimulates inositol lipid synthesis and enhances PDGF-induced inositol lipid breakdown, *J. Cell Biol.,* 121, 673–678.

Nishimura, S.L., Boylen, K.P., Einheber, S., Milner, T.A., Ramos, D.M., and Pytela, R. (1998) Synaptic and glial localization of the integrin αVβ8 in mouse and rat brain, *Brain Res.,* 791, 271–282.

Pabla, R., Weyrich, A.S., Dixon, D.A., Bray, P.F., McIntyre, T.M., Prescott, S.M., and Zimmerman, G.A. (1999) Integrin-dependent control of translation: engagement of integrin $\alpha_{IIb}\beta_3$ regulates synthesis of proteins in activated human platelets, *J. Cell Biol.,* 144, 175–184.

Parran, D.K., Mundy, W.R., and Barone, S., Jr. (2001) Effects of methylmercury and mercuric chloride on differentiation and cell viability in PC12 cells, *Toxicol. Sci.,* 59, 278–290.

Pinkstaff, J.K., Detterich, J., Lynch, G., and Gall, C. (1999) Integrin subunit gene expression is regionally differentiated in adult brain, *J. Neurosci.,* 19, 1541–1556.

Re, F., Zanetti, A., Sironi, M., Polentarutti, N., Lanfrancone, L., Dejana, E., and Colotta, F. (1994) Inhibition of anchorage-dependent cell spreading triggers apoptosis in cultured human endothelial cells, *J. Cell Biol.,* 127, 537–546.

Rossino, P., Gavazzi, I., Timpl, R., Aumailley, M., Abbadini, M., Giancotti, F., Silengo, L., Marchisio, P.C., and Tarone, G. (1990) Nerve growth factor induces increased expression of a laminin-binding integrin in rat pheochromocytoma PC12 cells, *Exp. Cell Res.,* 189, 100–108.

Sabo, S., Lambert, M.P., Kessey, K., Wade, W., Krafft, G., and Klein, W.L. (1995) Interaction of beta-amyloid peptides with integrins in a human nerve cell line, *Neurosci. Lett.,* 184, 25–28.

Santala, P. and Heino, J. (1991) Regulation of integrin-type cell adhesion receptors by cytokines, *J. Biol. Chem.,* 266, 23505–23509.

Schlaepfer, D.D., Jones, K.C., and Hunter, T. (1998) Multiple Grb2-mediated integrin-stimulated signaling pathways to ERK2/mitogen-activated protein kinase: summation of both cSrc- and focal adhesion kinase-initiated events, *Mol. Cell. Biol.,* 18, 2571–2585.

Selkoe, D.J. (1994) Cell biology of the amyloid β-protein precursor and the mechanism of Alzheimer's disease, *Annu. Rev. Cell. Biol.,* 10, 373–403.

Slack, B.E. (1998) Tyrosine phosphorylation of paxillin and focal adhesion kinase by activation of muscarinic m3 receptors is dependent on integrin engagement by the extracellular matrix, *Proc. Natl. Acad. Sci. U.S.A.,* 95, 7281–7286.

Sobel, R.A. (1998) The extracellular matrix in multiple sclerosis lesions, *J. Neuropathol. Exp. Neurol.,* 57, 205–217.

Song, X., Violin, J.D., Seidler, F.J., and Slotkin, T.A. (1998) Modeling the developmental neurotoxicity of chlorpyrifos *in vitro*: macromolecule synthesis in PC12 cells, *Toxicol. Appl. Pharmacol.,* 156, 78–80.

Staaz, W.D., Rajpara, S.M., Wayner, E.A., Carter, W.G., and Santoro, S.A. (1989) The membrane glycoprotein Ia-Iia (VLA-2) complex mediates the Mg^{++}-dependent adhesion of platelets to collagen, *J. Cell Biol.,* 108, 1917–1924.

Staubli, U., Chun, D., and Lynch, G. (1998) Time-dependent reversal of long-term potentiation by an integrin antagonist, *J. Neurosci.,* 18, 3460–3469.

Staubli, U., Vanerklish, P., and Lynch, G. (1990) An inhibitor of integrin receptors blocks long-term potentiation, *Behav. Neural Biol.,* 53, 1–5.

Storey, E., Beyreuther, K., and Masters, C.L. (1996a) Alzheimer's disease amyloid precursor protein on the surface of cortical neurons in primary culture co-localizes with adhesion patch components, *Brain Res.*, 735, 217–231.

Storey, E., Spurck, T., Pickett-Heaps, J., Beyreuther, K., and Masters, C.L. (1996b) The amyloid precursor protein of Alzheimer's disease is found on the surface of static but not actively motile portions of neurites, *Brain Res.*, 735, 59–66.

Tarone, G., Hirsch, T.G., Brancaccio, M., De Acetis, M., Barberis, L., Balzac, F., Retta, F., Botta, C., Altruda, F., and Silengo, L. (2000) Integrin function and regulation in development, *Int. J. Dev. Biol.*, 44, 725–731.

Tomaselli, K.J., Hall, D.E., Flier, L.A., Gehlsen, K.R., Turner, D.C., Carbonetto, S., and Reichardt, L.F. (1990) A neuronal cell line (PC12) expresses two β1-class integrins—α1β1 and β3β1—that recognize different neurite outgrowth-promoting domains in laminin, *Neuron*, 5, 651–662.

U.S. EPA (1998) *Guidelines for Neurotoxicity Risk Assessment (EPA/630/R-95/001F)*, EPA, Washington, D.C.

Van Gool, D., Carmeliet, G., Triau, E., Cassiman, J.J., and Dom, R. (1994) Appearance of localized immunoreactivity for the alpha 4 integrin subunit and for fibronectin in brains from Alzheimer's, Lewy body dementia patients and aged controls, *Neurosci. Lett.*, 170, 71–73.

Yamazaki, T., Koo, E.H., and Selkoe, D.J. (1997) Cell surface amyloid β-protein precursor colocalizes with β1 integrins at substrate contact sites in neural cells, *J. Neurosci.*, 17, 1004–1010.

Yanagida, H., Talnaka, J., and Maruo, S. (1999) Immunocytochemical localization of a cell adhesion molecule integrin alpha5beta1, in nerve growth cones, *J. Ortho. Sci.*, 4, 353–360.

Zhang, Z., Tarone, G., and Turner, D.C. (1993) Expression of integrin α1β1 is regulated by nerve growth factor and dexamethasone in PC12 cells, *J. Biol. Chem.*, 268, 5557–5565.

Zhang, Z., Turner, D.C., Drzewiecki, G.J., Hinshaw, D.B., and Hyslop, P.A. (1994) Impairment of integrin-mediated cell-matrix adhesion in oxidant-stressed PC12 cells, *Brain Res.*, 662, 189–197.

CHAPTER 33

Two-Photon Fluorescence Microscopy: A Review of Recent Advances in Deep-Tissue Imaging

Chen-Yuan Dong, Lily Hsu, Ki-Hean Kim, Christof Buehler, Peter D. Kaplan, Thomas D. Hancewicz, and Peter T. C. So

CONTENTS

INTRODUCTION

Noninvasive optical imaging of living tissues in three dimensions offers new research opportunities in biology, toxicology, and medicine. The two-photon microscopy is an important recent invention that addresses this tissue (Denk et al., 1990). Three-dimensional tissue imaging based on two-photon excitation has found applications such as studying cell growth in tissue engineering constructs (Agarwal et al., 1999, 2000, 2001), monitoring of chemical transport across the dermal epithelium (Yu et al., 2001), and investigating carcinogenesis processes in transgenic animals (Brown et al., 2001).

0-8493-1528-X/03/$0.00+$1.50
© 2003 by CRC Press LLC

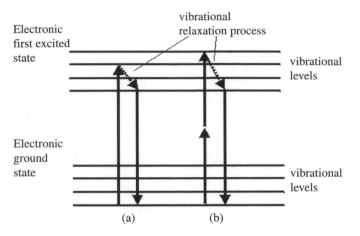

Figure 33.1 Jablonski diagrams for (a) one-photon and (b) two-photon excitation. One-photon excitation occurs through the absorption of a single photon. The two-photon process occurs through the simultaneous absorption of two lower energy photons. After either excitation process, the fluorophore relaxes to the lowest energy level of the first excited electronic state. The subsequent fluorescence emission process is independent of the mode of excitation.

Two-photon microscopy is a fluorescence imaging technique (Figure 33.1). Conventional one-photon fluorescence excitation results from the absorption of a single ultraviolet or visible photon that results in the electronic transition of a fluorescent molecule from the ground to the excited state. After vibrational relaxation, the fluorescent molecule returns to the ground state with the emission of a lower energy photon. For two-photon excitation, the excitation transition results from the fluorescent molecule simultaneously absorbing two photons. Energy conservation dictates that the two absorbed photons have energies that are approximately half the energy difference between the ground and the excited states. These photons are typically in the infrared spectral range. After vibrational relaxation, the fluorescent molecule resides in the same excited state independent of the excitation process. Therefore, the emission spectrum and the fluorescent lifetime are the same regardless whether the molecule is excited via one- or two-photon process. Multiphoton excitation is a more general term that describes the process in which the fluorescent molecule is excited by the absorption of two or more photons.

Two-photon microscopy has several key features. First, the excitation volume of two-photon microscopy is confined to a subfemtoliter focal volume greatly reducing off-focus background. Two-photon microscopy has inherent three-dimensional sectioning capability. The typical photoexcitation volume has a radial dimension of 0.3 μm and an axial dimension of 0.8 μm. Second, since the excitation is localized, photoexcitation induced damage is also limited to the same small volume. In contrast, one-photon confocal microscopy, another common three-dimensional optical imaging method that localizes the observation volume using a confocal pinhole, often produces greater specimen photodamage since the excitation volume is extended (Pawley, 1995). Third, two-photon microscopy allows the imaging of near-ultraviolet fluorescent molecules in tissues using infrared light that is absorbed and scattered significantly less than ultraviolet or visible photons used in one-photon microscopy. The tissue absorption extinction coefficient in the UV range can be two to three orders of magnitude higher than the infrared region. Rayleigh scattering cross-section is proportional to the inverse fourth power of the wavelength and is significantly reduced at longer wavelengths (Jackson, 1975). Therefore, two-photon excitation has greater depth penetration. In a recent study comparing imaging characteristics between one-photon and two-photon microscopy, it was shown that the two-photon technique can resolve structures at least twice as deep as the confocal approach (Centonze and White, 1998). Finally, the wide spectral separation between the two-photon excitation and fluorescence emission wavelengths allows high sensitivity detection. Unlike one-photon excitation where the excitation wavelengths are separated by around 50 nm, the multiphoton excitation wavelength is separated by about 200 nm or more from the fluorescence. The broader spectral separation ensures more sensitive detection of fluorescence emission while minimizing scattered excitation light contamination. Further, fluorescent spectroscopy studies of specimen biochemistry are easier because this spectral separation allows the entire emission spectrum to be measured.

This chapter provides an overview of two-photon imaging technology. We will subsequently review a number of recent advancements in this technology, including two-photon video rate imaging, resolution enhancement based on maximum likelihood deconvolution, and tissue biochemical assays based on two-photon spectroscopy.

BASIC TWO-PHOTON MICROSCOPY INSTRUMENTATION

There are two key components in a multiphoton instrument. First, an ultrafast, femtosecond laser source is essential for efficient two-photon excitation. Although two-photon excitation by picosecond and continuous wave lasers have been demonstrated (Booth and Hell, 1998; Hell et al., 1998), the narrow pulse width (around 100 fs) of femtosecond lasers ensures high temporal concentration of excitation photons needed for efficient two-photon excitation. The second major component is a scanning microscope system. A high-quality objective lens ensures diffraction-limited focusing of the excitation light. The spatial confinement of excitation photons further increases photon flux and enhances nonlinear photon absorption probability.

A typical two-photon microscope design is shown in Figure 33.2. Titanium Sapphire laser is one of the most convenient femtosecond light sources for two-photon microscopy (Mira 900, Coherent Inc., Mountain View, CA). The excitation light from the laser is guided toward an x-y galvanometric mirror scanner system (Model 6350, Cambridge Technology, Cambridge, MA). Raster scanning the laser beam using the galvanometric scanner allows two-dimensional imaging. The laser beam is reflected by a dichoric mirror toward the microscope. Additional optics for beam expansion is used to ensure overfilling the back aperture of the microscope objective. The uniform filling of the back aperture is necessary for diffraction-limited focusing at the specimen. Fluorescence is generated at the focal point and is collected by the same objective. Axial scanning of the specimen is achieved by a piezo-driven, objective positioner (P721 PIFOC®, Physik Instrumente (PI), Germany). Three-dimensional imaging is thus achieved by the combination of x-y scanner mirrors and an axial piezo positioner.

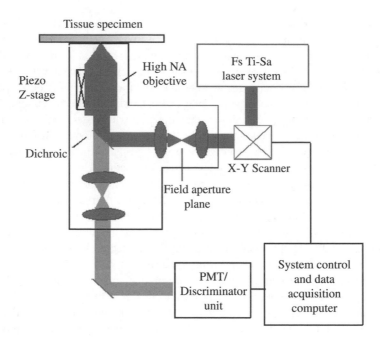

Figure 33.2 A schematic of two-photon fluorescence microscope design.

A wide range of high-quality objectives are available for two-photon imaging. High numerical aperture (NA) objectives are often chosen to minimize the excitation volume and tp optimize = image resolution. Oil-immersion objectives have higher numerical apertures and are efficient for thin specimens with thickness less than 10 μm. For thicker tissue specimens, water-immersion objectives are often used since they have refractive index better matched to many tissue specimens. Index matching minimizes image and signal deterioration due to spherical aberration.

The fluorescence signal passes through the dichroic mirror and additional barrier filters before reaching the detector. Either analog detection mode or single-photon counting detection mode can be used. Single-photon counting detection is illustrated in Figure 33.2. Individual photon burst is detected by high-sensitivity, low noise photomultiplier tubes (R7200, Hamamatsu, Bridgewater, NJ) and separated from detector noise using a discriminator circuit. The digitized signal is recorded by the data acquisition computer. The data acquisition computer is responsible for correlating the photon signal with positions of the *x-y* scanner and the axial piezo positioner.

DEEP TISSUE IMAGING BASED ON TWO-PHOTON MICROSCOPY

Although two-photon excitation allows microscopic resolution in living tissues with unprecedented depth, the performance of this technique is still limited due to complex, heterogeneous optical properties of tissue samples. For example, two-photon imaging of corneal structures, which is fairly transparent, can be accomplished down to a depth of hundreds of microns based on tissue autofluroescence

(Piston et al., 1995). The two-photon method has been used to image blood flow in neuronal tissues, which are slightly more opaque, using exogenous contrast agents down to a depth of over 500 μm (Kleinfeld et al., 1998). On the other hand, the skin is a much more complicated optical system. Optical coherence tomography has been used to measure the scattering coefficients and refractive index of skin. Both properties are found to change significantly from the surface stratum corneum down to the upper dermis (Tearney et al., 1995; Knuttel and Boehlau-Godau, 2000). In the stratum corneum, the refractive index is around 1.5 and the scattering coefficient is between 1 and 1.5 mm^{-1}. In the lower epidermis, the index of refraction decreases while the scattering coefficients increases; the refractive index is around 1.34 and the scattering coefficient is between 4 and 7 mm^{-1} in the basal layer. In the upper dermal layers, the refractive index and scattering coefficient are about 1.41 and 5–8 mm^{-1}. The refractive index variation prevents easy index matching and results in significant spherical aberration. Two-photon imaging of skin based on autofluorescence can only penetrate to a depth of about 200 μm (Masters et al., 1997; So et al., 1998). In two-photon microscopy, specimen absorption, scattering, and varying refractive indices all contribute to limit the useful penetration depths by restricting the reach of the incident photons and interfering with the collection of the fluorescence emission.

Since its invention a decade ago, two-photon fluorescence microscopy has been found to have applications in many diverse tissue imaging applications. This technology has been used in the study of tissue physiology (Piston et al., 1995; Masters et al., 1997; Bennett et al., 1996), neurobiology (Yuste et al., 1976–1987; Denk, 1994; Yuste and Denk, 1995; Svoboda et al., 1996, 1997, 1999), and embryology (Summers et al., 1996; Mohler et al., 1998, Mohler and White, 1998; Squirrell et al., 1999).

The use of two-photon microscopy for tissue imaging is well demonstrated in the study of dermal physiology based on autofluorescence. With two-photon microscopy, skin cellular and extracellular structures down to the dermal layer can be imaged nondestructively. Figure 33.3 shows the stratum corneum, the basal layer, and the upper dermis images based on tissue endogenous fluorescence. The observed structural features correspond well to known histology data.

RECENT ADVANCES IN TWO-PHOTON MICROSCOPY

Video Rate Two-Photon Microscopy

Typical two-photon microscopes have a frame rate on the order of a few seconds. While this scan rate is sufficient in many cases, it is inadequate to study some biological processes with fast kinetics such as calcium signaling (Fan et al., 1999). For the clinical applications, a faster scan rate allows efficient imaging of a macroscopic area of the tissue specimen, which is needed for thorough disease diagnosis. High-speed imaging also minimizes image degradation due to physiological motions with frequencies on the order of 1 Hz. Finally, high speed two-photon imaging allows the implementation of three-dimensional tissue image cytometry (Kim et al.,

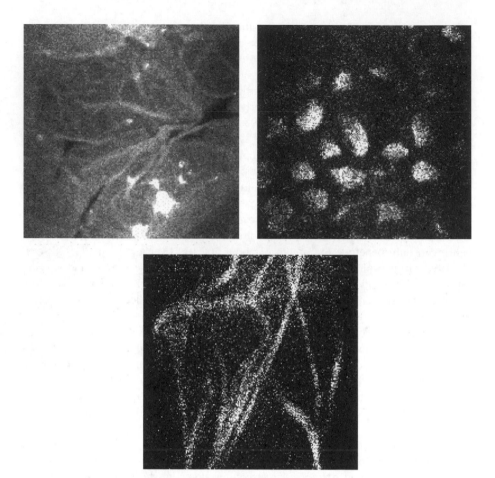

Figure 33.3 Two-photon autofluorescence images of human skin. Top left: stratum corneum. Top right: basal layer. Bottom: fibrous dermal layer (Zeiss Fluar 100× oil).

in press). Three-dimensional image cytometry allows *in situ* sampling of the cellular properties inside tissues. High-speed imaging ensures that a sufficiently large cell population can be sampled to provide statistically accurate measurement of cellular properties. The potential of two-photon three-dimensional image cytometry has been demonstrated in three-dimensional cell cultures where rare cells can be identified at ratios as low as 1 in 10^5.

One of the first video-rate two-photon microscopic systems is based on the line-scanning approach (Guild and Webb, 1995; Brakenhoff et al., 1996). Resonance mirror and multifocus scanning have also been implemented (Bewersdorf et al., 1996; Buist et al., 1998; Fan et al., 1999). Another way to achieve video-rate two-photon microscopy is to use a rotating polygonal mirror to replace one scanning axis (Kim et al., 1999).

The major limitation of a video-rate two-photon microscope is the inevitable reduction in signal-to-noise level. As the scan rate is increased, the number of excitation laser pulses available for excitation per pixel decreases. For a video-rate microscope (30 frames per second) generating 256×256 pixel images, the pixel residence time is 500 ns. There are approximately 40 laser pulses available for excitation during this time using a typical titanium-sapphire laser operating at 80 MHz repetition frequency. Within the residence time in a pixel, each fluorescent molecule at a given pixel can emit, at most, 10 photons without excitation saturation. Therefore, the low-signal photon flux is a key constraint for video-rate two-photon imaging. Possible solutions to circumvent this problem include increasing the laser repetition frequency, circularizing of the laser polarization, and using an analog detection scheme (Kim et al., 1999). The most promising approach is the parallelization of excitation and detection as implemented in multifocal multiphoton microscopes (Bewersdorf et al., 1996). As this technology is further developed, the utility of video-rate microscopes has been demonstrated in the study of cellular calcium signaling (Fan et al., 1999) and tissue physiology. Collagen/elastin fiber structures in the dermal layer of *ex vivo* human skin can be clearly seen based on autofluorescence at a frame rate of 12 Hz.

Enhancing Image Resolution Based on Maximum Likelihood Deconvolution

In addition to improving the image acquisition speed, it is also important to optimize the image resolution and signal level for deep tissue applications. Two-photon microscopy has good resolution, but its resolution is limited to 200–300 nm due to diffraction effect; numerical deconvolution methods allow further image resolution enhancement. Details of cellular and tissue structures with features smaller than the diffraction limit can sometimes be visualized based on numerical deconvolution. However, it should be noted that the resolution improvement beyond diffraction limit based on numerical deconvolution is rather modest due to signal-to-noise limitation. In deep tissue imaging, image resolution is often degraded due to spherical aberration and scattering effects. Numerical deconvolution allows some restoration of these images by partially negating aberration and scattering effects. Further, deconvolution based on maximum likelihood approach allows image restoration but also extracts the point spread function, a numerical quantification of the degree of image degradation in the specimen. The application of maximum likelihood blind deconvolution method to image heterogeneous, complex tissues allows a measure of its optical properties.

We have demonstrated the use of numerical deconvolution to further improve two-photon microscope images. Digital images were deconvoluted based on a maximum likelihood algorithm (Autodeblur™, AutoQuant Imaging, Inc., Watervliet, NY). Two-photon images were acquired of bovine pulmonary endothelial cells, labeled with BODIPY FL phallacidin (green F-actin) and DAPI (blue nucleus) (F-14780, Molecular Probes, Eugene, OR). Prior to deconvolution, the cross sections of the actin fiber bundles are elongated ovals due to the lower resolution of the two-photon microscope along the axial direction. This lower axial resolution does not allow individual fibers to be distinguished. The deconvolution process equalizes the resolutions along the axial and the radial directions and restores the cross sections

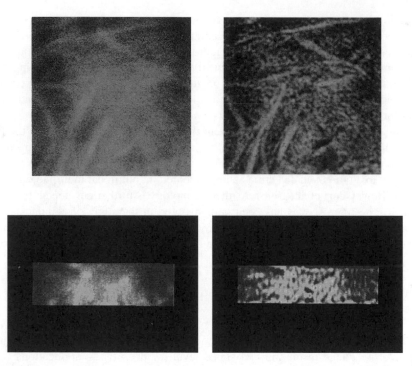

Figure 33.4 Image restoration of two-photon images of *ex vivo* human skin using maximum
likelihood approach. Autofluorescence (left) and blind deconvoluted (right) images
of human basal layer. Top: lateral view. Bottom: axial section (Zeiss Fluar 40× oil).

of the actin fiber bundles to an expected circular geometry allowing individual fibers
to be better resolved. The application of the deconvolution method to two-photon
tissue images was illustrated using data from *ex vivo* human skin. Figure 33.4 shows
the raw and deconvoluted images from the dermal layer of the skin. In the basal
layer, deconvolution allows the observation of melanin granules that are not visible
in the raw images. The individual elastin fibers are better resolved in the dermal
layer. The benefit of using deconvolution to further improve the resolution of two-
photon tissue images is being explored.

Two-Photon Spectral Characterization of Tissue Biochemistry

Two-photon microscopy imaging of endogenous fluorescent species or exogenous fluorescent probes has been shown to be a powerful method for the
quantification of tissue structure and biochemistry. Autofluorescence is observed
ubiquitously in many tissue types; the presence and the distribution of these
endogenous fluorescent species provide tissue functional information related to its
physiological and pathological states. Fluorescence spectroscopy has been used
to characterize different tissue types such as colon, lung, cervix, and skin (Zeng
et al., 1995; Nilsson et al., 1997). In addition to tissue type characterization,
spectroscopy has been used to monitor tissue physiological states (Cothren et al.,
1990; Richards-Kortum et al., 1991). The differences in tissue excitation spectra

have been used for disease diagnosis such as distinguishing between malignant and normal tissues (Glasgold et al., 1994; Schantz et al., 1997; Beauvoit and Chance, 1998; Licha et al., 2000). Tissue spectroscopy has also been used to study the effects of aging and photoaging (Yu et al., 1996). The use of exogenous probes have been applied to monitor a variety of tissue and cellular biochemical states such as the concentration of metabolites (pH, calcium, zinc, etc.) (Fan et al., 1999), the fluidity of the lipid membrane (Yu et al., 1996), and the distribution of oxygen (Helminger et al., 1997).

While autofluorescence is observed ubiquitously in many tissue types, the identities and distributions of these fluorescent molecules have not been completely characterized. The different fluorescent species are expected to have different fluorescence excitation and emission spectra. We have applied fluorescence excitation spectroscopy to identify autofluorescence biochemical species in *ex vivo* human skin. Total fluorescence emission intensity from 350 to 550 nm is measured at each pixel as a function of excitation wavelength from 720 to 920 nm. Spectral data is analyzed by self-modeling curve resolution (SMCR) approaches to extract spectroscopic components from these two-photon images.

The data to be analyzed are four-dimensional, including three spatial dimensions and an excitation wavelength dimension (x, y, z, λ). Ignoring possible correlation between pixels, the four-dimensional data set is converted into two dimensions (n, λ) for further analysis (two-way factor analysis) where n is the index of the pixels in a three-dimensional data set. We assume no correlation between pixels in the SMCR analysis. Therefore, the presence of a correlation of biochemical species distributions with physiological structural features in the tissue serves as an independent verification of the accuracy of this approach.

Two-way factor analysis assumes a bilinear data structure and attempts to separate the original data matrix of spectra, $\mathbf{D}$, into two submatrices, $\mathbf{C}$ and $\mathbf{S}$,

$$\mathbf{D} = \mathbf{C}\mathbf{S}^{\mathbf{T}} + \mathbf{E} \qquad (33.1)$$

where $\mathbf{C}$ is a matrix of coefficients related to the real concentration profiles (scores), $\mathbf{S}$ is a matrix of vectors related to the real spectra (factors), $\mathbf{E}$ is a matrix of spectral residuals, and $\mathbf{T}$ is the transpose operator.

The equation above describes the standard abstract principal component analysis solution. Alternative least square analysis with appropriate constraints is used to optimize the data fit by minimizing the error matrix. From the SMCR analysis, major factors (biochemical components) contributing autofluorescence in the human skin are identified. The SMCR analysis provides us with (1) the excitation spectrum of the individual component and (2) the three-dimensional distribution of each component, which can be reexpressed as a depth distribution profile for that component. The depth distribution profile describes the distribution of each component within the volume of skin as a function of depth. The distribution of each chemical component can be compared to the known histological structure of the skin.

In the analysis of skin excitation data, several autofluorescent components are identified by SMCR analysis. One of the components identified corresponds to

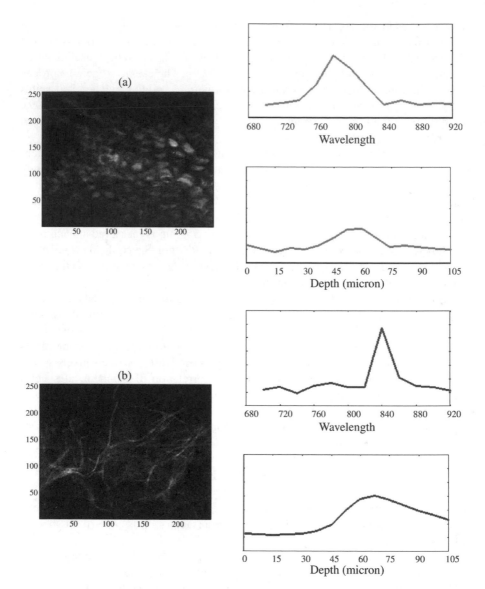

Figure 33.5 Two independent spectral components isolated in *ex vivo* human skin based on SMCR: (a) a spectral component corresponds to elastin fibers in the dermis and (b) a spectral component corresponds to melanin (or a fluorophore that colocalizes with melanin) in the epidermal–dermal junction. For (a) and (b): (left) a two-dimensional image of the concentration distribution of the spectral component; (right, top) the spectrum of this component; (right, bottom) the depth distribution profile of this component.

elastin fibers in the dermis (Figure 33.5A). An image reconstructed from the three-dimensional distribution of this component shows the well-defined morphology of elastin fibers in the dermis. The depth distribution profile shows that this component is not seen in the epidermis but only in the dermis. This observation is also consistent with skin physiology. Another component identified represents melanin or a bio-chemical component that colocalizes with melanin (Figure 33.5B). The reconstructed images from the distribution of this component have the typical morphology of the melanin caps at the basal layer. The distribution of this component is found to maximize at a depth between 40 and 60 μm corresponding to the epidermal–dermal junction of the skin as expected.

CONCLUSIONS

A decade after the invention of two-photon microscopy, this technique has become one of the most important techniques in modern optical microscopy. Two-photon microscopy has three-dimensional resolved imaging capability and enhanced depth penetration, and it is compatible with study tissue structure and biochemistry *in vivo*. Recent advances in high-speed imaging, resolution enhancement based on numerical deconvolution, and spectroscopic resolution allow further progress in tissue diagnosis. Three-dimensional image cytometry based on high-speed imaging measures cellular properties in tissues with high statistical precision through sampling a large cellular population. Numerical deconvolution methods provide higher resolution imaging of finer structures in cells and the extracellular matrix. Finally, the combination of two-photon spectroscopy and microscopy is a powerful method to simultaneously assay tissue function and structure.

REFERENCES

Agarwal, A. et al. (1999) Collagen remodeling by human lung fibroblasts in 3-D gels, *Am. J. Respir. Crit. Care Med.*, 159, A199.

Agarwal, A. et al. (2000) Two-photon scanning microscopy of epithelial cell-modulated collagen density in 3-D gels, *Faseb J.*, 14, A445.

Agarwal, A. et al. (2001) Two-photon laser scanning microscopy of epithelial cell-modulated collagen density in engineered human lung tissue, *Tissue Eng.*, 7, 191–202.

Beauvoit, B. and Chance, B. (1998) Time-resolved spectroscopy of mitochondria, cells, and tissues under normal and pathological conditions, *Mol. Cell. Biochem.*, 184, 445–455.

Bennett, B.D. et al. (1996) Quantitative subcellular imaging of glucose metabolism within intact pancreatic islets, *J. Biol. Chem.*, 271, 3647–3651.

Bewersdorf, J., Pick, R., and Hell, S.W. (1998) Mulitfocal multiphoton microscopy, *Opt. Lett.*, 23, 655–657.

Booth, M.J. and Hell, S.W. (1998) Continuous wave excitation two-photon fluorescence microscopy exemplified with the 647-nm ArKr laser line, *J. Microsc.*, 190, 298–304.

Brakenhoff, G.J. et al. (1996) Real-time two-photon confocal microscopy using a femtosecond, amplified Ti:sapphire system, *J. Microsc.*, 181, 253–259.

Brown, E.B. et al. (2001) *In vivo* measurement of gene expression, angiogenesis and physiological function in tumors using multiphoton laser scanning microscopy, *Nat. Med.*, 7, 864–868.

Buist, A.H. et al. (1998) Real time two-photon absorption microscopy using multipoint excitation, *J. Microsc.*, 192, 217–226.

Centonze, V.E. and White, J.G. (1998) Multiphoton excitation provides optical sections from deeper within scattering specimens than confocal imaging, *Biophys. J.*, 75, 2015–2024.

Cothren, R.M. et al. (1990) Gastrointentinal tissue diagnostic by laser-induced fluorescence spectroscopy at endoscopy, *Gastrointest. Endosc.*, 36, 105–111.

Denk, W. (1994) Two-photon scanning photochemical microscopy: mapping ligand-gated ion channel distributions, *Proc. Natl. Acad. Sci. U.S.A.*, 91, 6629–6633.

Denk, W., Strickler, J.H., and Webb, W.W. (1990) Two-photon laser scanning fluorescence microscopy, *Science*, 248, 73–76.

Fan, G.Y. et al. (1999) Video-rate scanning two-photon excitation fluorescence microscopy and ratio imaging with chameleons, *Biophys. J.*, 76, 2412–2420.

Glasgold, R. et al. (1994) Tissue autofluorescence as an intermediate endpoint in NMBA-induced esophageal carcinogenesis, *Cancer Lett.*, 82, 33–41.

Guild, J.B. and Webb, W.W. (1995) Line scanning microscopy with two-photon fluorescence excitation, *Biophys. J*, 68, 290a.

Hell, S.W., Booth, M., and Wilms, S. (1998) Two-photon near- and far-field fluorescence microscopy with continuous-wave excitation, *Opt. Lett.*, 23, 1238–1240.

Helmlinger, G. et al. (1997) Interstitial pH and pO2 gradients in solid tumors in vivo: high-resolution measurements reveal a lack of correlation, *Nat. Med.*, 3, 177–182.

Jackson, J.D. (1975) *Classical Electrodynamics*. John Wiley & Sons, New York.

Kim, K.H., Buehler, C., and So, P.T.C. (1999) High-speed, two-photon scanning microscope, *Appl. Opt.*, 38, 6004–6009.

Kim, K.H. et al. (in press) Three-dimensional image cytometry based on a high-speed two-photon scanning microscope, *SPIE Proc.*

Kleinfeld, D. et al. (1998) Fluctuations and stimulus-induced changes in blood flow observed in individual capillaries in layers 2 through 4 of rat neocortex, *Proc. Natl. Acad. Sci. U.S.A.*, 95, 15741–15746.

Knuttel, A. and Boehlau-Godau, M. (2000) Spatially confined and temporally resolved refractive index and scattering evaluation in human skin performed with optical coherence tomography, *J. Biomed. Opt.*, 5, 83–92.

Kollias, N. et al. (1998) Endogenous skin fluorescence includes bands that may serve as quantitative markers of aging and photoaging, *J. Invest. Dermatol.*, 111, 776–780.

Licha, K. et al. (2000) Hydrophilic cyanine dyes as contrast agents for near-infrared tumor imaging: Synthesis, photophysical properties and spectroscopic *in vivo* characterization, *Photochem. Photobiol.*, 72, 392–398.

Masters, B.R., So, P.T., and Gratton, E. (1997) Multiphoton excitation fluorescence microscopy and spectroscopy of in vivo human skin, *Biophys. J.*, 72, 2405–2412.

Mohler, W.A. and White, J.G. (1998) Stereo-4-D reconstruction and animation from living fluorescent specimens, *Biotechniques*, 24, 1006–1010, 1012.

Mohler, W.A. et al. (1998) Dynamics and ultrastructure of developmental cell fusions in the Caenorhabditis elegans hypodermis, *Curr. Biol.*, 8, 1087–1090.

Nilsson, A.M.K. et al. (1997) Near infrared diffuse reflection and laser-induced fluorescence spectroscopy for myocardial tissue characterization, *Spectrochim. Acta A*, 53, 1901–1912.

Pawley, J.B., Ed. (1995) *Handbook of Confocal Microscopy*, Plenum Press, New York.

Piston, D.W., Masters, B.R., and Webb, W.W. (1995) Three-dimensionally resolved NAD(P)H cellular metabolic redox imaging of the *in situ* cornea with two-photon excitation laser scanning microscopy, *J. Microsc.*, 178, 20–27.

Richards-Kortum, R. et al. (1991) Spectroscopic diagnosis of colonic dysplasia, *Photochem. Photobiol.*, 53, 777–786.

Schantz, S.P. et al. (1997) Native cellular fluorescence and its application to cancer prevention, *Environ. Health Perspect.*, 105, 941–944.

So, P.T.C., Kim, H., and Kochevar, I.E. (1998) Two-photon deep tissue ex vivo imaging of mouse dermal and subcutaneous structures, *Opt. Exp.*, 3, 339–350.

Squirrell, J.M. et al. (1999) Long-term two-photon fluorescence imaging of mammalian embryos without compromising viability, *Nat. Biotechnol.*, 17, 763–767.

Summers, R.G. et al. (1996) The orientation of first cleavage in the sea urchin embryo, Lytechinus variegatus, does not specify the axes of bilateral symmetry, *Dev. Biol.*, 175, 177–183.

Svoboda, K., Tank, D.W., and Denk, W. (1996) Direct measurement of coupling between dendritic spines and shafts, *Science*, 272, 716–719.

Svoboda, K. et al. (1997) *In vivo* dendritic calcium dynamics in neocortical pyramidal neurons, *Nature*, 385, 161–165.

Svoboda, K. et al. (1999) Spread of dendritic excitation in layer 2/3 pyramidal neurons in rat barrel cortex in vivo, *Nat. Neurosci.*, 2, 65–73.

Tearney, G.J. et al. (1995) Determination of the refractive-index of highly scattering human tissue by optical coherence tomography, *Opt. Lett.*, 20, 2258–2260.

Yu, B. et al. (2001) *In vitro* visualization and quantification of oleic acid induced changes in transdermal transport using two-photon fluorescence microscopy, *J. Invest. Dermatol.*, 117, 16–25.

Yu, W. et al. (1996) Fluorescence generalized polarization of cell membranes: a two-photon scanning microscopy approach, *Biophys. J.*, 70, 626–636.

Yuste, R. and Denk, W. (1995) Dendritic spines as basic functional units of neuronal integration, *Nature*, 375, 682–684.

Yuste, R. et al. (1999) Mechanisms of calcium influx into hippocampal spines: heterogeneity among spines, coincidence detection by NMDA receptors, and optical quantal analysis, *J. Neurosci.*, 19, 1976–1987.

Zeng, H. et al. (1995) Spectroscopic and microscopic characteristics of human skin autofluorescence emission, *Photochem. Photobiol.*, 61, 639–645.

Part VI

Role of Transgenics and Toxicogenomics in the Development of Alternative Toxicity Tests

Jerry Heindel

The astounding progress made in the science of genetics, especially the sequencing of the human and other species genomes, has also accelerated progress in many other scientific areas including that of developing alternative toxicity testing methods. Three areas developed from our new understanding of genetics that have the ability to revolutionize our thinking in the area of developing new toxicity tests and endpoints include the use of transgenic animals, genomics, and proteomics along with the bioinformatics and database development that goes along with these areas.

We now have the technology to manipulate the mammalian genome. A product of this technology is the development of transgenic animals (mainly mice). Genetically altered or transgenic animal models have been developed that contain activated oncogenes or inactivated tumor suppressor genes known to be involved in neoplastic processes both in animals and humans. This trait may allow them to respond to carcinogens more quickly than conventional rodent strains. In addition, the neoplastic effects of agents can be observed in transgenic models within a time frame in which few, if any, spontaneous tumors would arise. The use of target or reporter genes also allows for direct molecular and cellular analysis of a chemical's effects in these models and can provide additional mechanistic information about modes of action. Several transgenic mouse models have been proposed for use in carcinogenicity testing. These include p53 haploinsufficient mice that rapidly develop cancer to selected mutagenic carcinogens but not to selected nonmutagenic carcinogens. Another transgenic mouse model that is a candidate for use in carcinogenicity testing is the transgenic Tg.AC mouse with a mutation in the endogenous c-Ras gene. These models are in the beginning of a long process of experimentation and validation before they or others can be used to either supplement or replace the traditional 2-yr rodent cancer bioassay. The chapter by Frank Sistare discusses current data, efforts, and problems that need to be overcome in order to use the transgenic animals for carcinogenicity testing.

Genome-based technology has also lead to the development of the new fields of genomics and proteomics. The use of DNA microarray (genomics) and proteomic technologies to assess changes in gene and protein expression, respectively, is a rapidly growing research area that will have a large impact on many fields, including that of the development of alternative toxicity testing protocols. Global gene expression profiling using cDNA or oligonucleotide microarrays is a potentially powerful tool for recognizing chemical-induced effects. However proteomics, or the analysis of protein sequence, structure, and modification, provides advantages more clearly reflecting the actual current state of activity of the cell and therefore may actually be a more useful tool for the development of new biomarkers that may lead to the development of alternative toxicity tests.

The use of these technologies will allow a paradigm shift in biology and toxicology as they allow a global perspective on how an organism responds to a specific stress, drug, or toxicant. Data generated using these technologies will provide information on cellular networks of responding genes and proteins and help define important targets for toxicity, as well as providing future biomarkers and alternative testing procedures. Indeed, the use of genomics and proteomics in toxicology has led to the development of a new field called toxicogenomics. Toxicogenomics proposes to apply both gene expression changes and protein expression technologies to study chemical effects in biological systems. While the potential for toxicogenomics to revolutionize toxicity testing exists, at present this field is just developing the proof-of-principle data to show that the technologies can indeed detect gene expression and protein expression profiles of chemicals that can be used to permit the assignment of a chemical to a particular class with a specific mechanism. In addition, data are just accumulating to show that gene and protein expression data can be determined *in vivo* after exposure to toxicants and that these data can then be used to develop and validate *in vitro* alternative test systems and biomarkers based on the use of these technologies. Two authors in this section will discuss the use of genomic and proteomic data in toxicology with an eye to development of alternative test methods anchored in these technologies.

CHAPTER **34**

The Application of Genomics and Proteomics to Toxicological Sciences

Stephan Chevalier, William D. Pennie, and Ian Kimber

CONTENTS

INTRODUCTION

A major challenge facing toxicologists today is the development of new approaches to the identification and characterization of potential health or environmental hazards. Practical toxicologists have available numerous *in vitro* and *in vivo* assays to determine the potential of chemicals to cause adverse health effects. The hazards identified are often preceded by, and result from, alterations in gene and protein expression. Toxicant induced changes in gene expression are potentially so complicated that tools are required to allow multiple variables, such as mRNA and protein expression, to be considered simultaneously. Until recently, the standard approach was to examine the effects of chemicals on one or another gene or protein at a time by well-established technologies such as enzymatic assays, slot blots, or Northern or Western blotting. There have been very labor-intensive and heroic efforts to determine the various steps in biochemical pathways that are altered by toxicants. We are now entering a new phase in the biosciences where gene sequence information is no longer limiting (Waterston and Sulston, 1998), and new technologies are available to tackle the major challenges in toxicology, including the development of new *in vitro* assays. In the past five years there has been significant progress in large-scale genome sequencing and in the development of technical platforms to support this. Several genomes, such as the unicellular eukaryotic yeast *Saccharomyces cerevisiae* (DeRisi et al., 1996) and the multicellular nematode *Caenorhabditis elegans* (The *C. elegans* sequencing consortium, 1998), have now been completely sequenced, and sequencing of the entire human genome is anticipated to be complete soon as the result of significant international investment by both the academic and industrial sectors (Waterston and Sulston, 1998). As the full-length sequences of several mammalian genomes become available, new and exiting opportunities are emerging to develop a far more detailed appreciation of the ways in which cells and tissues respond to chemical challenges. The availability of both the sequence information for many thousands of mammalian genes and, in many cases, cDNA clones of the coding regions of these genes allows the simultaneous quantitative measurement of the transcriptional activity of potentially tens of thousands of genes in biological samples (Schena et al., 1996). Changes in mRNA or protein expression in a tissue may result from differences in physiology, developmental stage, differentiation status, pathology, chemical exposure, or environmental conditions. Recent advances in technology platforms facilitate evaluation of these changes by genomics and proteomics. The term genomics describes the use of genome scale DNA sequence information to investigate the response of the total gene complement of an animal or plant to a specific signal (Williams, 1999). The niche discipline of toxicogenomics is concerned with the application of genomic technologies to characterize changes in gene expression induced by chemicals to identify potential human and environmental toxicants and to determine the putative molecular mechanisms underlying their biological activity (Nuwaysir et al., 1999). Genomics clearly embraces many different technologies (Williams, 1999) and, here, we will focus on the application of DNA microarray analyses to toxicology and the anticipation that these new approaches will revolutionize the way some toxicological problems are investigated (Nuwaysir et al., 1999; Afshari, 1999; Khan, 1999). The application of genomics to the toxicological sciences (hereafter toxicogenomics) is anticipated to pay important dividends in a number of areas. These can be summarized as follows:

- Providing new research leads through identification of novel genes that display altered expression in response to xenobiotic challenge
- Identification of single genes, or patterns of genes, where altered expression provides robust markers of specific toxic processes that can be used as the basis for alternative approaches to hazard assessment
- The possibility, linked with the above, of applying novel hazard identification paradigms to high throughput screening and exclusion of potential toxicants from the development process
- Improved risk assessment resulting from a more detailed and more accurate extrapolation between species

Although the ultimate adaptation of a cellular system or an organism to a chemical, or a change in its environment, will necessarily be associated with the altered expression of genetic information, it is apparent that in many signal transduction systems, responses involving a large number of intracellular proteins occur without direct immediate induction of new mRNA synthesis. Although genomic analysis provides important data, it is informative also to measure individual protein levels directly, since steady state expression of mature gene products are subject to additional levels of control, and frequently mRNA and protein levels do not correlate directly ([Anderson and Seilhamer, 1997; Williams, 1999). Therefore, another key landmark will be to gain a comprehensive understanding of the identity and expression patterns of every protein that an organism can and may synthesize in any given set of circumstances, this being known as its proteome (Wilkins et al., 1997). The use of the term proteome is frequently restricted to describe the complete set of proteins that is expressed, or modified following expression by the entire genome of a cell at any one time. Since genome sequences can be used to predict the corresponding gene products, the wealth of information in this area provides an invaluable resource for understanding cellular function in mammals at the protein level. At the interface between molecular biology and protein biochemistry, proteomics is the large-scale screening of proteins expressed by a genome in an organism, a tissue, or a cell (Wilkins et al., 1997; Celis and Gromov, 1999). Proteomics is based on comparisons between different proteomes in order to determine patterns of protein expression that characterize a specific biological process (Celis and Gromov, 1999). Furthermore, this complements genomics-based approaches, since it can provide additional information on protein expression, protein turnover rate, and post-translational modifications, such as phosphorylation or acetylation, that alter the biological activity of proteins. An example is the vast number of combinations of post-translational modifications observed on histone proteins and their consequences for the regulation of gene expression (Strahl and Allis, 2000), which emphasizes the importance of taking into account the nature of mature gene products as well as levels of mRNA. In addition, it is probable that protein phosphorylation will be associated with consequential changes in gene expression, which will be detectable by genomic analysis. Although proteomics is not yet a highly automated process like toxicogenomics, the advantages and importance of directly analyzing proteins make a strong argument for combining these two approaches. In this review, we examine the current status in the toxicological sciences of these two highly complementary technologies.

MICROARRAY TECHNOLOGIES

DNA microarrays allow quantitative comparisons of the expression levels of potentially thousands of individual genes between different biological samples. This facilitates, for instance, comparisons of normal tissue with diseased and of control with chemical treated cell lines or tissues. Construction of microarrays involves the immobilization of known DNA sequences (either cDNA or oligonucleotides), which correspond to the coding sequence of genes of interest, on a solid support such as a glass slide or nylon membrane (Bowtell, 1999). The mRNA prepared from cells or tissues can be labeled and hybridized, usually in the form of a reverse transcribed cDNA copy, to a microarray and visualized using phosphorimager scanning. Alternatively, cDNAs from test and control sources can be labeled with two different fluorescent tags and hybridized concurrently with complementary sequences on the same microarray. Here fluorescence scanning is used to identify differential changes in mRNA expression. Changes in mRNA levels are normalized against housekeeping genes, the expression of which is assumed to be stable and independent of treatment, to reflect possible different levels of labeling of the test and control mRNA populations. Subsequent bioinformatic analyses using appropriate software allows determination of the extent of hybridization of the labeled probes to the corresponding arrayed cDNA spots, and a comparison of control with test samples permits quantitative assessment of changes in gene expression associated with treatment (Brown and Botstein, 1999). The development of specific DNA microarray analysis programs, data mining technologies, and reference databases is imperative for transcript profiling experiments to be practical and scientifically meaningful. Expression profiling could potentially focus on important marker genes for toxicity, permitting analysis of samples from both human and rodent cells, thereby revealing species-specific effects. Thus, the application of DNA microarray technology provides a powerful tool in identifying and characterizing changes in gene expression associated with specific toxicants or families of toxicants. Such analyses may reveal patterns of gene expression changes that would both assist our understanding of the possible mechanisms of toxicity and allow the identification of sensitive and specific early markers.

Many commercial microarrays are available, varying from those comprising several hundred genes (usually immobilized on a nylon membrane, and probed with radiolabeled cDNA) to those representing tens of thousands of oligonucleotide sequences (immobilized on glass slides and analyzed using dual fluorescent probe technology). The number of genes that should be represented on DNA microarrays will depend on whether the experimental intent is inductive or deductive. The inductive approach offers the opportunity to characterize novel genes and implicate them in a toxicological process. The strategy is to investigate the expression of large numbers of genes (ideally the whole genome of an animal) and expressed sequence tags (ESTs) on microarrays to provide molecular signatures for toxicants. For a deductive approach, the strategy is to investigate a particular biological or toxicological process, and selected genes of known function are incorporated on microarrays to provide a focused experimental design when some information on the biological pathways involved already exists. Of course, an alternative is to build DNA microarrays that include both genes of known functions and ESTs to tackle different toxicological issues. Therefore, DNA microarrays can either be broad spectrum or custom designed to profile particular tissues, biological pathways, or even disease states. In this regard, microarrays designed to profile genes involved in responses to toxic insult have been developed by commercial vendors, pharmaceutical and agrochemical companies, and academic institutions (Figure 34.1; Nuwaysir et al., 1999; Pennie, 2000).

PROTEOMIC TECHNOLOGIES

Proteomics can be defined as the simultaneous analysis of many proteins in order to understand the state of a cell or a tissue. It offers the possibility of identifying proteins regulated by xenobiotics without prior bias to class or function. There are two principal steps: the first is to separate proteins in a sample, usually using two-dimensional polyacrylamide gel electrophoresis (2D-PAGE). The total protein complement of cell extracts is analyzed according to isoelectric point (first dimension) and molecular weight (second dimension), allowing resolution of thousands of proteins on a single gel (Celis and Gromov, 1999). The second step is to identify the separated proteins, typically using advanced mass spectrometry techniques, bioinformatics, and database searching. With proteomic technologies, the effect of treatment of a cell or a tissue with chemicals can be addressed by direct and relatively high throughput studies at the protein level. Although the 2D-PAGE technology was developed 25 years ago (O'Farrell, 1975), higher resolution and reproducibility can now be achieved for three main reasons. First, commercially manufactured immobilized pH gradients, where the compounds used to set up the pH gradient are chemically immobilized, provide a stable and reproducible gradient. Second, improvements in the sensitivity of mass spectrometry permit the analysis of less abundant proteins. Third, the continuous development of powerful computers, computer analysis programs, and databases for 2D-PAGE protein gels and peptides allows the bioinformatic analysis of the 2D-PAGE and mass spectrometry data (Wilkins et al., 1997).

Silver staining and protein radiolabeling are currently the most popular methods of detection, and more sensitive protein fluorescent dyes, which will provide reliable quantitative analysis, have been developed recently. Each step involved in identifying proteins has limitations that make automation difficult. Therefore, proteomics is a new enabling technology, but there is a growing realization of its importance in the life sciences. This increased attention and investment will fuel the continued rapid advance of this technology and should allow proteomics to become a large-scale, highly automated process in the near future. In common with genomics, the availability of an increasingly comprehensive database has been critical to the development of proteomics. This technology has the potential to allow the comparison of all changes in protein expression, modification, and degradation between treated and untreated samples and to compare patterns of proteome changes induced by compounds with similar toxicological endpoints to identify expression profiles specific for families of toxicants (Wang and Hewick, 1999). The application of proteomics to the biology of rodents may help to identify signaling pathways involved in the mode of action of toxicants leading to more sophisticated *in vitro* assays for their activity. The advantages and importance of directly analyzing proteins make a strong argument for the value of proteomics. The shortcomings of throughput and sensitivity (including, for instance, the lack of a protein equivalent for the polymerase chain reaction) highlight the need for improved automation, enrichment, and detection methods. These technical challenges will undoubtedly be tackled and overcome with the increased awareness of the importance of proteomics (Figure 34.1).

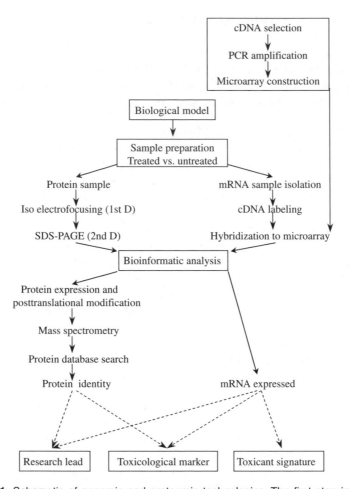

Figure 34.1 Schematic of genomic and proteomic technologies: The first step in toxicogenomics (right) is the construction of a microarray that involves the amplification
by PCR and the immobilization of known DNA sequences (either cDNA or
oligonucleotides) on a solid support. The mRNA prepared from a biological
model can be labeled and hybridized to the microarray and visualized using
phosphorimager scanning. Subsequent bioinformatic analyses using appropriate
software allows determination of the extent of hybridization of the labeled probes
to the corresponding arrayed cDNA spots, and a comparison of control with test
samples permits quantitative assessment of changes in gene expression associated with treatment. Total protein content from a biological model treated with
a toxicant is separated on two-dimensional gel electrophoresis according to
isoelectric point (first dimension) and molecular weight (second dimension),
allowing bioinformatic analysis of differences in protein expression of treated
versus untreated samples. Therefore, there is no preliminary work such as array
construction for proteomic studies (left), but proteins with altered expression
have to be identified subsequently. Individual proteins of interest are excised
from two-dimensional-gels, digested with trypsin, and applied to a mass spectrometer. Identification of these proteins is obtained by searching protein databases with mass spectrometry data.

TOXICOGENOMICS APPLICATIONS

As the full-length sequence of several mammalian genomes is revealed, there are increasing opportunities to determine how different mammalian genomes respond to toxicants. The application of DNA microarray technology provides a powerful tool in identifying and characterizing changes in gene expression associated with toxicity. In order for DNA microarray technology to be useful in toxicological sciences, the following two assumptions must be made. First, toxic insults are necessarily reflected directly or indirectly by changes in gene transcription. Second, the detectable pattern of induced changes in gene expression will be sufficiently comprehensive to permit the identification of important pathways and markers but not so complex that meaningful analysis is prohibited. Indeed, it has been proposed that in practice relatively few patterns of gene expression define elemental toxic responses (Farr and Dunn, 1999). Since mRNAs vary in their dynamic range and kinetics of induction, comprehensive and carefully designed studies should integrate the genomics approach with Northern blotting or RT-PCR of a short list of interesting candidates. Although DNA microarray is still a relatively new technology, it has already been used successfully to investigate altered gene expression in processes ranging from inflammatory disease to induction of senescence to cancer and tumor suppression (DeRisi et al, 1996; Heller et al., 1997; Shelton et al, 1999; Ross et al, 2000; Scherf et al, 2000).

The biological relevance of the experimental system for transcript profiling is clearly of major importance where a mechanistic understanding of a toxic process or a mode of action is required. Where the toxic endpoint is known in advance (at a physiological, histological, or biochemical level), an appropriate test system (*in vitro* or *in vivo*) can be designed to model the endpoint as closely as possible. As an example, nongenotoxic carcinogenesis is usually evaluated in the context of long term cancer bioassays in rodents (Chabra et al., 1990). Transcript profiling, as well as proteomic, applications may help to identify surrogate markers for the development of this phenotype, and indeed the exposure of rodent hepatocytes to the nongenotoxic carcinogen phenobarbital has been studied using both microarray and gel-based expression technologies. In excess of 300 genes have been identified where expression is modulated by this compound (Rodi et al., 1999).

In another study, a novel gene was discovered by using a 1046-element microarray of unknown human cDNAs to examine how treatment with the nongenotoxic carcinogen phorbol 12-myristate 13-acetate (phorbol ester, PMA) affects mRNA expression levels in human T (Jurkat) cells (Schena et al., 1996). The most highly induced genes by phorbol esters were the nuclear transcription factor-kappa B1 (NF-kB1) and PAC-1 tyrosine kinase, also involved in regulating transcription and cell cycle regulation (Schena et al., 1996). In our laboratory, Holden et al. examined the response of a human hepatoma cell line to the hepatotoxicant carbon tetrachloride (CCl_4) using a custom 600 genes DNA microarray (Holden et al., 2000). They have found that CCl_4 causes a rapid increase in interleukin 8 mRNA expression, and this was associated somewhat later by an increase in the level of the corresponding protein (Holden et al., 2000). Among the areas where transcript profiling is being applied in our laboratory are the following:

- Definition of marker genes that will permit the accurate identification and characterization of chemical allergens using *in vitro* approaches
- Characterization of the changes induced in rodent hepatocytes by nongenotoxic carcinogens with the purpose of identifying early markers and facilitating resolution at the molecular levels of species differences in susceptibility to nongenotoxic hepatocarcinogenesis
- Development of alternative *in vitro* approaches to the assessment of chemicals that are putative androgen or estrogen receptor agonists or antagonists based upon characterization of sex hormone responsive genes

These studies illustrate the potential of DNA microarray technology in the identification of novel gene changes associated with toxic processes (Pennie, 2000). Many other toxic endpoints could be profiled using this method, associated with combinatorial approaches, such as transgenic or knockout models (Ryffel, 1997), potentially providing insights into the role of specific genes.

PROTEOMICS APPLICATIONS

Despite the fact that genome sequences can be used to predict the corresponding gene products, it is apparent that the paradigm of one gene encoding a single protein is no longer tenable because of processes such as alternative mRNA splicing, RNA editing, and post-translational protein modification. The cell interior is a dynamic environment, where mRNA and proteins are perpetually being synthesized, modified, and eventually degraded. The number of genes in an individual mammal is static and fixed, but it is estimated that the average number of proteins per gene could be up to six for a predicted total of 140,000 genes in humans (Wilkins, 1996). In fact, it has been estimated that a single cell expresses 5000–10000 genes, with several-fold more proteins given the effects of post-translational modifications. Proteomics has already been used successfully to investigate altered protein expression in heart disease and cancer (Myers et al., 1997; Ostergaard et al., 1999; Dunn, 2000). Other examples of studies using proteomics have shown that many alterations in protein expression occur upon exposure of rodents to lead or JP-8 fuel used in the military environment, which suggests that biomarkers of complex toxic response could be uncovered by this technology (Witzmann et al., 1999a,b). Proteomic studies of drug effects have shown that proteins whose abundance or structure is strongly regulated by a compound provide direct indication of a plausible mechanism for drug action. For example, the toxic activity of cyclosporin A (CsA) (a drug successfully used in the treatment of some autoimmune diseases and as an immunosuppresent for renal transplantation) in rat kidney was investigated using proteomics (Steiner et al., 1996). Two-dimensional gel profiles of proteins isolated from a kidney treated with CsA have shown that one of the proteins down-regulated is calbindin, a molecule involved in calcium binding and transport. The loss of calbindin apparently accounts for failure to excrete calcium deposits in the kidney and could explain the nephrotoxicity of CsA in rodents (Aicher et al., 1998). Etomoxir, a reversible inhibitor of carnitine palmitoyltransferase, causes accumulation in liver of the adipocyte differentiation-related protein (ADRP), a protein thought to clothe the lipid droplets that accumulate as a result of the blocking effect of CsA on lipid metabolism (Steiner et al., 1996; Aicher et al., 1998).

The rodent liver response to nongenotoxic carcinogen peroxisome proliferators (PPs) involves changes in the expression of large numbers of liver proteins that have been studied by two-dimensional-gel electrophoresis (Watanabe et al., 1985; Witzmann et al., 1994; Anderson et al., 1996; Giometti et al., 1998; Edvardsson et al., 1999a,b; Chevalier et al., 2000). Among the rodent proteins whose expression has been shown to be altered upon treatment with PPs are the fatty acyl-CoA oxidase, the enoyl-CoA hydratase/3-hydroxyacyl-CoA dehydrogenase bifunctional enzyme (PBE), the cytosolic epoxide hydrolase, the 3-ketoacyl-CoA-thiolase peroxisomal, the hydroxy-methylglutaryl-CoA synthetase, the adipocyte fatty acid binding protein, and the cytochrome p450 4A1 (Desvergne and Wahli, 1999). Most of these proteins contain peroxisome proliferator responsive elements (PPREs) in the promoter regions of their genes and are known markers of PPARα activation and peroxisome proliferation. These proteins are involved directly in the peroxisomal metabolic response to PPs but appear not to be involved in hepatocyte proliferation and tumorigenesis (Chevalier and Roberts, 1998; Gonzalez et al., 1998). With proteomics, 32 proteins with altered expression in cultured rat hepatocytes treated with the hypolipidaemic PP nafenopin were identified, including the muscarinic acetylcholine receptor 3, intermediate filament vimentin and the β subunit of ATP synthase (Chevalier et al., 2000). It is not known yet whether the expression of the above proteins is regulated directly by PPARα or whether there exists a cascade of linked responses that regulate expression of these proteins as secondary events following initial PPARα-mediated alterations in protein expression. These non-peroxisomal protein targets may offer insights into the mechanisms of carcinogenesis in rodents by PPs and opportunities to identify markers to facilitate early identification of potential carcinogens. Another example is provided by the histamine H1 receptor antagonist methapyrilene, which was withdrawn from therapeutic use following discovery of its potent nongenotoxic hepatocarcinogenicity in rats. This drug causes covalent modification of a series of mitochondrial proteins, pointing to the action of a reactive drug metabolite in the mitochondria (Anderson et al., 1992; Cunningham et al., 1995). These proteome profiling experiments contribute to an enhanced understanding of the molecular mechanisms involved in the response to nongenotoxic carcinogens. These and other examples strongly imply functional relationships between drug treatment, protein expression detected by two-dimensional gels, and resulting pathophysiological effects. While proteomic studies are in their infancy, they could be applied to many toxicological issues and they are likely to result in the discovery of novel toxicological research leads and diagnostic markers.

THE CHALLENGE OF PATTERN RECOGNITION

The possibility that a specific group or class of compounds (as defined by toxic endpoint, mechanism, structure, or target organ) may induce signature patterns of changes in gene expression is one basis for the application of toxicogenomics to predictive toxicology. Exposure to different classes of toxicants is likely to result in

distinct patterns of altered mRNA and protein expression, and this offers the opportunity for fingerprinting toxicants of a particular type (Steiner and Anderson, 2000).
Transcript and proteome profiling studies can be used to categorize and classify
these effects through the direct comparison of mRNA or protein expression signatures in exposed and control samples. Potentially, mRNA or protein expression
patterns could be determined for various types of tissue-specific toxicants, allowing
candidate compounds to be screened for these characteristic patterns. Moreover,
such profiling experiments might be particularly useful to investigate the differences
in response to acute and chronic toxicity. Such investigations could assist in determining key parameters such as appropriate experimental models and choice of dose
and time-point to best elucidate mechanisms. Once an expression signature has been
characterized for known toxicants in a defined biological model, treatment of that
system with an unknown agent may activate a pattern of gene expression already
established and therefore identify this agent as a chemical belonging to a particular
toxic group.

   Moreover, it is possible to analyze sequence variations such as polymorphism
or DNA mutation with oligonucleotide-based microarrays to screen individuals that
may exhibit differential biological responses (Hacia and Collins, 1999). Therefore,
compiling data sets of toxicant exposures could allow estimation of the variability
in gene or protein expression between individuals in response to toxicants. Pattern
recognition may in turn allow the design and construction of customized miniarrays
to detect specific toxicity endpoints or pathways. If these systems were able to detect
potential adverse health effects of some development compounds, their application
in predevelopment toxicology screening would be of substantial benefit in providing
an early view of compound safety in advance of traditional studies. Development
of reference data sets to allow a pattern recognition approach to toxicology is likely
to require the application of complex computer algorithms and statistical approaches.
For example, statistical clustering techniques have been applied to microarray data
to analyze the temporal patterns of gene expression that characterize serum-respon-
siveness and wound repair (Iyer et al., 1999) and to distinguish cancerous tissue
from normal tissues and cell lines (Alon et al., 1999). The building of reference data
sets, possibly by comparison of microarray output across different laboratories, will
demand consistency in data analysis and format. A number of resources exist in
both the academic and commercial sectors for such purposes (Ermolaeva et al., 1998;
Bassett et al., 1999).

OPPORTUNITIES IN COMBINATION: A PERSPECTIVE

   There is an increasing desire and need to develop accurate and robust *in vitro*
methods for the identification and characterization of potential toxicants. Our
ability now to define in a more holistic fashion the molecular changes that are
induced in cells by trauma, damage, or other perturbations of physiological balance
provides exciting opportunities to explore new frameworks for alternative
approaches to safety assessment. Indeed, the development of biotechnology platforms and biological sciences is a major factor in the advancement of alternative

testing methodologies (Purchase et al., 1998). Responses of a cellular system or an organism to a chemical or a toxicant involve the expression of genetic information, but it is becoming increasingly clear that the behavior of gene products is difficult to predict from gene sequence. The combination of toxicogenomics and proteomics offers scientists the ability to integrate information from the genome, expressed mRNAs, and their respective protein products (Steiner and Anderson, 2000). Clearly, the possibility of toxicogenomics and proteomics giving an early alert to potential adverse effects at low levels of exposure, while powerful, raises many issues in the context of interpreting gene expression changes with respect to hazard and risk assessment. However, the examination of many genes in response to toxicants may help to determine their potential to induce adverse health effects that are difficult to predict currently in *in vitro* assays. It is reasonable to anticipate that in the first instance accurate interpretation of expression changes will only be possible when toxicogenomics and proteomics analyses are combined and conducted as part of a larger experimental design to understand observed toxicity at the physiological, histological, and biochemical levels and integrated with the vast amount of information already available on *in vivo* toxic responses to compounds in rodents.

Proteomics and toxicogenomics have the potential to encourage, and indeed require, toxicologists to consider biological responses in a more holistic fashion. It is inevitable that when opportunity to evaluate changes in the expression of only very few genes exists, those genes are selected carefully based upon our knowledge, expectations, or prejudice. What toxicogenomics and proteomics offer and demand of us is that consideration be given also to changes in the expression of genes that were believed to be of no apparent relevance. This may lead to the identification and consideration of new genes or proteins that have escaped previous consideration. One could predict that most exciting advances in defining toxicological mechanisms will derive from the interdisciplinary and more integrated toxicology that genomics and proteomics will undoubtedly encourage. With respect to *in vitro* toxicology, the careful and integrated interpretation of the vast amount of data generated using these powerful technologies will provide us with new information, in quality and quantity, and therefore new opportunities.

REFERENCES

Afshari, C.A., Nuwaysir, E.F., and Barrett, J.C. (1999) Application of complementary DNA microarray technology to carcinogen identification, toxicology and drug safety evaluation, *Cancer Res.*, 59, 4759–4760.

Aicher, L., Wahl, D., Arce, A., Grenet, O., and Steiner, S. (1998) New insights into cyclosporine A nephrotoxicity by proteome analysis, *Electrophoresis*, 19, 1998–2003.

Alon, U., Barkai, N., Notterman, D.A., Gish, K., Tbarra, S., Mack, D., and Levine, A.J. (1999) Broad patterns of gene expression revealed by clustering analysis of tumor and normal colon tissues probed by oligonucleotide arrays, *Proc. Natl. Acad. Sci. U.S.A.*, 96, 6745–6750.

Anderson, N.L. and Seilhamer, J. (1997) A comparison of selected mRNA and protein abundances in human liver, *Electrophoresis*, 18, 533–537.

Anderson, N.L., Copple, D.C., Bendele, R.A., Probst, G.S., and Richardson, F.C. (1992) Covalent protein modifications and gene expression changes in rodent liver following administration of methapyrilene: a study using two-dimensional electrophoresis, *Fundam. Appl. Toxicol.*, 18, 570–580.

Anderson, N.L., Esquer-Blasco, R., Richardson, F., Foxworthy, P., and Eacho, P. (1996) The effects of peroxisome proliferators on protein abundances in mouse liver, *Toxicol. Appl. Pharmacol.*, 137, 75–89.

Bassett, D.E.J., Eisen, M.B., and Boguski, M.S. (1999) Gene expression informatics—it's all in your mine, *Nat. Genet.*, 21, 51–55.

Bowtell, D.D. (1999) Options available, from start to finish, for obtaining expression data by microarray, *Nat. Genet.*, 21, 25–32.

Brown, P.O. and Botstein, D. (1999) Exploring the new world of the genome with DNA microarrays, *Nat. Genet.*, 21, 33–37.

C. elegans sequencing consortium (1998) Genome sequence of the nematode *C. elegans:* a platform for investigative biology, *Science*, 282.

Celis, J. and Gromov, P. (1999) 2D protein electrophoresis: can it be perfected? *Curr. Opin. Biotech.*, 10, 16–21.

Chabra, R.S., Huff, J.E., Schwetz, B.S., and Selkirk, J. (1990) An overview of prechronic and chronic toxicity/carcinogenicity experimental study designs and criteria used by the National Toxicology Program, *Environ. Health Perspect.*, 86, 313–321.

Chevalier, S. and Roberts, R.A. (1998) Perturbation of rodent hepatocyte growth control by non-genotoxic hepatocarcinogens: mechanisms and lack of relevance for human health, *Oncol. Rep.*, 5, 1319–1327.

Chevalier, S., Macdonald, N., Tonge, R., Rayner, S., Rowlinson, R., Shaw, J., Young, J., Davison, M., and Roberts, R.A. (2000) Proteomic analysis of differential protein expression in primary hepatocytes induced by EGF, TNFa or the peroxisome proliferator nafenopin, *Eur. J. Biochem.*, 267, 4624–4634.

Cunningham, M.L., Pippin, L.L., Anderson, N.L., and Wenk, M.L. (1995) The hepatocarcinogen methapyrilene but not the analog pyraline induces sustained hepatocellular replication and protein alterations in F344 rats in a 13-week feed study, *Toxicol. Appl. Pharmacol.*, 131, 216–223.

DeRisi, J., Penland, L., Brown, P.O., Bittner, M.L., Meltzer, P.S., Ray, M., Chen, Y., Su, Y.A., and Trent, J. (1996) Use of cDNA microarray to analyse gene expression patterns in human cancer, *Nat. Genet.*, 14, 457–460.

Desvergne, B. and Wahli, W. (1999) Peroxisome proliferator-activated receptor: nuclear control of metabolism, *Endocrine Rev.*, 20, 649–688.

Dunn, M.J. (2000) Studying heart disease using the proteomic approach, *Drug Discovery Today*, 5, 76–84.

Edvardsson, U., Alexandersson, M., Brockenhuus von Lowenhielm, H., Nystrom, A., Ljung, B., Nilsson, F., and Dahllof, B. (1999a) A proteome analysis of livers from obese (ob/ob) mice treated with the peroxisome proliferator WY14,643, *Electrophoresis*, 20, 935–942.

Edvardsson, U., Bergstrom, M., Alexandersson, M., Bamberg, K., Ljung, B., and Dahllof, B. (1999b) Rosiglitazone (BRL49653), a PPARg-selective agonist, cause peroxisome proliferator-like liver effects in obese mice, *J. Lipid Res.*, 40, 1177–1184.

Ermolaeva, O., Rastogi, M., Pruitt, K.D., Schuler, G.D., Bittner, M.I., Chen, Y., Simon, R., Meltzer, P., Trent, J.M., and Boguski, M.S. (1998) Data management and analysis for gene expression arrays, *Nat. Genet.*, 20, 19–23.

Farr, S. and Dunn, R.T.I. (1999) Concise review: gene expression applied to toxicology, *Toxicol. Sci.*, 50, 1–9.

Giometti, C.S., Tollaksen, S.L., Liang, X., and Cunningham, M.L. (1998) A comparison of liver protein changes in mice and hamsters treated with the peroxisome proliferator Wy-14,643, *Electrophoresis*, 19, 2498–2505.

Gonzalez, F.J., Peters, J.M., and Cattley, R.C. (1998) Mechanism of action of the nongenotoxic peroxisome proliferators: role of the peroxisome proliferator-activator receptor alpha, *J. Natl. Cancer Inst.*, 90, 1702–1709.

Hacia, J.G. and Collins, F.S. (1999) Mutational analysis using oligonucleotide microarrays, *J. Med. Genet.*, 36, 730–736.

Heller, R.A., Schena, M., Chai, A., Shalon, D., Redilion, T., Gilmore, J., Wooley, D.E., and Davis, R.W. (1997) Discovery and analysis of inflammatory disease-related genes using cDNA microarrays, *Proc. Natl. Acad. Sci. U.S.A.*, 94, 2150–2155.

Holden, P.R., James, N.H., Brooks, A.N., Roberts, R.A., Kimber, I., and Pennie, W.D. (2000) Identification by microarray technology of a possible association between carbon tetrachloride induced hepatotoxicity and interleukin 8 expression, *J. Mol. Biochem. Toxicol.*, 14, 283–290.

Iyer, V.R., Eisen, M.B., Ross, D.T., Schuler, G., Moore, T., Lee, J.C.F., Trent, J.M., Staudt, L.M., Hudson, J.J., Boguski, M.S., Lashkari, D., Sharon, D., Botstein, D., and Brown, P.O. (1999) The transcriptional program in the response of human fibroblasts to serum, *Science*, 283, 83–87.

Khan, J., Bittner, M.L., Chen, Y., Meltzer, P.S., and Trent, J.M. (1999) DNA microarray technology: the anticipated impact on the study of human disease, *Biochem. Biophys. Acta*, 1423, M27–M28.

Myers, T.G., Anderson, N.L., Waltham, M., Li, G., Buolamwini, J.K., Scudiero, D.A., Paull, K.D., Sausville, E.A., and Weinstein, J.N. (1997) A protein expression database for the molecular pharmacology of cancer, *Electrophoresis*, 18, 647–653.

Nuwaysir, E.F., Bittner, M., Trent, J., Barrett, J.C., and Afsharri, C.A. (1999) Microarrays and toxicology: the advent of toxicogenomics, *Mol. Carcinog.*, 24, 153–159.

O'Farrell, P.H. (1975) High resolution two-dimensional electrophoresis of proteins, *J. Biol. Chem.*, 250, 4007–4021.

Ostergaard, M., Wolf, H., Orntoft, T.F., and Celis, J.F. (1999) Psoriasin (S100A7): a putative urinary marker for the follow-up of patients with bladder squamous cell carcinomas, *Electrophoresis*, 20, 349–354.

Pennie, W.D. (2000) Use of cDNA microarrays to probe and understand the toxicological consequences of altered gene expression, *Toxicol. Lett.*, 112–113, 473–477.

Purchase, I.F.H., Botham, P.A., Bruner, L.H., Flint, O.P., Frazier, J.M., and Stokes, W.S. (1998) Workshop overview: scientific and regulatory challenges for the reduction, refinement, and replacement of animals in toxicity testing, *Toxicol. Sci.*, 43, 86–101.

Rodi, C.P., Bunch, R.T., Curtiss, S.W., Kier, L.D., Cabonce, M.A., Davila, J.C., Mitchell, M.D., Allen, C.L., and Morris, D.L. (1999) Revolution through genomics in investigative and discovery toxicology, *Toxicol. Pathol.*, 27, 107–110.

Ross, D.T., Scherf, U., Eisen, M.B., Perou, C.M., Rees, C., Spellman, P., Iyer, V., Jeffrey, S.S., Van de Rijn, M., Waltham, M., Pergamenschikov, A., Lee, J.C.F., Lashkari, D., Shalon, D., Myers, T.G., Weinstein, J.N., Botstein, D., and Brown, P.O. (2000) Systematic variation in gene expression patterns in human cancer cell lines, *Nat. Genet.*, 24, 227–235.

Ryffel, B. (1997) Impact of knock out mice in toxicology, *Crit. Rev. Toxicol.*, 27, 135–154.

Schena, M., Shalon, D., Heller, R., Chai, A., Brown, P.O., and Davis, R.W. (1996) Parallel human genome analysis: microarray-based expression monitoring of 1000 genes, *Proc. Natl. Acad. Sci. U.S.A.*, 93, 10614–10619.

Scherf, U., Ross, D.T., Waltham, M., Smith, L.H., Lee, J.K., Tanabe, L., Kohn, K.W., Reinhold, W.C., Myers, T.G., Andrews, D.T., Scudiero, D.A., Eisen, M.B., Sausville, E.A., Pommier, Y., Botstein, D., Brown, P.O., and Weinstein, J.N. (2000) A gene expression database for the molecular pharmacology of cancer, *Nat. Genet.*, 24, 236–344.

Shelton, D.N., Chang, E., Whittier, P.S., Choi, D., and Funk, W.D. (1999) Microarray analysis of replicative senescence, *Curr. Biol.*, 9, 939–945.

Steiner, S. and Anderson, N.L. (2000) Expression profiling in toxicology—potentials and limitations, *Toxicol. Lett.*, 112–113, 467–471.

Steiner, S., Aicher, L., Raymakers, J., Meheus, L., Esquerblasco, R., Anderson, N.L., and Cordier, A. (1996) Cyclosporine A mediated decrease in the rat renal calcium binding protein calbindin-D 28kDa, *Biochem. Pharmacol.*, 51, 253–258.

Strahl, B.D. and Allis, C.D. (2000) The language of covalent histone modifications, *Nature*, 403, 41–45.

Wang, J. and Hewick, R. (1999) Proteomics in drug discovery, *Drug Discovery Today*, 4, 129–133.

Watanabe, T., Lalwani, N.D., and Reddy, J.K. (1985) Specific changes in the protein composition of rat liver in response to the peroxisome proliferators ciprofibrate, Wy-14,643 and di-(2-ethylhexyl)phthalate, *Biochem. J.*, 227, 767–775.

Waterston, R. and Sulston, J. (1998) The human genome project: reaching the finish line, *Science*, 282, 55–57.

Wilkins, M.R. (1996) Current challenges and future applications for protein maps and post-translational vector maps in proteome projects, *Electrophoresis*, 17, 830–838.

Wilkins, M.R., Williams, K.L., Appel, R.D., and Hochstrasser, D.F.E. (1997) *Proteome research: new frontiers in functional genomics (principle and practice)*, Springer-Verlag, Berlin.

Williams, K.L. (1999) Genome and proteomes: towards a multidimensional view of biology, *Electrophoresis*, 20, 678–688.

Witzmann, F.A., Jarnot, B.M., Parker, D.N., and Clack, J.W. (1994) Modification of hepatic immunoglobulin heavy chain binding protein (BiP/Grp78) following exposure to structurally diverse peroxisome proliferators, *Fundam. Appl. Toxicol.*, 23, 1–8.

Witzmann, F.A., Fultz, C.D., Grant, R.A., Wright, L.S., Kornguth, S.E., and Siegel, F.L. (1999a) Regional protein alterations in rat kidneys induced by lead exposure, *Electrophoresis*, 20, 943–951.

Witzmann, F.A., Bauer, M.D., Fieno, A.M., Grant, R.A., Keough, T.W., Lacey, M.P., Siegel, F.L., Sun, Y., Wright, L.S., Young, R.S., and Witten, M.L. (1999b) Proteomic analysis of simulated occupational jet fuel exposure in the lung, *Electrophoresis*, 20, 3659–3669.

CHAPTER 35

Use of Transgenic Animals in Regulatory Carcinogenicity Evaluations*

Frank D. Sistare and Abigail C. Jacobs

CONTENTS

INTRODUCTION

Genetically engineered transgenic mice have been used in research for over 20 years (Palmiter and Brinster, 1986). Many models are now being created for drug discovery and development strategies to identify the critical biological role of the genetically modified molecule, to enhance understanding of pharmacological mechanisms, to study interactions with molecules impacting drug metabolism and distribution, and to gain insight into the likelihood for a drug under development for achieving efficacy and avoiding significant toxicity (Bolon and Galbreath, 2002; Elmquist and Miller, 2001; Harris et al., 1993; Livingston, 1999; Merlino, 1991).

* Authored in private capacity with no official support by the Food and Drug Administration intended or inferred.

A 1997 International Conference on Harmonization (ICH) agreement spurred intense interest in incorporating transgenic mice into a pivotal nonclinical safety regulatory evaluation for many human pharmaceuticals—assessment of carcinogenicity potential (ICH, 1997). With this agreement, sponsors now have an option to replace one of the two species (usually the mouse) needed for carcinogenicity assessments with a short- or medium-term alternative model with justification for their choice of model specified.

Transgenic mouse models have been genetically engineered to add or modify sequences coding for critical proteins that have been shown to play pivotal roles in human cancer development (van Dyke and Jacks, 2002). Advances in molecular medicine and greater scientific understanding of oncogenes, tumor suppressor genes, DNA repair enzymes, and regulators of genomic stability continue to provide a rich source of targets for the development of transgenic mouse models with accelerated tumor development responses to recognized carcinogens. When the models are engineered to modify pivotal proteins associated with mechanisms underlying human chemical carcinogenesis, then the models are expected to be more relevant to human mechanisms than are wild-type mice. If a protein is targeted that serves a pivotal role in a common pathway vital to producing tumors for every carcinogen relevant to humans, the model is expected to have great utility. However, if a protein is targeted that could not contribute to all mechanisms of chemical carcinogenesis relevant to humans, there would be legitimate concern in relying upon the general application of the model as a sole screen for identifying all potential human carcinogens (Johnson, 1999). Since chemical carcinogenesis can occur by such a variety of mechanisms, it is a great challenge to develop such an all-encompassing model. If a model is designed with a gene mutation targeted to a pathway that is not relevant or contributory to the carcinogenic process for a given test chemical, a false negative result is likely. The benefits of identifying universally applicable models are so great, that to accept the challenge and begin systematic testing with a prioritized selected list of chemicals is in everyone's best interest. While no single model is likely to identify all mechanisms of chemical carcinogenesis, if the strengths and limitations of several models can be specifically defined, then appropriate applications of alternatives for assessing defined issues relating to carcinogenic potential will need to be carefully selected on a case-by-case basis.

The targeted rewards for successfully developing genetically modified rodent models that will accurately identify human carcinogens under carefully specified and scientifically justified conditions of use are:

1. Outcomes are expected to be more relevant to human mechanisms of carcinogenesis than many of the species-specific mechanisms (MacDonald et al., 1994) that have surfaced in 2-year mouse bioassays. These models may reduce strain and species-specific tumor findings as many of these may derive from mechanisms that are generally adaptive and distally removed from a primary insult. However, tumor site specificity inherent across strains and visible as highly variable spectra of sporadic and susceptible tumors is not expected to be eliminated.
2. The genetic alterations are expected to accelerate the carcinogenic process. This acceleration is expected to: (a) reduce ambiguities and misinterpretations of rodent tumor findings that are prone to derive spontaneously in part from the effects of

aging; (b) avoid the expected attrition of animals during the normal conduct of a 2-year lifetime rodent bioassay, thereby allowing smaller initial animal numbers to be used and attaining a higher quality of animal health at study termination; (c) result in lower background tumor findings over a shorter study duration, so that signal-to-noise should be enhanced and fewer animals could provide statistical power similar to that currently in use; (d) allow earlier identification and reasonable options for assessing or alleviating sporadic situational drug development and regulatory concerns where, for example, waiting for the outcome of a repeat 2-year assay is impractical or mutually undesirable.

3. Molecular assessments of chemically induced tumors derived from genetically modified animal models provide a focused path forward for elucidating an understanding of how the carcinogen may have cooperated with the underlying genetic modification to result in tumor formation. Knowledge of how early gene and protein expression alterations could be interpreted to provide mechanistic information of drug action at target tumor tissue sites is rapidly evolving (Boley et al., 2002; Salleh et al., 2003; Hamadeh et al., 2002). Solving the puzzles to link early signal alterations with later appearing molecular fingerprints in more mature tumors is anticipated to provide, in the near future, an even more accurate assessment of tumorigenic mechanism and human relevancy.

If toxicologists are ever to evolve past total reliance on rodent lifetime bioassays for assessing a chemical's human carcinogenic potential, a careful assessment of novel models providing mechanistic insight, together with currently accepted traditional testing, is logical. As experience is gained and carefully considered adjustments and improvements are made to model systems, public health protection can be maintained while such testing paradigms can continue to develop and be further refined. Thus, the 1997 ICH agreement calling for maintained application of one traditional 2-year rodent (usually rat) study arm and a choice of either a short-term alternative or a second 2-year complementary rodent study is a reasonable path forward.

Based on logical scientifically supported thinking within the framework of studying the widely accepted multistep and multistage process of malignant tumor development (Fearon and Vogelstein, 1990), a number of genetically modified mouse lines have been derived for research purposes. Several of the models were judged to be suitable alternatives for carcinogenicity evaluation screening approaches. The models that were selected by a number of laboratories worldwide for specific evaluations of their abilities to distinguish carcinogens from noncarcinogens and to provide additional valuable information on mode as well as mechanism of action were (1) Tg.AC, (2) TgrasH2, (3) P53$^{+/-}$, and (4) XPA$^{-/-}$/P53$^{+/-}$ (Robinson and MacDonald, 2001).

Furthermore, additional bigenic and even trigenic (van Steeg, 2001) crosses have been derived, as well as additional transgenic models which are not generally commercially available (e.g., TGF alpha [Greten et al., 2001], TRAMP [Gingrich et al., 1996], p16(INK4A)$^{+/-}$ [Serrano et al., 1996], etc.), and others which are commercially available but have received more limited evaluation (PIM1 [van Lohuizen et al., 1989], XPC$^{-/-}$ [Sands et al., 1995]), and K6/ODC [Megosh et al., 1995]).

The criteria for an ideal short-term alternative tumor model for applications to regulatory decision-making would include:

1. Phenotypic and genetic stability allowing a high level of assay reproducibility
2. Relevant human exposures achieved and metabolism and tissue distribution mimicking that of humans
3. Reproducibly rapid and robust induction of statistically significant tumor numbers clearly associated with chemical carcinogen exposure without confounding sporadic background tumors
4. Broad tissue susceptibility useful for products with wide tissue exposures
5. Scientifically understood and easily identifiable mode or mechanistic basis of tumor induction
6. A performance record demonstrating appropriate sensitivity and specificity to discriminate human carcinogens from noncarcinogens

COMMERCIAL COMPLICATIONS

While government, academic, and commercial collaborators have succeeded in pursuing a pathway that has enabled a reasonably extensive evaluation and the continued availability of several transgenic models for pharmaceutical carcinogenicity evaluations, any identified needs for additional or further improved models may go unmet unless certain commercial complications can be resolved (Marshall, 2002). Broad patents currently exist on genetically modified mice that show enhanced cancer susceptibility (Gulezian, 1999; Swing, 2001). A license has been granted under these patents allowing commercial distribution of three of the genetically modified tumor endpoint models reviewed here: Tg.AC, TgrasH2, and P53[+/-]. Noncommercial research licenses to study tumor-susceptible genetically modified models are free to NIH scientists and NIH grantees but licenses for commercial applications with additional models must be negotiated on a user-by-user basis. The most restrictive patent extends to the year 2016 (Marshall, 2002). This situation has raised concerns that research to develop and evaluate additional improved models with genetic susceptibility to cancer development may be inhibited if commercial application strategies are not first resolved. Resource-intensive collaborative assessments like that completed recently (Robinson and MacDonald, 2001), but focused on new models perceived to have stronger or complementary attributes to those that are presently commercially available, may be difficult to coordinate unless, again, a broader licensing issue and sharing of intellectual property can be managed. Product sponsors appear to have been inhibited from using the XPA/P53 model in the United States, for example, until this licensing issue is resolved.

OVERVIEW OF INDIVIDUAL MODELS

More in-depth reviews of the currently available, most widely used transgenic models for carcinogenicity testing have recently been published (French et al., 2001; Storer et al., 2001; Tennant et al., 2001; Sistare et al., 2002; Eastin et al., 2001; Tamaoki, 2001; Usui et al., 2001; van Steeg et al., 2001; van Kreijl et al., 2001). A subset of those results has been summarized in Tables 35.1 to 35.4. We have found it helpful to construct the present overview of these transgenic mice by considering

Table 35.1 IARC Class I or 2A Human Carcinogen, or NTP Reasonably Anticipated Human Carcinogen

	Tg.AC Topical	TgrasH2	p53+/–	XPA–/–/p53+/–
Genotoxic				
Benzene	+	+	+	nd*
Benzo(a)pyrene	+	nd	+	+
Cyclophosphamide	–	+	+	nd
7,12-Dimethylbenzanthracene	+	nd	+	+**
Melphalan	–	+/–	+	nd
Phenacetin	–	+	–	–
Procarbazine	nd	+	nd	nd
Nongenotoxic				
Cyclosporin A	+	+/–	+	+
Diethylstilbestrol	+	+	+	+
17-β-estradiol (or ethinyl estradiol#)	+#	–	+/–	+
Oxymetholone	+	nd	–	nd
2,3,7,8-TCDD	+	nd	–	nd

* nd: no adequate data available on the performance of the compound in that model.
**Positive in 6 month XPA–/– and positive in 6 month p53+/–; not tested in XPA–/–/P53+/– bitransgenic.

Table 35.2 Genotoxic Trans-Species Rodent Carcinogens

	Tg.AC Topical	TgrasH2	P53+/–	XPA–/–/P53+/–
p-Cresidine	–	+	+	+
2,4-Diaminotoluene	+	nd	–	nd
Diethylnitrosamine	nd	+	nd	nd
Dimethylnitrosamine	nd	+	+	nd
N-Ethylnitrosourea	nd	+	+	nd
Glycidol	–	+	–	nd
N-Methylnitrosourea	nd	+	+	nd
Phenolphthalein	nd	–	+	nd
Thiotepa	nd	+	nd	nd
Urethane	nd	+	+	nd
4-Vinyl-1-cyclohexene-diepoxide*	–	+	+	nd

* Applied dermally to each model tested.

the specific genetic modification for each model in the context of the three generally accepted stages encompassing the multistep and multistage complex process driving the development of a single normal cell into progeny of malignant tumor cells: initiation, promotion, and progression.

Tg.AC

The Tg.AC (v-Ha-ras) mouse developed by Leder et al. (1990) is regarded as genetically initiated. Since the *ras* family of proteins are common transducers for diverse growth stimulatory receptor signaling pathways, an activating mutation in a

Table 35.3 Nongenotoxic Rodent Carcinogens and Human Carcinogenicity Unlikely or Uncertain

	Tg.AC Topical	TgrasH2	P53+/−	XPA−/−/P53+/−
Chlorpromazine	nd	−	nd	nd
Clofibrate	+	+	−	nd
Dieldrin	nd	nd	−	nd
Diethylhexylphthalate	−	+	+/−	−
Haloperidol	nd	−	−	−
D-Limonene	nd	nd	−	nd
Metaproterenol	nd	−	−	nd
Pentachlorophenol	+	nd	−	nd
Phenobarbital	−	−	−	−
Reserpine	−	−	−	−
Sulfamethoxazole	−	−	−	−
WY-14643	−	+	−	+*

* Positive in 6 month XPA−/−, not tested in XPA−/−/p53+/− bitransgenic.

Table 35.4 Rodent Noncarcinogens

	Tg.AC Topical	TgrasH2	P53+/−	XPA−/−/P53+/−
Genotoxic				
p-Anisidine	−	−	−	nd
2-Chloroethanol	−	nd	nd	nd
1-Chloro-2-propanol	−	nd	−	nd
2,6-Diaminotoluene	−	nd	−	nd
8-Hydroxy-quinoline	−	−	−	nd
Nongenotoxic				
Ampicillin	nd	−	nd	nd
Benzethonium chloride	−	nd	nd	nd
D-Mannitol	nd	−	nd	−
Oleic acid diethanolamine	−	nd	−	nd
Phenol	−	nd	nd	nd
Resorcinol	+	−	−	nd
Rotenone	−	−	−	nd
Sulfisoxazole	−	−	nd	nd

ras protein is likely to generate a sustained proliferative signal capable of driving tumorigenesis. An expressed mutation in a *ras* protein might be expected, then, to convey to a cell properties of both initiation and sustained growth promotion. However, if the model is designed such that the expression of this mutated gene is repressed or severely restricted, no tumor might be expected unless and until the gene is activated, or the very limited permissive cell population is relieved of all growth-repressive forces within its local cellular environment. The Tg.AC hemizygous mouse contains at least one inverted repeat and approximately 40 tandem repeat integrated copies of a microinjected DNA construct consisting of a mouse fetal zetaglobin promoter linked to v-Ha-ras with activating mutations in codons 12 and 59, followed by an SV-40 polyadenylation tail (Leder et al., 1990; Thompson et al., 1998). The expression of transgene is restricted to only certain tissue sites, presumably because of the high tissue specificity of the zetaglobin promoter sequence. The reliable transgene-dependent chemically inducible site of tumorigenesis in the mature mouse appears to be certain stem cells of the dermal hair follicle (Hansen and Tennant, 1994) favoring evaluations of dermal exposures with test compounds.

Topical applications of certain chemicals or full-thickness wounding (Cannon et al., 1997) result in tumor growth that is associated with transgene expression. Interestingly, a critical inverted repeat orientation of two copies of transgene in a head-to-head orientation appears to be essential for generating a tumor response to chemical treatment (Thompson et al., 1998; Honchel et al., 2001). The interaction of this inverted repeat with integration site sequence at the 3' end appears to be optimal for transgene sequence function (Leder et al., 2002). Mice harboring as many copies of transgene but with a critical inherited spontaneous germ cell-derived deletion of sequence at or near the inverted repeat junction are resistant to tumor induction. Tumors derived from sensitive mice show varying degrees of instability in this same region (Thompson et al., 2001). Increasing genomic instability favors tumor formation (Leder et al., 2002) and thus may be a component of the properties of the chemical tumorigens that are positive in Tg.AC. However, there remains a lack of clarity currently in the mechanisms underlying initial events triggered by chemical exposure leading to chemical tumorigenesis in this model.

Experience with the set of chemicals summarized in Tables 35.1 and 35.2 indicates that direct DNA reactive mechanisms are not likely either to trigger activation of transgene expression or to clonally expand the rare follicular stem cell that can express transgene. Understanding the cellular events that can trigger either process is important to many investigators who ponder the practical utility of this model. The failure of this model to identify, at the dermal site of application, the majority of genotoxic carcinogens tested, including melphalan, cyclophosphamide, p-cresidine, phenacetin, and glycidol, raises concerns that genotoxic mechanisms of carcinogenesis are not likely to be reliably detected with Tg.AC dermal dosing. Generation of forestomach tumors or systemic neoplastic endpoints following oral dosing of Tg.AC with carcinogens appears to be unreliable (Sistare et al., 2002).

There are precautions to carefully consider with the conduct of a Tg.AC study. Test compounds with high aqueous solubility and poor solubility in ethanol, methanol, or acetone may pose practical dosing limitations since assuring uniform skin exposures of repeated dosings may be difficult with solutions that exceed an aqueous content of 14% (Sistare et al., 2002). The addition of solvent components such as dimethylsufoxide (DMSO) and olive oil (Sistare et al., 2002; Stoll et al., 2001) to improve the solubility of hydrophilic compounds has been shown to compromise assay performance. The model appears to develop tumors in response to dermal toxicity and inflammation (e.g., 2,4-dinitro-1-fluorobenzene (DFNB) [Albert et al., 1996] and resorcinol [Eastin et al., 2001]), while low levels of inflammation observable microscopically appear to be tolerated (Moser et al., 2001; Nylander-French and French, 1998). A careful definition of the upper dose limit in study design is essential to avoid confounding interpretations of test results.

The model appears to have value for testing, using a dermal route of exposure, for nongenotoxic mechanisms of compounds intended for either topical or systemic administration. As shown in Tables 35.1 and 35.2, the model responds to agents that may involve estrogen, aryl hydrocarbon, or androgen receptor-mediated pathways contributing to tumorigenesis. Furthermore, the known skin tumor promoters TPA, benzoyl peroxide, and o-benzyl-p-chlorophenol have also tested positive following dermal dosing of Tg.AC mice (Eastin et al., 2001), providing further indications that activation of tumor growth-promoting pathways leads rapidly to skin tumorigenesis in Tg.AC mice. If it is not important to further investigate that a test compound may be a genotoxic carcinogen, but rather more important to assess potential to activate nongenotoxic pathways leading to tumorigenesis, this model appears to be useful. It may be difficult to distinguish relying upon Tg.AC study findings, a pure tumor promotor from a complete carcinogen working through a nongenotoxic mechanism, but this could be an important distinction for product development decision-making. Furthermore, it is not clear from available testing data that if a compound has both potent mutagenic as well as tumor promotional/proliferative activity, whether the mutagenic activity might actually interfere with and reduce apparent tumorigenicity in Tg.AC. Would, for example, a mixture of melphalan with phorbol 12-myristate 13-acetate (TPA) reduce the tumor signal produced by TPA alone? Could this account for the negative findings with WY-14643 which have been shown to be clastogenic (Galloway et al., 2000), as compared to the positive findings observed in this model with clofibrate? If such were truly the case, a negative Tg.AC study finding with an agent yielding positive relevant findings in a genotoxicity assay may be uninformative and possibly misleading. More thorough investigation of this issue is warranted. Situations sometimes arise when a compound is intended for human systemic administration, but human exposure levels cannot be achieved in the mouse by systemic dosing routes. Achieving high local concentrations at the skin site of application could add value over the performance of a systemic low exposure 2-year mouse assay in such circumstances.

TgrasH2

For the TgrasH2 model, unlike with Tg.AC, the transgene *ras* sequence is not mutated. TgrasH2 mice contain three copies of constitutively expressed human c-Ha-ras sequence under transcriptional control of its own promoter (Suemizu et al., 2002). The model is not initiated, therefore, and expression of the transgene is not tissue restricted. The model may be conceptualized, then, as pre-promoted through the actions of a sustained elevated steady-state expression of the growth stimulatory signal transducing *ras* protein. The simplistic consideration, then, is that this model's tissues are receiving a sustained growth-promoting influence. This leads to the logical prediction that a genotoxic insult resulting in a stable mutation in the transgene, in a cooperating oncogene, or in a tumor suppressor gene could result in a rapid rise in tumor burden.

These predictions appear accurate since exposures to genotoxic agents including benzene, cyclophosphamide, phenacetin, p-cresidine, diethylnitrosamine, dimethylnitrosamine, N-ethylnitrosourea (ENU), glycidol, N-methylnitrosourea (MNU), procarbazine, thiotepa, and 4-vinyl-1-cyclohexene-diepoxide result in significantly increased tumor burdens within 6 months of dosing (Tables 35.1 and 35.2). The one unexpected equivocal finding observed with melphalan dosing deserves careful consideration (Usui et al., 2001). In that study 3 of 8 surviving female mice developed forestomach papillomas after dosing with 1.5 mg/kg melphalan I.P. weekly. Seven of the 15 females died as a result of I.P. injection-induced abdominal cavity adhesion. In contrast, Tg.AC mice have tolerated oral and topical dosing with 4 mg/kg/week, and male, but not female, P53$^{+/-}$ mice tolerated 4.5 mg/kg/week delivered as 3× per week I.P. dosing with 1.5 mg/kg melphalan in propylene glycol. In the P53$^{+/-}$ study, males showed a statistically significant increase in tumors at this high dose, while no statistically significant increases were noted in either sex at the next lower dose tested — 0.3 mg/kg 3× per week (Storer et al., 2001).

These data underscore two fairly consistent and noteworthy trends in the data with this as well as with other transgenic models:

1. The transgenic mouse models are not "super sensitive" to carcinogens. Aggressive dosing is important and identifying the correct maximally tolerated dose is critical for optimizing accuracy of assay outcome. Important decisions must be made regarding dose, dosing route, and dosing frequency to maximize and optimize exposures while avoiding dose-limiting toxicities.
2. A narrow decrement in dosing levels (i.e., twofold, rather than fivefold) seems prudent for high and mid-dose selections. This would provide greater confidence in study interpretation for those instances when the number of animals remaining in the high dose group at study termination may be significantly reduced and the outcome of the mid-dose group must assume prime importance. The positive control MNU used for TgrasH2 studies is negative when administered to TgrasH2 mice at a dose of 18.75 mg/kg, a dose equivalent of 1.4 g for a 75-kg human. However, only a twofold higher dose yields forestomach tumors in 27 of 28 mice and 75 mg/kg appears to be very close to the maximally tolerated dose in this model (Usui et al., 2001).

A "pre-promoted" model might not be expected to develop an accelerated tumor burden in response to indirect acting, nor nongenotoxic carcinogens nor tumor promoters. However, the liver tumors seen following exposures to the peroxisome proliferators clofibrate, diethylhexylphthalate, and WY-14643 suggest that indirect mechanisms of carcinogenesis are detectable that may involve oxidative DNA damage and may additionally involve altered growth deregulation (Table 35.3). Ethylene thiourea, 1,4-dioxane, and ethylacrylate represent examples of additional nongenotoxic trans-species rodent carcinogens that tested positive in TgrasH2 (Usui et al., 2001). The expectations for this model to detect all human relevant nongenotoxic carcinogens are somewhat dimmed by the negative findings reported with 17-β-estradiol (Table 35.1). Other nongenotoxic mechanisms which have not been evaluated in this model include, for example, activators of growth promotion by agents such as phorbol esters, mezerein, or mirex and other mechanisms involving additional nuclear receptor-mediated pathways such as those activated by androgen receptor and aryl hydrocarbon receptor agonists.

While the human liver relevance of the positive peroxisome proliferator liver tumor findings is legitimately questioned (Gonzalez, 2002; Peters et al., 1997; Ward et al., 1998), these findings are not unreasonable and not so surprising in such a mouse model. If humans were similarly endowed with a higher density of high affinity peroxisome proliferator-activated alpha receptors in liver or other tissue sites, we might be expected to be similarly at high risk to liver or other tumor inductions under such chronic exposure conditions with this class of agents, and this would be important to know. This finding also serves as a good example that the human relevance of all positive tumor findings in transgenic models should not be assumed in cases when there is a clear understanding of the likely mechanisms and accurate knowledge of pivotal species differences. Empirical assessments are often insufficient and experimental strategies providing improved understanding of mechanisms will always be important.

The inconsistency of positive responses with TgrasH2 mice to nongenotoxic carcinogens indicates the potential for the model to respond to certain nongenotoxic carcinogens and help with assessments of nongenotoxic mechanisms, but further testing of nongenotoxic carcinogens would be helpful. This model may be the most widely encompassing as a screen to identify more modes of chemical carcinogenesis than either Tg.AC, P53$^{+/-}$, or XPA$^{-/-}$/P53$^{+/-}$. On the other hand, since the model is quite efficient at identifying genotoxic carcinogens, without further information that might be derived, for example, from molecular analyses of resultant tumors, it may be difficult to draw conclusions regarding carcinogen mode of action.

Investigations of tumors derived from TgrasH2 mice exposed to the genotoxic carcinogens ENU, MNU, and urethane as well as investigations of sporadic tumors provide an indication that mutations in the transgene are not obligatory to tumor induction in this model, but rather overexpression of the human H-ras transgene is consistently observed (Tamaoki, 2001; Maruyama et al., 2001). While not obligatory, however, transgene human H-ras mutations are consistently observed in MNU and urethane-induced tumors, while mutations in endogenous murine H-ras are seen in tumors induced by urethane but not MNU. Expansion of similar tumor analyses for mutations and for alterations in DNA methylation in other critical oncogenes and in tumor suppressor genes across collections of sporadic tumors, and in tumors induced by genotoxic and nongenotoxic agents could be illuminating and practically useful for regulatory decision-making. Further research in this area is encouraged.

This model deserves further investigation of utility using dermal exposure routes. Since Tg.AC has been developed as a skin dosing model, other models such as TgrasH2 and P53$^{+/-}$ have generally not been evaluated very much with compounds dosed by the dermal route. Such use of these models is worth further consideration for chemicals that will be components of dermal products and, as discussed above, perhaps under circumstances when sufficiently high exposures cannot be achieved in rodents following systemic dosing routes.

P53$^{+/-}$ MODEL

The role of the p53 protein to maintain genomic stability and serve as "the guardian of the genome" (Lane, 1992; Morris, 2002) is well appreciated. Proper function of the protein is critical to maintaining appropriate regulation of cell cycle, apoptosis, DNA repair, and cellular differentiation. It is not so surprising, then, that (1) mutations in the p53 gene are seen in 50% of human cancers (Hollstein et al., 1991; Greenblatt et al., 1994); (2) numerous animal and cellular models with engineered or natural defects in p53 function are prone to dysregulation of cell cycle, apoptosis, DNA repair, and cellular differentiation; and (3) chemical- or radiation-induced DNA damaging events or genetically engineered cellular oncogene imbalance will lead to an apparent homeostatic activation of p53.

Cells with deficient p53 protein function have been shown (Donehower et al., 1992) to traverse the cell cycle more quickly and to spend less fractional time in G_o, the stage of the cell cycle when DNA damage is known to be repaired. Furthermore, since the cellular machinery responsible for shunting damaged cells toward apoptotic death is compromised, more damaged cells are prone to survive through a shorter cell cycle and enter cell division. Such cells might then be conceptualized as classically "pre-promoted" and prone to chemical initiation. Mutational or other genetically modifying initiating events are more likely to be retained and thus tumors are more likely to develop in response to genotoxic agents as opposed to those that are more growth stimulatory or tumor promoting. Animals with knockout of both p53 genes quickly develop spontaneous tumors (Donehower et al., 1992), suggesting that normal background genotoxic insults and editing errors that cannot be processed efficiently lead to tumorigenesis. Furthermore, additional experimental evidence suggests that reduction in p53 gene dosage also contributes to enhancement of malignant progression (Kemp et al., 1993).

This model uses a fifth generation backcross onto C57BL/6 mice of a founder line derived from p53 genetically modified AB1 (129Sv) embryonic mouse cells. These mice are heterozygous, containing a wild type p53 tumor suppressor gene and a null allele that is not transcribed or translated (Donehower et al., 1992; Harvey et al., 1993). Study findings confirm the expectations for this model with few exceptions. Genotoxic agents known to cause deletions or mutations such as benzene, cyclophosphamide, melphalan, p-cresidine, N-methylnitrosourea, etc. (see Tables 35.1 and 35.2) are positive tumorigens in the P53[+/-] model. Critical tests of sensitivity to agents with nongenotoxic carcinogenic mechanisms (see Tables 35.1 and 35.3) including exposures to 2,3,7,8-tetrachlorodibenzo-para-dioxin (TCDD), oxymetholone, WY-14643, and clofibrate were negative, while 17-β-estradiol test results were equivocal. The model's high reliability for identifying genotoxic carcinogens and for not identifying nongenotoxic carcinogens adds confidence to study interpretations where an appreciation for whether a genotoxic or nongenotoxic mechanism may be underlying a tumorigenic response is important to regulatory and product development decision-making. This can be especially helpful when genotoxicity testing battery results are inconsistent or findings are marginally positive and proposed patterns of clinical use and expected systemic exposures would benefit from such knowledge.

Recent data (Recio et al., 2000) taken in context with other published findings (Donehower et al., 1992; Storer et al., 2001) have generated interest in a more carefully staged assessment of P53 model performance with dosing of study compounds for 9 as compared to 6 months. While the study was not specifically designed to compare 6- and 9-month tumor data, the results (Recio et al., 2000) indicate, in accordance with earlier data (Donehower et al., 1992), that background tumor findings remain low for 9 months. Furthermore, benzene inhalation resulted in a tumor incidence that exceeded that previously seen at 6 months using maximally tolerated oral dosing. The results across 19 studies in male and female p53[+/-] mice treated with the positive control *p*-cresidine at a dose of 400 mg/kg/day by gavage indicate that only 1 of the 19 studies was judged to be negative (Storer et al., 2001). Upon closer examination of the data, however, if the male and female arms of each study are considered separately, and a statistical threshold rather than the less stringent rare tumor threshold is considered for this positive control compound, then 6 of 38 study arms failed to meet statistical significance, and an additional 6 of 38 study arms just met statistical significance. After 6 months of exposure to a maximally tolerated dose, the bladder tumor response of P53$^{+/-}$ mice to the *p*-cresidine positive control has not been consistently robust.

Since the P53$^{+/-}$ model represents the fifth generation backcross onto C57Bl/6 mice of the original founder strain derived using the 129Sv embryonic stem cell line, only 3% of original 129Sv DNA is retained except for the genetically selected chromosome 11 containing the genetically modified p53 allele. The linkage of retained 129Sv sequence flanking the modified 129Sv p53 locus allows researchers opportunities to investigate molecular clues in this region of tumors that can be contrasted with the wild type allele and used to provide insight into potential mechanisms of genetic damage (Hulla et al., 2001). Such molecular investigations of genetic alterations focused on this region have demonstrated, for example, that phenolphthalein-induced thymic lymphomas are associated with loss of p53 heterozygosity, which appears to involve homologous recombination (Hulla et al., 2001); that benzene-induced tumors are also associated with loss of p53 heterozygosity appearing to involve nonhomologous end-joining (Boley et al., 2000); and that *p*-cresidine bladder tumors do not involve loss of heterozygosity nor point mutations in p53 but rather show evidence of point mutations at alternate genetic loci, certain of which presumably cooperate with the phenotypic effects of the reduced p53 gene dosage (Venkatachalam et al., 2001). Further development of such molecular analyses is encouraged to improve understanding of chemical tumorigenesis and potentially to assist with differential diagnosis of spontaneous tumors from statistically insignificant but biologically important chemically induced tumors. Futhermore, the negative findings with glycidol and 2,4-diaminotoluene (Table 35.2) indicate that further efforts are needed to either better understand the model's limitations and apparent resistance to those mutagenic carcinogens, or to investigate improved sensitivity of the model to these compounds under a modified protocol study design (e.g., 9-month dosing with 25 animals per group at well-defined maximally tolerated doses and optimized dosing schedules).

XPA$^{-/-}$/P53$^{+/-}$

The protein encoded by the xeroderma pigmentosum complementation group A (XPA) gene is involved in the recognition of DNA damage and is critical for proper nucleotide excision repair function. Humans with xeroderma pigmentosum with a specific inherited loss of the XPA gene are hypersensitive to UV light-induced skin tumors and development of other internal neoplasias (Kraemer et al., 1984). The XPA$^{(-/-)}$ knockout mice, like XPA patients, demonstrate increased susceptibility to UV light-induced skin tumors (De Vries et al., 1995; Nakane et al., 1995).

DNA strand breaks, DNA adduct formation, DNA nucleotide dimerization, and cross-linking reactions by chemical genotoxic carcinogens or damaging UV light are known to result in gene mutations. Inefficient cellular repair mechanisms for these forms of DNA damage would be expected to result in increased rates of mutation incorporation. Indeed, adduct formation, mutation frequencies, and tumor development following exposures with directly genotoxic chemical carcinogens such as benzo[a]pyrene (de Vries et al., 1997a; de Vries et al., 1997b) and 7,12-dimethylbenzanthracene (de Vries et al., 1995; Nakane et al., 1995), known to cause bulky DNA adducts normally repaired via a functional nucleotide excision repair (NER) pathway, are elevated in XPA$^{-/-}$ mice as compared to wild-type mice. These mice, then, are not chemically initiated but are certainly prone to becoming chemically initiated if exposed to a direct DNA damaging agent. Agents devoid of such activity that may produce neoplasia through tumor-promoting, cellular proliferative, and even indirect DNA damaging mechanisms might be expected, then, to go undetected by such a model.

Further evaluations of the XPA$^{-/-}$ model with other known directly genotoxic chemical carcinogens led investigators to extend the protocol dosing duration from 6 to 9 months to improve statistical power to an acceptable level (van Steeg et al., 2001). To broaden the range of tissue susceptibility and carcinogen sensitivity beyond those that are dependent specifically upon NER pathways, the XPA$^{-/-}$ model was cross-bred with the P53$^{+/-}$ mouse. The P53$^{+/-}$ model chosen was not the same as that described above, but rather derived from a different genetically engineered embryonic stem cell line (Jacks et al., 1994). Both this chosen P53$^{+/-}$ model and the XPA$^{-/-}$ model had been derived from C57Bl/6 backgrounds, which is the same background used for the P53$^{+/-}$ model described above. Crossing these two transgenic lines was found, as was hoped, to improve the speed and robustness of tumorigenesis, for example, following exposures to benzo[a]pyrene (van Oostrom et al., 1999). Such modifications were incorporated more recently, however, and the number and variety of compounds that have been evaluated are not as great as those for the other three models (Tables 35.1 to 35.4). Within our informal discussion of initiation/promotion/progression, this model could be considered pre-promoted and progression enhanced owing to p53 insufficiency, and even further prone to chemical initiation by certain mutagens owing to the loss of XPA.

Since the bigenic XPA$^{-/-}$/P53$^{+/-}$ model would be expected to perform similarly to the P53$^{+/-}$ model following exposure to genotoxic and nongenotoxic agents, any differences might be attributable to either the extended 3-month assay design, to the loss of XPA function, or to the slightly different p53 genotype. As shown in Tables 35.1 to 35.4, every genotoxic agent that tested positive in P53$^{+/-}$ similarly tested positive in XPA$^{-/-}$/P53$^{+/-}$. The human genotoxic carcinogen phenacetin was tested at a top dose half that of the dose used for evaluating the P53$^{+/-}$ 6-month assay. At the dose of 0.75% in diet, the XPA$^{-/-}$/P53$^{+/-}$ assay was considered negative. However, a rare renal adenoma was reported with dose-dependent hyperplasia seen in all animals. Nongenotoxic rodent carcinogens that tested negative in P53$^{+/-}$ generally tested negative, as well, in XPA$^{-/-}$/P53$^{+/-}$. Among these nongenotoxic agents, the somewhat unexpected P53$^{+/-}$ positive finding with the immunosuppressant cyclosporin was replicated in XPA$^{-/-}$/P53$^{+/-}$. The peroxisome proliferator di(2-ethylhexyl)phthalate

(DEHP), which produced equivocal findings in P53$^{+/-}$, yielded an unequivocal negative result in XPA$^{-/-}$/p53$^{+/-}$, suggesting that the P53$^{+/-}$ equivocal finding may represent a true negative. On the other hand, the peroxisome proliferator WY-14643, which tested negative in P53$^{+/-}$, yielded positive findings in XPA$^{-/-}$ after only 6 months. Finally, while producing equivocal findings in P53$^{+/-}$, 17-β-estradiol produced an unequivocal positive result in XPA$^{-/-}$/P53$^{+/-}$ in 9 months. Genotoxic rodent noncarcinogens remain to be tested in XPA$^{-/-}$/P53$^{+/-}$. Collectively, these few sets of additional data suggest, but have not yet established, that this bigenic model may retain the high specificity of the P53$^{+/-}$ model to avoid noncarcinogens and indirect carcinogens with pure nongenotoxic modes of action, but appear to have gained additional sensitivity. The positive findings with WY-14643 and with 17-β-estradiol and diethylstilbestrol (DES) in this model suggest that DNA adducts that have been reported with DES (Bhat et al., 1994) and estrogens (Cavalieri et al., 2000; Shimomura et al., 1992), and the clastogenic positive findings reported with WY-14643 (Galloway et al., 2000) may be contributing to the observed tumorigenic activity of these molecules. It is unclear if the extended 9-month protocol duration in the single transgenic knockout P53$^{+/-}$ model would yield similar results.

REGULATORY EXPERIENCE

By the end of 2002, the Food and Drug Administration's Center for Drug Evaluation and Research (CDER) had received about 90 protocols proposing alternative carcinogenicity assay alternatives and had received final results for about two dozen of these assays. These results supplement what has been learned from the ILSI collaborative program and other published data. Issues that are still being evaluated include criteria for selection of the best model, protocol issues for the various assays, and integration of the results of the alternative assays into the overall assessment of carcinogenicity potential.

Two thirds of alternative assay results received by CDER have been for the P53 model. Although all but two of the products studied in the P53$^{+/-}$ assay were considered to be genotoxic, results in the P53$^{+/-}$ assay have been uniformly negative thus far. Positive genotoxic results associated with these compounds were predominately *in vitro* clastogenicity in either Chinese hamster ovary (CHO) cells, Chinese hamster lung (CHL) cells, or human lymphocytes. One product was positive in *Salmonella typhimurium* strain TA 1537. Several products were positive in more than one test in the standard ICH genotoxicity battery. Several were positive in the *in vivo* micronucleus assay, as well as in other assays for mutagenicity or clastogenicity.

Positive results have been seen in traditional 2-year rat carcinogenicity studies for products that were negative in the P53$^{+/-}$ mouse assay. Neoplasms seen in the few 2-year rat carcinogenicity studies that have been completed for products that were negative in the P53$^{+/-}$ mouse assay include hibernomas, urinary bladder carcinomas, enterochromaffin-like cell neoplasms, thyroid neoplasms, renal neoplasms, lymphomas, and testicular neoplasms.

The performance of the positive control for the P53$^{+/-}$ studies, *p*-cresidine, was variable with no clear explanation. Some studies yielded bladder neoplasms in 90%

of treated animals, while others yielded tumors in less than 10%. Of eight complete study data sets comprising 16 study arms (8 male/8 female), 1 study was considered negative, while overall, 3 study arms failed to reach rare tumor criteria. Three study arms just met rare tumor criteria (2 of 15 animals with tumors associated with hyperplasia). On the other hand, in 6 of the 16 study arms, the incidence of bladder tumors exceeded 50%. Additional questions remaining about the P53$^{+/-}$ protocol include the ideal duration of the study, age of animals at study initiation, and associated historical background neoplasm issues.

The Tg.AC assay has primarily been used in CDER to test dermally applied products, but study protocols have been reviewed and approved for products not intended for dermal use. Although 26 Tg.AC protocol proposals have been reviewed by CDER, results from only five studies had been received by the end of 2002. Findings of urogenital tumors following topical exposure in one study were not considered reliably relevant indicators of human tumor risk. With these criteria, three of the five studies were considered positive. Two of these three positive studies had negative results in traditional 2-year rat carcinogenicity assays, and traditional carcinogenicity studies have not been completed for the third product. None of the products was positive in the standard genotoxicity battery; one of the products with negative results in the Tg.AC assay was positive in the Syrian hamster embryo (SHE) cell assay. Product-related skin squamous papillomas occurred in the absence or presence of inflammation, hyperkeratosis, or hyperplasia. When inflammation, hyperkeratosis, or hyperplasia was present, the severity was similar to that for the positive control TPA.

SUMMARY AND CONCLUSIONS

Great progress has been made by investigators worldwide who have contributed vast resources to evaluate these transgenic mouse models and advance the science of carcinogenicity evaluation. Our understanding of these models has evolved and the utility of these models is becoming clearer. Important advances always lead to more questions and even further advances. The results conforming with predicted outcomes together with the unexpected results are challenging the toxicology community to design further important mechanistic research approaches to clarify the underlying early and late appearing molecular signals in these models responsible for the observed tumor outcomes. Further investigation of the patterns of molecular alterations in DNA, RNA, or proteins from mature tumors, coupled with investigations of alterations in these molecules at earlier preneoplastic stages of exposures, is likely to help clarify mechanisms, establish human relevance of rodent tumor findings, and accelerate reduced dependence on 2-year rodent bioassays.

The data are also challenging toxicologists to consider critical study design modifications that could serve to optimize the confidence that is critical for stakeholders to accept and integrate interpretations and conclusions from transgenic model carcinogenicity studies. Protocol refinement issues that could be considered might include (1) the numbers of animals per dosing group to optimize study statistical power, e.g., Morton et al. (2002) have indicated that 25 animals per dosing group is optimal for TgrasH2; (2) study duration, for example, the issue of whether 9 months vs. 6 months may be optimal for the P53$^{+/-}$ model; (3) closely spaced top doses and strong evidence that maximally tolerated doses and optimal dosing schedules have been used; (4) avoiding confounding influences of vehicle components in Tg.AC; (5) carefully defining the maximally tolerated topical skin dosing inflammatory endpoint in the Tg.AC model that will not confound tumorigenicity interpretations; (6) avoiding use of subcutaneous transponder implants in P53$^{+/-}$ and XPA$^{-/-}$/P53$^{+/-}$ mice (Blanchard et al., 1999); (7) addition of an appropriate wild type high dose study arm to assess the contribution of the model's specific genetic modification to tumor outcome; (8) assessing the utility of TgrasH2, P53$^{+/-}$, and XPA$^{-/-}$/P53$^{+/-}$ models for topical routes of application.

Over the past 2 years 25% of the proposed mouse carcinogenicity study protocols that have been received by the FDA's Center for Drug Evaluation and Research's Executive Carcinogenicity Assessment Committee have opted for an alternative model. Data from approximately two dozen completed transgenic mouse alternative assays have been received and evaluated. The value that these assays are adding to the safety assessment process can be categorized as one of the following: (1) to add important information relating to mode of action that will impact on pattern of product use considerations; (2) to specifically address the implications for carcinogenic potential based on genotoxicity findings and provide early information that will impact drug development go/no-go decision-making; (3) to help resolve ambiguities when the adequacy of a 2-year study is questionable and repeating a 2-year study is mutually undesirable; (4) to help resolve ambiguities when a 2-year rat study is adequate but the findings are equivocal; (5) as a rapid early assessment to address genotoxicity study concerns prior to initiation of a clinical trial. To help decide which model will best address regulatory concerns and reduce uncertainties, the model chosen has depended upon knowledge of the drug's mechanisms, anticipated patterns of human use, the specific profile of *in vitro* and *in vivo* battery of genotoxicity studies, and knowledge of the drug's absorption distribution, metabolism, and excretion (ADME) and exposure profiles relative to anticipated human use.

A recent analysis indicates that combined use of alternative transgenic mouse models, when considered together with a 2-year rat assay, would result in no loss of carcinogen detection sensitivity while gaining significant improvement in specificity over the use of the 2-year mouse assay (Pritchard et al., 2002). However, when any of the transgenic models are considered alone, or when several combinations of transgenic mouse models alone are considered, without taking into account the supplemental information provided by the 2-year rat bioassay, several human carcinogens would have been missed. This analysis provides strong support for the 1997 ICH decision reflecting current regulatory practice in FDA's Center for Drug Evaluation and Research, and Center for Biologics Evaluation and Research.

The data of TgrasH2 together with P53$^{+/-}$ presently appear to provide the greatest combined coverage for detecting relevant carcinogens. Data are missing, however, for oxymetholone, TCDD, and 2,4-diaminotoluene in TgrasH2, and estradiol, 2,4-diaminotoluene, glycidol, diethylnitrosamine, and even *p*-cresidine may be worthy of investigation in a 9-month P53$^{+/-}$ assay design. To further evaluate the utility of applications of alternative transgenic models for carcinogenicity testing, more experience with agents that are clastogenic but not mutagenic and are known or strongly suspected to be relevant carcinogens would be very helpful. Results from such investigations may encourage further confidence, utilization, and evolution of short-term alternatives and less reliance on 2-year assay study durations.

REFERENCES

Albert, R., French, J., Maronpot, R., Spalding, J., and Tennant, R. (1996) Mechanism of skin tumorigenesis by contact sensitizers: the effect of the corticosteroid fluocinolone acetonide on inflammation and tumor induction by 2,4-dinitro-1-fluorobenzene in the skin of the Tg.AC (v-Ha-ras) mouse, *Environ. Health Perspect.*, 104, 1062–1068.

Bhat, H.K., Han, X., Gladek, A., and Liehr, J.G. (1994) Regulation of the formation of the major diethylstilbestrol–DNA adduct and some evidence of its structure, *Carcinogenesis*, 15, 2137–2142.

Blanchard, K.T., Barthel, C., French, J.E., Holden, H.E., Moretz, R., Pack, F.D., Tennant, R.W., and Stoll, R.E. (1999) Transponder-induced sarcoma in the heterozygous p53(+/–) mouse, *Toxicol. Pathol.*, 27, 519–527.

Boley, S.E., Anderson, E.E., French, J.E., Donehower, L.A., Walker, D.B., and Recio, L. (2000) Loss of p53 in benzene-induced thymic lymphomas in p53+/– mice: evidence of chromosomal recombination, *Cancer Res.*, 60, 2831–2835.

Boley, S.E., Wong, V.A., French, J.E., and Recio, L. (2002) p53 heterozygosity alters the mRNA expression of p53 target genes in the bone marrow in response to inhaled benzene, *Toxicol. Sci.*, 66, 209–215.

Bolon, B. and Galbreath, E. (2002) Use of genetically engineered mice in drug discovery and development: wielding Occam's razor to prune the product portfolio, *Int. J. Toxicol.*, 21, 55–64.

Cannon, R.E., Spalding, J.W., Trempus, C.S., Szczesniak, C.J., Virgil, K.M., Humble, M.C., and Tennant, R.W. (1997) Kinetics of wound-induced v-Ha-ras transgene expression and papilloma development in transgenic Tg.AC mice, *Mol. Carcinog.*, 20, 108–114.

Cavalieri, E., Frenkel, K., Liehr, J.G., Rogan, E., and Roy, D. (2000) Estrogens as endogenous genotoxic agents — DNA adducts and mutations, *J. Natl. Cancer Inst. Monogr.*, pp. 75–93.

De Vries, A., van Oostrom, C.T.H., Hofhuis, F.M.A., Dortant, P.M., Berg, R.J.W., De Gruijl, F.R., Wester, P.W., Van Kreijl, C.F., Capel, P.J.A., Van Steeg, H., and Verbeek, S.J. (1995) Increased susceptibility to ultraviolet-B and carcinogens of mice lacking the DNA excision repair gene XPA *Nature*, 377, 169–173.

De Vries, A., van Oostrom, C.T.H., Dortant, P.M., Beems, R.B., Van Kreijl, C.F., Capel, P.J.A., and Van Steeg, H. (1997a) Spontaneous liver tumours and benzo[a]pyrene-induced lymphomas in XPA-deficient mice, *Mol. Carcinog.*, 19, 46–53.

De Vries, A., Dolle, M.E., Broekhof, J.L., Muller, J.J., Kroese, E.D., van Kreijl, C.F., Capel, P.J., Vijg, J., and van Steeg, H. (1997b) Induction of DNA adducts and mutations in spleen, liver and lung of XPA-deficient/lac Z transgenic mice after oral treatment with benzo[a]pyrene: correlation with tumour development, *Carcinogenesis*, 18, 2327–2332.

Donehower, L.A., Harvey, M., Slagle, B.L., McArthur, M.J., Montgomery, C.A.J., Butel, J.S., and Bradley, A. (1992) Mice deficient for p53 are developmentally normal but susceptible to spontaneous tumors, *Nature*, 356, 215–221.

Eastin, W.C., Mennear, J.H., Tennant, R.W., Stoll, R.E., Braustetter, D.G., Bucher, J.R., McCullough, B., Binder, R.L., Spalding, J.W., and Mahler, J.F. (2001) Tg.AC genetically altered mouse: assay working group overview of available data, *Toxicol. Pathol.*, 29(Suppl.), 60–80.

Elmquist, W.F. and Miller, D.W. (2001) The use of transgenic mice in pharmacokinetic and pharmacodynamic studies, *J. Pharm. Sci.*, 90, 422–435.

Fearon, E.R. and Vogelstein, B. (1990) A genetic model for colorectal tumorigenesis, *Cell*, 61, 759–767.

French, J., Storer, R.D., and Donehower, L.A. (2001) The nature of the heterozygous Trp53 knockout model for identification of mutagenic carcinogens, *Toxicol. Pathol.*, 29(Suppl.), 24–29.

Galloway, S.M., Johnson, T.E., Armstrong, M.J., and Ashby, J. (2000) The genetic toxicity of the peroxisome proliferator class of rodent hepatocarcinogen, *Mutat. Res.*, 448, 153–158.

Gingrich, J.R., Barrios, R.J., Morton, R.A., Boyce, B.F., DeMayo, F.J., Finegold, M.J., Angelopoulou, R., Rosen, J.M., and Greenberg, N.M. (1996) Metastatic prostate cancer in a transgenic mouse, *Cancer Res.*, 56, 4096–4102.

Gonzalez, F.J. (2002) The peroxisome proliferator-activated receptor alpha (PPARalpha): role in hepatocarcinogenesis, *Mol. Cell Endocrinol.*, 193, 71–79.

Greenblatt, M.S., Bennett, W.P., Hollstein, M., and Harris, C.C. (1994) Mutations in the p53 tumor suppressor gene: clues to cancer etiology and molecular pathogenesis, *Cancer Res.*, 54, 4855–4878.

Greten, F.R., Wagner, M., Weber, C.K., Zechner, U., Adler, G., and Schmid, R.M. (2001) TGF alpha transgenic mice. A model of pancreatic cancer development, *Pancreatology*, 1, 363–368.

Gulezian, D. (1999) Managing intellection property rights for improved access to transgenic technology, *Lab. Animal*, 28, 28–32.

Hamadeh, H.K., Bushel, P.R., Jayadev, S., Martin, K., DiSorbo, O., Sieber, S., Bennett, L., Tennant, R., Stoll, R., Barrett, J.C., Blanchard, K., Paules, R.S., and Afshari, C.A. (2002) Gene expression analysis reveals chemical-specific profiles, *Toxicol. Sci.*, 67, 219–231.

Hansen, L.A. and Tennant, R.W. (1994) Follicular origin of epidermal papillomas in v-Ha-ras transgenic Tg.AC mouse skin, *Proc. Natl. Acad. Sci. U.S.A.*, 91, 7822–7826.

Harris, S., Davis, N.K., Jowett, M.I., Rees, E.S., and Topps, S. (1993) Transgenic animals as tools in drug development, *Agents and Actions*, 38, c57–c58.

Harvey, M., McArthur, M.J., Montgomery, C.A.J., Butel, J.S., Bradley, A., and Donehower, L.A. (1993) Spontaneous and carcinogen-induced tumorigenesis in p53-deficient mice, *Nat. Genet.*, 5, 225–229.

Hollstein, M., Sidransky, D., Vogelstein, B., and Harris, C.C. (1991) p53 mutations in human cancers, *Science*, 253, 49–53.

Honchel, R., Rosenzweig, B., Thompson, K.L., Blanchard, K.T., Furst, S.M., Stoll, R,E,, and Sistare, F.D. (2001) Loss of palindromic symmetry in Tg.AC mice with a nonresponder phenotype, *Mol. Carcinog.*, 30, 99–110.

Hulla, J.E., French, J.E,, and Dunnick, J.K. (2001) Chromosome 11 loss from thymic lymphomas induced in heterozygous Trp53 mice by phenolphthalein, *Toxicol. Sci.*, 60, 264–270.

International Conference on Harmonization, Expert Working Group on Safety (1997) Guidance for Industry SIB Testing for Carcinogenicity of Pharmaceuticals, www.fda.gov/cder/guidance/index.htm.

Jacks, T., Remington, L., Williams, B.O., Schmitt, E.M., Halachmi, S., Bronson, R.T., and Weinberg, R.A. (1994) Tumor spectrum analysis in p53-mutant mice, *Curr. Biol.*, 4, 1–7.

Johnson, F.M. (1999) Carcinogenic chemical-response "fingerprint" for male F344 rats exposed to a series of 195 chemicals: implications for predicting carcinogens with transgenic models, *Environ. Mol. Mutagenesis*, 34, 234–245.

Kemp, C.J., Donehower, L.A., Bradley, A., and Balmain, A. (1993) Reduction of p53 gene dosage does not increase initiation or promotion but enhances malignant progression of chemically induced skin tumors, *Cell*, 5, 813–822.

Kraemer, K.H., Lee, M.M., and Scotto, J. (1984) DNA repair protects against cutaneous and internal neoplasia: evidence from xeroderma pigmentosum, *Carcinogenesis*, 5, 511–514.

Lane, D.P. (1992) Cancer: p53, guardian of the genome, *Nature*, 358, 15–16.

Leder, A., Kuo, A., Cardiff, R., Sinn, E., and Leder, P. (1990) v-Ha-ras transgene abrogates the initiation step in mouse skin tumorigenesis: effects of phorbol esters and retinoic acid, *Proc. Natl. Acad. Sci. U.S.A.*, 87, 9178–9182.

Leder, A., Lebel, M., Zhou, F., Fontaine, K., Bishop, A., and Leder, P. (2002) Genetic interaction between the unstable v-Ha-RAS transgene (Tg.AC) and the murine Werner syndrome gene: transgene instability and tumorigenesis, *Oncogene*, 21, 6657–6668.

Livingston, J.N. (1999) Genetically engineered mice in drug development, *J. Internal Med.*, 245, 627–635.

MacDonald, J.S., Lankas, G.R., and Morrissey, R.E. (1994) Toxicokinetic and mechanistic considerations in the interpretation of the rodent bioassay, *Toxicol. Pathol.*, 22, 124–140.

Marshall, E. (2002) DuPont ups ante on use of Harvard's Oncomouse, *Science*, 296, 1212–1213.

Maruyama, C., Tomisawa, M., Wakana, S., Yamazaki, H., Kijima, H., Suemizu, H., Ohnishi, Y., Urano, K., Hioki, K., Usui, T., Nakamura, M., Tsuchida, T., Mitsumori, K., Nomura, T., Tamaoki, N., and Ueyama, Y. (2001) Overexpression of human H-ras transgene is responsible for tumors induced by chemical carcinogens in mice, *Oncol. Rep.*, 8, 233–237.

Megosh, L., Gilmour, S.K., Rosson, D., Soler, A.P., Blessing, M., Sawicki, J.A., and O'Brien, T.G. (1995) Increased frequency of spontaneous skin tumors in transgenic mice which overexpress ornithine decarboxylase, *Cancer Res.*, 55, 4205–4209.

Merlino, G.T. (1991) Transgenic animals in biomedical research, *FASEB J.*, 5, 2996–3001.

Morris, S.M. (2002) A role for p53 in the frequency and mechanism of mutation, *Mutat. Res.*, 511, 45–62.

Morton, D., Alden, C.L., Roth, A.J., and Usui, T. (2002) The TgrasH2 mouse in cancer hazard identification, *Toxicol. Pathol.*, 30, 75–79.

Moser, G.J., Trempus, C.S., Mahler, J.F., Ward, S.M., Wilson, R., M. Streicker, M., Tice, R.R., Goldsworthy, T.L., and Tennant, R.W. (2001) Topical exposure of v-Ha-ras Tg.AC mice to the insecticide rotenone, *Toxicologist*, 60, 278.

Nakane, H., Takeuchi, S., Yuba, S., Saijo, M., Nakatsu, Y., Murai, H., Nakatsuru, Y., Ishikawa, T., Hirota, S., Kitamura, Y., Kato, Y., Tsunoda, Y., Miyauchi, H., Horio, T., Tokunaga, T., Matsunaga, T., Nikaido, O., Nishimune, Y., Okada, Y., and Tanaka, K. (1995) High incidence of ultraviolet-B or chemical-carcinogen-induced skin tumors in mice lacking the xeroderma pigmentosum group A gene, *Nature*, 377, 165–168.

Nylander-French, L.A. and French, J.E. (1998) Tripropylene glycol diacrylate but not ethyl acrylate induces skin tumors in a twenty-week short-term tumorigenesis study in Tg.AC (v-Ha-ras) mice, *Toxicol. Pathol.*, 26, 476–483.

Palmiter, R.D. and Brinster, R.L. (1986) Germ-line transformation of mice, *Ann. Rev. Genet.*, 20, 465–499.

Peters, J.M., Cattley, R.C., and Gonzalez, F.J. (1997) Role of PPAR alpha in the mechanism of action of the nongenotoxic carcinogen and peroxisome proliferator Wy-14,643, *Carcinogenesis*, 18, 2029–2033.

Pritchard, J.B., French, J.E., Davis, B.J., and Haseman, J.K. (2002) Transgenic models: their role in carcinogen identification, *Environ. Health Perspect.*, doi: 10.12.89/ehp. 5778 (available at http://dx.doi.org).

Recio, L., Boley, S., Everitt, J., James, R.A., Janszen, D., Healy, L., Roberts, K., Walker, D., Pluta, L., and French, J.E. (2000) Cancer bioassay and genotoxicity of inhaled benzene in P53$^{+/-}$ and C57Bl6 mice, *Toxicologist,* 54, 222.

Robinson, D.E. and MacDonald, J.S. (2001) Background and framework for ILSI's collaborative evaluation program on alternative models for carcinogenicity assessment, *Toxicol. Pathol.*, 29(Suppl.),13–19.

Salleh, M.N., Caldwell, J., and Carmichael, P.L. (2003) A comparison of gene expression changes in response to diethylstilbestrol treatment in wild-type and p53(+/–) hemizygous knockout mice using focussed arrays, *Toxicology*, 185, 49–57.

Sands, A.T., Abuin, A., Sanchez, A., Conti, C.J., and Bradley, A. (1995) High susceptibility to ultraviolet-induced carcinogenesis in mice lacking XPC, *Nature*, 377, 162–165.

Serrano, M., Lee, H., Chin, L., Cordon-Cardo, C., Beach, D., and DePinho, R.A. (1996) Role of the INK4a locus in tumor suppression and cell mortality, *Cell*, 85, 27–37.

Shimomura, M., Higashi, S., and Mizumoto, R. (1992) ^{32}P-postlabeling analysis of DNA adducts in rats during estrogen-induced hepatocarcinogenesis and effect of tamoxifen on DNA adduct level, *Jpn. J. Cancer Res.*, 83, 438–444.

Sistare, F.D., Thompson, K.L., Honchel, R., and DeGeorge, J. (2002) Evaluation of the Tg.AC transgenic mouse assay for testing the human carcinogenic potential of pharmaceuticals — practical pointers, mechanistic clues, and new questions, *Int. J. Toxicol.*, 21, 65–79.

Stoll, R.E., Furst, S.M., Stoltz, J.H., Lilly, P.D., and Mennear, J.H. (2001) Dermal carcinogenicity in transgenic mice: effect of vehicle on responsiveness of hemizygous Tg.AC mice to phorbol 12-myristate 13-acetate (TPA), *Toxicol. Pathol.*, 29, 535–540.

Storer, R.D., French, J.E., Haseman, J., Hajian, G., LeGrand, E.K., Long, G.G., Mixson, L.A., Ochoa, R., Sargartz, J.E., and Sopor, K.A. (2001) P53$^{+/-}$ hemizygous knockout mouse: overview of available data, *Toxicol. Pathol.*, 29(Suppl.), 30–50.

Suemizu, H., Muguruma, K., Maruyama, C., Tomisawa, M., Kimura, M., Hioki, K., Shimozawa, N., Ohnishi, Y., Tamaoki, N., and Nomura, T. (2002) Transgene stability and features of rasH2 mice as an animal model for short-term carcinogenicity testing, *Mol. Carcinog.*, 34, 1–9.

Swing, S. (2001) Intellectual property issues involving transgenic rodent models, *Am. Genomic/Proteomic Technol.*, 1, 25–26.

Tamaoki, N. (2001) The rasH2 transgenic mouse: nature of the model and mechanistic studies on tumorigenesis, *Toxicol. Pathol.*, 29(Suppl.), 81–89.

Tennant, R.W., Stasiewicz, S., Eastin, W.C., Mennear, J.H., and Spalding, J.W., (2001) The Tg.AC (v-Ha-ras) transgenic mouse: nature of the model, *Toxicol. Pathol.*, 29(Suppl.), 51–59.

Thompson, K., Rosenzweig, B., and Sistare, F. (1998) An evaluation of the hemizygous transgenic Tg.AC mouse for carcinogenicity testing of pharmaceuticals. II. A genotypic marker that predicts tumorigenic responsiveness, *Toxicol. Pathol.*, 26, 548–555.

Thompson, K.L., Rosenzweig, B.A., Honchel, R., Cannon, R.E., Blanchard, K.T., Stoll, R.E., and Sistare, F.D. (2001) Loss of critical palindromic transgene promoter sequence in chemically induced Tg.AC mouse skin papillomas expressing transgene-derived mRNA, *Mol. Carcinog.*, 32, 176–186.

Usui, T., Mutai, M., Hisada, S., Takoaka, M., Soper, K.A., McCullough, B., and Alden, C. (2001) CB6F1-rasH2 mouse: overview of available data, *Toxicol. Pathol.*, 29(Suppl.), 90–108.

Van Dyke, T. and Jacks, T. (2002) Cancer modeling in the modern era: progress and challenges, *Cell*, 108, 135–144.

Van Kreijl, C.F., McAnulty, P.A., Beems, R.B., Vynckier, A., van Steeg, H., Frausson-Steen, R., Alden, C.L., Forster, R., van der Laan, J.W., and Vandenberghe, J. (2001) Xpa and Xpa/p53$^{+/-}$ knockout mice: overview of available data, *Toxicol. Pathol.*, 29(Suppl.), 117–127.

Van Lohuizen, M., Verbeek, S., Krimpenfort, P., Domen, J., Saris, C., Radaszkiewiczs, T., and Berns, A. (1989) Predisposition to lymphomagenesis in pim-1 transgenic mice: cooperation with c-myc and N-myc in murine leukemia virus-induced tumors, *Cell*, 56, 673–682.

Van Oostrom, C.T., Boeve, M., van Den Berg, J., de Vries, A., Dolle, M.E., Beems, R.B., van Kreijl, C.F., Vijg, J., and van Steeg, H. (1999) Effect of heterozygous loss of p53 on benzo[a]pyrene-induced mutations and tumors in DNA repair-deficient XPA mice, *Environ. Mol. Mutagen.*, 34, 124–130.

Van Steeg, H. (2001) The role of nucleotide excision repair and loss of p53 in mutagenesis and carcinogenesis, *Toxicol. Lett.*, 120, 209–19.

Van Steeg, H., de Vries, A., van Oostrom, C.T., van Benthem, J., and Beems, R.B., van Kreijl, C.F. (2001) DNA repair-deficient Xpa and Xpa/p53$^{+/-}$ knock-out mice: nature of the models, *Toxicol. Pathol.*, 29(Suppl.), 109–116.

Venkatachalam, S., Tyner, S.D., Pickering, C.R., Boley, S., Recio, L., French, J.E., and Donehower, L.A. (2001) Is p53 haplo insufficient for tumor suppression? Implications for the p53+/– mouse model in carcinogenicity testing, *Toxicol. Pathol.*, 29(Suppl.), 147–154.

Ward, J.M., Peters, J.M., Perella, C.M., and Gonzalez, F.J. (1998) Receptor and nonreceptor-mediated organ-specific toxicity of di(2-ethylhexyl)phthalate (DEHP) in peroxisome proliferator-activated receptor alpha-null mice, *Toxicol. Pathol.*, 26, 240–246.

CHAPTER 36

Changes in Gene Expression after Exposure to Organophosphorus (OP) Agents

Jennifer W. Sekowski, Kevin P. O'Connell, Akbar S. Khan, James J. Valdes, Maryanne Vahey, Martin Nau, Maha Khalil, and Mohyee E. Eldefrawi

CONTENTS

INTRODUCTION

Soldiers operating in a chemical or biological warfare environment face the possibility of exposure resulting in incapacitating symptoms or death. The mechanisms by which chemical weapons cause acute injury are well understood, thanks to an exhaustive study of these compounds during much of the 20th century. However, personnel involved in decontaminating equipment or destroying chemical weapons, as well as personnel on the periphery of an attack, may also face exposure at low levels that may not induce obvious immediate damage. In addition, soldiers face a toxicological risk from exposure to toxic industrial chemicals (TICs) and toxic industrial materials (TIMs) during deployment in areas of the world where environmental regulations are lacking, and such compounds may also be used as weapons of opportunity against U.S. personnel and the civilian population. Scientists have been assessing the effects of chemical weapons, TICs, and TIMs on living systems for nearly 80 years. For most of that time, toxicology research both inside and outside the Army has consisted of chemical exposures to animals followed by observations of a limited number of physiological changes, including death. This work has provided a unique and valuable body of immediate, practical solutions to battlefield toxicological problems: decontamination, personal protection, and antidotes for acute exposures. However, exposure to chemical weapons, TICs, or TIMs that does not result in immediate injury may yet predispose soldiers to ailments that arise much later and whose origins are difficult to determine. Traditional toxicological methods lack the power to determine the mechanisms of action of toxic agents at the most fundamental level, that is, how the very genes that determine how we function respond to toxic insults, and how these changes become manifest as pathology over time.

This study investigates gene expression changes caused by exposure to a compound that is directly relevant to military personnel for two important reasons. Chlorpyrifos (CPF; commercially sold under the names Lorsban or Dursban) is one of the most commonly used OP insecticides in the agricultural industry outside of the U.S. It has been banned for agricultural and home use in the U.S., but it remains in use in many other parts of the world. As such, military personnel encounter it during the course of military activity in agricultural areas. Second, as an OP compound, it may mirror the molecular mechanism of action of low-level exposures of OP chemical warfare agents such as GB (Sarin) and GD (Soman). In mammals, CPF and other OP compounds exert their primary toxic effect by inhibiting the activity of acetyl- and butylcholinesterase (AchE and BChE). After secondary metabolism in the liver, the OP compound is converted into its oxon metabolite (e.g., CPF oxon), which binds irreversibly to AChE and BChE (Whitney et al., 1995). This action of both CPF and CPF oxon has the effect of increasing the available concentration of the neurotransmitter acetylcholine (ACh) in the synapse and thereby inducing a host of cholinergic hyperstimulatory effects.

There is significant evidence in the literature, however, to suggest that OP compounds also exert a range of important, but subtler, noncholinergic effects on the body (Song et al., 1997; Bagchi et al., 1997; Lieberman et al., 1998; Crumpton et al., 2000). Such molecular and subcellular effects disrupt the normal cellular metabolism and have the potential to create long-term damage to the body (Song et al., 1997). The processes whereby signals are translated from the cell surface to intracellular targets are sensitive to perturbation by chlorpyrifos (Huff et al., 1994; Ward and Mundy, 1996; Song et al., 1997). These complex chemical pathways influence many other factors that trigger the regulation of the expression of genes, for example. The regulation of the production of gene products also fundamentally influences the health and metabolic status of the cell. The inappropriate induction or down-regulation of the expression of specific genes can lead to the over or under production of a critical polypeptide or protein that ultimately leads to cell injury, disease, or death. By gaining insight into the patterns of altered gene expression in response to a particular toxicant, it is possible to begin building a database of exposure "signatures." These signatures of exposure can be used in monitoring potentially exposed personnel, monitoring biomass from the environment, and forensic analyses. Furthermore, the discovery of the identity and function of these altered genes can yield important clues into the molecular mechanism of toxicity and point to potential targets for preventative and therapeutic intervention.

The advent of DNA microarrays facilitates these types of analyses. With gene arrays it is possible to measure the expression level of hundreds to thousands of genes simultaneously. Briefly, the mRNA (genetic transcript or RNA copy of a gene) is extracted from the exposed and control samples, enzymatically converted to cDNA, labeled with a fluorescent tag, and hybridized to the microarray. After washing the chip, only those mRNA transcripts for which there is a complementary sequence (a gene) on the chip will remain. The chip reader apparatus then detects the fluorescent signal from each gene spot. Through bioinformatics software, the quantitated fluorescent data can be normalized to the control and patterns of gene expression can be compared. From the identity of genes whose expression has been altered, we can begin to infer the effects of OP agents on cells at the molecular level and the identity and function of those altered genes can be determined (Figure 36.1).

METHODS

Dosing Regimen

Sprague-Dawley rats were chosen as a model system because of the wealth of traditional toxicological data available on that species and because of the ready availability of commercial DNA microarrays displaying rat gene sequences. CPF was administered intraperitoneally (IP) to three 200-g male rats at an LD_{30} dose (125 mg/kg body weight). Three additional rats (controls) received HEPES-buffered saline (HBS). Rats given CPF or HBS exhibited no obvious symptoms such as miosis or tremors at any time during the experiment.

Collection of Tissue

To examine the effect of the treatment on the gene expression in the central nervous system and in the organ that carries out the most detoxification, the brain

Figure 36.1 Rat toxicology U34 gene array. This gene expression display was created by GeneSpring® (Silicon Genetics) gene array analysis software from our data (rat brain RNA 1 h postexposure to CPF) read from an Affymetrix Rat Toxicology U34 GeneChip®. In the original display (depicted in gray tones here), red and purple blocks represented up-regulated genes and the blue represented down-regulated genes. Gray blocks represented genes whose expression is essentially the same as in the control animal.

and the liver of one rat per treatment were obtained at periods of 1, 4, and 24 hr postexposure. Each brain and liver was immediately frozen in liquid nitrogen and stored at –80°C until the RNA extraction.

Preparation of Total RNA and mRNA

Briefly, the brain and liver tissue samples (0.5 mg liver and 0.6 to 0.9 mg whole brain) were homogenized in 5 ml volumes of TRIzol reagent (Gibco BRL Life Technologies) using a polytron, and the homogenate was immediately placed on ice. The total RNA extraction and precipitation steps were carried out essentially as described by Chomczynski and Sacchi (1987). In order to increase the level of messenger RNA available to the GeneChip from the liver samples, liver mRNA was purified from the total RNA using Ambion's Poly(A)Pure™ mRNA isolation kit.

Synthesis of Biotin-Labeled cRNA and Target Preparation

The *in vitro* synthesis and purification of biotin-labeled antisense cRNA (target) was carried out according to Affymetrix instructions, with modifications as described in Vahey et al. (2000). The biotin-labeled cRNA was fragmented using 5× fragmentation buffer (200 m*M* Tris-acetate, pH 8.1; 500 m*M* KOAc; 150 m*M* MgOAc) as described in Nau et al. (2000).

Hybridization, Staining, and Washing of DNA Microarray

The hybridization, washing, and staining steps were carried out according to Affymetrix instructions and as described in Nau et al. (2000).

Probe Array Scan

The Affymetrix Gene Chips® were scanned according to the protocol described in Nau et al. (2000).

Analysis of DNA Microarray Data

Analysis of the data obtained was performed using GeneSpring® array analysis software.

Measurement of Butylcholinesterase (BChE) Activity

The BChE activity in the blood of exposed and control rats (drawn at 1, 4, and 24 hr postexposure) was measured using the Ellman procedure as described by Ellman et al. (1961).

RESULTS

Selection of Genes to Measure

In order to most efficiently focus our "first pass" search for altered gene expression in the rat, we chose two high-quality commercially available DNA microarrays. The Rat Neurobiology U34 GeneChip contains a subset of the total rat genome, containing the sequences of over 1200 genes and expressed sequence tags (ESTs) known to be expressed in a variety of neuronal cell types. ESTs are DNA sequences that are expressed by an organism for which there is no ascribed function or gene name. The Rat Toxicology U34 GeneChip is also a subset of the total rat genome. This array contains sequences of over 850 genes and ESTs known to play a role in the mammalian response to toxic compounds.

Analysis of Gene Expression Patterns

In order to more objectively classify the up- and down-regulation of gene expression of time, we grouped the genes into the six most common patterns observed in the data. Nearly all of the gene expression data from the DNA microarrays fit into one of six categories (Figure 36.2).

Quantification of Gene Expression Patterns in the Brain

In order to quantify the types of alterations in gene expression induced by exposure to CPF, we assigned nearly all of the genes for which we had sufficient data to one of the six most common patterns observed in the data. The analysis of the brain gene expression levels in the CPF exposed rat using the Rat Neurobiology U34 GeneChip reveals that 411 genes and ESTs (33%) out of the 1200 genes and ESTs on the chip fall into the A pattern, 280 genes and ESTs (23%) fall into the B pattern, 155 genes and ESTs (13%) fit into the C pattern, 79 genes and ESTs (7%) fit into the D pattern, 83 genes and ESTs (7%) fit into the E pattern, and 50 genes and ESTs (4%) fit into the F pattern. The remaining 12% of genes and ESTs have been excluded from analysis due to incomplete data or due to outlier status of one or more of the data points.

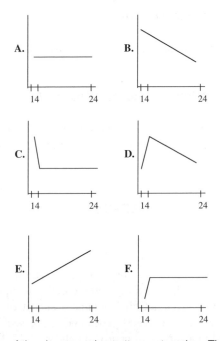

Figure 36.2 Illustrations of the six expression pattern categories. The numerals under the x-axis represent hours after CPF exposure. Y-axis represents relative gene expression level. (A) No alteration of gene expression; (B) initial up-regulation, then return to normal by 24 h; (C) initial up-regulation, then return to normal by 4 h; (D) delayed up-regulation by 4 h, then return to normal by 24 h; (E) delayed up-regulation by 24 h; (F) rapid down-regulation, then return to normal by 4 h.

The rat brain genes analysis performed using the Rat Toxicology U34 Gene Chip reveal that 293 genes and ESTs (34%) of the total 850 genes and ESTs on the chip fall into the A pattern, 43 genes and ESTs (5%) fall into the B pattern, 97 genes and ESTs (11%) fit into the C pattern, 56 genes and ESTs (7%) fit into the D pattern, 83 genes and ESTs (10%) fall into the E pattern, and 82 genes and ESTs (10%) fall into the F pattern. The remaining 23% of genes and ESTs on the chip have been excluded from analysis due to incomplete data on the chip or due to the outlier status of one or more of the data points.

Quantification of Gene Expression Patterns in the Liver

Gene expression levels in the exposed rats' livers were measured on the Rat Toxicology U34 GeneChip and analyzed using the GeneSpring software. It was revealed that 282 (33%) of the genes were expressed at levels similar to those detected in the control animals (pattern A). Of the remaining genes, 76 (9%) fit into the B pattern, 41 (5%) fit into the C pattern, 119 (14%) into the D pattern, 52 (6%) fit into the E pattern, and 38 (4%) fit into the F pattern. As was found during the brain gene expression analysis on the toxicology gene chip, a significant number of liver genes (29%) also did not have a complete set of data, due to missing and outlier data points detected on the Gene Chip (Figures 36.3 and 36.4).

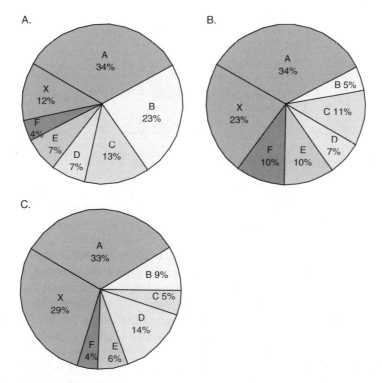

Figure 36.3 The relative percentages of the six patterns of gene expression detected in the CPF-exposed rats.

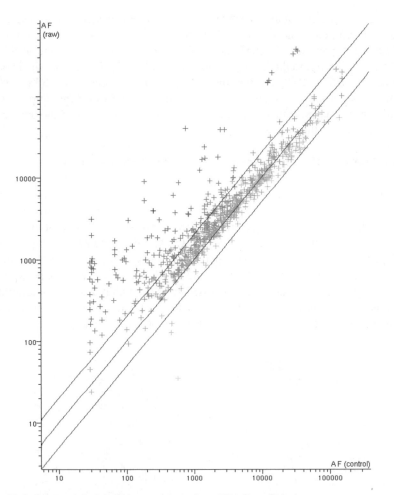

Figure 36.4 Scatterplot of data from rat toxicology U34 GeneChip.

Identification of Up-Regulated Genes Involved in Key Cellular Functions and Biochemical Pathways

In order to begin to link the altered genes to cellular functions and biochemical pathways, we grouped the induced genes (expression patterns B–E) into functional classes. To date, we have identified three such functional classes of genes. The first group is involved with phosphorylation events. Included in this group are genes coding for extracellular signal related kinase 2 (ERK2), mitogen-activated protein (MAP) kinase, and protein kinase C (PKC). The second functional group includes genes coding for neurotransmitter receptors, transporters, and their subunits. Gene products in this group include the glutamate/aspartate transporter (GLAST), two subunits of the GABA-A and GABA-B receptors, and the D1 Dopamine receptor protein. The third grouping includes several genes involved in the metabolism and detoxification of compounds. These include cytochrome P450 and cytochrome b5.

Identification of Down-Regulated Genes Involved in Key Cellular Functions and Biochemical Pathways

We also separated the down-regulated genes into rough functional classes. To date, we have identified two functional classes of genes down-regulated as a result of CPF exposure. The first class includes several genes that code for enzymes important in metabolism and detoxification. In this class are cytochrome p450 ISF/BNF, cytochrome p450 2B15, cytochrome p450 4F6, nitric oxide synthase, plasma glutathione peroxidase, liver arginase, aldose reductase, and monoamine oxidase. The second class of down-regulated genes contributes to the protection, development, and regeneration of the nervous system and includes brain-1 (BRN-1) and brain-derived neurotrophic factor (BDNF).

Measurement of BChE Activity in Blood of CPF-Exposed Rats

In order to correlate our gene expression data with a known metric of OP exposure, we analyzed the BChE activity from the OP-exposed and control rats. BChE activity of the blood from rats exposed to CPF demonstrates a predicted decrease in activity as a function of postexposure time. At the 1 hr postexposure time the BChE activity was decreased by 17% (±0.25%), by 4 hr the BChE activity decreased by 36% (±0.25%), and by 24 hr the activity decreased by 64% (±0.25%) (Figure 36.5).

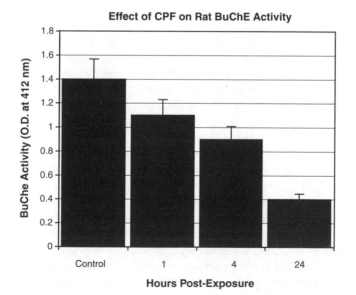

Figure 36.5 *In vivo* effects of CPF on BuChE activity.

DISCUSSION

Since the description of Gulf War syndrome, there has been increased interest in the effects of subacute and low-level exposure to chemical agents, including OP compounds. While the acute and overt effects of OP agent toxicity have been extensively studied, the subtle and molecular level alterations that occur in response to these agents are not well understood. Agent-induced damage and alterations occurring at the molecular level have been implicated in the etiology of injury and disease that may present itself weeks, months, and even years after the initial toxicant exposure (NRC, 1997; Jamal, 1998; McDiarmid et al., 2000). This study indicates that exposure to the OP insecticide, chlorpyrifos, may cause significant alterations in the expression of many genes, and that induction of several of these genes persist to (and presumably beyond) 24 hr postexposure. Furthermore, this observation was made in exposed animals presenting no overt physical symptoms.

Gene expression analysis using DNA microarrays has permitted the identification of six chief patterns of gene expression in the rat model exposed to CPF. We have begun to investigate the connection of the identified genes' critical cellular functions and involvement in key biochemical pathways. Three main functional classes describe the majority of the induced (by the 4 hr postexposure time point) genes. Interestingly, within the first functional grouping we see in the expression of several genes those products have been linked to exposure to pesticides. Within the first group of genes are those that code for products that participate in phosphorylation-related events. ERK2 appears to be up-regulated in response to CPF exposure. ERK2 and other MAP kinases have been shown to have enhanced activity in cells exposed to the organochlorine insecticide heptachlor and are also postulated to play important roles in the alteration of many cellular signal cascades (Chuang and Chuang, 1998). Phosphokinase C (PKC), whose expression also appears to be induced by CPF, has been shown to mediate the oxidative stress effects of CPF in the brains and livers of exposed animals (Bagchi et al., 1997). Overall, these and other kinases participate in altering the activity of a wide variety of signal transduction pathways. Further investigation into the mechanisms underlying the increased expression and role of kinases in the toxicity of CPF is necessary.

The second group of induced genes contains those that participate in forming neuronal transporters and receptors. For example, the gene product of the GLAST gene, the glutamate-aspartate transporter, has been reported to be important in maintaining homeostasis of neurotransmitter concentration in the synapse (Storck et al., 1992). The amino acids glutamate and aspartate are both potent excitatory molecules found in high concentrations in diverse regions of the brain (Cotman et al., 1994). Thus, induction of GLAST expression may serve to increase the reuptake of the excitatory amino acids in the synapses.

The last functional group of induced genes includes those that code for metabolic and detoxification enzymes. Induction of genes such as cytochrome b5 and other p450 isoforms is most likely a general detoxification response to the presence of the OP compound. The same response could have been elicited by any of several other toxicants. Cytochrome b5 is suggested to have a role in reactive oxygen species production and programmed cell death (apoptosis) via modulation of microsomal monooxygenase (Katsutani et al., 2000; Nakamura et al., 2000; Davydov, 2001).

The genes identified as down-regulated (i.e., expression pattern F in Figure 36.2) in response to CPF have been divided into several functional classes as well. The largest contains genes that code for polypeptides that participate directly in toxicant metabolism and detoxification. Specifically, these include genes that code for p450 ISF/BNF, cytochrome 2B15, cytochrome 4F6, nitric oxide synthase (NOS), plasma glutathione peroxidase (GSHPx), liver arginase, aldose reductase, and monoamine oxidase (MAO). p450 ISF/BNF, for example, has been shown to be important in the detoxification reaction of furylfuramide (a peroxisome proliferator) in the liver microsomes of rat and human (Shimada et al., 1990). This suggests that a decrease in the expression of the protein could lead to a delayed clearance of the compound from the body and increased toxicity. Cytochrome 2B15 is a member of the large heterogeneous family of uridine diphosphate glucuronyltransferases (UDP-glucuronyltransferases). The glucuronylation reaction (phase II conjugation) mediated by this enzyme converts its substrate to a water-soluble glucuronide conjugate suitable for elimination by urine or bile. While the main endogenous function of cytochrome 2B15 is to glucuronylate steroids, it also has a high affinity for morphine, phenobarbitol, and a few other xenobiotics (Turgeon et al., 2001). A decreased expression of this enzyme could be the result of interrupted cell signaling and/or transcription factor activity or could be due to a feedback inhibition in response to a decrease in available substrate. Overall, reduced availability of the cytochrome 2B15 could lead to delayed clearance and increased toxicity of its substrates in the body. More research is required to determine what role this enzyme plays in the metabolism of organophosphate compounds.

CYP4F6 is a member of the large cytochrome p450 family of metabolic enzymes and is expressed in both brain and liver (Kawashima and Strobel, 1995). Like all of the cytochrome p450 family members, CYP4F6 is involved in biotransformation of drugs and toxicants. It is usually induced in response to exposure to drugs and toxicants in order to carry out a hydroxylation reaction. However, inhibition of expression in response to toxicant exposure has also been reported. For example, cDNA expression of CYP4F6 is decreased in the presence of clofibrate, a peroxisome proliferator (Kawashima et al., 1997). Since it appears that CPF also causes an inhibition of CYP4F6 expression, reduction in available CYP4F6 may lead to prolonged availability of CPF in the body and increased toxicity of CPF and other substrates. More research is necessary to determine the role CYP4F6 plays in the metabolism and toxicity of CPF and other OP compounds.

Plasma glutathione peroxidase (hpGSH-Px) is a selenocysteine-containing protein expressed in a variety of tissues including brain and liver. It plays a complementary role with selenoprotein P in antioxidant defense. Specifically, it helps reduce lipid hydroperoxides and plasma hydrogen peroxide concentrations. Thus, a decrease in pGSH-Px could lead to an overall increase in reactive oxygen species and the many forms of cellular and tissue damage caused by those reactive molecules.

Nitric oxide synthase (NOS) is widely recognized as an important regulator of vascular and inflammatory responses (Snyder and Dawson, 1994). Constitutively expressed in neurons, capillary endothelial cells, and macrophages, reports show that NOS is involved in such diverse functions as long-term potentiation, glutamate (NMDA)-mediated neurotoxicity, guanylyl cyclase activation, and neurotransmitter release and reuptake (Bloom, 1994). The constitutive induction of NOS cDNA is subject to a variety of feedback mechanisms including kinases and NO itself. To date, it is not known by which mechanism(s) CPF exposure decreases NOS gene transcription.

Liver arginase appears to serve multiple metabolic and regulatory functions. Unlike the type II arginase produced by monocytes, liver arginase (type I) is produced solely in hepatic tissue. Its main function is to metabolize L-arginine to L-ornithine and urea. In addition to its role in urea production, it also catalyzes the production of nitric oxide radicals (NO-). Its role in NO- synthesis, and the fact that it is found in high quantities in ischemic and diseased liver tissue, have lead to the conclusion that liver arginase plays a key role in wound healing and cell repair (Waddington and Cattell, 2000; Ikemoto et al., 2001). Liver arginase expression is regulated by cytokines, substrate competition, and the products of NO- metabolism (Waddington and Cattell, 2000). Since liver arginase and NOS expression are both regulated by this set of intercellular signals, it is likely their reduced expression is the result of the same CPF-induced mechanism. The observed reduction in the expression of liver arginase could lead to increased susceptibility to tissue damage and reduced ability to carry out cellular repair.

Aldose reductase is a broad specificity aldo-ketoreductase. It is expressed at different levels in individuals and may predispose those with reduced levels to increased risk of toxicity of certain drugs and toxicants. It follows that the observed decrease in aldose reductase expression associated with CPF exposure could lead to decreased clearance and increased toxicity of certain types of CPF and other toxicants.

Monoamine oxidase (MAO) is the chief degradative enzyme for the neurotransmitters serotonin (5-HT), epinephrine (E), norepinephrine (NE), and dopamine (DA). A decrease in the availability of MAO leads to a decrease in the degradation (and removal) of these neurochemicals from the synapses in the brain (and in the peripheral nervous system). The concomitant increase in the availability of these neurochemicals leads to a host of altered brain functions caused by the disrupted neurochemical homeostasis. A myriad of functions are affected by the concentration of the neuromodulator and neurotransmitter 5-HT, including sensory perception, sleep, cognition, pain perception, mood, appetite, sexual behavior, hormone secretion, and temperature regulation. Epinephrine (adrenaline), the chief agonist of both α and β adrenergic receptors, has, as such, diverse effects on its target organs. The main affected target organ systems are the vascular and respiratory systems and the smooth and skeletal muscle. Adrenaline is one of the chief effector molecules of the sympathetic ("fight or flight") nervous system reaction. Its action results in increased blood pressure, elevated heart rate, constricted cutaneous capillaries, dilated bronchi, relaxed gastrointestinal smooth muscle, and increased glucose metabolism. Without the normal degradative reaction mediated by MAO, an overabundance of epinephrine may result in restlessness, anxiety, tenseness, tremors, weakness, throbbing headache, dizziness, and pallor. Norepinephrine (NE) is the chemical mediator released by mammalian postglanglionic adrenergic nerves, and it has most of the same properties as epinephrine. As such, an overavailability would lead to many of the same symptoms described for epinephrine. It differs only in that it has little effect on cerebral and skeletal muscle blood flow and little to no effect on overall metabolism. Dopamine (DA), the immediate precursor of NE and epinephrine, is a central neurotransmitter most directly involved with the regulation of movement. Inhibition of its degradation and an increase in its availability in the brain leads to a variety of effects including headaches, tremors, and even seizures.

A decrease in available MAO in humans may have the same overall effect as MAO inhibitors (i.e., phenelzine (Nardil); clorgyline, a MAO-A inhibitor for major depression; and selegiline (Eldepryl), a MAO-B inhibitor (MAO-BI) for Parkinson's disease). The antidepressant effect in clinically depressed individuals is generally assumed to be due to the overall increase in the availability of one or more monoamines in the central nervous system (CNS), although this assumption has been difficult to demonstrate. Although MAO inhibition may have a mood-elevating effect on otherwise normal (nonclinically depressed) individuals, the stimulant effects could possibly lead to restlessness, sleeplessness, and anxiety. A second functional group of down-regulated genes includes those that produce neuroprotective and neurotrophic factors. For example, brain derived neurotrophic factor (BDNF) is known to play a critical neuroprotective role in the developing and adult brain in response to hypoxia–ischemia and other neurotoxic brain injuries (Hyman et al., 1991; Beck et al., 1992; Kokaia et al., 1996; Han et al., 2000). Mechanistically, it appears that the BDNF is dependent on the phospatidylinositol 3-kinase (PI-3K)–MAPK (ERK1 and ERK2) pathway to mediate its neuroprotective effects. It appears that BDNF decreases the activity of caspase–3, a protein involved in promoting programmed cell death (apoptosis) (Han et al, 2000). Thus, BDNF appears to play a direct role in preventing apoptotic cell death in response to a toxic injury. The observed decrease in available BDNF mRNA may provide insight into a neuronal environment that is more vulnerable to apoptosis and other permanent neuronal and cognitive damage as a result of OP intoxication.

Another down-regulated gene, brain-1 (BRN-1), has also been reported to be important for the development and regeneration of the CNS, PNS, and glial cells (Josephson et al, 1998). Decreased expression of BRN-1 protein may contribute to longer term neurological damage due to the lack of this normal regenerative and repair mechanism. Decreased BRN-1 could also greatly interfere with developmental neurotrophic events, thereby contributing to key learning and memory deficits in young animals exposed to CPF. A study is underway to examine the functional consequences of these and other genes on learning and memory (D. Jett, 2001, personal communication).

Thus far, the results of this pilot study demonstrate the utility of the DNA microarray technology to identify alterations of gene expression induced by OP agents. The study has also yielded some important insight into genes and gene products that may play roles in mediating the effects of CPF exposure. While the results from the BChE activity assay were sufficient to suggest that the acute toxic response of the rats to CPF exposure occurred as predicted, future studies will include multiple animals for each time and dose point in order to decrease the possibility of interanimal variability in gene expression response. Furthermore, collection of data at lower doses of OP agents and at time points closer to and farther from the initial dose point will be required in order to begin to build a more complete understanding of lower dose and exposure duration to OP agents.

This pilot study represents an important first step toward designing and implementing future toxicogenomic studies that will build understanding of the molecular effects of OP agents and other important TICs and TIMs. This study has also clearly demonstrated the ability of the DNA microarray technology to identify genetic components underlying OP toxicity. Future toxicogenomic studies will use multiple animals per dosage and time point so that statistically valid gene expression observations can be made. Recently, we have begun to assess the effect of a low-level exposure of the OP agent Sarin to identify genetic changes unique to OP nerve agent intoxication. Overall, the future of toxicogenomics promises to yield information critical to designing better material for detection, personal protection, and decontamination that will serve to protect both the performance and the health of military and industrial personnel.

REFERENCES

Bagchi, D., Bagchi, M., Tang, L., and Stohs, S.J. (1997) Comparative *in vitro* and *in vivo* protein kinase C activation by selected pesticides and transition metal salts, *Toxicol. Lett.*, 91, 31–37.

Beck, K.D., Knusel, B., Winslow, J.W., Rosenthal, A., Burton, L.E., Nikolics, K., and Hefti, F. (1992) Pretreatment of dopaminergic neurons in culture with brain-derived neurotrophic factor attenuates toxicity of 1-methyl-4-phenylpyridinium, *Neurodegeneration*, 1, 27–36.

Bloom, F. (1994) Neurotransmission and the Central Nervous System, in *Goodman and Gilman's The Pharmacological Basis of Therapeutics*, Hardman J.G. and Limbrid, L.E., Eds., McGraw-Hill, New York, p. 286.

Chomczynski, P. and Sacchi, N. (1987) Single step method of RNA isolation by acid guanidinium thiocyanate-phenol-chloroform extraction, *Anal. Biochem.*, 162, 156–159.

Chuang, L.F. and Chuang, R.Y. (1998) Heptachlor and the mitogen-induced protein kinase module in human lymphocytes, *Toxicology*, 128, 17–23.

Cotman, C.W., Kahle, J.S., Miller, S., Ulas, J., and Bridges, R.J. (1994) Excitatory amino acid neurotransmission, in *Psychopharmacology: The Fourth Generation of Progress*, Bloom, F.E. and Kupfer, D.J., Eds., Raven Press, New York, pp. 75–85.

Davydov, D.R. (2001) Microsomal monooxygenase in apoptosis another target for cytochrome c signaling?, *Trends Biochem. Sci.*, 26, 155–160.

Ellman, G.L., Courtney, K.D., Andres, V., Jr., and Featherstone, R.M. (1961) A new rabbit colorimetric acetylcholinesterase activity assay, *Biochem. Pharmacol.*, 7, 88–95.

Han, B.H., D'Costa, A., Back, S.A., Parsadanian, M., Patel, S., Shah, A.R., Gidday, J.M., Srinivasan, A., Deshmukh, M., and Holtzman, D.M. (2000) BDNF blocks Caspase-3 activation in neonatal hypoexia-ischemia, *Neurobiol. Dis.*, 7, 38–53.

Hyman, C., Hofer, M., Barde, Y.A., Juhasz, M., Yancopoulos, G.D., Squinto, S.P., and Lindsay, R.M. (1991) BDNF is a neurotrophic factor for dopaminergic neurons of the substantia nigra, *Nature*, 350, 230–232.

Ikemoto, M., Tsunekawa, S., Toda, Y., and Totani, M. (2001) Liver-type arginase is a highly sensitive marker for hepatocellular damage in rats, *Clin. Chem.*, 47, 946–948.

Jamal, G.A. (1998) Gulf War syndrome—a model for the complexity of biological and environmental interaction with human health, *Adverse Drug React. Toxicol. Rev.*, 17, 1–17.

Josephson, R., Muller, T., Pickel, J., Okabe, S., Reynolds, K., Turner, P.A., Zimmer, A., and McKay, R.D. (1998) POU transcription factors control expression of CNS stem cell-specific genes, *Development,* 125, 3087–3100.

Katsutani, N., Sekeido, T., Aoki, T., and Sagami, F. (2000) Hepatic drug metabolic enzymes induced by clofibrate in rasH2 mice, *Toxicol. Lett.,* 115: 223–229.

Kawashima, H., Husunose, E., Thompson, C.M., and Strobel, H.W. (1997) Protein expression, characterization, and regulation of CYP4F4 and CYP4F5 cloned from rat brain, *Arch. Biochem. Biophys.,* 347, 148–154.

Kawashima, H. and Strobel, H.W. (1995) cDNA cloning of three new forms of rat brain cytochrome P450 belonging to the CYP4F subfamily, *Biochem. Biophys. Res. Commun.,* 217, 1137–1144.

McDiarmid, M.A., Keogh, J.P., Hooper, F.J., McPhaul, K., Squibb, K., Kane, R., DiPino, R., Kabat, M., Kaup, B., Anderson, L., Hoover, D., Brown, L., Hamilton, M., Jacobson Kram, D., Burrows, B., and Walsh, M. (2000) Health effects of depleted uranium on exposed Gulf War veterans, *Environ. Res.,* 82, 168–180.

Nakamura, T., Okada, K., Nagata, K., and Yamazoe, Y. (2000) Intestinal cytochrome p450 and response to rifampicin in rabbits, *Jpn. J. Pharmacol.* 82, 232–239.

Nau, M.E., Emerson, L.R., Martin, R.K., Kyle, D.E., Wirth, D.F., and Vahey, M. (2000) Technical assessment of the affymetrix yeast expression GeneChip YE6100 platform in a heterologous model of genes that confer resistance to anti-malarial drugs in yeast, *J. Clin. Microbiol.,* 38, 1901–1908.

NRC (1997) National Research Council's Committee on Toxicology: The First 50 Years 1947–1997, *Natl. Acad. Sci.,* 1–38.

Snyder, S.H. and Dawson, T.M. (1994) Nitric oxide and related substances as neuronal messengers, in *Psychopharmacology: The Fourth Generation of Progress,* Bloom, F.E. and Kupfer, D.J., Eds., Raven Press, New York, pp. 609–618.

Steiner, S. and Anderson, N.L. (2000) Expression profiling in toxicology-potentials and limitations, *Toxicol. Lett.,* 112–113, 467–471.

Storck, T., Schulte, S., Hofmann, K., and Stoffel, W. (1992) Structure, expression, and function of Na+ dependent glutamate/aspartate transporter from rat brain, *Proc. Natl. Acad. Sci. U.S.A.,* 89: 10955–10959.

Turgeon, D., Carrier, J., Levesque, E., Hum, D.W., and Belanger, A. (2001) Relative enzymatic activity, protein stability, and tissue distribution of human steroid-metabolizing UGT2B subfamily members, *Endocrinology,* 142, 778–787.

Waddington, S.N. and Cattell, V. (2000) Arginase in glumerulonephritis, *Exp. Nephrol.,* 8, 128–134.

PART VII

Recent Innovations in Alternatives

HARRY SALEM AND SIDNEY A. KATZ

Included in this section are chapters on the archival and computational resources for animal alternatives, as well as applications of low-frequency vibrational spectrometry and the tropoblast toxicity assay for evaluating mutagenicity *in vitro*.

The focus of Chapter 37, by Millard Mershon, is the reassessment of existing data as an alternative to collecting new information from living subjects. In Chapter 38, T.B. Worobec describes the extensive collections of material available at the Library of Congress. Chapter 40, by Martin Béliveau and Kannan Krishnan, reviews biologically based algorithms for estimating physiologically based pharmacokinetic models and shows how these models can be applied in human health risk assessment. In Chapter 41, by William White, the application of quantum mechanical methods for relating toxicity to chemical reactivity with computational techniques is described. The chapter by C.K. Zoltani and S.I. Baskin, Chapter 42, describes the use of computational methods for analyzing information on biological processes and identifying potential therapeutic agents.

The chapter contributed by Globus and his collaborators describes measurement of conformational changes in DNA from its low-frequency internal vibrations and possible predictions of mutation. Harvey Kliman's chapter, Chapter 44, describes the development of an *in vitro* tropoblast toxicity assay for evaluating potential adverse effects therapeutic drugs and environmental toxins may have on the placenta (and hence fetus) during human gestation.

These recent innovations make use of computer technology, instrument technology, and biotechnology to provide alternative toxicological methods for the new millennium.

CHAPTER 37

Archival Data in Toxicology: Minimizing Need for Animal Experiments

Millard M. Mershon

CONTENTS

0-8493-1528-X/03/$0.00+$1.50
© 2003 by CRC Press LLC

INTRODUCTION

Perspective

Use of animal surrogates in prediction of human responses to toxic substances is based upon the concept that human and animal subjects have physiological and biochemical systems likely to show qualitatively similar responses. This idea underlies preclinical studies for dose–response estimations. Such studies are typically designed to reduce experimental variables as much as is possible. Accordingly, test conditions are carefully controlled. Standardized animal models and procedures are used if possible. This means that many investigators are conditioned to avoid melding of data from dissimilar sources. However, similarities of physiological function for human and animal organs may justify projection of superficially dissimilar animal responses to permit approximation of human responses (Mershon and Callahan, 1975). Various biological common denominators support use of archived animal data for modeling of human responses if human or animal experimentation is precluded and best estimates must suffice. Animals may be used as surrogate persons, i.e., they are models. Here it is suggested that fragments of human and animal data can be combined to improve modeling of human responses if suitable data are available.

PROBLEM SOLVING

Modeling does not create data. It follows that the modeler must collect useful data. Modelers use existing data to extrapolate and interpolate on the basis of some unifying characteristics or principle. Accordingly, a modeler needs to have or acquire an understanding of relationships between experimental subjects and required estimates. A preliminary understanding of the problem and relevant archival resources must precede the collection of useful data; given such understanding, a modeler can (1) look for useful literature or other sources; (2) review documents for detail and data relevant to the given problem; (3) try to understand mechanisms or rationales that underlie results; (4) assemble pieces of data to fit rationales; (5) create draft pictures or concepts, (6) seek and use constructive criticism; (7) compare predicted values with known examples; (8) refine new concepts, and (9) smooth projections to construct a reasonable model of reality. Exact methods must be varied to fit the problems and data at hand.

Three examples illustrate unconventional applications of data from some conventional experiments or observations that are unlikely to be repeated or redesigned. Hopefully these examples will suggest other ways to analyze existing data in lieu of collecting new data with experimental animals. The first example involved estimation of lethal human dosages for inhaled hydrogen cyanide (HCN). These estimates were based on observed animal and human intravenous doses of NaCN or equivalent inhaled HCN dosages. Another example shows how data from human eye exposures to diethyldichlorosulfide (mustard) vapor were compiled for prediction of eye effects from unknown mustard dosages. The last example shows how delayed incapacitating effects of enterotoxigenic *Escherichia coli* (ETEC) were projected from observed consequences of "Montezuma's Revenge" in a diverse group of persons attending a medical convention.

INHALATION TOXICOLOGY OF HYDROGEN CYANIDE

Modeling Approaches

The sponsoring agency wanted to know whether a proposed drug pretreatment could provide enough protection against an unexpected HCN exposure to justify drug development. A set of modeling methods can be used to answer such questions if (1) the lethal and/or incapacitating dosages and probit slopes are known for the toxic substance and (2) at least one protection level is stipulated as effective. In this case, doubling of the lethal HCN dosage by the candidate drug was stipulated as significant protection. However, there were no accepted dosage/effect values or probit slopes for inhaled HCN in human subjects.

To obtain the required estimates, it was necessary to start the nine-step process described in the Introduction. Results from step one suggested that no simple answer, such as discovery of complete data from one surrogate species, was available. Apparent gaps in the available data suggested that biological common denominators should be sought. It was hoped that support could be found for melding of data from dissimilar species. However, step two revealed major influences of species differences and HCN features in modification of responses to HCN inhalation dosages.

Relevant Toxicological Features and Methodology

Aviado and Salem (1987) have outlined fundamental principles of inhalation pharmacology and toxicology as follows: (1) receptors in the upper and lower respiratory tract respond to chemical inhalants, therapeutic or otherwise; (2) bronchial muscles respond to chemical inhalants and drugs by releasing humoral agents, activating bronchopulmonary nerve structures, or both; (3) the uptake of inspired chemical substances is determined by chemophysical properties of the inhalant and corresponding vascular responses in the respiratory system; and (4) oronasal inhalation is the only acceptable experimental procedure simulating human exposure, whereas direct tracheal inhalation and installation are research techniques for identifying mechanisms, and they may or may not relate to the human respiratory system.

Features of HCN are compared with relevant features of nerve gas in Figure 37.1. It was observed that inhaled HCN induces involuntary hyperventilation in man, dog, and pig—but not in rats used to provide much of the reported data. It was also observed that endogenous detoxification mechanisms act rapidly enough to skew results, as usually calculated. This means that multiplication of the agent concentration (C) in air by the time (t) of exposure is inappropriate to find a lethal inhaled dosage (LCt_{50}) for HCN. This approach (Haber, 1924) works well with agents that cause additive toxic effects if concentrations remain constant during exposures. This

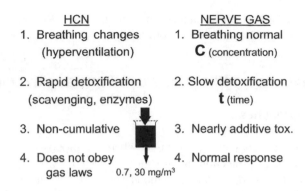

Figure 37.1 Comparison of toxicological features of HCN and nerves gases, such as sarin. The larger arrow represents inhaled HCN. The smaller arrow represents the effective dosage, after detoxification and loss of the 30% of inhaled HCN that is exhaled (Moore and Gates, 1946), leaving 0.7 retained. HCN concentrations up to 30 mg/m³ are normally neutralized by human detoxification systems before effects become observable (Prentiss, 1937).

is usually true for relatively brief nerve agent exposures but is much less likely for exposures with tiny HCN molecules; the HCN is rapidly degraded and diffuses more rapidly than Boyle's gas law would indicate. It is also noteworthy that effective dosages are reduced (×0.7) by the 30% of HCN exhaled (Moore and Gates, 1946) and by its detoxification. HCN, at concentrations up to 30 mg/m³, is normally detoxified without producing observable effects (Prentiss, 1937).

Ballantyne (1987) recognized the problem of measuring HCN toxicity with varying time factors and the consequent changing impacts of detoxification. In place of studies with a fixed HCN concentration and varied exposures times, he changed HCN concentrations and fixed the exposure duration. A plot of the 50% lethal concentration (LC_{50}) of HCN (Ballantyne, 1987) is represented on the left side of Figure 37.2. This plot reveals a precipitous decline of lethal concentration with rat exposure times exceeding 10 sec. This shows the role of high HCN concentrations during the inhalation of lethal dosages if few respiratory cycles are possible during an exposure. The slope is steep when there is insufficient time for detoxification of HCN. An abrupt change of slope is found with scavenging and degradation of HCN during exposures longer than 5 min.

The right side of Figure 37.2 represents Ballantyne's (1987) replot of his LC_{50} data. This plot shows that LCt_{50} dosages must rise, with increasing exposure time, to offset losses of HCN by detoxification. The steeply rising line would tend to parallel the baseline if Ct values were constant, as has been assumed for LCt_{50} determinations with nerve agents.

Analysis of Ballantyne's approach led modelers to exclude data based on Haber's approach. This left one other source of rat data. Levin et al. (1985) employed the Ballantyne approach, but a different strain of rat, to determine both HCN LC_{50} values and incapacitating concentration (IC_{50}) values. They found their LC_{50} and IC_{50} data to have parallel slopes. However, a glance at Figure 37.3 shows differing probit slopes and line equations for Ballantyne and Levin data sets. Modelers did not know whether one strain better represents man, so they made an arbitrary decision. The

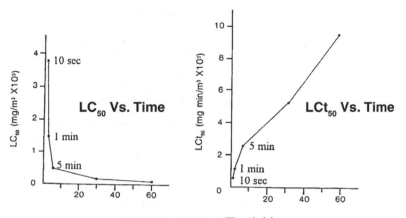

HCN Vapor Exposure Time (min)

Figure 37.2 Contrasting plots of data from the same rat exposures to HCN (after Ballantyne, 1987). One plot (left) reflects use of exposures with fixed duration and varied HCN concentrations. The steep initial slope shows that HCN must be very concentrated for a small number of breaths to deliver a lethal dosage. The second plot presents the data results as customarily displayed, given a fixed toxic gas concentration and varied exposure durations. LCt_{50} values tend to increase as more time becomes available for detoxification.

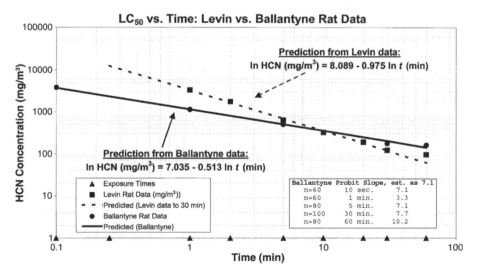

Figure 37.3 Comparison of responses from different strains of rats under similar HCN exposure conditions (after Levin et al., 1985). Log–log plots of the data reveal differences of effective HCN concentrations and probit slopes of lines but do not show which strain better represents the human race.

line equation from the Levin data, the more conservative choice, was combined with the probit slope of the Ballantyne data. This chimera was tentatively chosen to represent HCN dosage responses in the absence of hyperventilation, which is minimal in rats. However, hyperventilation could not be disregarded since it is critical in human HCN toxicology.

SEQUENCE	MECHANISMS
1. Lung ← **HCN** :	Un-ionized → Absorbed
↓	↓
2. Pulmonary artery	Scavenging (Hbg, albumen)
↓	↓
3. Carotid body	Low O_2 sensor
↓	↓
4. Respiratory centers	Stimulation: 10-15 sec
↓	↓
5. Involuntary	5x Dose/t : 15 sec → 2 min
hyperventilation	
↓	↓
6. Disoriented → Unconcious	15 → 30 sec (mask??)

↓   ↗ gasping -------- 3 → 5 min → Incapacitation

7.   Apnea ↘

convulsions --- Lethal : 5 ± min

Figure 37.4 Relationships of anatomical and pharmacological factors leading to lethality for mammals that inhale HCN. Nonionized HCN is rapidly absorbed into blood to move the short distance from alveoli to the sensor. The sensor response (or lack of a signal) communicates a need for oxygen to respiratory neurones that initiate hyperventilation. Increased minute volumes multiply HCN intake until respiratory center poisoning leads to apnea.

Mechanisms and Rationales

In accord with modeling step three (above), pathophysiology of HCN was reviewed and outlined in Figure 37.4. It was observed that nonionized HCN rapidly diffuses from lung alveoli into blood en route to the carotid body oxygen sensor. Bodansky and Helm (1944) estimated that respiratory stimulation begins within 5 to 10 sec after cyanide reaches the pulmonary capillaries. It appears that poisoning of the oxygen sensor alters signals via the vagus nerve to inform the respiratory center that oxygen is not being detected. Until the respiratory center is poisoned, it induces involuntary hyperventilation that briefly boosts the minute volume. This increased ventilation multiplies the HCN dosage absorbed two to six times (Mershon and Fanzone, 1998) during at least three to six deep inspirations (Bodansky and Helm, 1944), confounding any LCt_{50} determination based upon assumed constancy of uptake. A subsequent interval of apnea (e.g., 15 sec to 2 min) briefly stops uptake. The uptake pattern is further disrupted when gasping follows apnea. This analysis suggested that the dosage threshold for human hyperventilation would be a crucial value for modeling purposes.

Extrapolations of Human Data

Three human studies of hyperventilation were identified, but each was found to involve intravenous dosing with sodium cyanide (NaCN), not inhaled HCN. A single dose (0.11 mg/kg) bolus injection within 1 sec induced hyperventilation in 11 subjects during World War II (Bodansky and Helm, 1944). Another single dose study, with a 0.10-mg/kg dose given within 2 sec, was said to induce hyperventilation in "most subjects" (Cope and Abramovitz, 1960). When doses were given slowly, within a 15-sec interval, a 0.11-mg/kg dose "frequently failed to stimulate

Table 37.1 Hydrogen Cyanide Concentrations and Effects Associated with Various HCN Exposure Conditions in Animals and Man

Mg/m³	Effects	Ref.
30,000[a]	Rat, inhalation LC_{50}	Levin et al., 1985
9,300[b]	Men, 11/11 hyperventilate	Bodansky and Helm, 1944
7,740[b]	Men, "most hyperventilate"	Cope and Abramovitz, 1959
4,000[a]	Rat, inhalation LC_{50}	Ballantyne, 1987
3,200[b]	Men, "50% hyperventilate"	Wexler et al., 1947
2,230	Pig, LC_{50} within 2 min of inhalation	Stemler et al., 1994

[a] Lethal concentration for 50% of subject rats, 0.1 min inhalation exposure.
[b] Equivalent HCN mg/m³ dosage calculated for intravenous sodium cyanide solution.

respiration," and 0.15-mg/kg doses produced fractional responses (Wexler et al., 1947). These authors reported that a larger dose, 0.20 mg/kg, was 100% effective.

The described human NaCN data might be considered too imprecise for use in conventional toxicology, but they were the best available. Therefore, assumptions were applied in an effort to improve their usefulness. As shown in Table 37.1, it was assumed that the rapid injections were equivalent to single breath dosages and that the subjects might inhale three times during the 15-sec deliveries. Applications of accepted tidal volume values and molecular weight values were used in calculations of HCN concentrations (mg/m³) that might be expected to produce the various degrees of hyperventilation reported with NaCN doses. In Table 37.1 these values are compared with an estimated value, 9,300 mg/m³, given in a summary of World War II studies (Moore and Gates, 1946). A further comparison shows that these human value estimates are, in general, bracketed by the rat single breath LC_{50} values derived from line equations shown in Figure 37.3 for both sets of rat results.

It might be concluded that neither rat strain properly represents man, since the implied single breath lethal concentrations of HCN for the two rat strains appear to bracket values projected for man. However, the values associated with bolus dosing (8,824 and 7,740 mg/m³) of men by Bodansky and Helm (1944) appear to be higher (Table 37.1) than the values (3,200 and 2,230 mg/m³) associated with deliveries made in 15-sec (Cope and Abramovitz, 1960) and 2-min (Wexler et al., 1947) periods, respectively. The available data do not support conclusions as to whether one rat strain resisted the inhalation of a foreign substance more capably than the other, or prove that essential experimental conditions were totally identical. The data do show that small differences in exposure conditions or individual responses are associated with a broad range of dosages when exposure conditions are brief.

A Biological Common Denominator

The divergence of estimated rat LC_{50} values fostered the desire to find a biological common denominator for HCN effects in hyperventilating species. Figure 37.5 illustrates the following: (1) an apparent candidate, the aortic blood HCN concentration, (2) an overlay of respiratory and HCN parameters from two figures (after Stemler et al., 1994), (3) that death was associated with a 4-µg/ml aortic blood level

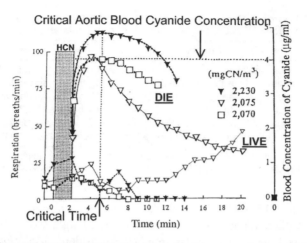

Figure 37.5 Observed breathing rates and blood cyanide concentrations of three miniature pigs exposed to HCN for 2 min (after Stemler et al., 1994). Values for blood concentrations of cyanide, at the top and right side of Figure 37.5, are presented with the corresponding respiratory rate values. Although data acquired after the onset of HCN exposure for 2 min are very limited, they are consistent with other indicators that an aortic blood HCN concentration of 4 mg/m³ at 5 min is a threshold value for a lethal outcome.

of HCN at 3 min after 2 min of exposure to HCN at 2,230 mg/m³, and (4) only two deaths and one recovery suggest 4 μg/ml as the live or die level in aortic blood of miniature pigs. However, this value is consistent with levels estimated for 2 HCN inhalation victims (Harper and Goldhaber, 1997) and reported by Ballantyne (1987) in rabbit, rat, monkey, and a different strain of pig. The same value was found in dogs (Vick et al., 2000) after use of a challenge method similar to the intravenous dosing used with human volunteers. The results with several dogs are represented in Figure 37.6 and appear to be consistent with data shown in Figure 37.5. Therefore,

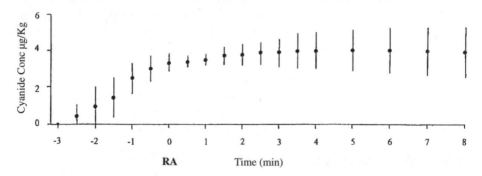

Figure 37.6 Average whole blood cyanide levels in dogs after four continuous intravenous slow infusion trials (1 mg/kg/min) with NaCN solution at 4.0 mg/ml (after Vick et al., 2000). RA indicates respiratory arrest and cessation of NaCN infusion. Methemoglobin formation by 20 mg/ml hydroxylamine hydrochloride solution was initiated 30 sec after RA. Although 3.6 μg/kg was the average value observed at RA, it appears that survival is dependent upon avoidance of blood cyanide concentrations above 4 μg/kg.

it is suggested that the 4 μg/ml HCN aortic blood concentration may represent the blood threshold level for irreversible damage to the respiratory center neurons of animals and man. If this is true, it follows that differences of inhalation dosage may largely reflect species differences of detoxification rates and susceptibility to induction of hyperventilation.

Acute and Peracute Exposures

The preceding analysis suggested that the threshold level of HCN for induction of hyperventilation would delineate two different populations of cyanide casualties. People might become acutely ill but would probably survive without treatment when the threshold is not exceeded during relatively brief, i.e., 2 to 5 min, acute exposures. It was suggested that such acute exposures could be modeled with the line equation calculated from the data of Levin et al. (1985) and a probit slope of 7.1 derived from the data of Ballantyne (1987). For dosages that are well above the critical threshold, Bodansky and Helm (1944) suggested that rapid disorientation and incapacitation would render a soldier unable to don a gas mask. It appears unlikely that self-treatment would occur after such peracute exposures. Therefore, for modeling purposes, it was assumed that induction of hyperventilation is equivalent to inhalation of a fatal HCN dosage when the HCN level is very high or persists for 2 min. Hyperventilation leads to peracute exposures.

Peracute lethal exposures are rare, in part because noxious inhalants typically induce apneic defensive reflexes. Aviado and Salem (1987) describe, as follows, sets of human receptors that respond in sequential order to inhaled chemicals, beginning with the Kratchmer reflex receptors of the upper respiratory tract. Kratchmer receptors induce apnea, bradycardia, and initially falling blood pressure. Next, lower respiratory tract receptors initiate cough reflexes. Then the Kratchmer reflex protective responses are reinforced by cardiopulmonary receptors for the Bezold-Hirt reflex and by aortic arch and carotid sinus baroreceptors, all acting to reduce respiratory intake.

In the case of HCN inhalation, it appears that energy-releasing mechanisms of receptors fail so swiftly that reflex signals are compromised. Intact energy transfer mechanisms are essential for the maintenance of electrochemical gradients needed for transmitter releases and responses at nerve endings (Mershon, 1964). Peracute lethal exposures may also represent levels of potency that permit poisoning with one or few respiratory excursions and low multiples of circulation time. It might be expected that persons could perceive the distinctive odor of HCN and voluntarily suspend respiration while donning a mask or seeking fresh air. However, half of a population would not notice the odor (Hall, 1997), and HCN can induce involuntary hyperventilation (Bodansky and Helm, 1944).

An exposure to HCN at 2,230 mg/m^3 for 2 min (Figure 37.5) may represent the lethal threshold value for miniature pigs (Table 37.1). Analysis of all values in Table 37.1 suggests that human hyperventilation threshold values could readily fall between 2,230 and 8,824 mg/m^3, depending on the exposure duration and individual detoxifying capabilities. This range is consistent with the steepness of the curves plotted by Ballantyne (1987), as seen in Figure 37.3. These data have been applied during the modeling of human toxicity estimates for HCN (Mershon, 1998) and assessment of the prophylactic potential of methemoglobin-forming drugs against HCN poisoning (Mershon and Fanzone, 1998).

Lessons Learned

One lesson was relearned. Mershon and Fanzone (1998) found that much of the enthusiasm for methemoglobin-forming drugs was apparently based upon reports of early experimental results. Seemingly relevant data were obtained by successful titration of intravenously administered sodium cyanide with a methemoglobin-forming drug in dogs. This experiment is considered misleading because it did not factor in hyperventilation, and consequent increased dosage levels, that would be induced by inhaled HCN. For the reasons outlined by Aviado and Salem (1987), oronasal inhalation is the only acceptable experimental procedure for simulating human inhalation exposure.

Successful application of the described nine-step strategy is not simple. Although modeling can succeed when it is not possible to design and execute a new experiment or find the record of an old experiment meeting all criteria, there are many constraints. Valid relationships must exist between fragments of data from different sources and the reality being modeled. Unless some biological common denominator(s) is identified, the risk of making an apples-and-oranges comparison may be great. It appears that careful and creative matching of physiological features and pathological consequences is one key to recognition of data fragments that might be matched appropriately.

Human data or nonhuman data that provide a direct link with human beings should be located, if possible. If such data cannot be located, the modeler may be able to estimate key quantities, set plausible intervals, and parameterize to outline best/worst or most likely outcomes. However, for modeling success, it is essential to avoid feeding garbage into the dreaded modeler's equation: "garbage in, garbage out."

PROJECTION OF DELAYED EYE EFFECTS OF MUSTARD EXPOSURES

Vive la Difference!

In the manner of public opinion polls, most experiments in the laboratory involve selection of a few subjects that are supposed to represent a population. Subject difference variations are limited in pursuit of statistical significance, or numbers are increased to achieve statistical power. An experiment is usually designed to exclude diversity. Sometimes it may be necessary to reverse this bias: to seek a few unifying factors to shape deductions about nonmeasurable conditions and a fundamentally diverse population. We have all learned to compare differing results; modelers compare both data and results that differ. For example, one may consider the pros and cons of sorting and analyzing inputs from all available experimental findings reported for human eye exposures with mustard vapor since the early days of World War I.

Dose Responses—with Time

Sponsor requirements dictated predictions of mustard lesion severity or degrees of recovery on successive days after unexpected exposure of human military populations to a range of mustard vapor dosages. In accordance with the described modeling strategy, review and evaluation of available literature were initiated. It was found that many of the useful observations were made during World Wars I and II, but some followed accidents or Iraqi attacks on Iranians (Deverill et al., 1994).

During attempts to understand mechanisms or rationales, it was observed that the various human organ systems show both qualitative and quantitative differences of response to mustard vapor. Accordingly, implementation of modeling step four led to assembly of data according to organ systems, such as skin or eye. More than one hundred sets of observations on eye responses were found (Deverill et al., 1994). Although they were often imprecise, comments about the duration of particular symptoms were made in 22 cases. The times from exposure to the onset of described symptoms were recorded in 18 cases. Comments on both onset and recovery times were found in 13 records. Unfortunately, such emphasis on dose/response relationships and inattention to the extended time course is common both in old reports and more recent ones.

Dosage-Degree-Duration

One experimental report (Unde and Dumphy, 1944) provided correlation of the extended time course of effects noted (signs as observed, symptoms as reported) with a single mustard vapor concentration (90 mg/m^3) and an assumed exposure duration of 1 min. Effects were graded in six severity categories according to a subjective grading scale. The triple correlation of data provided the key to conceptualization of a picture, as per modeling step five. The 90-mg/m^3 dosage is associated with the reported effects; the combination is represented as a heavy dashed line in Figure 37.7. The airfoil shape of this line, with peak effect at less than one third of the chord, is based on the reported data as plotted. This shape is consistent with the observation that, in general, onset times were reported with relative precision in hours while recovery times were given by the day. Accordingly, the time scale is altered from hours to days after 24 hr. This shape is also consistent with illustration of response curves with steep initial slopes near onset and gradually receding slopes during recovery.

Onsets were observed earlier, and recoveries noted later, as exposure dosages and effect severity increased. This pattern is evident in Figure 37.7, which was constructed by plotting reported data points at appropriate sites in the dosage/time/severity frame. Each dosage rib was constructed individually, with distances plotted from the baseline representing severity levels at elapsed times. Dosage ribs were stacked according to their positions on a linear dosage scale. Lines were drawn to connect data points of similar severity. As per step four, these pieces of data were assembled to fit the Haber rationale that mustard vapor concentration and exposure time determine dosage and degree of damage at a given time after exposure. The initial picture was critiqued, checked for consistency of differing data sources, refined

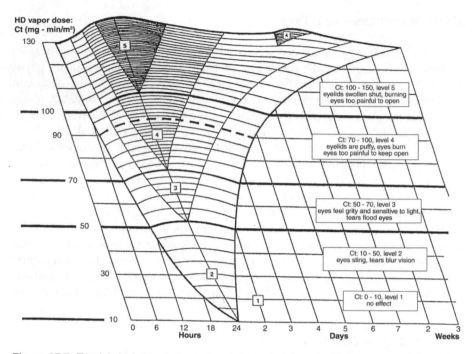

Figure 37.7 Triaxial depiction that was hand drawn to integrate (1) time course information reported hourly or by the day; (2) mustard vapor dosage information; and (3) levels of human effect severity for the given time and dosage. The dashed line represents data from one particularly relevant experiment (Unde and Dunphy, 1944) among more than 100 experimental reports that were considered.

with ribs marking arbitrary dosage bands, and smoothed to make Figure 37.7. Heavy lines mark ribs for dosages of 10, 50, 70, and 100 mg-min/m³. These lines represent boundaries of convenience for designation of dosage bands that were used later in estimates (Deverill et al., 1994) of casualty rates with time.

Values associated with symptoms, listed in legend blocks of Figure 37.7, are distinctly different from those used in the final casualty estimation. This is because the blocks of Figure 37.7 describe peak effects (worst case symptoms) observed in the more susceptible members of exposed groups. However, casualty estimates are based on averaged/mean responses to be expected in an entire population over time. The nature of this distinction can be observed in Figure 37.7. At the exposure level of 50 mg-min/m³, Figure 37.7 shows little time at effect level two, with regard to the entire time scale. For estimation of casualties over the whole time span, level three was assumed to apply only for populations exposed at levels above 50 mg-min/m³. Accordingly, "eyes feel gritty and sensitive to light, tears flood eyes" was assumed to be a typical, but not universal, response of men exposed to mustard concentrations near 70 mg-min/m³.

Applications of Figure 37.7

This unpublished figure (Mershon, 1994) was used, with similar figures for estimating responses of other human organs, in the construction of a bar chart published by Deverill et al. (1994) and a table used in a medical planning guide (OTSG, 1998). Although the original purpose for construction of Figure 37.7 was to support casualty estimation, it might be used to show how individual data points that are relatively meaningless may be assembled to make a meaningful nomogram. Exposure dosage levels are rarely measured during accidents or wartime exposures, but the earliest exposure time is usually known. Therefore, the elapsed time from an exposure can be estimated. Figure 37.7 shows how this parameter might be used. By following the line for 6 hr up to its intersection with the curve for onset of level two symptoms, one sees that the corresponding exposure level appears to exceed 90 mg-min/m³. At that concentration, victims are likely to notice stinging eyes with tears about 6 hr after exposure. However, it is probably more clinically relevant to observe that this figure can be used to predict onset of responses at effect level four to occur between 12 and 18 hr after the mustard exposure.

The described methodology produced a surprise, as represented by the secondary peak at level four on the top line of Figure 37.7. Although scattered descriptions of delayed relapses following initial brief recoveries were found during a literature review (Mershon, 1994), the phenomenon has received little attention in textbooks. Some eye exposure victims were described as briefly recovering from day two to day five before suffering temporary relapses. Similar relapses were observed in skin of volunteers exposed to mustard vapor, as reported by a former medical officer (Sinclair, 1948) shortly after World War II. Such delayed relapses have been noted in skin after thermal and radiation burns. Compilation of related information from various sources led to the hypothesis that such relapses represent antigen–antibody reactions. It appears that the antigens are derived from proteins denatured by chemical reactions with mustard (or coagulation from thermal or radiation burns). Formation of antibodies that react with such antigens in eyes can be expected after 5 days of activity by the immune system. However, skin responses may be delayed and/or prolonged (Sinclair, 1948).

ESTIMATION OF PERFORMANCE DEGRADATION BY "FOOD POISONING"

Traveler's Diarrhea

Mexican physicians (Cesarman et al., 1993) have observed that, "Although it is true that Moctezuma (not Montezuma) can strike travelers with a vengeance ... a lot of us get traveler's diarrhea in Manhattan." The common denominator may be ingestion of organisms for which the recipient has not developed effective immunity, as was suspected more than 25 years ago. At that time, an extraordinary prospective study (Merson et al., 1976) was designed to characterize clinical patterns, epidemiology, and infective agents in a population with varying degrees of resistance. A group of 73 physicians, 44 spouses, and 4 children traveled to Mexico City, where 59 persons (49%) developed traveler's diarrhea. Enterotoxigenic *Escherichia coli* (ETEC) coliform bacteria were isolated from 21 persons, of whom 19 were diagnosed with traveler's diarrhea.

From Cases to Predictions

Historically, far more soldiers have died of disease than wounds. It remains true that diseases cause greater losses of military strength, i.e., casualties, than battle injuries. It is also true that armies tend to travel into areas populated with bacteria for which they lack immunity. Therefore, modelers were asked if they could estimate how many soldiers might be disabled on each given day after exposure to food or water contaminated with ETEC. Modeling step one revealed the prospective study report (Merson et al., 1976), which incorporated several of the other modeling steps. The report even provided a figure that showed cases of traveler's diarrhea per day from arrival in Mexico. That figure indicates numbers of cases with cultures of *E. coli* strains, *Salmonella* strains, both, or neither. The data for depiction of three severity levels were derived from information given in the text. For example, it was stated that "Nineteen percent were confined to bed, and 39 percent changed activities because of their illness...." Conveniently, a table provided data on days in bed or with changed activity for stated numbers of persons with positive ETEC cultures.

The available pieces of information were integrated to yield a picture, as per modeling step five. This was the basis for Figure 37.8, which shows comparisons of severity and persistence of illness for the affected population. A review of other reports on ETEC infections suggested that the observed group might reasonably be considered to represent a military population with diverse levels of resistance to a variety of ETEC strains. Table 37.2 shows how the published data for the particular population were transformed into a generalized form. Table 37.2 provided the modeler's answer to the military question, "How many soldiers might be disabled on each given day after exposure to food and water contaminated with ETEC?" (Fischer and Mershon, 1994, unpublished data)

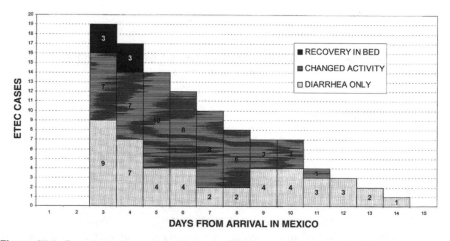

Figure 37.8 Bar chart designed to illustrate relative severity of enteric disease effects as correlated with time after arrival of a mixed population in Mexico City. Each of the 19 represented cases involved isolation of enterotoxigenic *Escherichia coli* organisms that accounted for 45% of traveler's diarrhea cases observed during this prospective study (Merson et al., 1976).

Table 37.2 Estimates of Percent of Military Personnel with Indicated Degree of Performance-Degradation per Day after Onset of Gastrointestinal Symptoms/Signs from Infection with Enterotoxigenic *Escherichia coli* Bacteria[a]

Day of Onset[b]	Percentage of cases with degraded military performance				
	% New Cases[c]	No.[d] (25%)[c]	No.[e] (50%)[c]	No.[f] (100%)[c]	Recovered[g] (%)[c]
1	(14.6)	9 (47.4)	7 (36.8)	3 (15.5)	0 (0)
2	(19.0)	7 (36.8)	7 (36.8)	3 (15.8)	2 (10.5)
3	(19.3)	4 (21.1)	10 (52.6)	(0)	5 (26.3)
4	(17.1)	4 (21.1)	8 (42.1)	(7)	(36.8)
5	(9.8)	2 (10.5)	8 (42.2)	(9)	(47.4)
6	(6.1)	2 (10.5)	6 (31.6)	(11)	(57.9)
7	(4.1)	4 (21.1)	3 (15.8)	(12)	(63.2)
8	(2.9)	4 (21.1)	2 (10.5)	(13)	(68.4)
9	(2.0)	3 (15.8)	1 (5.3)	(15)	(78.9)
10	(1.5)	3 (15.8)	(0)	(16)	(84.2)
11	(1.3)	2 (10.5)		(17)	(89.5)
12	(1.1)	1 (5.3)		(18)	(94.7)
13	(0.7)	0.5 (2.6)		(18.5)	(97.4)
14	(0.5)	(0)		(19)	(100.0)

[a] Percentages based upon data from 19 proven cases of enterotoxigenic *Escherichia coli* infection acquired in Mexico City (Merson et al., 1976).
[b] Onset day 1 is day 3 from exposure to infection.
[c] Calculated from daily rate curve (Fischer and Mershon, 1994).
[d] Cases (9) with uncomplicated traveler's diarrhea, performance 25% degraded on day 1.
[e] Cases (7) with changed activities, performance 50% degraded during onset day 1.
[f] Cases (3) with recovery time in bed; performance 100% degraded during onset day 1.
[g] Cases (19) all had some degree of incapacitation during onset day 1.

SUMMARY

Three examples are provided to show how archival data may be used in the place of experimental data collection. Nine steps found to facilitate the use of archival data are listed and demonstrated. The overall modeling process is illustrated by an archeological analogy presented as Figure 37.9. First, one must recognize the potential value of doing a lot of digging and sorting. Next, one must decide which material is worth keeping and analyze possible relationships. The assembly of the final product requires creative interpolation, extrapolation, and careful interpretation. However, a modeling approach may offer the only way to get a product when "they don't make 'em like that anymore!"

ACKNOWLEDGMENTS

Research was funded under contract DAMD17-93-C-3141 by the U.S. Army Medical Research and Materiel Command, Medical Chemical Biological Defense Research Program, Fort Detrick, MD 21702–5012, or DNA contract 001-90-C-0164 by the Defense Nuclear Agency (now: Defense Threat Reduction Agency, Fort Belvoir, VA 22060–6201).

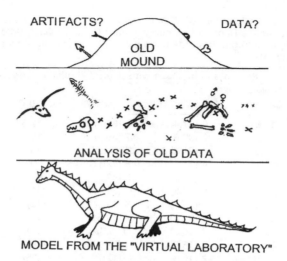

ARTIFACTS?   DATA?

OLD
MOUND

ANALYSIS OF OLD DATA

MODEL FROM THE "VIRTUAL LABORATORY"

Figure 37.9 This cartoon is included to suggest that modeling represents a combination of art and science. The art of modeling methodology is applied when conventional testing methods are not applicable for collection of experimental results. In each case, previously collected data were reacquired and analyzed to provide a best possible estimate of reality.

REFERENCES

Aviado, D. and Salem, H. (1987) Respiratory and bronchomotor reflexes in toxicity studies, in *Inhalation Toxicology. Research Methods, Applications, and Evaluation,* Marcel Dekker, Inc., New York, pp.135–151.

Ballantyne, B. (1987) Toxicology of cyanides, in *Clinical and Experimental Toxicology of Cyanides,* Ballentyne, B. and Marrs, T., Eds., Wright, Bristol, England, pp. 41–126.

Bodansky, O. and Helm, J. (1944) The inability of man to inhibit respiration after the injection of sodium cyanide, *Report MRL-EA-15, Jan 15, 1944,* Edgewood Arsenal, MD (AD-E471963).

Cesarman, C., Cesarman, E., and Lagos, G. (1993) Prevention and treatment of traveler's diarrhea, *New Engl. J. Med.,* 329, 1584.

Cope, C. and Abramovitz, S. (1960) Respiratory responses to intravenous sodium cyanide, a function of the oxygen-cyanide relationship, *Am. Rev. Respir. Dis.,* 81, 321–328.

Deverill, A., Metz, D., Mershon, M., and Gavlinsi, K. (1994) Defense Nuclear Agency Improved *Casualty Estimation (DICE) Chemical Insult Program: Acute Chemical Agent Exposure Effects,* Defense Nuclear Agency Technical Report 93-162, Defense Nuclear Agency, Alexandria, VA, p. 57.

Fischer, B. and Mershon, M. (1994) Unpublished data.

Haber, F. (1924) Funf Vortrage aus den Jahren 1920–1923, Springer-Verlag, Berlin, Germany.

Hall, A., (1997), Personal communication.

Harper, C. and Goldhaber, S. (1997) Inhalation exposure, in *Toxicological Profile for Cyanide (Update),* U.S. Department of Health and Human Services, Agency for Toxic Substance and Disease Registry, Atlanta, pp. 13–21.

Levin, B., Faabo, M., Gurman, J., Baier, L., and Braun, E. (1985) An acute inhalation toxicological study of incapacitating and lethal concentrations of hydrogen cyanide atmospheres, *Report of Phase I and Phase II to the U.S. Army Medical Research Institute of Chemical Defense*, Levin, B., Ed., Edgewood Area, Aberdeen Proving Ground, MD.

Mershon, M. (1964) Biochemical and nutritional aspects of tetany in cattle, paper presented in Scientific Proceedings, 101st Annual Meeting, American Veterinary Medical Association, Schaumburg, IL, pp. 47–70.

Mershon, M. (1994) Review reported in Deverill, et al., ibid, 1994.

Mershon, M. (1998) New human estimates for hydrogen cyanide, paper presented in Proceedings of the 1997 ERDEC Scientific Conference on Chemical and Biological Defense Research, Edgewood Research, Development and Engineering Center Special Publication 063, Berg, D., Ed., Aberdeen Proving Ground, MD, pp. 61–68.

Mershon, M. and Callahan, J. (1975) Exploiting the differences: animal models in dermatology, in *Animal Models in Dermatology*, Maibach, H., Ed., Churchill Livingstone, New York, pp. 41–73.

Mershon, M. and Fanzone, J. (1998) Can hydrogen cyanide threats be neutralized with methemoglobin formers? in *Proceedings of 1998 Bioscience Review* (on CD), U.S. Army Medical Research Institute of Chemical Defense, Aberdeen Proving Ground, MD, pp. 1–7.

Merson, M., Morris, G., Sack, D., Wells, J., Feeley, J., Sack, R., Creesh, W., Kapikian, A., and Gangarosa, E. (1976) Traveler's diarrhea in Mexico: a prospective study of physicians and family members attending a congress, *New Engl. J. Med.*, 294, 1299–1305.

Moore, S. and Gates, M. (1946) Hydrogen cyanide and cyanogen chloride, in *Summary Technical Report of Division 9, Part I*, National Defense Research Committee, Washington, D.C.

OTSG (Office of the Surgeon General) (1998) Ratification Draft, Medical Planning Guide of NBC Battle Casualties, Chemical, AMedP-8(A), Vol. III, Office of the Surgeon General (OTSG), Washington, D.C., 2–21.

Prentiss, A. (1937) *Chemicals in War: A Treatise on Chemical War*, McGraw Hill, New York, pp. 170–174.

Sinclair, D. (1948) The clinical features of mustard gas poisoning in man, *Br. Med. J.*, 2, 290–294.

Stemler, F., Kaminskis, A., Tezak-Reid, T., Stotts, R., Moran, T., Hurt, H., and Ahle, N. (1994) Correlation of Atmospheric and Inhaled Blood Cyanide Levels in Miniature Pigs, Chapter 21 in *Fire and Polymers II. Materials and Tests for Hazard Prevention and American Chemical Society Symposium Series 59*, American Chemical Society, Washington, D.C.

Unde, G. and Dunphy, E. (1944) The effect of oily drops on eyes exposed to mustard vapor, *Porton Report 2800, August 9, 1944*, British Chemical Establishment, Porton Down, England.

Vick, J., Marino, M., Von Bredow, J., Kaminskis, A., and Brewer, T. (2000) A reproducible nonlethal animal model for studying cyanide poisoning, *Military Med.*, 12, 967–972.

Wexler, J., Whittenberger, J., and Dumke, P. (1947) The effect of cyanide on the electrocardiogram of man, *Am. Heart J.*, 34, 163–173.

CHAPTER 38

Information Management at the Library of Congress: An Overview with Special Reference to Biomedicine*

Roman B. Worobec

CONTENTS

---

* The views expressed in this chapter are solely those of the author and do not necessarily reflect the official views of the Library of Congress.

INTRODUCTION

Casual visitors to the Library of Congress (LC) are often surprised to learn that LC houses extensive collections of materials on science and technology, including life sciences; they expect an institution dedicated to works dealing with the humanities and social sciences.

The underlying philosophy for this universality of LC's holdings is embodied in the following revealing quote:

"... there is, in fact, no subject to which a Member of Congress may not have occasion to refer."

Thomas Jefferson
1814, in a letter to S.H. Smith (Mearns, 1990)

The impetus for this paper was the response that a poster presentation on information analysis at LC elicited at a recent toxicology meeting [Worobec, 2000). The poster attracted a respectable level of interest, challenging questions, insightful commentary, and, again, surprise that LC collects and analyzes items falling into all branches of science and technology. Rather surprisingly, there was considerable interest in how the Library manages its vast holdings and, to an even greater extent, how LC goes about ensuring access to specialized biomedical information. This paper follows up on this interest in the Library and in the manner in which it manages information.

The discourse commences with a cursory historical survey of the Library and the growth of its collections. The intention is to introduce LC as a national information resource center covering virtually all spheres of knowledge. Discussion of information processing practices shall emphasize subject analysis of medical sciences, and provide a behind-the-scenes glimpse of the effort that underlies the bibliographic records seen by those seeking information.

The views expressed in this paper are entirely personal and based on the experience and perceptions of a medical scientist in a library setting. It would certainly be surprising if a professional librarian did not take exception to some of these interpretations and assertions.

A HISTORICAL SKETCH

Although LC is a *de facto* national library and serves a global clientele, as a legislative library its first and foremost obligation is to Congress. In addition to serving as a national knowledge and cultural resource center and as a copyright depository, the Library has also been called upon to fulfill international missions in advancing democracy in the world. For example, in 1947 a *Library of Congress Mission to Japan* provided guidance for the establishment of the National Diet Library, and in the early 1990s, with the collapse of communism, the Library played a similar role vis-à-vis the parliamentary libraries of Central and Eastern Europe (Cole, 1993).

The Library was established by an act of Congress in 1800, after a decade or so of on-and-off deliberations. Among the key players actively supporting the creation of the Library were Thomas Jefferson, John Adams, and James Madison. The initial appropriation consisted of $5,000 for purchasing books "and for fitting up a suitable apartment in the new Capitol as a library."

The first purchase order on behalf of the Library was placed with a London book vendor on June 20, 1800. By May 2, 1801, the contents of a shipment of 11 hair trunks from the dealer— consisting of 152 works in 740 volumes and 3 maps—were ensconced in the Office of the Clerk of the Senate which at that time served as the home of the nascent library.

During the War of 1812 British forces captured Washington and burned the Capitol with its Library on August 24, 1814. By that time the holdings of the Library had grown to over 3,000 volumes and more than 50 maps. Most history books and encyclopedic articles assert that the Library's collection was completely destroyed in the conflagration. Nevertheless, some historical records indicate that Assistant Librarian J. T. Frost and a house clerk, S. Burch, working under extremely adverse conditions, succeeded in saving a number of books and later claimed that the books that were lost "… were all duplicates of those which have been preserved" (Johnston, 1904).

Shortly thereafter, on September 21, 1814, Thomas Jefferson took the initiative to "recommence" the Library by offering to sell his extensive personal library to Congress. A bill was eventually passed on January 30, 1815 by a narrow margin (81 to 71) to purchase Jefferson's library of 6,487 books for $23,950. What made this particular acquisition so unique was that Jefferson's books constituted the largest and the finest library in America at that time, consisting of a multilingual collection encompassing a wide range of topics. As noted in the bill, Congress had indeed secured "a most admirable substratum for a National Library" (Conaway, 2000; Mearns, 1990).

The Library sustained another major loss in 1851 when a fire in the Capitol destroyed most of Jefferson's original library. The surviving 2,465 books are now valued at $5,000 to $50,000 each because of their provenance, and the Library is attempting to reconstitute the original collection through purchases and donations (Gewalt, personal communication).

Despite occasional setbacks the Library's collections, staff, and services continued to expand. In 1897 the Library relocated to its new building across from the Capitol in order to serve its clientele better and accommodate holdings that had grown to about 1 million items. Today, most of the Library's offices and 22 reading rooms are located in three large buildings on Capitol Hill. The total floor space of the three buildings comes to approximately 71 acres.

The Library is headed by the Librarian of Congress, a presidential appointment that became subject to Senate confirmation in 1897. The first Librarian, John J.

Beckley, was appointed by President Thomas Jefferson in 1802. To date, there have been 13 librarians with various backgrounds, including businessmen, political scientists, politicians, journalists, authors, poets, lawyers, historians, a physician (appointed by Abraham Lincoln), and one professional librarian (Cole, 1993).

LC's development and growth are also reflected in its finances. On December 21, 2000, President Clinton signed into law a budget of $547.2 million that had been approved by Congress 6 days earlier. This sum, together with revolving funds, gift and trust funds, reimbursable programs, etc., brings the amount currently available to the Library to $699.2 million (LC Budget, 2001). Another indicator of the Library's importance is the size of its staff. In 1802, the first librarian had one assistant, while the present librarian, Dr. James H. Billington, and the deputy librarian, General Donald C. Scott, oversee a staff of more than 4,200 (Public Affairs Office, 2000).

CURRENT HOLDINGS

LC's holdings at the beginning of the present millennium consist of almost 119 million items in more than 470 languages and various formats, occupying approximately 530 miles of shelf space. This number includes over 18 miillionn cataloged books and more than 9.4 million other printed items, including periodicals, incunabula, dissertations, technical reports, newspapers, etc. Moreover, the Library's special collections house over 90 million maps, manuscripts, visual materials, computer programs, music scores, and so forth. While exact figures are unavailable, it has been estimated that 60 to 70% of the materials are in languages other than English.

Current receipts at the Library run to some 22,000 items each working day, of which approximately 10,000 are selected for addition to the collections (Public Affairs Office, 2000).

SCIENCE AND TECHNOLOGY

It may be of particular interest to scientists to know that LC serves as the repository for one of the largest and most diverse collections of scientific and technical information in the world. The number of books, journals, reprints, dissertations, and other resources in this category is on the order of 5 million items. In addition, the Library also maintains this country's largest collections of technical reports and standards, a figure that now stands at some 4.4 million foreign and domestic items (Public Affairs Office, 2000).

As a historical antecedent it is interesting to note that Jefferson's original library included almost 500 books on various aspects of science and technology. It was from this nucleus that the science collections expanded at an exponential rate and, by the 1940s, had acquired the reputation of being the most diversified and possibly the largest in the United States. The prominence of these holdings led the then-Librarian of Congress Luther H. Evans to describe the Library of Congress as "the National Library of Science as well as the National Library generally" (Evans, 1948).

CLIENT SERVICES STATISTICS

In 1999 the various reference and research arms of the Library and the Copyright Office handled nearly 2 miillion requests for information made in person, by regular mail and e-mail, and by telephone. This figure includes over 545,000 service transactions for Congress carried out by the Congressional Research Service (CRS). CRS is a unit that works exclusively for Congress, providing conventional reference support, confidential consultations, and analytical studies in support of policy decisions.

The Library's global reach is further confirmed by statistics showing that the Library's public Web sites recorded an average of 80 million transactions per month in 1999–2000, while the number of on-site domestic and foreign researchers, readers, and visitors exceeded 2 million annually (Public Affairs Office, 2000).

INFORMATION MANAGEMENT

In the Beginning...

People have been concerned since antiquity with keeping a permanent record of their thoughts, literature, historical events, and business transactions. In the Middle East tens of thousands of Sumerian clay tablets, some dating back to 3000 B.C., attest to the propensity of humans for creating a permanent record of their activities and their ideas. Information retrieval was obviously a problem even then, and one approach was to use the opening words of a text as a title to identify a tablet.

Some larger Babylonian libraries relied on an indexing system to indicate what tablets, appropriately tagged, were stored in a room. In that early information managing system special clay tablets inscribed with the first few words of text from the tagged tablets, i.e., index terms, were kept near the entrance to the room housing the tablets with the full text. Other descriptive information often included the scribes' names, the owner's name, tablet number, and so forth (Strout, 1956). In pharaonic Egypt, lists of titles written on the walls of temples and pyramids indicated which papyri were stored inside. In Mesopotamia the practice was to use the opening words of a text and the names of scribes and their patrons to identify an item, while usually ignoring the names of authors (Johnson and Harris, 1976; Glaister,1979; Eisenstein, 1983).

It seems particularly fitting to note that a 5,000-year-old catalog in Ur anticipated some modern information retrieval concepts. Rather than listing the first few words of a text, the catalog relied on keywords selected from the first two lines of the text to identify a tablet (Dalby, 1986).

In time, scrolls became the medium of choice for record-keeping, to be eventually supplanted by codices in the 4th century A.D. The appearance of the codex was a major breakthrough in written communication because one could easily navigate within a text from page to page. In the Middle Ages, European librarians kept inventories of books arranged by author, title, title catchwords, the first line of a text, or combinations thereof (Johnson and Harris, 1976). Although taken for granted today, a seminal event in bibliographic control was the appearance of the first title page in 1476. By 1500 the title page was firmly established as a convention in publishing. The 16th century witnessed the appearance of tables of contents, summaries, and various indices. These developments facilitated the creation of book lists, catalogs, and other forms of "secondary literature" that ensured access to primary sources of information (Eisenstein, 1983).

Current LC Practices

In its 200 years of existence LC has evolved into the largest research library in the world with vast and complex collections. Recognizing that information that cannot be accessed is lost, the Library developed an elaborate cataloging system to control its collections and ensure subject-based access to information in individual bibliographic items. These practices enable the Library to fulfill its mission " ... to make its resources available and useful to the Congress and the American people and to sustain and preserve a universal collection of knowledge and creativity for future generations" (LC Mission Statement, 2000).

The following discussion shall deal with written works, whether at the hardcopy galley stage, an electronic file, or a *bona fide* publication. In brief, cataloging — or access-facilitating activity — consists of the creation of a specific bibliographic record for each publication. The resultant record consists of a number of *data fields,* each containing distinct information (author, title, publisher, etc.). In modern terminology these various elements of information are referred to as *access points*. Selective searching of access points in a single field or a combination of fields leads to retrieval of a specific publication, or a group of related items that have some access point(s) in common.

In cataloging two categories of information are used to define an item. The more familiar information is that represented by descriptive elements derived from the title page and physical characteristics of a publication, i.e., the author's name, title, etc. The other category is represented by *subject headings*, which are controlled, thematic indicators assigned to reflect the intellectual content of an item (*Library of Congress Subject Headings*, 2000; Chan, 1995). Each category is regulated by codified, time-tested practices and policies to ensure the authority, consistency, and reliability of LC's bibliographic databases.

In functional terms, the present cataloging stream at LC— simplified for convenience — can be distilled into the following five, somewhat arbitrary and overlapping, stages: *preliminary processing, descriptive cataloging, subject cataloging, classification,* and *shelflisting*. The first two stages are concerned with descriptive elements, while the subsequent stages concentrate on the subject matter.

The following is a brief description of the different cataloging stages:

1. *Preliminary processing,* as used here, is not part of cataloging per se, but is carried out at the acquisition stage and is intended to identify a new receipt and place it under immediate control. It involves the assignment of an LC control number and a limited number of descriptive elements.
2. *Descriptive cataloging* is the stage at which an item receives detailed bibliographic description, including information on the author/creator (personal or corporate), editor, publisher, title, edition, language, pagination, presence of illustrations, etc.

This stage also addresses problematic issues related to mis-attributions, different versions of a publication, translations, variant titles, publication conventions in different countries, multipart items, multivolume works, accompanying materials, work-within-a-work materials, name changes, disambiguation of authors, etc. The primary purpose of descriptive cataloging is to identify and provide access to a specific bibliographic entity.

3. *Subject cataloging* is the stage at which an item undergoes subject analysis and assignment of subject headings. This stage will be covered in more detail later. The purpose of subject cataloging is to provide access to the information contained in a bibliographic entity.

4. *Classification*, a component of subject cataloging, entails the assignment of an alphanumeric class number that consigns the item to an appropriate niche in LC's subject classification scheme. For example, the specific number for works on genetic toxicology is RA1224. In the online environment, browsing through class numbers is another easy option to determine what materials a database contains on a given subject. This feature is particularly valuable when access to stacks is denied.

5. *Shelflisting* represents the end stage of cataloging. In shelflisting a class number is transformed into a unique document number based on the author's name, title, year, edition, etc. The item then occupies a unique physical location on a library shelf. For example, RA1224.3.G457 1991 is the specific book number for *Genetic Toxicology*, edited by A.P. Li and R.H. Heflich, and published in 1991.

The alphanumeric classification scheme used at LC was implemented in 1900. It employs letters of the alphabet (A to Z) to indicate broad classes that cover all categories of knowledge, e.g., N for Fine Arts, Q for Science, R for Medicine, T for Technology, etc. Narrower disciplines (subclasses) are indicated by two letters, e.g., QR for Microbiology and Immunology, RB for Pathology, RC for Internal Medicine, and so forth.

A separate division assigns Dewey Decimal Classification numbers to certain LC records for the convenience of institutions that do not use LC classification.

A Historical Perspective

Until mid-1992, the descriptive and subject functions were carried out in different administrative units of the cataloging operation in recognition of the fact that they required staff with markedly different educational backgrounds and competencies. There were two divisions responsible for descriptive cataloging. These were staffed by professional librarians and organized, for the most part, into language-based sections. Although dealing with the seemingly more transparent data in English and other languages, the processing of descriptive information is, nevertheless, a time-consuming and very complex activity controlled in great detail by hundreds of pages of rules, supplemented by hundreds more on "rule interpretations."

Another division in existence at that time, the Subject Cataloging Division (SCD), specialized in subject analysis and classification, and was organized mostly into subject-oriented sections. Publications in the biological and medical sciences, for example, were handled by the Life Sciences Section. SCD included professional staff with educational credentials and experience in various subject areas, and in most cases with high-level competency in the foreign language(s) required for their particular assignment(s). SCD was formed in a 1940 reorganization when the Library recognized the need for "subject specialists, each with a wide range of foreign languages" in the hope of making headway against a backlog of approximately 1.5 million partially processed publications awaiting subject analysis. The need for reorganization was all the more compelling because the backlog was increasing at a rate of 30,000 items per year (*Annual Report of the Librarian of Congress for the Fiscal Year Ending June 30, 1941*, 1942).

In 1992 the cataloging operation was again restructured to resume a holistic approach to information management by combining descriptive and subject functions in one position description. A vision for the future holds that descriptive duties will eventually devolve to library technicians, while the subject-related functions will remain the purview of the professional staff.

The present Cataloging Directorate is one of LC's larger units, and at the end of fiscal year 2000 employed 550 full-time equivalent staff members. It is also the largest cataloging operation in the world and its policies and practices have an international impact. In addition, the number of LC staffers with subject and language expertise exceeds that at any other library anywhere. In fiscal year 2000 the output of the entire cataloging operation exceeded 200,600 items. Publications in biomedicine, biotechnology, and ancillary disciplines are processed within the Medical Sciences and Biotechnology Team (MSBT). With a current staff of eight, MSBT processes 10,000 to 13,000 items per year in various European languages, although nearly 70%of the receipts are in English.

It is an interesting fact that until 1900 the classification scheme employed at LC was essentially that which Thomas Jefferson had used for his library. Jefferson's classification was based on Francis Bacon's ideas for the organization of knowledge; however, LC had modified his scheme for its own use to be more pragmatic and user friendly (LaMontagne, 1961).

Due to the preeminence of its bibliographic resources, funding, and staffing, LC assumed a lead role in developing cataloging and classification practices and standards in the United States more than a century ago. The Library's willingness to share its data with other libraries relieved many of them of the need to do their own original cataloging. This program was so successful that by 1915 the Library was responsible for approximately 75% of the cataloging done in the United States (Bishop, 1916).

SUBJECT-BASED ACCESS TO INFORMATION

Preamble

Information retrieval is a concept of paramount importance in the Information Age. In an ideal world an efficient information retrieval system would retrieve records containing precisely the information that was being sought. In order for information retrieval to be as efficient as possible at LC, information in individual items is tagged with subject descriptors that can be used to formulate highly specific queries.

The first step in providing subject-based access to information is obviously *subject analysis,* or the determination of the theme, scope, and intellectual level of a publication. The salient elements of information are summarized, and the key concepts translated into *subject headings,* i.e., subject descriptors/access points that are assigned to the work at hand. *Subject cataloging,* which by definition consists of subject analysis, assignment of subject headings, and classification, is the primary method employed by LC to provide access to specific information in its collections (Chan, 1995; Foskett, 1996; *Subject Cataloging Manual,* 1996; Hjørland, 1997; Langridge, 1989).

Subject Headings: General Information

Subject headings at LC constitute a controlled vocabulary published annually in hard copy and online formats as the *Library of Congress Subject Headings* (LCSH; 2000). This list is a hierarchical system of concepts that has been in development for over 100 years, and in 1988 was recast into the form of a thesaurus. The 2000 print edition of LCSH consists of five massive, foot-high volumes with a total of 6,677 pages and more than 250,000 entries, of which 30,000 to 35,000 are estimated to be biomedical. LCSH has gained international acceptance and to date has been adopted or adapted for use in Canada, France, England, Switzerland, Iran, Portugal, Belgium, and Brazil, and work along these lines is in progress in several other countries. In addition, LCSH is used extensively by bibliographic utilities and commercial information retrieval services such as DIALOG, WILSONLINE, and others.

LCSH is not a perfect system and never will be, but it has withstood the test of time as an effective tool for accessing information. Despite the overall stability of LCSH, the vocabulary is constantly revised and updated, growing in the past decade at the rate of 6,000 to 10,000 new terms per year. Inconsistencies and shortcomings in LCSH, and occasional baroque terminology, are in many cases a reflection of more than a century of practices and then-prevalent social and political views and fads. Whether internally generated or in response to suggestions and/or pressure from outside interests, archaic or otherwise inappropriate terms are adjusted or replaced. Updating LCSH may be labor-intensive and costly in the case of complicated subject headings with numerous links to other terms. Furthermore, updating of bibliographic records to reflect changes in subject headings may be problematic if a large number of records is involved because of the lack of a global update capability at this time.

Because LC is a comprehensive general library, popular usage in LCSH is favored over scientific designations whenever possible. On the whole, American spelling is preferred, although *sulfur* is spelled *sulphur,* and most sulfur derivatives are spelled with *ph* rather than *f.* This practice reflects conventions dating to the 19th century. Another policy is not to use trademarks as subject headings for drugs and chemicals, relying instead on nonproprietary designations. Thus, the alternate chemical name *Polytef* is used as a subject heading for Teflon®, and *Adrenaline* is employed rather than Adrenalin® (with the appropriate cross-references).

Finally, because of its long history, LCSH contains many quaint and outdated terms. For example, the ill-defined subject heading *Spinal irritation* was first assigned to an item published in 1832, and was last used on a work appearing in 1877.

Rationale for Subject Headings

The rationale for subject headings is to have an agreed-upon, standard, controlled vocabulary to express ideas and concepts found in the literature, regardless of what nomenclature and terminology individual authors may employ (McRay et al., 1994; McRay, 1998). For example, LCSH employs only the term *Congresses* for works that authors may describe as congresses, meetings, conferences, symposia, or colloquia. The strategy in subject cataloging is to use the authorized terms and their allowed permutations in an eclectic and economic manner to express the subject matter of a publication. In a sense, the subject headings system constitutes a terse, stilted, language with its own grammar, syntax, and definitions specifically designed for information access and retrieval. This practice is somewhat analogous to the way sound bites are used to get information across in politics, newscasts, and commercials.

Therefore, the subject heading *Cancer* will always be assigned to works on cancer, although the author may prefer to use malignancy, malignant neoplasia, malignant tumor, or even archiplasm. This heading will also identify publications on cancer in foreign languages that deal with *pistriak, cancro, gan, rak, Krebs, kanker, rakovina,* or *aizheng.* Similarly, *Medical education* will be assigned to general works on medical education, and *Medicine–Study and teaching* will cover publications on the methods of instruction and curricula in the teaching of medicine. Likewise, a journal dedicated to the history of medicine will be found under *Medicine–History–Periodicals,* while a history of medical journals should be sought under *Medicine–Periodicals–History.*

Although access to a publication and, to some extent, subject matter can obviously be attained by searching via descriptive access points, searching by subject headings is generally the most precise and efficient approach to specific information at LC. The search can be fine-tuned through the use of combinations of headings, as well as via "subject strings." The latter involves assigning certain verbal elements (*subdivisions*) to a primary heading to bring out special aspects of a particular topic (*vide infra*). Nevertheless, an appropriate caveat is that any controlled vocabulary system has its limitations and disadvantages, particularly one that covers all subjects and embodies over a century of variable practices.

LC's basic policy is to establish a new subject heading when a work at hand concerns a new topic or a novel concept. This means that in the case of print and electronic galleys a new subject heading may be established for an item before it is published. Comments on the proposed subject heading are solicited from interested parties, and the proposal is redacted at an editorial meeting to ensure appropriate terminology and relationships with existing concepts in LCSH. Finally, an official *subject authority record* is created, authorizing the use of the new term as a subject heading. The final decision on a new heading — and whether a proposal merits discussion — is usually in the hands of a group of cataloging policy specialists rather than the subject specialists. This arrangement ensures invaluable lay input into the entire process in keeping with LC's role as a general library.

The Subject Authority Record

The structure of the subject authority record for *Immunotoxicology* is depicted below to show the basic structure of an uncomplicated record. Each field of information is identified by a numerical tag; explanations have been added to this record for didactic purposes (Figure 38.1).

The **010** tag in Figure 38.1 contains the subject heading authority record identification number (**sh85064594**), with the first two numbers showing that the heading was established in or before 1985. The **053** tag indicates the classification number (**RC582.17**) where works on this topic are classed, and the **150** tag identifies the subject heading. The two **450** tags (*Use For*) list the alternate expressions that guide the searcher to the authorized form of the heading. Anyone entering a search for *Immunotoxicity* in the subject file, for example, would be directed to *Immunotoxicology* as the authorized subject heading. Finally, there are two **550** tags that list *Immunopathology* and *Toxicology* as hierarchically broader subject headings (*Broader Term*), and one **550** field giving *Immunopharmacology* as a related heading (*Related Term*). The record also shows that the different kinds of **550** fields are differentiated by different codes within the **550** field. In their turn, the authority records for *Immunopathology* and *Toxicology* have *Narrower Term* references to *Immunotoxicology* as a subordinate topic, while *Immunopharmacology* has a reciprocal *Related Term* reference to *Immunotoxicology*.

In some cases LCSH still retains "see also" references under a broad or generic heading that directs users to a related group of individual subject headings, a practice that is being phased out. For example, a *see also* notation under the subject heading *Heart* calls the user's attention to *"headings beginning with the words Cardiac or Cardiogenic."* Finally, a number of headings are accompanied by scope notes that may provide cursory explanations and guidance on their consistent application.

Subject Analysis: General Principles

The principles and practices of subject analysis are covered extensively in several excellent monographs (Chan, 1995; Foskett, 1996; Hjørland, 1997; Langridge,

Tag	Field Data	Explanations
010	_a sh 85064594	Record Number
053	_a RC582.17	Class Number
150	_a Immunotoxicology	Subject Heading
450	_a Immunologic toxicology	UF (Use For Term)
450	_a Immunotoxicity	UF (Use For Term)
550	_w g _a Immunopathology	BT (Broader Term)
550	_w g _a Toxicology	BT (Broader Term)
550	_a Immunopharmacology	RT (Related Term)

Figure 38.1 LC authority record for *Immunotoxicology*, supplemented with explanatory notations.

1989). In addition, the concepts of subject analysis have also been addressed by the International Organization for Standardization, which has published guidelines for examining documents and assigning subject headings (ISO No. 5963; International Organization for Standardization, 1985).

The five fundamental principles of subject analysis at LC, especially as applied to MSBT, are outlined here to provided a foundation for the examples of subject heading usage to follow:

1. The purpose of subject analysis is to summarize the content of the item as a whole rather than index all the concepts contained in a work.
2. For a subject access point to be assigned for a given topic, the topic should account for at least 20% of the subject matter in the item.
3. Subject headings should be as precise as possible, neither too broad nor too narrow.
4. New subject headings are established when needed to cover new concepts and topics.
5. Subject headings are always assigned for ground-breaking concepts and advances in biomedicine, no matter how minor a component they may be of the work as a whole.

In the final analysis, successfull subject analysis in the biomedical sciences is dependent on the following factors: (1) broad, high-level subject competency; (2) ability to rapidly identify, interpret, and succinctly conceptualize relevant information; (3) a high degree of familiarity with LCSH in general and with medical subject headings in particular; (4) skill in representation of information by subject headings; (5) facility in rapidly refocusing from topic to disparate topic while remaining productive; and, as in everything else, (6) common sense in formulating subject strings.

In addition to subject expertise, individuals working with foreign language materials should have excellent command of the target language in general, and as it applies to their subject area in particular.

Since LCSH contains many terms that serve as patterns for special situations and provides for subject strings, the number of potential headings reaches into the millions, well beyond the basic 250,000 terms listed in LCSH. A tongue-in-cheek comparison is that the lexicon that the subject specialist has to contend with exceeds even Shakespeare's working vocabulary of some 25,000 words by a wide margin.

Without embarking on a philosophical statement, it seems safe to state that a half century ago the various facets of the health sciences were still fairly well defined and information analysis was relatively uncomplicated. Today, however, the progressive obliteration of barriers among formerly distinct specialties has been accompanied by a rise in interdisciplinary publications. Analyzing and interpreting complex interdisciplinary information that is remote to one's professional background and range of knowledge is a rather daunting proposition. This quandary is further compounded when dealing with multifaceted works that may span medicine, other natural sciences, social sciences, and/or the humanities (Cravens et al., 1996).

For the subject heading approach to information to be valid there has to be a high level of consistency in the independent assignment of subject headings to the same document by different, equally qualified individuals. Unfortunately, robust studies addressing this issue seem to be lacking. Nevertheless, a reanalysis of several papers points to a consistency on the order of 80% in the assignment of subject headings to works on nonmedical topics, as opposed to 10 to 20% for the assignment of uncontrolled keywords (Mann, 1997). A concordance approaching 90% was observed in terms of the first subject heading assigned at LC to high-priority galleys in narrowly focused basic medical disciplines (Worobec, 1996). Considering that one is dealing with subjective factors in assigning subject headings, a concordance on the order of 80% seems quite good. Therefore, based on the available evidence, one can intuit that querying via properly constructed subject headings is likely to yield a four- to eightfold better chance of accessing the desired information than if uncontrolled keywords are used.

Finally, while the overarching principles governing subject analysis are the same for all branches of knowledge, distinctions in the subject matter of the humanities, social sciences, and the natural sciences frequently require different analytical approaches and practices, as well as the use of different sets of subject headings (Foskett, 1996; Hjørland, 1997; Langridge, 1989).

Subject Headings: Select Biomedical Examples

The following are intended to offer a few sample subject headings — largely biomedical — to illustrate their various forms (*Library of Congress Subject Headings*, 2000).

Subject headings may consist of a single word to cover a single topic or discipline: *Immunotoxicology; Apoptosis; Obesity; Glucocorticoids; Toxins; Endocrinology; Psychoneuroimmunology*; *Poly-beta-hydroxybutyrate; Oncogenes; Organotherapy; Psychiatry; Biophysics; Prodrugs.*

Subject headings may consist of multiword terms for concepts that cannot be readily expressed by a single word: *Pulmonary ventilation; Alternative toxicity testing; Writer's cramp; Toxicological interaction; Natural childbirth; Molecular toxicology; Tumescent local anesthesia; Toxic epidermal necrolysis; Computational neuroscience; Drug-nutrient interactions; Antigen-presenting cells; Ukrainian American physicians; African American surgeons; Jewish pharmacists; Internet addiction.*

Popular terms are preferred whenever possible, with appropriate cross-references from unused terms: *Alcohol* (not ethanol); *Adrenaline* (not epinephrine); *Mustard gas* (not dichlorodiethyl sulfide); *Salt* (not sodium chloride).

Headings may include parenthetical qualifiers when needed for clarification or to avoid ambiguities: *Iris (Eye); Iris (Plant); AIDS (Disease); Cold (Disease); AZT (Drug); Free radicals (Chemistry); Crack (Drug); Medical laws and legislation (Canon law); Crowns (Dentistry); Neural networks (Neurobiology); Neural networks (Computer science); Relative biological effectiveness (Radiobiology); High throughput screening (Drug development); Infants (Newborn); Infants (Premature); Organizer (Embryology); Residents (Medicine); Institutional review boards (Medicine); Bases (Chemistry); Bases (Architecture); Bases (Linear Topological Spaces).*

Headings may consist of phrases to encompass complex, multiple-concept themes that would otherwise be difficult to express in an efficient manner: *AIDS (Disease) in old age; Medicine and the humanities; Child sexual abuse by clergy; Medical personnel–caregiver relationships; Physician and patient in literature; Communism and medicine; Fuzzy systems and medicine; Physicians on postage stamps; Hypnotism in ophthalmology.*

Select Subdivision Examples

The use of *subdivisions* in creating subject strings for expressing the special facets of a topic and the format of a work is illustrated by the following examples from bibliographic records: for example, the proceedings of a congress on computer simulation of cardiac pathophysiology received the heading *Heart–Pathophysiology–Computer simulation–Congresses,* where the three verbal elements after the primary subject heading *Heart* are examples of subdivisions. An atlas on myocardial infarction received the heading *Heart–Infarction–Atlases.* A work dealing with the involvement of concerned citizens in AIDS prevention in the United States was described by the following subject string: *AIDS (Disease)–United States–Prevention–Citizen participation.* Likewise, a publication on mathematical modeling of dose-response relationships in toxicology received *Toxicology–Dose-response relationships–Mathematical models.* An item on testing dental materials for toxicity was described by *Dental materials–Toxicity testing,* while a publication dealing with the toxicity of such materials in general received the string *Dental materials–Toxicity.*

Finally, a publication designed to provide information on "best" medical care in the Chicago area, *How to Find the Best Doctors: Metropolitan Chicago,* 1999, received the following array of headings: (1) *Physicians–Chicago Metropolitan Area–Directories*; (2) *Physicians–Rating of–Chicago Metropolitan Area–Directories*; (3) *Medicine–Specialties and specialists–Chicago Metropolitan Area–Directories*; (4) *Hospitals–Chicago Metropolitan Area–Directories*; (5) *Medical centers–Chicago Metropolitan Area–Directories.* This combination of subject strings clearly indicates the type of information included in the publication, serving in effect as an indicative abstract of the work.

Because subdivisions are essential for specificity in subject analysis and the information retrieval system at LC, the following are some additional examples of the flexibility and specificity they impart to subject strings: *Brain–Localization of functions–Research–History*; *Drugs–Generic substitution*; *German language–Medical German–Word formation*; *Artificial intelligence–Medical applications–Periodicals–Indexes*; *Gentamicin–PMMA chains*; *Human beings–Effect of environment on*; *Antipsychotic drugs–Dose-response relationship*; *Drugs–Structure-activity relationships*; *Diagnosis–Decision making*; *Molecular biology–Computer network resources*; *Extreme environments–Physiological effect–Congresses–Abstracts*; *Harvard Medical School–Humor.*

The purpose of these examples was to reinforce the view that LC subject headings and subdivisions constitute a flexible, yet disciplined linguistic environment that can be quite effective in subject analysis and information retrieval.

LCSH: Coda

The medical component of LCSH constitutes one of the earlier examples of a general controlled medical vocabulary, and has served as a model for other efforts along these lines. The proliferation of health sciences literature has triggered the appearance of numerous general and specialized biomedical databases. Most of them are accompanied by controlled vocabularies to provide an infrastructure for the biomedical concepts and disciplines they cover. The development of new controlled vocabularies in various disciplines may be regarded as further proof of their acceptance by scientific and library communities as effective information retrieval tools for analog and digital databases (Anderson et al., 2000; Malet et al., 1999; Markovitz, 2000; National Library of Medicine, 2001; Rogers, 1968).

INFORMATION RETRIEVAL

It should be kept in mind that the search strategies discussed here are within the context of the LC online public-access bibliographic system. As noted earlier, a subject heading-based search can be fine-tuned through the use of specific headings, combinations of headings, and by further refinement of each primary heading by subdivisions. This approach, in combination with the availability of truncation, wildcat characters, Boolean operators *(AND, OR, NOT)*, and the opportunity to search by selected data fields and field combinations, makes for a very powerful, efficient, and consistent information retrieval system. Subject-based searching, in addition to accessing information in foreign languages, also obviates problems posed by nonstandard terminology, variable spellings, typographic errors, variant word orders, and singular and plural verbal forms.

Although search strategies based on natural language querying are conceptually appealing, the complexity of English and its rich vocabulary may pose problems in selecting appropriate search terms since there may be only a 10 to 20% agreement among individuals when thinking of keywords to describe a topic (Mann, 1997). Moreover, keywords generally require more time and considerably more tweaking for acceptable results. Nonetheless, keywords and fixed phrases are often valuable and common sense adjuncts to subject heading-based searches (Foskett, 1996; Hjørland, 1997).

In the final analysis, however, successful searching at LC for information via subject headings depends on four factors: (1) high-quality subject analysis and assignment of appropriate subject headings; (2) good understanding of LCSH and its use in the domain of interest; (3) concise, precise, and logical formulation of a query; and (4) a more than perfunctory familiarity with the LC information retrieval system.

While the first factor is beyond the control of the information-seeking client, and the second may not be practicable, the third and fourth may also pose barriers to successful information retrieval and be an occasion for embarrassment. There are studies indicating that while most users of online systems prefer to access information via subject searching, the majority run into difficulties because of unfamiliarity and inexperience with this modality (Markey, 1984; Drabenstott and Visine-Goetz, 1994). On balance, then, the best approach usually is to rely on a reference professional who is well versed in controlled vocabulary searching in the area of interest, and experienced in subtle and refined forms of interrogation that reveal what information the client actually desires. Reference librarians have compiled many anecdotes about patrons who may be leading experts in their own fields, yet cannot find the information they desire in their particular discipline. As a librarian at Harvard put it decades ago, " ... they will choke to death and die with the secret in them rather than tell you what they want ..." (Wilcox, 1922).

An uncomplicated example should suffice to illustrate the difference between keyword and specific subject heading searches, as well as the need for understanding LC's controlled vocabulary in designing specific queries.

One familiar with the structure and operation of LCSH and interested in works on the general history of medicine would formulate his or her subject heading query as *Medicine–History*. Currently, this search yields 658 works in various languages either wholly devoted to the general history of medicine, or in which medical history is a significant component. Materials on particular countries, conference proceedings, specific time periods, or any other special aspect would not be retrieved because they were not specified. For example, publications on the history of medicine in 18th century Germany would not be retrieved, but the query *Medicine–Germany–History–18th century* would yield seven relevant records. Similarly, the search *Medicine–Japan–History* yields 32 documents on the history of medicine in Japan, but anyone specifically interested in the history of medicine in Kyoto needs to search *Medicine–Japan–Kyoto–History* to readily access the six documents concentrating on that specific topic. Of course, there is always the longer option of browsing through all 212 records dealing with the history of medicine in Japan to target publications of interest.

On the other hand, a keyword search in the subject heading field with the words *history* and *medicine* yields a barrage of over 5,000 hits because both terms were found in the subject field, but not necessarily in the sense of "history of medicine." Keyword searches limited to titles are also hit-or-miss propositions because the wording may be nonspecific or in a foreign language. For example, the following works with information on the history of medicine — as indicated by a subject search — would be missed in title searches: *Rekishi no naka no yamai to igaku, From Witchcraft to Antisepsis: A Study in Antithesis, Magic and Healing, The Patient's Progress, Od kamennoho noze ke skalpu,* and *Progress and Regress!*

The Futility Point

While much is being written about efficient searching strategies, relevance, recall, precision, Venn diagrams for overlapping hits, and search engines, the concept of the *futility point* (FP) is often neglected. FP refers to the number of hits that searchers are actually likely to read before rejecting large retrievals as impractical and useless. Consequently, FP has direct bearing on the importance of specificity in subject searching because high specificity limits retrieval to the most relevant items. Although it depends on an individual's perseverance, need, and commitment to scholarship, there are studies pointing to different FP limits among the different branches of learning. In engineering the average FP has been reported to be about 10 hits, in social studies around 30, and in medicine approximately 60 (Blair, 1980; Lantz, 1981).

The concept embodied in FP, as a common sense parameter, should be juxtaposed with the large numbers of hits that Web search engines are prone to generate (Peterson, 1997). One anecdote circulating among information professionals is about a Zen librarian getting 28 million hits while searching for "nothing" on the Internet. Furthermore, some search engines have been reported to be programmed to give preferential "ranking" to some Web sites regardless of their merits (Corn, 1996). Accordingly, in order to bring some order out of chaos in this electronic soup, it has been suggested that subject cataloging of the high-quality information resources on the Web may prevent their being swamped by resources of dubious value (Peterson, 2001; Gorman, 1998; Coiera, 2000).

THE MARC RECORD*

For those who may be interested in arcane minutiae, this section offers a look at the raw bibliographic record as it exists in the Information Age. To begin with, a traditional LC catalog card (Figure 38.2) will be compared with its modern counterpart, the so-called MARC record (Figure 38.3). In both figures the records have been slightly simplified to eliminate undue clutter.

MARC formats, MARC records, MARC standards, and *MARC-compatible* are phrases that have acquired prominence in information and library science with the transition to the online environment. Accordingly, a cursory explanation of the MARC paradigm and comparison with the traditional catalog card may be of some interest to those who still remember the old days. The catalog card began life during the French Revolution when the libraries of the nobility were confiscated, and the

---

Genetic toxicology / editors, Albert P. Li, Robert H. Heflich. --
Boca Raton : CRC Press, cl991.
x, 493 p. : ill. ; 24 cm.

Includes bibliographical references.
Includes index.
ISBN 0-8493-8815-3

1. Genetic toxicology.   I. Li, A. P.   II. Heflich, Robert U., 1946-

[DNLM: 1. Carcinogens. 2. Chromosome Abnormalities--chemically induced. 3. Mutagens--adverse effects. 4. Mutation.   QH 465.C5 G328]
RA1224.3.G457   1991   615.9'02--dc20   90-11279
   DNLM/DLC
   for Library of Congress

Figure 38.2 Traditional LC catalog card for *Genetic Toxicology,* Li, AP, and Heflich, RH, editors, 1991.

* MARC Web site: http://lcweb.loc.gov/marc/umb (3 January 2001).

Tag	Ind I	Ind 2	Field Data
000			01037pam__2200325_a_4500
001			996520
005			9910520155750.7
008			900824sl991____njua____b____001_0_eng_c
035			_9 (DLC) 90011279
906			_a 7 _b cbc _c orignew _d 1 _e ocip _f 19 _g y-gencatlg
955			_a CIP ver. ea10 to SL 05-13-91
010			_a 90011279
020			_z 0849388153
040			_a DNLM/DLC _c DLC _d DLC
050	0	0	_a RA1224.3 _b .G457 1991
060			_a QH 465.C5 G328
082	0	0	_a 615.9/02 _2 20
245	0	0	_a Genetic toxicology / _c editors, Albert P. Li, Robert H. Heflich.
260			_a Boca Raton : _b CRC Press, _c cl991.
300			_a x, 493 p. : _b ill. ; _c 24 cm.
504			_a Includes bibliographical references.
500			_a Includes index.
650		0	_a Genetic toxicology.
650		2	_a Carcinogens.
650		2	_a Chromosome Abnormalities _x chemically induced.
650		2	_a Mutagens _x adverse effects.
650		2	_a Mutation.
700	1		_a Li, A. P.
700	1		_a Heflich, Robert H., _d 1946-
991			_b c-GenColl _h RA1224.3 _i .G457 1991 _t Copy 1 _w

Figure 38.3 LC MARC record for *Genetic Toxicology*, Li, AP, and Heflich, RH, editors, 1991.

revolutionaries started keeping track of books on the backs of playing cards. The rest is history, and the catalog card remained at the center of information retrieval in libraries until about two decades ago.

MARC stands for *MA*chine-*R*eadable *C*ataloging record, with "machine-readable" referring to the fact that a computer armed with the appropriate software can recognize and process the bibliographic data in a MARC record. In today's world, the online display of a MARC record has generally replaced the traditional 3×5 catalog card. The MARC format was designed for automated control of bibliographic data via data storage, manipulation, and retrieval, as well as for efficient interinstitutional transmission of information.

The MARC format was developed at LC in the 1960s. The Library continues to maintain the basic documentation, but changes and revisions are made in concert with other libraries, information centers, professional and scholarly associations, commercial vendors, and bibliographic utilities.

The level of bibliographic data may vary among libraries and countries, thus the existence of different, mutually intelligible versions designated as LCMARC, USMARC, UKMARC, CANMARC, UNIMARC (UNIversal MARC), etc. (The acronyms may also reveal the country of origin of a given MARC standard.) However, the differences among them are minor and MARC 21, created by merging USMARC and CANMARC, has been designated the 21st century standard.

The most important advantage of a single global standard is that it fosters information sharing, prevents duplication of work, and promotes quality control because a record may be scrutinized by many more professionals. Furthermore, because MARC is an industry-wide standard, libraries and information services are free to select commercial automation systems that best meet their individual needs while retaining data compatibility.

Finally, the old card catalog was inefficient in that it had to utilize multiple, alphabetically filed cards for one publication to bring out various access points (author, title, subject). The MARC record, on the other hand, is a single source of far more information.

The MARC record consists of a standardized system of numbers, letters, and other symbols that specify individual elements and sub-elements of bibliographic information. This information is contained in various *fields* that are identified by three-digit numerical *tags*. The tagging structure enables software to identify and interpret each of these elements. For example, topical subject headings are found in fields identified by the **650** tag, while the **856** field is reserved for Electronic Location and Access information such as e-mail addresses and URLs (Uniform Resource Locators).

Most of the elements in the two versions of the record are self-explanatory. However, the more extensive information in the MARC record (Figure 38.3) tells us that this book was originally cataloged at the galley stage, i.e., before it was published. This fact is indicated by the **_d 1** and **_e ocip** codes in the **906** field. The data also show that the record was part of a cooperative program and contains classification numbers and subject headings assigned by LC and the National Library of Medicine (NLM). The LC class number **(RA1224.3.G457 1991)** is indicated by the **050** field, and its subject heading **(Genetic toxicology)** in the **650** field is identified by the **0** value in the second indicator position **(Ind 2)**. The classification number assigned by NLM **(QH465.C5 G328)** is found in the **060** field, while the four NLM subject headings in the **650** field are identified by the value **2** in the second indicator position. In the old catalog card the NLM data were included in the two bracketed lines in lower portion of the card (Figure 38.2).

At this point it should be noted that the catalog card (Figure 38.2) and the MARC record (Figure 38.3) for the publication under discussion are atypical as they contain NLM data. Only a small fraction of LC records contains information contributed by other institutions.

The Library's OPAC (Online Public Access Catalog) offers several options in viewing retrieved records. Most patrons appear to prefer the *Full Record* display (Figure 38.4), which contains the type of information found in Figure 38.2, but with line-by-line explanations. However, LC and NLM subject headings are not differentiated if both are present. The OPAC also offers the *MARC Tags* option that displays the information depicted in Figure 38.3, but in a somewhat different format. It is safe to assume that few library patrons would willingly elect the last option.

Finally, the *Genetic Toxicology* record used here also exemplifies the LC policy of assigning a single, specific subject heading that summarizes the entire scope of an item. In this case, the LC subject heading and the subject matter of the work form a perfect match.

Genetic toxicology / editors, Albert P. Li, Robert H. Heflich	
LC Control Number:	90011279
Main Title:	Genetic toxicology / editors, Albert P. Li, Robert H. Heflich
Published/Created:	Boca Raton : CRC Press, c1991.
Related Names:	Li, A. P.
	Heflich, Robert H., 1946-
Description:	x, 493 p.,: ill.; 24 cm.
ISBN:	0849388153
Notes:	Includes index.
	Includes bibliographical references.
Subjects:	Genetic toxicology.
	Carcinogens.
	Chromosome Abnormalities--chemically induced.
	Mutagens--adverse effects.
	Mutation.
LC Classification:	RA1224.3 .G457 1991
NLM Class No.:	QH465.C5 G328
Dewey Class No.:	615.9/02 20

Figure 38.4 LC OPAC Full Record display for *Genetic Toxicology*, AP Li, and RH Heflich, editors, 1991.

EPILOGUE

Much of the language employed in librarianship and information science originated in the "book" world, and is now supplemented by neologisms reflecting the Digital Age. Thus, the expression *cataloging data* is now joined by *metadata,* the latter applied to electronic formats. Metadata is popularly defined as data about data, or more explicitly as information about the structure and content of a record. Computers have dramatically changed the manner in which information is processed, analyzed, rendered accessible, and delivered. Availability of computational support also led to the replacement of the catalog card by the machine- or computer-readable cataloging record in the online environment. As a result, the very term *cataloging* — so intimately connected with books and volumes and beloved by librarians — seems to have acquired a somewhat antiquated connotation in this day and age, and may be due for replacement with a term more in tune with information analysis and informatics.

Today, many of the practices LC developed over the years to manage its collections and provide access to information are being challenged by digital reality as LC enters the 21st century. As part of its response to the new reality, LC has implemented a digitization program and recently hosted a conference to assess methods of providing "improved access to Web resources through library catalogs and application of metadata" (*Bicentennial Conference on Bibliographic Control for the New Millennium*, 2000). To keep up with the phenomenal growth of information and the variety of formats in which it is being packaged, LC's use of advanced information technologies is being complemented by cooperative ventures with partners sharing similar interests.

The issues faced by LC involve assessing and developing the technological infrastructure for capturing, saving, analyzing, preserving, and ensuring access to collections derived from selected Web sites. These so-called "born digital" resources are created in electronic form and usually lack an analog counterpart, i.e., a hard-copy or print format. Additional complications arise from the copyright implications of archiving such materials and providing access to their contents. These problems are exacerbated by the inherent fluidity of Web sites, with the need to contend with constantly changing formats and revised information (Coiera, 2000; Gorman, 1998; Markovitz, 2000; Morris, 2000).

A National Research Council study commissioned by the Library in 1998 has addressed these issues. The study recommended that the Library approach these challenges by classifying collectable digital resources into four categories: (1) materials that would be owned and archived/preserved by the Library, (2) materials that would be owned but not permanently archived, (3) materials that would mirror remote access materials on the Library's Web site, and (4) remote-access materials to which the Library would provide links from its Web site (*LC21: A Digital Strategy for the Library of Congress*, 2000). A recent agreement that falls under the first recommendation commits LC to owning, serving, and permanently archiving the electronic journals of the American Physical Society (Morris, 2000).

The online *Science* journal produced by the American Association for the Advancement of Science exemplifies the type of complications posed by the dynamic nature of electronic resources. To begin with, the online version is a much larger and a more complex entity than the weekly print copy and, unlike the fixed information in the print copy, the information in the corresponding online issue is subject to periodic revisions. Moreover, further variability is introduced because the contents of online *Science* may be customized to satisfy the interests of individual subscribers via links to a current awareness service (Morris, 2000; *Science* online, 2000).

While some librarians are concerned with the practical side of the here-and-now and adaptation to ongoing changes in technology, others take a more futuristic stance and see the Internet and advanced computers as a panacea for knowledge management and information retrieval. They feel that increasingly powerful Internet search engines, with their capacity to scour the estimated 3 billion Web sites that have been created to date, will provide the solution to the global information glut. One LC consultant has predicted that "brute force computing — simple algorithms plus immense computing power — may outperform human intelligence" and will render MARC and other standards obsolete, although allowing that human intelligence itself cannot be replaced by computers (Arms, 2000).

Because of their number-crunching power in manipulating and representing data, computers are of inestimable value in information retrieval via access points. But what are the implications of computer power and artificial intelligence for subject analysis, if any? Will it be possible to scan an entire text or selected portions into a computer and have an expert system determine the topic(s) and assign appropriate, coordinated subject headings and subject strings? Decades of attempts have shown that no expert system can match the human brain when it comes to the type of reasoning and decision-making required for high-caliber information extraction, conceptualization, subject analysis, or foreign language translation. Current expert systems that have been spoon-fed specific baseline information offer speed, automate the more routine decision-making, and function very well indeed within restricted domains according to "if-then" rules (Association for Machine Translation in the Americas, 1998; Krings, 2001; Pazienza, 1999; Sabourin, 1994; Schwarzl, 2001; Whitelock and Kilby, 1995). However, in a broad realm of limitless, diverse information — a domain that is not artificially constrained and predefined — expert systems may provide, at best, some inkling as to what a document is all about. This level of *topic spotting* has given prominence to the now widely used neologism *gisting*. In fact, the Defense Intelligence Agency (DIA) has developed an efficient machine translation program appropriately named *Gister* to indicate its functionality. At a recent DIA meeting addressing these issues, the keynote theme cautioned the attendees not to "give up on the brain," since there is nothing better on the horizon (Defense Intelligence Analysis Center, 2001).

REFERENCES

Anderson, C.A., Copestake, P.T., and Robinson, L. (2000) A specialist toxicity database (TRACE) is more effective than its larger, commercially available counterparts, *Toxicology,* 151, 37–43.

Arms, W.Y. (2000) quoted in Fineberg, G. and Arcaro, T. Interpreting the past, shaping the future: library hosts symposium on national libraries, *Library of Congress Information Bulletin,* 59, 290–292, 307.

Association for Machine Translation in the Americas (1998) Machine translation and the information soup, in *3rd Conf. of the AMTA, AMTA '98,* October 28–31, 1998, Farwell, D. et al., Eds., Springer, New York.

Bicentennial Conference on Bibliographic Control for the New Millennium: Confronting the Challenges of Networked Resources and the Web (2000) Library of Congress, Washington, D.C., http://lcweb.loc.gov/catdir/bibcontrol/.

Bishop, W.W. (1916) *Cataloging as an Asset: An Address to the New York State Library School, May 1, 1915,* The Waverly Press, Baltimore, MD.

Blair, D.C. (1980) Searching biases in large interactive document retrieval systems, *J. Am. Soc. Inform. Sci.,* 17, 271–277.

Chan, L.M. (1995) *Library of Congress Subject Headings: Principles and Application,* 3rd Ed., Libraries Unlimited, Inc., Englewood, CO.

Coiera, E. (2000) Information economics and the Internet, *J. Am. Inform. Assoc.,* 7(3), 215–221.

Cole, J.Y. (1993) Jefferson's Legacy: A Brief History of the Library of Congress, Library of Congress, Washington, D.C., 1993.

Conaway, J. (2000) *America's Library: The Story of the Library of Congress, 1800–2000,* Yale University Press in association with the Library of Congress, New Haven, CT.

Corn, D. (1996) Anatomy of a netscam: why your Internet search may not be as honest as you think, *Washington Post,* July 7, p. C5.

Cravens, H., Marcus, A.I., and Katzman, D.M. (1996) *Tehcnical Knowledge in American Culture: Science, Technology, and Medicine Since the Early 1800s,* University of Alabama Press, Tuscaloosa.

Dalby, A. (1986) The Sumerian catalogs, *J. Library Hist.,* 21, 475–487.

Defense Intelligence Analysis Center (July 16, 2001) 2nd Foreign Language and Technology Day, Bolling Air Force Base, Washington, D.C.

Drabenstott, K.M. and Visine-Goetz, D. (1994) *Using Subject Headings for Online Retrieval*, Academic Press, San Diego, CA.

Eisenstein, E.L. (1983) *The Printing Revolution in Early Modern Europe*, Cambridge University Press, Cambridge.

Evans, H.E. (1948) The Library of Congress as the National Library of Science, *The Scientific Monthly*, 66, 405–412.

Foskett, A.C. (1996) *The Subject Approach to Information*, 5th Ed., Library Assoc. Publishing, London.

Gawalt, G.W. (January 12, 2001) Manuscript Historian, Library of Congress, personal communication.

Glaister, J.S. (1979) *Glaister's Glossary of Books*, 3rd ed., George Allen & Unwin, London.

Gorman, M. (1998) The future of cataloguing and catalogers, *Int. Catalog Bibl. Control*, 27(4), 68–71.

Hjørland, B. (1997) *Information Seeking and Subject Representation: An Activity-Theoretical Approach to Information Sciences*, Greenwood Press, London.

ISO Standard No. 5963 (1985) International Organization for Standardization, Methods for Examining Documents, Determining Their Subjects, and Selecting Indexing Terms, International Organization for Standardization, Geneva.

Johnson, E.D. and Harris, M.H. (1976) *History of Libraries in the Western World*, 3rd ed., Scarecrow Press, Metuchen, NJ.

Johnston, W.D. (1904) History of the Library of Congress, 1800–1864, Vol. 1, Library of Congress, Washington, D.C.

Krings, H.P. (2001) Repairing Texts: Empirical Investigations of Machine Translation Post-Editing Processes, translated from German by Koby, J.S. et al., Kent State University Press, Kent, OH.

LaMontagne, L.E. (1961) *American Library Classification, with Special Reference to the Library of Congress*, Shoe String Press, Hamden, CT.

Langridge, S.W. (1989) *Subject Analysis: Principles and Procedures*, Bowker-Saur, London.

Lantz, B.E. (1981) The relationship between documents read and relevant references retrieved as effectiveness measures, *J. Document*, 37(3), 134–145.

LC (1942) Annual Report of the Librarian of Congress for the Fiscal Year Ending June 30, 1941, Library of Congress, Washington, D.C.

LC Budget (2001) Public Affairs Office Information Sheet, Library of Congress, Washington, D.C.

LC Mission Statement (December 27, 2000) http://lcweb.loc.gov/ndl/mission.html.

Library of Congress Subject Headings, 23rd ed. (2000) Library of Congress, Washington, D.C., 5 vols.

Malet, G., Munoz, F., Appleyard, R., and Hersh, W. (1999) A model for enhancing Internet medical document retrieval with "Medical Core Metadata," *J. Am. Med. Inform. Assoc.*, 6, 163–172.

Mann, T. (1997) "Cataloging must change!" and indexer consistency studies: misreading the evidence at our peril, *Cataloging & Classification Q.*, 23(3/4), 3–45.

MARC Web site (January 3, 2001) http://lcweb.loc.gov/marc/umb.

Markey, K. (1984) *Subject Searching in Library Catalogs: Before and After the Introduction of Online Catalogs*, OCLC, Dublin, OH.

Markovitz, B.P. (2000) Biomedicine's electronic publishing paradigm shift: copyright policy and PubMed Central, *J. Am. Med. Inform. Assoc.*, 7, 222–227.

McRay, A.T. (1998) The nature of lexical knowledge, *Methods Inf. Med.*, 37(4–5), 353–360.

McRay, A.T., Srinivasan, S., and Browne, A.C. (1994) Lexical methods for managing variation in biomedical terminologies, *Proc. Annu. Symp. Comput. Appl. Med. Care*, 235–239.

Mearns, D.C. (1990)*The Story Up to Now: The Library of Congress 1800–1946*, Library of Congress, Washington, D.C.

Morris, S. (2000) Born digital planning retreat, *Library Services News*, 8(1), 8–9.

National Library of Medicine (January 30, 2001) Fact Sheet: Unified Medical Language System, http://www.nlm.nih.gov/pubs/factsheets/umls.html.

NRC (July 26, 2000) *LC21: A Digital Strategy for the Library of Congress*, Prepublication Copy, National Research Council, Washington, D.C.

Pazienza, M.T., Ed. (1999) *Information Extraction: Towards Scalable, Adaptable Systems*, Springer-Verlag, New York.

Peterson, R.E. (January 2, 1997) Eight Internet search engines compared, *First Monday*, 2(2), http://www.firstmonday.dk/issues/issue2_2/peterson/.

Public Affairs Office, Library of Congress (1999, 2000) *Fascinating Facts about LC*.

Rogers, F.B. (1968) Problems of medical subject cataloging, *Bull. Med. Libr. Assoc.*, 56, 355–364.

Sabourin, C. (1994) *Computational Linguistics in Information Science: Information Retrieval (Full-Text or Conceptual). Automatic Indexing, Text Abstraction, Content Analysis, Information Extraction, Query Languages*, Infolingua, Montreal.

Schwarzl, A. (2001) *The (Im)Possibilities of Machine Translation*, Peter Lang, New York.

Science online (December 1, 2000) http://www.scienceonline.org/.

Strout, R.F. (1956) The development of the catalog and catalog codes, *Library Q.*, 26, 254–275.

Subject Cataloging Manual, 5th ed. (1996) Library of Congress, Washington, D.C., 4 vols.

Whitelock, P. and Kilby, K. (1995) *Linguistic and Computational Techniques in Machine Translation System Design*, 2nd ed., UCL Press, London.

Wilcox, E.V. (1922) Why do we have librarians? *The Harvard Graduates' Mag.*, 30, 477–491.

Worobec, R.B. (1996) Consistency in medical subject analysis: evaluation of 300 pharmacology, toxicology, and biochemistry CIPs, unpublished findings.

Worobec, R.B. (2000) *Subject Analysis and Intellectual Access to Biomedical Information at the Library of Congress (Poster)*, paper presented at the 2000 Alternative Toxicological Methods Symposium, November 28–December 1, U.S. Army Center for Health Promotion and Preventive Medicine, Aberdeen Proving Ground, MD, p. 17.

CHAPTER 39

World Wide Web Biomedical, Chemical, and Toxicological Information Resources from the National Library of Medicine

George C. Fonger, James Knoben, Stephanie Publicker, Philip Wexler, and Georgette Whiting

CONTENTS

INTRODUCTION AND BACKGROUND

The National Library of Medicine (NLM), on the campus of the National Institutes of Health, is the world's largest medical library. Its collections number approximately 6 million items, among which are many materials relating to toxicology. The origin of providing toxicological databases dates to 1967, when the Toxicology Information Program was formed at NLM in response to recommendations in the report, *Handling of Toxicological Information,* prepared by the President's Science Advisory Committee.

For more than 30 years, the NLM's division of Specialized Information Services (SIS) has managed the Toxicology and Environmental Health Information Program (TEHIP). TEHIP (see homepage, Figure 39.1) has been at the forefront in designing and implementing publicly accessible databases in toxicology and related disciplines. Its major information initiative is the creation of the Toxicology Data Network, or TOXNET, which consists of computerized databases that cover diverse subjects related to the health effects of chemicals in humans and animals, as well as their effects upon the environment.

The introduction of the TOXNET system revolutionized the methods by which bibliographic files and factual databases could be created, maintained, and updated (Wexler, 2001). TOXNET, which began life on a minicomputer, went through a number of system migrations over the years (Vasta and Wexler, 1985). Currently, TOXNET and its resident files are available via the World Wide Web. These databases are made available to users free of charge, and no registration is required to use the web-based system (NLM/SIS, 2002). Figure 39.2 displays a search on TOXNET's page.

BIBLIOGRAPHIC DATABASES

TOXLINE provides about 3 million bibliographic citations to numerous journals that specialize in the broad scope of toxicology, environmental health, pharmacology, metabolism, carcinogenesis, epidemiological studies, and occupational medicine. TOXLINE references can be searched using the Chemical Abstracts Service Registry Number (CAS RN), chemical name, or subject-related terms.

TOXLINE is divided into two major parts: (1) TOXLINE core, which is comprised of standard literature citations and is a limit subset of the MEDLINE database that is searchable on PubMed, and (2) TOXLINE special, found on the TOXNET system, which includes special technical reports, notices of research projects, and collections with historical significance. Both components may be searched through TOXNET, with results displayed separately or together (Wexler, 2001).

DART/ETIC (Developmental and Reproductive Toxicology/Environmental Teratology Information Center) provides bibliographic data on the effects of chemicals, drugs, and physical agents that may have adverse effects on reproductive systems and fetal development.

FACTUAL DATABASES

The Hazardous Substances Data Bank (HSDB) is an important TOXNET database. HSDB now contains over 4,500 chemical-specific records, including high-production and high-volume chemicals, acutely toxic chemicals, fungicides, herbicides, pesticides, and rodenticides, as well as solvents, chemical intermediates, plant and animal toxins, and drugs with adverse effects on humans and the environment. HSDB is divided into the following broad subject categories:

- Administrative information
- Substance identification
- Manufacturing/use information
- Chemical and physical properties
- Safety and handling
- Toxicity/biomedical effects
- Pharmacology
- Environmental fate/exposure potential
- Exposure standards and regulations

- Monitoring and analysis methods
- Additional references

HSDB is a factual database that is fully referenced and scientifically reviewed by the scientific review panel (SRP), an advisory group that examines the chemical records for accuracy. The SRP is made up of nationally and internationally known specialists in general toxicology, as well as industrial hygiene, pharmacology, teratogenesis, medical surveillance, and other subject areas, such as environmental chemistry, regulatory requirements, and engineering, including treatment, clean up, and disposal of hazardous chemicals (Fonger et al., 2000).

Through its TOXNET system, NLM complements HSDB by offering databases in special topic areas of toxicology including the following:

The Chemical Carcinogenesis Research Information System (CCRIS) is funded and produced by the National Cancer Institute (NCI). CCRIS provides fully referenced citations and data on carcinogenicity, mutagenicity, tumor promotion, and tumor inhibition studies. The data found in CCRIS are reviewed by NCI scientists and advisors for scientific accuracy.

The GENE-TOX database is a peer-reviewed database that details mutagenicity data from highly respected journals. GENE-TOX is funded and built by the Environmental Protection Agency (EPA).

The Integrated Risk Information System (IRIS) is also built and maintained by the EPA. Data found in this factual databank cover the carcinogenic and noncarcinogenic risks from chemical exposure. The data are referenced and undergo review by EPA scientists and other advisory panels (Wexler, 2001).

The Toxics Release Inventory (TRI files) are built and maintained by the EPA. They contain estimated releases of toxic chemicals to the environment (air, soil, water, and underground injection) by industry. TRI details the name of the facility, addresses, contact points, and pollution prevention measures, such as chemical treatment and offsite disposal and recycling (Bronson, 1991).

Because the vast majority of toxicology research is concerned with the effects of chemicals, ChemID*plus* (Chemical Identification File) is of tremendous value for accurately identifying chemicals by their names, molecular formulae, structures, and Chemical Abstracts Service Registry Numbers. This file provides factual data in chemical-specific records for names, synonyms, molecular formulae, and structure proximity searching and includes active links to regulatory data and other information resources at the substance level.

SIS/TEHIP also maintains specialized bibliographies about environmental justice and herbal medicines. AltBib, another World Wide Web resource, is an extensive, searchable bibliographic database of citations and abstracts concerning alternatives to the use of live vertebrates in biomedical research and testing. AltBib includes abstracts taken from TOXLINE and other scientific information sources and covers the years 1992 through June 2002. In addition, the AltBib database is available in downloadable quarterly compilations. AltBib is easily searched by author names and special categories, which include the following: carcinogenesis; cytotoxicity; dermal toxicity; ecotoxicity; mutagenesis; hepatic, renal, ocular, and pulmonary toxicology; and immunotoxicity studies.

National Library of Medicine
Specialized Information Services
About • Contact • Search
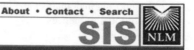

Toxicology and Environmental Health

TOXNET
Databases in toxicology and environmental health.

TOXLINE	HSDB	ChemIDplus
DART	TRI	IRIS
GENE-TOX	CCRIS	

Special Topics
Evaluated links to Internet resources on current issues such as arsenic or chemical warfare.

Haz-Map
Database on hazardous chemicals and occupational diseases.

AltBib
References about alternatives to the use of live animals in biomedical research and testing.

Toxicology Tutor
Three self-guided tutorials on toxicology.

News and Events
Links to news items on the web site, outreach activities and a calendar of events.

Consumer Health
MEDLINEplus
     Poisoning,Toxicology and
     Environmental Health
DIRLINE
     Over 10,000 health organizations.
Health Hotlines
     Toll-free numbers to 300 organizations.

MEDLINE/PubMed
References from more than 4,600 biomedical journals, including the
     Toxicology Subset.

Other Resources
Chemical Information
Selected Toxicology Links
Reference Material
     Bibliographies, glossary, reports.
Database descriptions
Lecture guides
Locatorplus
     The NLM catalog of books, journals, and audiovisuals.
NLM Gateway
     Search multiple retrieval systems at NLM.

U.S. National Library of Medicine, 8600 Rockville Pike, Bethesda, MD 20894,
National Institutes of Health, Department of Health & Human Services
Copyright and Privacy Policy, Freedom of Information Act, Accessibility
Customer Service: tehip@teh.nlm.nih.gov.
Last modified on August 6, 2002

Figure 39.1 TEHIP homepage.

About • Contact • Search

National Library of Medicine
Specialized Information Services

SIS NLM

TOXNET ▷ Tox. & Env. Health ▷ TOXNET

Welcome to TOXNET, a cluster of databases on toxicology, hazardous chemicals, and related areas.

Databases

HSDB	ⓘ
IRIS	ⓘ
GENE-TOX	ⓘ
CCRIS	ⓘ
Multi-Databases	ⓘ
TOXLINE	ⓘ
DART/ETIC	ⓘ
TRI	ⓘ
ChemIDplus	ⓘ

Search All Databases

acrylamide

Search Clear

Search Results:

Database	Records found ⓘ
TOXLINE Special	2050
DART Special	64
HSDB	36
IRIS	1
GENETOX	2
CCRIS	8
TRI	91
CHEMIDplus	1

Other NLM Resources

DIRLINE
Haz-Map
Tox Weblinks
MEDLINEplus
  Tox/Env. Health subset
PubMed
NLM Gateway
Locatorplus

Support Pages

Help
Database Descriptions
News
Recent TOXNET
Survey Results

U.S. National Library of Medicine, 8600 Rockville Pike, Bethesda, MD 20894,
National Institutes of Health, Department of Health & Human Services
Copyright and Privacy Policy, Freedom of Information Act, Accessibility
Customer Service: tehip@teh.nlm.nih.gov.
Last modified on May 8, 2002.

Figure 39.2 TOXNET's page search on "acrylamide."

REFERENCES

Bronson, R.J. (1991) Toxic chemical release inventory information, *Med. Ref. Serv. Q.*, 10, 17–34.

Fonger, G.C., Stroup, D., Thomas, P.L., and Wexler, P. (2000) TOXNET: a computerized collection of toxicological and environmental health information, *Toxicol. Indust. Health,* 16, 4–6.

NLM/SIS (2002) Fact Sheet Toxicology Data Network, http://www.nlm.nih.gov/pubs/fact-sheets/toxnetfs.html

Vasta, B.M. and Wexler, P. (1985) NLM's new Toxicology Network, *The NLM Technical Bulletin,* 193, 6–11.

Wexler, P. (2001) TOXNET: an evolving web resource for toxicology and environmental health information, *Toxicology,* 157, 3–10.

NIH/NLM URL PAGES

National Institutes of Health http://www.nih.gov
National Library of Medicine http://www.nlm.nih.gov

CHAPTER **40**

In Silico Approaches for Physiologically Based Pharmacokinetic Modeling

Martin Béliveau and Kannan Krishnan

CONTENTS

INTRODUCTION

Physiologically based pharmacokinetic (PBPK) models are increasingly being used for conducting dose extrapolations, route extrapolations, species extrapolations, and exposure scenario extrapolations required for risk assessments (Andersen et al., 1987). PBPK models are basically mechanism-based mathematical descriptions of the processes of absorption, distribution, metabolism, and excretion in the intact organism (Krishnan and Andersen, 2001). The algebraic and differential equations constituting the PBPK models are solved with the knowledge of various input parameters, namely, physiological (tissue volumes, blood flow rates, cardiac output, alveolar ventilation rate), physicochemical (blood:air partition coefficients, tissue:blood partition coefficients, absorption rate constants, permeability coefficients), and biochemical (maximal velocity, Michaelis affinity constant) parameters. Whereas the information on physiological parameters can be obtained from the biomedical literature (Arms and Travis, 1988), this is frequently not the case for physicochemical (partition coefficients, absorption constants, and permeability coefficient) and biochemical parameters (hepatic or renal clearances, maximal velocity of metabolism, and Michaelis affinity constant).

The physicochemical and biochemical parameters needed for constructing chemical-specific PBPK models can be obtained using *in vivo* or *in vitro* approaches. *In vivo* approaches involve collection of pharmacokinetic data in exposed animals and analysis of such data using a PBPK model. By adjusting the model simulations to match the experimental data, the numerical values of the missing parameters can be estimated. Such a procedure is reliably applied for estimating one or two parameters at a time. Parameter estimation using *in vivo* studies, particularly for nonvolatiles, can be tedious and can require extensive use of animals (Krishnan and Andersen, 2001).

The *in vitro* methods, facilitating reduced animal use, have been proven to be useful only for estimating partition coefficients. The *in vitro* derived metabolism constants cannot be directly incorporated within PBPK models, even though freshly isolated hepatocytes and postmitochondrial fractions appear to hold some promise (Krishnan and Andersen, 2001). The considerations of cost effectiveness as well as reduction/replacement of animal use have led to the development of other alternative approaches, particularly *in silico* approaches, for estimating PBPK model parameters. Two kinds of *in silico* approaches are useful in this context. The first one involves the use of available data for various PBPK parameters in order to develop equations that associate characteristics of chemicals to the magnitude of the parameters. An example of this category is the classical quantitative structure-activity relationship (QSAR) approach. Another *in silico* approach involves the development of mechanistic algorithms based on an understanding of the interrelationships among certain biological and chemical determinants in order to predict the numerical value of PBPK model parameters. The objectives of this chapter are (1) to review the state-of-the art of *in silico* approaches (QSARs, biologically based algorithms) for estimating PBPK model parameters, and (2) to illustrate how the *in silico*–based PBPK models can be used in human health risk assessment applications.

METHODOLOGICAL BASIS OF *IN SILICO* APPROACHES

The following paragraphs provide a brief description of the methodological basis of the two types of *in silico* approaches, namely, QSARs and biologically based algorithms.

QSARs

The QSARs typically relate a biological activity or, more specifically, a *property* in this context, to structural features specific to chemicals through a mathematical function (*f*):

$$\text{Biological property} = f(\text{structural feature}) \tag{40.1}$$

Since empirical data are used to derive the mathematical function fulfilling the above relationship, depending upon the nature of the data the functions can be linear, multilinear, or supralinear. Two types of QSARs have been used to estimate the value of PBPK model parameters: linear-free energy (LFE) models and Free–Wilson models.

LFE-Type Models

LFE-type models are quantitative relationships that describe activity as a function of chemical structure, relying upon the principles of thermodynamics (Hansch and Fujita, 1964). The basis of the commonly used Hansch approach is that the differences in magnitude of a given biological activity within a series of chemicals correspond to changes in the free energy (ΔG) during the processes involved. As the difference in biological activity and the change in free energy are likely to be linearly related, the resulting mathematical relationships are referred to as "linear free energy relationships." Because it is very difficult to directly determine ΔG in biological systems, its thermodynamic components such as the energy (ΔE), enthalpy (ΔH), and entropy (ΔS) are used instead and are represented by a series of structural descriptors that can be derived for any given molecule (Seydel and Schaper, 1982). The coefficients for these descriptors (i.e., slopes and intercepts) are then regressed using standard statistical techniques. In this type of approach, structural descriptors can be broadly classified into three general types: electrostatic, steric, or hydrophobic. LFE models can incorporate one or many of these categories of structural descriptors, based on the statistical significance of each feature in the final model.

Electrostatic Features in LFE-Type Models

Electronic effects typically include electron donating and withdrawing tendencies, partial atomic charges, and electrostatic field densities as defined by Hammett sigma (σ) values, resonance parameters (R values), inductive parameters (F values), and Taft substituent values (ρ^*, σ^*, E_s). Because ionized molecules cannot pass through biological membranes and electrostatic effects, constants are derived from ionization characteristics of the molecule, relating pharmacokinetic behavior of all chemicals to only electrostatic features is not totally relevant. Abraham and Weathersby (1994) used dipolarity/polarizability, among others, as electrostatic descriptors for relating structure to the numerical values of tissue:air and blood:air partition coefficients of a series of chemicals. They observed that water, plasma, blood, lung, kidney, muscle, brain, fat, and olive oil progressively became less dipolar/polarizable due to increasing lipid content (0 to 100%). Thus, the electrostatic descriptor is relevant only for functionally substituted compounds such as 1-propanol. Lewis and Dickins (2002) have shown the importance of electrostatic descriptors such as ionization potential and pK_a in relating structure of various drugs to metabolic rates and binding to CYP450. Correlations were improved with the incorporation of these descriptors, especially for ionizable or polar drugs. This is probably related to the binding site of the compound on the CYP protein, which contains polar amino acids.

Steric Features in LFE-Type Models

Steric effects are conventionally represented by values calculated for molar refractivity and the Taft steric parameter. However, since steric effects describe the "bulkiness" of the molecule, they can include molecular volume, molecular weight, surface area, carbon chain branching, etc. Molecular connectivity indices and features derived from three-dimensional QSAR can also be considered as being of a steric nature, although the relationship between structure and these features is often obscure and not as intuitive, in certain instances. Furthermore, obtaining the chemical-specific values for these features often requires the use of specialized chemical modeling software.

Gargas et al. (1988) used steric descriptors in order to relate structure to PBPK model parameter values, and they suggested that a LFE equation combining connectivity indices and *ad hoc* descriptors (such as the number of halogens in a compound) provided better descriptions for tissue:air partition coefficients than using either descriptors alone. Use of connectivity indices is limited because the relationship between these descriptors and structure is not informative in a transparent and direct manner. For example, the first order valence connectivity index represents both structural and electronic features of a compound, in a complex way. Order indices represent multiple substitution patterns of the halogens on the carbons in the compounds, flexibility in polymers, or halogen substitution patterns. More intuitive is the other descriptor used by Gargas et al. (1988), namely, the number of halogen atoms present in the molecule, although it may not always be relevant for all molecules of interest. Gargas et al. (1988) also used steric parameters to relate structure to maximal velocity of metabolism (V_{max}), but because of the level of electronic information contained in the connectivity indices used in the descriptions, the authors suggested that more accurate modeling of V_{max} could be attempted by using both steric descriptors and more specific electronic information such as charge distribution.

Hydrophobic Features in LFE-Type Models

Hydrophobic features in LFE-type equations are frequently represented by using the log octanol:water partition coefficient (log $P_{o:w}$) or the hydrophobic parameter,

π, which is derived from $P_{o:w}$. However, other partition coefficients (e.g., water:air [$P_{w:a}$], oil:air [$P_{o:a}$], oil:water, n-hexadecane:air [$P_{he:a}$] partition coefficients) and solubility parameters have also been used. Hydrophobic parameters (namely, octanol:air, oil:air, or water:air) have been extensively used for relating structure and PBPK model parameters. The use of various datasets and experimental data in multiple species (rat, human, or fish) in the regressions have led to varied coefficient values for $P_{o:w}$, $P_{o:a}$, or $P_{w:a}$. Because blood:air and tissue:air partition coefficients (PC) represent distribution between a biological matrix (consisting of lipid and water) and air, it is logical that reasonably good correlations are obtained using a partition measure for another relevant matrix and air (i.e., $P_{w:a}$ or $P_{o:a}$). Furthermore, since tissue is composed of water, lipids, and protein, the coefficients of these descriptors have been suggested to reflect tissue composition (Abraham and Weathersby, 1994). Recently, Meulenberg and Vijverberg (2000), after an extensive review of the literature, found that values of the coefficients obtained following regression analysis using $P_{w:a}$, $P_{o:a}$, and the experimental PC values for rats and humans were essentially the same as the tissue lipid water and lipid content, highlighting the importance of tissue composition in the partitioning process.

Free–Wilson Type Models

Although the relationships between pharmacokinetic parameters and hydrophobic determinants have been explored frequently, the development of such relationships using other determinants in the LFE approach is not as straightforward. Furthermore, it is often unclear how these determinants as used in LFE equations relate to PK processes, and in order to successfully explore all relevant structural combinations, a substantial dataset is required and is often unavailable. Because of this, alternatives to the LFE approach have been explored. In this regard, Free and Wilson (1964) developed a series of substituent constants by relating biological activity with the nature and frequency of occurrence of specific functional groups in the parent molecule. This methodological approach is reflected by the following equation:

$$\text{Activity} = A + \Sigma_i\Sigma_j G_{ij}X_{ij} \qquad (40.2)$$

where A is defined as the average biological activity for the series, G_{ij} is the contribution to activity of a functional group i in the jth position and X_{ij} the presence (1.0) or absence (0.0) of the functional group i in the jth position.

The Free–Wilson approach requires that the contributions of substituents be additive and that a sufficiently large database be available to facilitate the determination of the contribution of various substituents. In the pharmacokinetic arena, the Free–Wilson type QSARs have been developed for the rate of oral absorption ($K_{a(oral)}$) of sulfonamides (Seydel and Schaper, 1982). Based on the fragment constants derived, it was possible to predict the compound with the highest $K_{a(oral)}$ value by combining the fragments with the highest contributions. More recently, Free–Wilson algorithms for relating structure to PBPK model parameters for a series of chloroethanes in rats, humans, and fish have been developed (Fouchécourt and Krishnan, 2000; Fouchécourt et al., 2000). These algorithms were then successfully integrated into a PBPK model in order to simulate the kinetics of these chemicals in the various species. The limiting factor of such an approach, however, is that the Free–Wilson model developed for chloroethanes could not be used to predict the parameter values for chemicals lacking the common structure and substituents. Such a limitation can be overcome with the development and use of biologically based algorithms.

Biologically Based Algorithms

Contrary to the *in silico* methods described above, biologically based algorithms do not require *a priori* knowledge of experimental data. Here, information on specific biological processes that determine the magnitude of a PBPK parameter is gathered, and a predictive mathematical relationship between the PBPK parameter and biological determinants is developed. The predictions of the algorithm are then compared with experimental data for validation purposes. Uncertainty regarding the prediction of parameter values for *de novo* compounds is somewhat reduced because the algorithm is based on known biological mechanisms. In cases where predicted values differ from experimental data, hypotheses concerning other plausible mechanisms can be generated and incorporated within the algorithm for further verification. Theoretically, these types of algorithms can be developed for any PBPK parameter regardless of the chemical class or molecular structure. The development and application of such algorithms is only limited by the current level of understanding of the mechanistic basis and phenomena that determine the magnitude of the PBPK model parameters.

At the present time, several QSARs (LFE and Free–Wilson) and biologically based algorithms are available to facilitate the prediction of chemical-specific PBPK model parameters. All of these *in silico* approaches, as detailed in the following section, have been uniquely applied to estimate the PBPK model parameters of organic substances.

IN SILICO APPROACHES FOR PBPK MODEL PARAMETERS

In Silico Approaches for Tissue:Air Partition Coefficients

Tissue:air PCs describe the relative concentrations of volatile organic chemicals (VOCs) in tissues and air at steady-state. Both LFE-type QSAR models and biologically based algorithms have been developed for predicting tissue:air partition coefficients of a variety of chemicals (Table 40.1).

In developing a LFE-type QSAR for human tissue:air PCs, Abraham and Weathersby (1994) observed that nonpolar solutes only needed hexadecane:air partitioning (a hydrophobic descriptor), whereas an electrostatic descriptor (π_2^H) was important for functionally substituted compounds such a 1-propanol. Abraham and Weathersby (1994) correctly underscore the importance of limiting the use of these equations

Table 40.1 *In Silico* Approaches for Estimating the Tissue:Air Partition Coefficients (*P*) of Chemicals

Approach[a]	Species[b]	Chemical Class[c]	Reference
QSARs: LFE-type equations			
Electrostatic descriptors			
$\log P_{adipose:air} = -0.294 - 0.172R_2 + 0.729\,\pi_2^H + 1.7474\,\alpha_2^H + 0.219\,\beta_2^H + 0.895 \log P_{he:a}$	H	Inert Gases; LMWVOCs	Abraham and Weathersby (1994)
$\log P_{brain:air} = -1.074 + 0.427R_2 + 0.286\,\pi_2^H + 2.781\,\alpha_2^H + 2.787\,\beta_2^H + 0.609 \log P_{he:a}$	H	Inert Gases; LMWVOCs	Abraham and Weathersby (1994)
$\log P_{heart:air} = -1.208 + 0.128R_2 + 0.987\,\pi_2^H + 0.643\,\alpha_2^H + 1.783\,\beta_2^H + 0.597 \log P_{he:a}$	H	Inert Gases; LMWVOCs	Abraham and Weathersby (1994)
$\log P_{kidney:air} = -1.084 + 0.417R_2 + 0.226\,\pi_2^H + 3.624\,\alpha_2^H + 2.926\,\beta_2^H + 0.534 \log P_{he:a}$	H	Inert Gases; LMWVOCs	Abraham and Weathersby (1994)
$\log P_{liver:air} = -1.031 + 0.059R_2 + 0.774\,\pi_2^H + 0.593\,\alpha_2^H + 1.049\,\beta_2^H + 0.654 \log P_{he:a}$	H	Inert Gases; LMWVOCs	Abraham and Weathersby (1994)
$\log P_{lung:air} = -1.300 + 0.667R_2 + 0.680\,\pi_2^H + 3.539\,\alpha_2^H + 3.35\,\beta_2^H + 0.458 \log P_{he:a}$	H	Inert Gases; LMWVOCs	Abraham and Weathersby (1994)
$\log P_{muscle:air} = -1.14 + 0.544R_2 + 0.216\,\pi_2^H + 3.4714\,\alpha_2^H + 2.924\,\beta_2^H + 0.578 \log P_{he:a}$	H	Inert Gases; LMWVOCs	Abraham and Weathersby (1994)
Steric descriptors			
$\log P_{adipose:air} = (0.734^1 x^v) - (0.029\ x_s^v) - (1.57(1/^1 x)) - (0.559(1/^1 x^v)) - 0.0983\ x_c^v + 2.213$	R	Haloalkanes	Gargas et al. (1988)

(continued)

Table 40.1 (continued) In Silico Approaches for Estimating the Tissue:Air Partition Coefficients (P) of Chemicals

Approach[a]	Species[b]	Chemical Class[c]	Reference
log $P_{adipose:air}$ = 0.734$^1X^v$ − 0.0291 x_s^v − 1.570/$^1X^v$ − 0.559$^1X^v$ − 0.098$^4 x_c^v$ + 2.213	R	Haloalkanes	Csanady and Laib (1990)
log $P_{adipose:air}$ = 0.563N_{Cl} + 1.028N_{Br} + 0.467N_C + 0.270Q_H − 0.199N_F − 0.097	R	Haloalkanes	Gargas et al. (1988)
log $P_{adipose:air}$ = 1.037$^1x^v$ − (0.007(1/x_s^v)) + 0.022Q_H − 0.177$^3 x_c^v$ − 0.199N_F − 0.0036	R	Haloalkanes	Gargas et al. (1988)
log $P_{liver:air}$ = (1.072$^1x^v$) − (0.021(1/x_s^v)) + (0.647(1/$^1x^v$)) − (0.304$^4 x_c^v$) − 1.212	R	Haloalkanes	Gargas et al. (1988)
log $P_{liver:air}$ = 0.366N_{Cl} − 0.588N_{Br} + 0.345Q_H − 0.179N_F − 0.007	R	Haloalkanes	Gargas et al. (1988)
log $P_{liver:air}$ = −0.685$^1x^v$ − (0.020(1/x_s^v)) + 0.232Q_H + (0.298(1/$^1x^v$)) + 0.104N_{Cl} − 0.726	R	Haloalkanes	Gargas et al. (1988)
log $P_{liver:air}$ = 1.072$^1X^v$ − 0.021/x_s^v + 0.647/$^1X^v$ − 0.304$^4 x_c^v$ − 1.212	R	Haloalkanes	Csanady and Laib (1990)
log $P_{muscle:air}$ = 0.379Q_H − 0.278N_{Cl} + 0.536N_{Br} − 0.190N_F + 0.169N_{Cl} − 0.439	R	Haloalkanes	Gargas et al. (1988)
log $P_{muscle:air}$ = 0.399$^1x^v$ − (0.007(1/x_s^v)) + 0.295Q_H + 0.259$^4 x_{pc}^v$ − 0.194N_F − 0.217	R	Haloalkanes	Gargas et al. (1988)
log $P_{muscle:air}$ = (0.995$^1x^v$) − (0.018(1/x_s^v)) − (0.424$^4 x_c^v$) − (0.559(1/$^1x^v$)) + (0.602(1/$^1x^v$)) − 1.334	R	Haloalkanes	Gargas et al. (1988)

Hydrophobic descriptors

log($P_{adipose:water}$ − V_{wt}) = 0.9$P_{o:w}$ + 0.31	F	Chloroethanes; Benzene	Bertelsen et al. (1988)
log($P_{kidney:water}$ − V_{wt}) = 0.72$P_{o:w}$ − 0.56	F	Chloroethanes; Benzene	Bertelsen et al. (1988)
log($P_{liver:water}$ − V_{wt}) = 1.06$P_{o:w}$ − 1.43	F	Chloroethanes; Benzene	Bertelsen et al. (1988)
log($P_{muscle:water}$ − V_{wt}) = 0.63$P_{o:w}$ − 0.60	F	Chloroethanes; Benzene	Bertelsen et al. (1988)
ln $P_{adipose:air}$ = 0.032T_b − 5.456	H	Haloalkanes	Csanady and Laib (1990)

Equation		Reference
$\ln P_{liver:air} = 0.022 T_b - 4.638$	H Haloalkanes	Csanady and Laib (1990)
$\log P_{adipose:air} = 0.209 + 0.0628 \log P_{w:a} + 0.8868 \log P_{o:a}$	H Inert gases; LMWVOCs	Abraham et al. (1985)
$\log P_{adipose:air} = 0.21 \log P_{o:a} + 0.24 \log P_{w:a}$	H Hydrophilic VOCs	Tichy (1991b)
$\log P_{adipose:air} = 0.782 \log P_{o:a} + 0.201 \log P_{w:a} + 0.432$	H Hydrophobic VOCs	Tichy (1991a)
$\log P_{adipose:air} = 0.901 \log P_{o:a} + 0.150$	H LMWVOCs	Fiserova-Bergerova et al. (1984)
$\log P_{adipose:air} = 0.174 + 0.910 \log P_{o:a}$	H Inert gases; LMWVOCs	Abraham et al. (1985)
$\log P_{brain:air} = -0.16 \log P_{o:a} + 0.82 \log P_{w:a} + 0.47$	H Hydrophilic VOCs	Tichy (1991b)
$\log P_{brain:air} = 0.274 + 0.537 \log P_{w:a} + 0.444 \log P_{o:a}$	H Inert gases; LMWVOCs	Abraham et al. (1985)
$\log P_{brain:air} = 0.394 + 1.096 \log P_{w:a}$	H Inert gases; LMWVOCs	Abraham et al. (1985)
$\log P_{brain:air} = 0.471 \log P_{o:a} + 0.630 \log P_{w:a} - 0.305$	H Hydrophobic VOCs	Tichy (1991a)
$\log P_{brain:air} = 0.844 \log P_{o:a} - 1.124$	H LMWVOCs	Fiserova-Bergerova et al. (1984)
$\log P_{brain:air} = -0.850 + 0.773 \log P_{o:a}$	H Inert gases; LMWVOCs	Abraham et al. (1985)
$\log P_{brain:air} = -3.692 + 1.253 R_G$	H Inert gases; LMWVOCs	Abraham et al. (1985)
$\log P_{kidney:air} = -0.18 \log P_{o:a} + 0.82 \log P_{w:a} + 0.53$	H Hydrophilic VOCs	Tichy (1991b)
$\log P_{kidney:air} = 0.277 + 1.111 \log P_{w:a}$	H Inert gases; LMWVOCs	Abraham et al. (1985)
$\log P_{kidney:air} = 0.466 \log P_{o:a} + 0.379 \log P_{w:a} - 0.332$	H Hydrophobic VOCs	Tichy (1991a)
$\log P_{kidney:air} = 0.700 \log P_{o:a} - 0.877$	H LMWVOCs	Fiserova-Bergerova et al. (1984)
$\log P_{kidney:air} = -0.920 + 0.764 \log P_{o:a}$	H Inert gases; LMWVOCs	Abraham et al. (1985)
$\log P_{liver:air} = -0.388 + 0.502 \log P_{w:a} + 0.497 \log P_{o:a}$	H Inert gases; LMWVOCs	Abraham et al. (1985)
$\log P_{liver:air} = 0.432 + 1.064 \log P_{w:a}$	H Inert gases; LMWVOCs	Abraham et al. (1985)
$\log P_{liver:air} = 0.746 \log P_{o:a} + 0.178 \log P_{w:a} - 0.767$	H Hydrophobic VOCs	Tichy (1991a)
$\log P_{liver:air} = 0.871 \log P_{o:a} - 1.044$	H LMWVOCs	Fiserova-Bergerova et al. (1984)
$\log P_{liver:air} = -0.875 + 0.773 \log P_{o:a}$	H Inert gases; LMWVOCs	Abraham et al. (1985)
$\log P_{lung:air} = -0.21 \log P_{o:a} + 0.91 \log P_{w:a} + 0.41$	H Hydrophilic VOCs	Tichy (1991b)
$\log P_{lung:air} = -0.057 + 0.870 \log P_{w:a} + 0.146 \log P_{o:a}$	H Inert gases; LMWVOCs	Abraham et al. (1985)
$\log P_{lung:air} = 0.057 + 0.978 \log P_{w:a}$	H Inert gases; LMWVOCs	Abraham et al. (1985)

(continued)

Table 40.1 (continued) *In Silico* Approaches for Estimating the Tissue:Air Partition Coefficients (*P*) of Chemicals

Approach[a]	Species[b]	Chemical Class[c]	Reference
$\log P_{lung:air} = 0.373 \log P_{o:a} + 0.416 \log P_{w:a} - 0.216$	H	Hydrophobic VOCs	Tichy (1991a)
$\log P_{lung:air} = 0.644 \log P_{o:a} - 0.815$	H	LMWVOCs	Fiserova-Bergerova et al. (1984)
$\log P_{lung:air} = -0.833 + 0.911 \log P_{o:a}$	H	Inert gases; LMWVOCs	Abraham et al. (1985)
$\log P_{muscle:air} = -0.19 \log P_{o:a} + 0.82 \log P_{w:a} + 0.54$	H	Hydrophilic VOCs	Tichy (1991b)
$\log P_{muscle:air} = 0.49 \log P_{o:a} + 0.39 \log P_{w:a} - 0.31$	H	Hydrophobic VOCs	Tichy (1991b)
$\log P_{muscle:air} = -0.263 + 0.575 \log P_{w:a} + 0.423 \log P_{o:a}$	H	Inert gases; LMWVOCs	Abraham et al. (1985)
$\log P_{muscle:air} = 0.351 + 1.108 \log P_{w:a}$	H	Inert gases; LMWVOCs	Abraham et al. (1985)
$\log P_{muscle:air} = 0.652 \log P_{o:a} - 0.702$	H	LMWVOCs	Fiserova-Bergerova et al. (1984)
$\log P_{muscle:air} = -0.852 + 0.768 \log P_{o:a}$	H	Inert gases; LMWVOCs	Abraham et al. (1985)
$\log P_{muscle:air} = -3.247 + 0.965 R_G$	H	Inert gases; LMWVOCs	Abraham et al. (1985)
$P_{adipose:air} = 0.447 P_{o:a} + 0.075 P_{w:a} + 6.59$	H	LMWVOCs; CFCs	Meulenberg and Vijverberg (2000)
$P_{brain:air} = (0.026 S_o + 0.51 S_w)/S_a$	H	LMWVOCs	Paterson and Mackay (1989)
$P_{brain:air} = 0.020 P_{o:a} + 0.380 P_{w:a} + 0.94$	H	LMWVOCs; CFCs	Meulenberg and Vijverberg (2000)
$P_{kidney:air} = (0.014 S_o + 0.51 S_w)/S_a$	H	LMWVOCs	Paterson and Mackay (1989)
$P_{kidney:air} = 0.011 P_{o:a} + 0.400 P_{w:a} + 0.69$	H	LMWVOCs; CFCs	Meulenberg and Vijverberg (2000)
$P_{kidney:air} = -0.391 + 0.550 \log P_{w:a} + 0.440 \log P_{o:a}$	H	Inert gases; LMWVOCs	Abraham et al. (1985)
$P_{liver:air} = (0.028 S_o + 0.51 S_w)/S_a$	H	LMWVOCs	Paterson and Mackay (1989)
$P_{liver:air} = 0.028 P_{o:a} + 0.79$	H	LMWVOCs; CFCs	Meulenberg and Vijverberg (2000)
$P_{muscle:air} = 0.014 P_{o:a} + 0.384 P_{w:a} + 0.94$	H	LMWVOCs; CFCs	Meulenberg and Vijverberg (2000)
$\ln P_{adipose:air} = 0.032 T_b - 5.456$	R	LMWVOCs	Csanady and Laib (1990)
$\ln P_{liver:air} = 0.022 T_b - 4.638$	R	LMWVOCs	Csanady and Laib (1990)
$\log P_{adipose:air} = 0.920 \log P_{o:a} + 0.136$	R	LMWVOCs	Gargas et al. (1989)
$\log P_{adipose:air} = 0.927 \log P_{o:a} - 0.032 \log P_{w:a} + 0.120$	R	LMWVOCs	Gargas et al. (1989)

Equation	Species	Chemical	Reference
$\log P_{adipose:air} = 1.027 \log P_{o:a} - 0.046 \log P_{w:a} - 0.119$	R	Haloalkanes	Gargas et al. (1988)
$\log P_{liver:air} = 0.574 \log P_{o:a} + 0.302 \log P_{w:a} - 0.278$	R	Haloalkanes	Gargas et al. (1988)
$\log P_{liver:air} = 0.730 \log P_{o:a} + 0.128 \log P_{w:a} - 0.550$	R	LMWVOCs	Gargas et al. (1989)
$\log P_{muscle:air} = 0.477 \log P_{o:a} + 0.365 \log P_{w:a} - 0.374$	R	Haloalkanes	Gargas et al. (1988)
$\log P_{muscle:air} = 0.644 \log P_{o:a} + 0.180 \log P_{w:a} - 0.725$	R	LMWVOCs	Gargas et al. (1989)
$P_{adipose:air} = 0.594 P_{o:a} + 0.085 P_{w:a} + 9.40$	R	LMWVOCs; CFCs	Meulenberg and Vijverberg (2000)
$P_{brain:air} = 0.054 P_{o:a} + 0.832 P_{w:a}$	R	LMWVOCs; CFCs	Meulenberg and Vijverberg (2000)
$P_{kidney:air} = 0.097 P_{o:a} + 0.826 P_{w:a}$	R	LMWVOCs; CFCs	Meulenberg and Vijverberg (2000)
$P_{liver:air} = 0.026 P_{o:a} + 0.878 P_{w:a} + 2.36$	R	LMWVOCs; CFCs	Meulenberg and Vijverberg (2000)
$P_{muscle:air} = 0.010 P_{o:a} + 0.772 P_{w:a} + 0.29$	R	LMWVOCs; CFCs	Meulenberg and Vijverberg (2000)

Biologically based algorithms

Equation	Species	Chemical	Reference
$P_{tissue:air} = (S_s V_{wt} + S_v V_{nt} + 0.7 S_s V_{pt} + 0.3 S_v V_{pt})/S_a$	R, H	LMWVOCs	Poulin and Krishnan (1996a)
$P_{tissue:air} = P_{o:w} P_{w:a}(V_{nt} + 0.3 V_{pt}) + P_{w:a}(V_{wt} + 0.7 V_{pt})$	R, H	LMWVOCs	Poulin and Krishnan (1996c)

a π_2^H = dipolarity/polarizability, α_2^H = overall hydrogen-bond acidity, β_2^H = overall hydrogen-bond basicity, $^1X^v$, x_s^v, $^3x_c^v$, ^1X, $^4x_c^v$, $^4X_{ypc}$ = connectivity indices, N_{Br} = number of bromide atoms in the molecule, N_C = number of carbon atoms in the molecule, N_{Cl} = number of chloride atoms in the molecule, N_F = number of fluoride atoms in the molecule, $P_{he:a}$ = hexadecane:air partition coefficient, $P_{o:a}$ = *n*-octanol:air partition coefficient (or vegetable oil:air), $P_{o:w}$ = n-octanol:water partition coefficient (or vegetable oil:water), $P_{w:a}$ = water:air partition coefficient, R_g = average solubility in entire set of solvent systems, S_a = solubility in air, S_o = solubility in n-octanol (or vegetable oil), R_2 = Excess molar refraction, S_v = solubility in vegetable oil, S_w = solubility in water, T_b = boiling point, Q_H = variable dependant on the polarity of the molecule due to the presence of hydrogen atoms, S_s = solubility in saline, V_{pt} = volume fraction of phospholipids in tissues, V_{nt} = volume fraction of neutral lipids in tissues, and V_{wt} = volume fraction of water in tissues.

b F = fish, H = human, and R = rats.

c CFCs = chlorofluorocarbons, LMWVOCs = low molecular weight volatile organic chemicals, and VOCs = volatile organic chemicals.

for interpolation, particularly for the kinds of chemicals considered during model development. Gargas et al. (1988) used connectivity indices in order to correlate structure with the rat tissue:air PCs of a series of haloalkanes. Because of the electronegativity of halogen atoms (F > Cl > Br), it was suggested that these atoms increased the solubility in tissues via dispersion interactions. In other words, these atoms increase lipophilicity characteristic of the molecule, and it is therefore difficult to separate the purely "steric" from the purely "hydrophobic" influence because of the interdependency of these parameters as they relate to tissue solubility. As listed in Table 40.1, most of the published studies have established the quantitative relationship between tissue:air PCs and descriptors such as $P_{w:a}$ and $P_{o:a}$, due to the importance of the solubility of chemicals in tissue water and tissue lipids. Currently, there do not exist any Free–Wilson type models for tissue:air PCs of VOCs.

Mechanistic algorithms for predicting tissue:air PCs have, however, been developed on the basis of the determinants of two components, namely, tissue water:air PC and tissue lipid:air PC. Whereas the tissue water:air PC is considered to be the same as the inverse of the Henry's law constant, the tissue lipid:air PC is assumed to be equivalent to $P_{o:w}$. Along these lines, Poulin and Krishnan (1996c) developed the following algorithm to predict tissue:air partition coefficients ($P_{t:a}$):

$$P_{t:a} = [P_{o:w}P_{w:a}(V_{nt} + 0.3V_{pt})] + [P_{w:a}(V_{wt} + 0.7V_{pt})] \qquad (3)$$

where $P_{o:w}$ = n-octanol:water partition coefficient, $P_{w:a}$ = water:air partition coefficient, V_{nt} = volume fraction of neutral lipid in tissue, V_{pt} = volume fraction of phospholipid in tissue, and V_{wt} = volume fraction of water in tissue.

In the above equation, $P_{o:w}$ and $P_{w:a}$ can be directly estimated from knowledge of molecular structure (Hine and Mookerjee, 1975; Hansch and Leo, 1979), whereas the volume fractions of tissue components can be found in the literature for a number of species (Poulin et al., 1999) or established experimentally. The above equation has been used to predict rat and human $P_{t:a}$ (liver, muscle, fat) of several alkanes, haloalkanes, and aromatic hydrocarbons. For oxygen-containing VOCs (alcohols, esters, ethers), using vegetable oil instead of n-octanol as the lipid surrogate provides better estimates of their tissue solubility (Poulin and Krishnan, 1996c).

In Silico Approaches for Blood:Air PCs

The blood:air PC is an important parameter since it influences the extent and rate of absorption, distribution, and elimination of VOCs. Table 40.2 presents the various LFE-type and Free–Wilson-type QSAR models, as well as mechanistically based *in silico* approaches that have been developed so far for the prediction of blood:air PCs of VOCs.

The LFE-type QSARs have benefited from the numerous studies involving anesthetic gases in humans (Eger and Larson, 1964; Cowles et al., 1971; Steward et al., 1973; Saraiva et al., 1977; Laass, 1987). Since anaesthetic-like compounds are relatively lipophilic, the best regression equations are mostly those that contain

Table 40.2 *In Silico* Approaches for Estimating the Blood:Air Partition Coefficients (*P*) of Chemicals

Approach[a]	Species[b]	Chemical Class[c]	Reference
QSARs: LFE-type equations			
Electrostatic descriptors			
$\log P_{bloodair} = -1.269 + 0.612R_2 + 0.916\,\pi_2^H + 3.614\,\alpha_2^H + 3.381\,\beta_2^H + 0.362 \log P_{heair}$	H	Inert Gases; LMWVOCs	Abraham and Weathersby (1994)
$\log P_{plasmaair} = -1.48 + 0.490R_2 + 2.04\,\pi_2^H + 3.5074\,\alpha_2^H + 3.911\,\beta_2^H + 0.157 \log P_{heair}$	H	Inert Gases; LMWVOCs	Abraham and Weathersby (1994)
Steric descriptors			
$\log P_{bloodair} = 0.0072MW + 0.197$	H	Trihalomethanes	Batterman et al. (2002)
$\log P_{bloodair} = 0.321N_{Br} + 1.06$	H	Trihalomethanes	Batterman et al. (2002)
$P_{bloodair} = 0.07MW + 5.59$	H	Aliphatic hydrocarbons	Perbellini et al. (1985)
$\log P_{bloodair} = 0.443Q_H - 0.303N_F + 0.225N_{Cl} + 0.510N_{BR} + 0.155N_C - 0.104$	R	Haloalkanes	Gargas et al. (1988)
Hydrophobic descriptors			
$\log (P_{bloodwater} - V_{wb}) = 0.7P_{ow} - 0.75$	F	Chloroethanes; benzene	Bertelsen et al. (1998)
$\ln P_{bloodair} = 0.038T_b - 13.3$	H	Aliphatic hydrocarbons	Csanady and Laib (1990)
$\log P_{bloodair} = 0.0109T_b - 2.584$	H	Trihalomethanes	Batterman et al. (2002)
$\log P_{bloodair} = -0.14 \log P_{oa} + 0.86 \log P_{wa} + 0.47$	H	Hydrophilic VOCs	Tichy (1991b)
$\log P_{bloodair} = 0.685 \log P_{oa} - 0.6565$	H	Trihalomethanes	Batterman et al. (2002)
$\log P_{bloodair} = 0.45 \log P_{wa} + 1.21$	H	VOCs	Laass (1987)
$\log P_{bloodair} = -0.003 \log P_{wa} + 1.47$	H	VOCs	Laass (1987)
$\log p_{bloodair} = -0.074 + 0.802 \log P_{wa} + 0.218 \log P_{oa}$	H	Inert gases; LMWVOCs	Abraham et al. (1985)
$\log P_{bloodair} = -0.07 \log S_w + 1.21$	H	VOCs	Laass (1987)

(continued)

Table 40.2 (continued) *In Silico* Approaches for Estimating the Blood:Air Partition Coefficients (P) of Chemicals

Approach[a]	Species[b]	Chemical Class[c]	Reference
$\log P_{blood:air} = -0.09 \log P_{o:a} + 2.45$	H	VOCs	Laass (1987)
$\log P_{blood:air} = -0.102 + 0.675 \log P_{w:a} + 0.315 \log P_{o:a}$	H	Inert gases; LMWVOCs	Abraham et al. (1985)
$\log P_{blood:air} = -0.295 + 0.588 \log P_{w:a} + 0.411 \log P_{o:a}$	H	Inert gases; LMWVOCs	Abraham et al. (1985)
$\log P_{blood:air} = -0.338 \log P_{o:a} + 3.121$	H	Halogenated hydrocarbons	Tichy et al. (1984)
$\log P_{blood:air} = -0.6737 + 0.5319 \log P_{o:a} \log P_{w:a}$	H	VOCs	Sato and Nakajima (1979)
$\log P_{blood:air} = 0.695 \log P_{o:a} - 1.076$	H	LMWVOCs	Fiserova-Bergerova et al. (1984)
$\log P_{blood:air} = -0.820 + 0.754 \log P_{o:a}$	H	Inert gases; LMWVOCs	Abraham et al. (1985)
$\log P_{blood:air} = 0.09 \log S_w + 8.25 \log V_o - 11.09$	H	VOCs	Laass (1987)
$\log P_{blood:air} = 0.11 \log S_w + 1.91$	H	VOCs	Laass (1987)
$\log P_{blood:air} = 0.180 \log P_{o:a} + 0.889 \log P_{w:a} + 0.054$	H	Hydrophobic VOCs	Tichy (1991a)
$\log P_{blood:air} = 0.20 \log S_w + 1.29$	H	VOCs	Laass (1987)
$\log P_{blood:air} = 0.22 \log P_{w:a} + 0.67 \log P_{o:a} - 0.98$	H	VOCs	Laass (1987)
$\log P_{blood:air} = 0.22 \log S_w + 10.78 \log V_w - 40.99$	H	VOCs	Laass (1987)
$\log P_{blood:air} = 0.262 + 0.996 \log P_{w:a}$	H	Inert gases; LMWVOCs	Abraham et al. (1985)
$\log P_{blood:air} = 0.27 \log 1000/P + 5.10 \log V_o - 6.67$	H	VOCs	Laass (1987)
$\log P_{blood:air} = 0.31 \log S_w + 3.90 \log V_o - 4.53$	H	VOCs	Laass (1987)
$\log P_{blood:air} = 0.35 \log 1000/P + 1.01$	H	VOCs	Laass (1987)
$\log P_{blood:air} = 0.35 \log S_w + 0.79 \log 1000/P + 1.34 \log V_o - 2.23$	H	VOCs	Laass (1987)
$\log P_{blood:air} = 0.37 \log S_w + 10.09 \log V_w - 38.40$	H	VOCs	Laass (1987)
$\log P_{blood:air} = 0.38 \log S_w + 0.91 \log 1000/P - 0.45$	H	VOCs	Laass (1987)
$\log P_{blood:air} = 0.45 \log S_w + 0.81 \log 1000/P - 0.40$	H	VOCs	Laass (1987)
$\log P_{blood:air} = 0.48 \log S_w + 0.75 \log 1000/P + 1.67 \log V_o - 2.77$	H	VOCs	Laass (1987)
$\log P_{blood:air} = 0.51 \log 1000/P + 0.37$	H	VOCs	Laass (1987)
$\log P_{blood:air} = 0.581 \log P_{o:a} + 0.332 \log P_{w:a} - 0.599$	H	LMWVOCs	Gargas et al. (1989)
$\log P_{blood:air} = 0.63 \log 1000/P + 0.38$	H	VOCs	Laass (1987)
$\log P_{blood:air} = 0.65 \log P_{o:a} - 0.84$	H	VOCs	Laass (1987)
$\log P_{blood:air} = 0.851 \log S_w + 1.78$	H	VOCs	Laass (1987)

Equation		Category	Reference
$\log P_{blood:air} = 0.984 \log P_{w:a} + 0.053$	H	Ketones; ethers; gases	Tichy et al. (1984)
$\log P_{blood:air} = 1.07 \log P_{w:a} + 0.27 \log P_{o:a} - 0.79$	H	VOCs	Laass (1987)
$\log P_{blood:air} = 1.21 \log V_o - 0.17$	H	VOCs	Laass (1987)
$\log P_{blood:air} = 3.05 - 0.34 P_{o:n}$	H	Ketones	Cabala et al. (1992)
$\log P_{blood:air} = -3.922 + 1.369 R_G$	H	Inert gases; LMWVOCs	Abraham et al. (1985)
$\log P_{blood:air} = 5.89 \log V_w - 21.43$	H	VOCs	Laass (1987)
$\log P_{blood:air} = 7.86 \log V_o - 10.40$	H	VOCs	Laass (1987)
$\log P_{blood:air} = 8.90 \log V_w - 33.40$	H	VOCs	Laass (1987)
$\log P_{milk:air} = 0.900 \log P_{o:a} - 1.095$	H	Trihalomethanes	Batterman et al. (2002)
$\log P_{plasma:air} = -0.079 + 0.896 \log P_{w:a} + 0.149 \log P_{o:a}$	H	Inert gases; LMWVOCs	Abraham et al. (1985)
$\log P_{plasma:air} = -0.082 + 0.894 \log P_{w:a} + 0.152 \log P_{o:a}$	H	Inert gases; LMWVOCs	Abraham et al. (1985)
$\log P_{plasma:air} = -0.848 + 0.890 \log P_{o:a}$	H	Inert gases; LMWVOCs	Abraham et al. (1985)
$\log P_{plasma:air} = -3.696 + 1.208 R_G$	H	Inert gases; LMWVOCs	Abraham et al. (1985)
$\log P_{plasma:air} = 0.038 + 1.019 \log P_{w:a}$	H	Inert gases; LMWVOCs	Abraham et al. (1985)
$P_{blood:air} = 0.0072 P_{o:a} + 0.898 P_{w:a} + 0.03$	H	LMWVOCs; CFCs	Meulenberg and Vijverberg (2000)
$P_{blood:air} = 0.08 e^{0.0308 Tb}$	H	Aliphatic hydrocarbons	Perbellini et al. (1985)
$P_{blood:air} = 0.00442 P_{o:a}$	H	Aliphatic hydrocarbons	Perbellini et al. (1985)
$P_{blood:air} = 0.88 P_{w:a} + 0.012$	H	VOCs	Feingold (1976)
$P_{blood:air} = 0.89 P_{w:a} + 0.011 P_{o:a}$	H	LMWVOCs	Tichy et al. (1984)
$P_{blood:air} = 0.90 \log P_{w:a} - 461$	H	Esters; alcohols	Kaneko et al. (1994)
$P_{blood:air} = P_{w:a} + (P_{o:a}/100)$	H	Anaesthetics	Eger and Larson (1964)
$P_{blood:air} = S_w(1 + 0.0035 P_{o:w})/S_a$	H	LMWVOCs	Paterson and Mackay (1989)
$\log P_{blood:air} = P_{w:a}[V_{lb} P_{o:w}^{0.85} + V_{prb}(86.2/P_{o:w} + 3.70)] + V_{wb}$	H, R	LMWVOCs	Connell et al. (1993)
$\log P_{blood:air} = 0.426 \log P_{o:a} + 0.515 \log P_{w:a} - 0.070$	R	Haloalkanes	Gargas et al. (1988)
$\log P_{blood:air} = 0.553 \log P_{o:a} + 0.351 P_{w:a} - 0.286$	R	LMWVOCs	Gargas et al. (1989)
$P_{blood:air} = 0.0054 P_{o:a} + 0.931 P_{w:a} + 1.16$	R	LMWVOCs; CFCs	Meulenberg and Vijverberg (2000)

(continued)

Table 40.2 (continued) In Silico Approaches for Estimating the Blood:Air Partition Coefficients (P) of Chemicals

Approach[a]	Species[b]	Chemical Class[c]	Reference
QSARs: Free–Wilson-type equations			
$P_{blood:water} = BS_{(C-C)}(28.4) + nCL_2(-12.9) + nCL_3(12.9)$	F	Chloroethanes	Fouchécourt et al. (2000)
$P_{blood:air} = BS_{(C-C)}(26.2) + nH_3(-34.9) + nCL(-4.51) + nCL_2(29.4) + nCL_3(11.5)$	H	Chloroethanes	Fouchécourt and Krishnan (2000)
$P_{blood:air} = BS_{(C-C)}(45.6) + nH_3(-51.5) + nCL(-8.86) + nCL_2(36.4) + nCL_3(11.1)$	R	Chloroethanes	Fouchécourt and Krishnan (2000)
Biologically based algorithms			
$P_{blood:air} = P_{o:a}P_{w:a}(V_{nb} + 0.3V_{pb}) + P_{w:a}(V_{wb} + 0.7V_{pb})$	R, H	LMWVOCs	Poulin and Krishnan (1996c)
$P_{blood:air} = [f_e(S_sV_{we} + S_vV_{ne} + 0.7S_sV_{pe} + 0.3S_vV_{pe}) + f_p(S_sV_{wp} + S_vV_{np} + 0.7S_sV_{pp} + 0.3S_vV_{pp})]/S_a$	R, H	LMWVOCs	Poulin and Krishnan (1996b)

a π_2^H = dipolarity/polarizability, α_2^H = overall hydrogen-bond acidity, β_2^H = overall hydrogen-bond basicity, BS = Basic structure, f_e = fraction of erythrocytes in blood, f_p = fraction of plasma in blood, MW = molecular weight, N_{Br} = number of bromide atoms in the molecule, N_C = number of carbon atoms in the molecule, N_{Cl} = number of chloride atoms in the molecule, nCL = number of CL fragments, nCL_2 = number of CL$_2$ fragments, nCL_3 = number of CL$_3$ fragments, N_F = number of fluoride atoms in the molecule, nH_3 = number of H$_3$ fragments, P = vapor pressure, P_{hea} = hexadecane:air partition coefficient, $P_{o:a}$ = n-octanol:air partition coefficient (or vegetable oil:air), $P_{o:n}$ = vegetable oil:nitrogen partition coefficient, $P_{o:w}$ = n-octanol:water partition coefficient (or vegetable oil:water), $P_{w:a}$ = water:air partition coefficient, Q_H = variable dependant on the polarity of the molecule due to the presence of hydrogen atoms, R_2 = excess molar refraction, R_g = parameters relative to the solvent, S_a = solubility in air, S_s = solubility in saline, S_v = solubility in vegetable oil, S_w = solubility in water, T_b = boiling point, V_{lb} = volume fraction of lipids in blood, V_{nb} = volume fraction of neutral lipids in blood, V_{ne} = volume fraction of neutral lipids in erythrocytes, V_o = surface tension, V_{np} = volume fraction of neutral lipids in plasma, V_{pb} = volume fraction of phospholipids in blood, V_{pe} = volume fraction of phospholipids in erythrocytes, V_{pp} = volume fraction of phospholipids in plasma, V_{prb} = volume fraction of proteins in blood, V_w = heat released due to evaporation of the substance at boiling temperature, V_{wb} = volume fraction of water in blood, V_{we} = volume fraction of water in erythrocytes, and V_{wp} = volume fraction of water in plasma.

b F = fish, H = human, and R = rats.

c CFCs = chlorofluorocarbons, LMWVOCs = low molecular weight volatile organic chemicals, and VOCs = volatile organic chemicals.

hydrophobic parameters such as $P_{o:a}$ and $P_{w:a}$ or measures of solubility in lipids and water. Batterman et al. (2002) related the human blood:air PCs of trihalomethanes to various descriptors, including molecular weight and number of bromine atoms in the compound. Since these descriptors also tend to be correlated with lipophilicity (i.e., increases in molecular weight or number of bromine tend to increase $P_{o:w}$), these types of correlations, especially for such a reduced dataset, are to be expected. DeJongh et al. (1997) and Meulenberg and Vijverberg (2000) used the hydrophobic descriptors $P_{o:w}$, $P_{o:a}$, and $P_{w:a}$ to relate rat blood:air PC to the structure of VOCs. However, contrary to the regression with tissue:air PCs, they could only derive adequate regressions when a significant intercept was included. Since partitioning into lipids and water was taken into account by the hydrophobic descriptors, presence of an intercept was interpreted as being the result of significant binding to blood proteins. To date, there have not been any attempts to correlate the magnitude of this binding intercept to LFE-type descriptors.

Free–Wilson-type QSARs have recently been developed for a series of chloroethanes. Each chemical in the chloroethane family was described with a common basic structure (BS) of two carbons (C-C), as well as a set of substituent groups. The working hypothesis was that each substituent group in the structure had an additive and constant contribution to the blood:air PC (P_b) as reflected by the following equation (Free and Wilson, 1964):

$$P_b = BS + \sum fs \times Cs \qquad (40.4)$$

where BS = contribution of the basic structure to P_b, fs = frequency of occurrence of the substituent S in the chemical, and Cs = contribution of the substituent S to P_b.

The frequency and identity of each fragment in a given molecule was provided as input, along with rat and human experimental values of P_b for each chloroethane, and multiple linear regression analyses on the experimental data were conducted to identify the contribution of the basic structure and the substituent groups (Fouché-court and Krishnan, 2000). Group contribution to blood:air PC values, however, is different from one species to another, as can be seen in Table 40.2.

Biologically based algorithms for predicting blood:air PCs should be able to account for chemical solubility in blood lipids (phospholipids and neutral lipids), solubility in blood water fraction, as well as protein binding. Poulin and Krishnan (1996c) proposed the following algorithm for predicting P_b of VOCs:

$$P_{b:a} = [P_{o:w}P_{w:a}(V_{nb} + 0.3V_{pb})] + [P_{w:a}(V_{wb} + 0.7V_{pb})] \qquad [40.5]$$

where V_{nb} = volume fraction of neutral lipid in blood, V_{pb} = volume fraction of phospholipid in blood, and V_{wb} = volume fraction of water in blood.

The predictions of rat blood:air partition coefficient obtained using the above equation were found to be adequate for relatively hydrophilic organics (e.g., alcohols, ketones, acetate esters), but not for relatively lipophilic organic chemicals for which the predicted P_b was significantly lower than the experimental values. The blood:air partition coefficient of a chemical is a composite number that can represent two processes occurring in the blood, namely, solubility and binding. Whereas chemical solubility is likely to be determined by the neutral lipid, phospholipid, and water contents in blood, the binding would appear to be associated with plasma proteins or hemoglobin. For alcohols, acetate esters, and ketones, rat and human blood:air partition coefficients appear to be adequately predicted using solubility based algorithms. For more lipophilic VOCs (e.g., alkanes, haloalkanes, aromatic hydrocarbons), however, the blood:air partition coefficients obtained using the solubility based algorithm are lower than the experimental data. The fact that the rat blood:air partition coefficient of lipophilic VOCs is underpredicted has been explained by the potential binding of these substances to blood proteins (Poulin and Krishnan, 1996b). However, such a discrepancy between predicted and experimental data is less pronounced in humans. Given that differences in blood lipid composition between rat and human are minor, interspecies differences in binding to blood components (either affinity constants or number of binding sites) can possibly be the basis for this difference (Wiester et al. 2002). At the present time, there are no validated mechanistic algorithms for predicting association constants for blood protein binding of organic chemicals. However, a qualitative approach for identifying VOCs that can bind to blood proteins has been developed on the basis of the consideration of structural features and lipophilic characteristics (Poulin et al. 1999).

In Silico Approaches for Tissue:Blood PCs

Tissue:blood PCs are fundamental parameters required for the construction of PBPK models. These parameters not only determine the tissue concentration at steady-state, but also influence the time taken to attain steady-state. In the case of VOCs, the tissue:blood PCs can be computed by dividing the tissue:air PCs with the blood:air PC. It is useful, however, to develop approaches for predicting tissue:blood PCs directly. The in silico approaches published to date for the purpose of estimating tissue:blood PCs of organic chemicals are presented in Table 40.3. Among the available in silico approaches, the LFE-type QSARs have mainly focused on using steric or hydrophobic descriptors. Abraham and Weathersby (1994) developed equations for many tissues using the McGowan volume (V_x), an indicator of compound bulkiness. The brain:blood PCs of a series of CNS-acting pharmaceutical agents (most notably H_2R antagonists) have been extensively studied and related to the steric descriptors V_x, molar volume (V_m), molecular weight (MW), and polar surface area (PSA). Parham et al. (1997) also developed QSARs, using steric descriptors, for estimating adipose tissue:blood PCs of a series of polychlorinated biphenyls (PCBs) congeners. These descriptors included some that described planarity, position of chlorines, and the effect of the chlorines on the adjacent carbons. It was shown that the PC depended mostly on the presence or absence of adjacent non-chlorine-substituted meta and para carbons. Since PCB congeners without unsubstituted meta–para pairs tend to be more slowly eliminated than those with such pairs, it is suggested that the reason for this slower elimination might be the higher adipose tissue:blood PC, which leads to a greater storage of PCBs in this tissue. Most of the work relating to hydrophobic descriptors has involved a series of basic drugs in rabbit tissues, for which tissue:blood (or plasma) PCs were related to $P_{o:w}$ using an

Table 40.3 *In Silico* Approaches for Estimating the Tissue:Blood Partition Coefficients (*P*) of Chemicals

Approach[a]	Species[b]	Chemical Class[c]	Reference
QSARs: LFE-type equations			
Steric descriptors			
$\log P_{adipose:blood} = 0.168 + 0.198R_2 + 0.130\,\pi_2^H - 1.211\,\alpha_2^H - 3.267\,\beta_2^H + 2.275V_x$	H	Inert gases; LMWVOCs; CFCs	Abraham and Weathersby (1994)
$\log P_{brain:blood} = -0.166 + 0.239R_2 - 0.626\,\pi_2^H - 0.368\,\alpha_2^H - 0.615\,\beta_2^H + 1.072V_x$	H	Inert gases; LMWVOCs; CFCs	Abraham and Weathersby (1994)
$\log P_{brain:blood} = -0.0148\text{PSA} + 0.152\log P_{o:w} + 0.139$	H	Inert gases; HMWOCs; LMWVOCs	Clark (1999)
$\log P_{brain:blood} = 1.359 + 0.338\log P_{cyh} - 0.00618V_m$	H	H_2-R antagonists	Kalizan and Markuszewski (1996)
$\log P_{heart:blood} = -0.346 + 0.204\,\pi_2^H - 2.150\,\alpha_2^H - 0.853\,\beta_2^H + 0.931V_x$	H	Inert gases; LMWVOCs; CFCs	Abraham and Weathersby (1994)
$\log P_{kidney:blood} = -0.188 + 0.226R_2 - 0.559\,\pi_2^H - 0.433\,\beta_2^H + 0.832V_x$	H	Inert gases; LMWVOCs; CFCs	Abraham and Weathersby (1994)
$\log P_{liver:blood} = -0.270 + 0.233R_2 - 0.375\,\pi_2^H - 1.004\,\alpha_2^H - 1.118\,\beta_2^H + 0.832V_x$	H	Inert gases; LMWVOCs; CFCs	Abraham and Weathersby (1994)
$\log P_{lung:blood} = -0.150 - 0.195\,\pi_2^H + 0.389V_x$	H	Inert gases; LMWVOCs; CFCs	Abraham and Weathersby (1994)
$\log P_{muscle:blood} = -0.222 - 0.479\,\pi_2^H - 0.517\,\beta_2^H + 0.999V_x$	H	Inert gases; LMWVOCs; CFCs	Abraham and Weathersby (1994)
$P_{adipose:plasma} = 1.9988 - 0.5004\text{UNS} + 0.1793\text{NPL} + 0.05931\text{DIFF}^2$	H	PCBs	(48)
$\log P_{brain:blood} = 0.088 + 0.264R_2 - 0.966\,\pi_2^H - 0.705\Sigma\,\alpha_2^H - 0.756\Sigma\,\beta_2^H + 1.189V_x$	R	H_2-R antagonists	Norinder and Haeberlein (2002)

(continued)

Table 40.3 (continued) In Silico Approaches for Estimating the Tissue:Blood Partition Coefficients (P) of Chemicals

Approach[a]	Species[b]	Chemical Class[c]	Reference
$\log P_{brain:blood} = -0.088 + 0.272 \log P_{o:w} - 0.00116MW$	R	H_2-R antagonists	Kalizan and Markuszewski (1996)
$\log P_{brain:blood} = 0.00116MW + 0.272 \log P_{o:w} - 0.088$	R	Inert gases; volatile hydrocarbons	Norinder and Haeberlein (2002)
$\log P_{brain:blood} = -0.01V_m + 0.35 \log P_{o:w} + 0.99I_3 + 1.25$	R	Drug-like molecules	Norinder and Haeberlein (2002)
$\log P_{brain:blood} = -0.021PSA - 0.003MV + 1.643$	R	Inert gases; HMWOCs; LMWVOCs	Clark (1999)
$\log P_{brain:blood} = -0.0322DPSA + 1.33$	R	HMWOCs	Norinder and Haeberlein (2002)
$\log P_{brain:blood} = -0.038 + 0.198R_2 - 0.687 \pi_2^H - 0.715\Sigma \alpha_2^H - 0.698\Sigma \beta_2^H + 0.995V_x$	R	H_2-R antagonists; Inert gases; SOMs	Norinder and Haeberlein (2002)
$\log P_{brain:blood} = -0.218(N_N + N_O) + 0.235 \log P_{o:w} - 0.027$	R	HMWOCs	Norinder and Haeberlein (2002)
$\log P_{brain:blood} = 0.476 + 0.541 \log P_{o:w} - 0.00794MW$	R	H_2-R antagonists	Kalizan and Markuszewski (1996)
$\log P_{brain:blood} = 1.296 + 0.309 \log P_{oyh} - 0.00570MW$	R	H_2-R antagonists	Kalizan and Markuszewski (1996)

Hydrophobic descriptors

$\log P_{brain:blood} = 0.39 \log P_{o:w} + 0.68$	H	Drugs, hormones	Seydel and Schaper (1982)
$\log P_{brain:blood} = 0.054G^o + 0.43$	H	H_2-R antagonists; LMWVOCs	Lombardo et al. (1996)
$P_{adipose:blood} = [(V_{lt} P_{o:w}^{A1} + V_{wt})/(V_{lb} P_{o:w}^{A2} + V_{wb})] + B$	H, R	LMWVOCs	DeJongh et al. (1997)
$P_{brain:blood} = [(V_{lt} P_{o:w}^{A1} + V_{wt})/(V_{lb} P_{o:w}^{A2} + V_{wb})] + B$	H, R	LMWVOCs	DeJongh et al. (1997)
$P_{kidney:blood} = [(V_{lt} P_{o:w}^{A1} + V_{wt})/(V_{lb} P_{o:w}^{A2} + V_{wb})] + B$	H, R	LMWVOCs	DeJongh et al. (1997)
$P_{liver:blood} = [(V_{lt} P_{o:w}^{A1} + V_{wt})/(V_{lb} P_{o:w}^{A2} + V_{wb})] + B$	H, R	LMWVOCs	DeJongh et al. (1997)

	H, R		
$P_{muscle:blood} = [(V_{ft} P_{o:w}^{A1} + V_{wt})/(V_{lb} P_{o:w}^{A2} + V_{wb})] + B$		LMWVOCs	DeJongh et al. (1997)
Ln $P_{kidney:blood} = 0.0065\Sigma o$	R	HMWOCs	Yamaguchi et al. (1996)
Ln $P_{liver:blood} = 0.025\Sigma i$	R	HMWOCs	Yamaguchi et al. (1996)
Ln $P_{muscle:blood} = 0.0069\Sigma i$	R	HMWOCs	Yamaguchi et al. (1996)
log $P_{brain:blood} = 0.035\Delta G_{solv} + 0.259$	R	H_2-R antagonists; LMWVOCs	Norinder and Haeberlein (2002)
log $P_{brain:blood} = 0.4275 - 0.3873 n_{acc,solv} + 0.1092 \log P_{o:w} - 0.0017 A_{pol}$	R	Drugs; LMWVOCs; anaesthetics	Feher et al. (2000)
log $P_{brain:blood} = 1.979 + 0.373 \log P_{cyh} - 0.00275 V_{wav}$	R	H_2-R antagonists	Kalizan and Markuszewski (1996)
log $P_{brain:plasma} = -0.48 \Delta\log P_{oct-cyc} + 0.89$	R	H_2-R antagonists	Testa et al. (2000)
ln $P_{adipose:blood} = 0.05\Sigma i + 0.021$	R	HMWOCs	Yamaguchi et al. (1996)
$P_{adipose:blood} = 0.915\, P_{o:w}^{0.573}$	Rb	Basic drugs	Yokogawa et al. (1990)
$P_{adipose:plasma} = 0.016\, P_{o:w}^{1.225}$	Rb	Basic drugs	Yokogawa et al. (2002)
$P_{bone\ marrow:blood} = 1.975\, P_{o:w}^{0.273}$	Rb	Basic drugs	Yokogawa et al. (1990)
$P_{bone:plasma} = 0.036\, P_{o:w}^{0.947}$	Rb	Basic drugs	Yokogawa et al. (2002)
$P_{brain:blood} = 3.157\, P_{o:w}^{0.312}$	Rb	Basic drugs	Yokogawa et al. (1990)
$P_{brain:plasma} = 0.062\, P_{o:w}^{0.984}$	Rb	Basic drugs	Yokogawa et al. (2002)
$P_{gut:blood} = 3.002\, P_{o:w}^{0.346}$	Rb	Basic drugs	Yokogawa et al. (1990)
$P_{gut:plasma} = 0.058\, P_{o:w}^{1.02}$	Rb	Basic drugs	Yokogawa et al. (2002)
$P_{heart:blood} = 1.678\, P_{o:w}^{0.422}$	Rb	Basic drugs	Yokogawa et al. (1990)
$P_{heart:plasma} = 0.032\, P_{o:w}^{1.098}$	Rb	Basic drugs	Yokogawa et al. (2002)
$P_{kidney:plasma} = 0.075\, P_{o:w}^{1.037}$	Rb	Basic drugs	Yokogawa et al. (2002)

(continued)

Table 40.3 (continued) *In Silico* Approaches for Estimating the Tissue:Blood Partition Coefficients (*P*) of Chemicals

Approach[a]	Species[b]	Chemical Class[c]	Reference
$P_{\text{liver:plasma}} = 0.064\ P_{\text{o:w}}^{0.884}$	Rb	Basic drugs	Yokogawa et al. (2002)
$P_{\text{lung:blood}} = 1.158\ P_{\text{o:w}}^{0.565}$	Rb	Basic drugs	Yokogawa et al. (1990)
$P_{\text{lung:plasma}} = 0.031\ P_{\text{o:w}}^{1.236}$	Rb	Basic drugs	Yokogawa et al. (2002)
$P_{\text{muscle:blood}} = 4.928\ P_{\text{o:w}}^{0.221}$	Rb	Basic drugs	Yokogawa et al. (1990)
$P_{\text{muscle:plasma}} = 0.099\ P_{\text{o:w}}^{0.889}$	Rb	Basic drugs	Yokogawa et al. (2002)
$P_{\text{skin:blood}} = 2.997\ P_{\text{o:w}}^{0.256}$	Rb	Basic drugs	Yokogawa et al. (1990)
$P_{\text{skin:plasma}} = 0.058\ P_{\text{o:w}}^{0.927}$	Rb	Basic drugs	Yokogawa et al. (2002)
$P_{\text{spleen:blood}} = 3.002\ P_{\text{o:w}}^{0.346}$	Rb	Basic drugs	Yokogawa et al. (1990)

QSARs: Free–Wilson-type equations

Approach[a]	Species[b]	Chemical Class[c]	Reference
$P_{\text{adipose:blood}} = BS_{(C-C)}(94.5) + nCL_2(-29.2) + nCL_3(29.2)$	F	Chloroethanes	Fouchécourt et al. (2000)
$P_{\text{liver:blood}} = BS_{(C-C)}(2.93) + nCL_2(-0.238) + nCL_3(0.238)$	F	Chloroethanes	Fouchécourt et al. (2000)
$P_{\text{muscle:blood}} = BS_{(C-C)}(3.02) + nCL_2(-0.175) + nCL_3(0.175)$	F	Chloroethanes	Fouchécourt et al. (2000)
$P_{\text{adipose:blood}} = BS_{(C-C)}(49.2) + nH_3(-0.440) + nCL(-14.54) + nCL_2(-6.65) + nCL_3(26.5)$	H	Chloroethanes	Fouchécourt and Krishnan (2000)
$P_{\text{liver:blood}} = BS_{(C-C)}(2.64) + nH_3(-0.61) + nCL(-0.66) + nCL_2(-0.18) + nCL_3(1.68)$	H	Chloroethanes	Fouchécourt and Krishnan (2000)
$P_{\text{muscle:blood}} = BS_{(C-C)}(1.11) + nH_3(0.08) + nCL(-0.02) + nCL_2(-0.21) + nCL_3(0.15)$	H	Chloroethanes	Fouchécourt and Krishnan (2000)
$P_{\text{adipose:blood}} = BS_{(C-C)}(30.1) + nH_3(-9.88) + nCL(-6.02) + nCL_2(-3.90) + nCL_3(17.3)$	R	Chloroethanes	Fouchécourt and Krishnan (2000)
$P_{\text{liver:blood}} = BS_{(C-C)}(1.79) + nH_3(-0.9) + nCL(-0.38) + nCL_2(-0.21) + nCL_3(1.27)$	R	Chloroethanes	Fouchécourt and Krishnan (2000)

Algorithm	Species[b]	Chemical class[c]	Reference
$P_{muscle:blood} = BS_{(C-C)}(0.69) + nH_3(-0.12) + nCL(0.04) + nCL_2(-0.12) + nCL_3(0.17)$	R	Chloroethanes	Fouchécourt and Krishnan (2000)

Biologically based algorithms

Algorithm	Species[b]	Chemical class[c]	Reference
$P_{tissue:blood} = (S_o V_{nt} + S_w 0.7 V_{pt} + S_o 0.3 V_{pt} + S_w V_{wt})/(S_o V_{nb} + S_w 0.7 V_{pb} + S_o 0.3 V_{pb} + S_w V_{wb})$	H	LMWVOCs	Poulin and Krishnan (1995a)
$P_{tissue:blood} = (P_{o:w} V_{nt} + V_{wt} + P_{o:w} 0.3 V_{pt} + 0.7 V_{pt})/[f_e(P_{o:w} V_{ne} + V_{we} + P_{o:w} 0.3 V_{pe} + 0.7 V_{pe}) + f_p(P_{o:w} V_{np} + V_{wp} + P_{o:w} 0.3 V_{pp} + 0.7 V_{pp})]$	R	Ketones; Alcohols; Esters	Poulin and Krishnan (1995b)
$P_{tissue:blood} = [P_{o:w}(V_{nt} + 0.3 V_{pt}) + (V_{wt} + 0.7 V_{pt})]/[P_{o:w}(V_{nb} + 0.3 V_{pb}) + (V_{wb} + 0.7 V_{pe})]$	R, H	LMWVOCs	Poulin and Krishnan (1996b)

[a] π_2^H = dipolarity/polarizability, α_2^H = overall hydrogen-bond acidity, β_2^H = overall hydrogen-bond basicity, ΔG_{solv} = free energy of solvation in hexadecane, Σi = molecular structure Fujita value, A_1, A_2 = Collander-type coefficient, A_{pol} = polar surface area, B = correction factor, BS = basic structure, DIFF = variable dependant on the number of chloride atoms in the aromatic cycle, DPSA = dynamic polar surface area, f_e = fraction of erythrocytes in blood, f_p = fraction of plasma in blood, l_3 = variable dependant on the presence of an amino nitrogen or carboxyl group, MV = molecular volume, MW = molecular weight, $n_{acc,solv}$ = number of solvated hydrogen-bond acceptors, nCL = number of CL fragments, nCL_2 = number of CL_2 fragments, nCL_3 = number of CL_3 fragments, nH_3 = number of H_3 fragments, N_N = number of nitrogens, N_O = number of oxygens, NPL = variable dependant on the number of chloride atoms in the molecule in ortho position, ^oG = Gibbs free energy related to the solvation of the substance in water, P_{cyh} = cyclohexane:water partition coefficient, $P_{o:w}$ = n-octanol:water partition coefficient (or vegetable oil:water), $P_{oct-cyc}$ = octanol-cyclohexane, PSA = polar surface area, R_2 = Excess molar refraction, S_o = solubility in n-octanol (or vegetable oil), S_w = solubility in water, UNS = variable dependant on the number of atoms in the molecule that are not chlorides, V_{lb} = volume fraction of lipids in blood, V_{lt} = volume fraction of lipids in tissue, V_m = molar volume, V_{nb} = volume fraction of neutral lipids in blood, V_{ne} = volume fraction of neutral lipids in erythrocytes, V_{np} = volume fraction of neutral lipids in plasma, V_{nt} = volume fraction of neutral lipids in tissues, V_{pb} = volume fraction of phospholipids in blood, V_{pe} = volume fraction of phospholipids in erythrocytes, V_{pp} = volume fraction of phospholipids in plasma, V_{pt} = volume fraction of phospholipids in tissues, V_{wav} = volume of water needed in order to solubilize the substance, V_{wb} = volume fraction of water in blood, V_{we} = volume fraction of water in erythrocytes, V_{wp} = volume fraction of water in plasma, V_{wt} = volume fraction of water in tissue, V_{wt} = volume fraction of water in tissues, and V_x = McGowan characteristic volume.

[b] F = fish, H = human, and R = rats.

[c] CFCs = chlorofluorocarbons, HMWOCs = high molecular weight organic chemicals, LMWVOCs = low molecular weight volatile organic chemicals, PCBs = polychlorobiphenyls, and VOCs = volatile organic chemicals.

exponential function (Yokogawa et al., 1990, 2002). For rat tissue:blood PCs, incorporation of $P_{o:w}$ data in regression equations has necessitated significant intercepts (DeJongh et al.,1997), due to the blood protein binding of these chemicals.

Free–Wilson-type QSARs have also been developed for the tissue:blood PCs of chloroethanes in rats, humans, and fish (Table 40.3). Because experimental PCs for fish were limited to three chemicals (instead of the possible nine in the series, as for rats and humans), the number of fragments in rats and humans is not the same as in fish (four vs. two, respectively). The statistical power of the fish model is, therefore, low compared to other LFE-type QSARs.

Regarding the biologically based algorithms for the estimation of tissue:blood partition coefficients, the following published by Poulin and Krishnan (1995a,b) is of use with VOCs that do not exhibit significant binding to blood proteins:

$$P_{t:b} = \frac{P_{o:w}(V_{nt} + 0.3V_{pt}) + (V_{wt} + 0.7V_{pt})}{P_{o:w}(V_{nb} + 0.3V_{pb}) + (V_{wb} + 0.7V_{pb})} \tag{40.6}$$

If blood protein binding is important (as is the case for lipophilic VOCs), then it should be additionally accounted for.

In Silico Approaches for Protein Binding

Some chemicals bind to specific transport proteins. For example, various drugs (e.g., warfarin) bind to serum albumin. Other chemicals bind to tissue proteins. In these cases, partitioning of a compound in that tissue will depend not only on solubility in tissue water and lipids, but also on the binding to protein. Since only unbound chemical can freely distribute across tissue membranes, determination of the fraction unbound (f_u) becomes important. For chemicals that reversibly bind to proteins, f_u is related to the binding affinity constant (K_a) as follows:

$$1/f_u = 1 + K_a(nC_p - C_b) \tag{40.7}$$

where n = number of binding sites on the protein, C_p = molar concentration of binding protein, and C_b = molar concentration of bound chemical.

The available *in silico* approaches for estimating f_u and K_a are listed in Table 40.4. These approaches have mainly relied upon the use of hydrophobic descriptors in LFE-type equations. For example, Nestorov et al. (1998) related the ratio of fraction bound to fraction unbound for various tissues in rats to the $P_{o:w}$ in LFE-type QSARs for a series of barbituric acids. The number of binding sites was assumed to be one for all tissues. The K_a or f_u in human blood for penicillins, organic acids, cephalosporins, and aromatic acids have also related to hydrophobic descriptors. These observations seem to suggest that nonspecific reversible binding to tissue protein is mostly a lipophilic process, probably because of the intrinsic hydrophobic nature of the binding site. To date there have been no Free–Wilson-type QSARs developed to describe tissue or blood protein binding.

Table 40.4 In Silico Approaches for Estimating Protein Binding of Chemicals[a]

Approach[b]	Species[c]	Chemical Class	Reference
QSARs: LFE-type equations			
Hydrophobic descriptors			
$\log (1/f_{u(\text{plasma})} - 1) = 0.994 \log P_{\text{o:w}} - 1.10$	H	Aromatic acids	Testa et al. (2000)
$\log (1/f_{u(\text{plasma})} - 1) = 0.994 \log P_{\text{o:w}} - 1.10$	H	Organic acids	Laznicek et al. (1987)
$\log (1/K_{a(\text{plasma})}) = -3.91 \log P_{\text{o:w}}^2 + 13 \log P_{\text{o:w}} - 13.7$	H	Cephalosporins	Testa et al. (2000)
$\log (1 - f_{u(\text{brain})}) = 0.36 \log P_{\text{o:w}} - 1.07$	H	Barbiturates	Seydel and Schaper (1982)
$\log (1 - f_{u(\text{plasma})}) = 0.276 \log P_{\text{o:w}} + 1.2$	H	Penicillins	Seydel and Schaper (1982)
$\log (1 - f_{u(\text{plasma})}) = 0.30 \log P_{\text{o:w}} - 1.03$	H	Barbiturates	Seydel and Schaper (1982)
$\log (1 - f_{u(\text{plasma})}) = 0.33 \log P_{\text{o:w}} + 1.94$	H	Tetracyclines	Seydel and Schaper (1982)
$\log 1/K_{a(\text{albumin binding})} = -0.85 \log P_{\text{o:w}} + 2.73$	H	Sulfapyrimidines; sulfapyridines	Seydel and Schaper (1982)
$\log 1/K_{a(\text{albumin binding})} = -0.97 \log P_{\text{o:w}} + 3.24$	H	Sulfapyridines	Seydel and Schaper (1982)
$\log 1/K_{a(\text{albumin binding})} = -0.97 \log P_{\text{o:w}} - 0.70I + 3.24$	H	Sulfapyrimidines; sulfapyridines	Seydel and Schaper (1982)
$\log 1/K_{a(\text{albumin binding})} = -0.99 \log P_{\text{o:w}} + 2.49$	H	Sulfapyrimidines	Seydel and Schaper (1982)
$\log K_{\text{albumin binding}} = 0.89 \log P_{\text{o:w}} + 1.47$	H	Sulfapyrimidines	Seydel and Schaper (1982)
$\log K_{\text{albumin binding}} = 1.15 \log P_{\text{o:w}} + 1.23$	H	Sulfonamides	Seydel and Schaper (1982)
$\log K_{\text{albumin binding}} = 1.23 \log P_{\text{o:w}} - 0.056$	H	Steroid bisguanylhydrazones	Seydel and Schaper (1982)
$\log K_{\text{albumin binding}} = 1.32 \log P_{\text{o:w}} + 0.37$	H	Penicillins	Seydel and Schaper (1982)
$\log K_{\text{albumin binding}} = 1.39 \log P_{\text{o:w}} - 1.19$	H	Cardenolides	Seydel and Schaper (1982)
$\log K_{\text{albumin binding}} = 1.65 \log P_{\text{o:w}} - 2.57$	H	Steroid hormones	Seydel and Schaper (1982)
$\log K_{\text{plasma protein binding}} = 0.73\Delta R_{\text{mui}} + 1.46$	H	Sulfapyridines	Seydel and Schaper (1982)
$\log K_{a(\text{blood protein binding})} = 0.504\Sigma\pi - 0.665$	H	Penicillins	Bird and Marshall (1967)
$\log (1/f_{u(\text{plasma})} - 1) = 1.011 \log P_{\text{o:w}} - 1.745$	R	Organic acids	Laznicek et al. (1987)
$\log (1 - f_u)/f_{u(\text{adipose})} = \log 0.750 + 0.936 \log P_{\text{o:w}}$	R	Barbituric acids	Nesterov et al. (1998)
$\log (1 - f_u)/f_{u(\text{brain})} = \log 0.073 + 0.860 \log P_{\text{o:w}}$	R	Barbituric acids	Nesterov et al. (1998)

(continued)

Table 40.4 (continued) *In Silico* **Approaches for Estimating Protein Binding of Chemicals**[a]

Approach[b]	Species[c]	Chemical Class	Reference
$\log (1 - f_u)/f_{u(\text{gut})} = \log 0.099 + 0.824 \log P_{\text{o:w}}$	R	Barbituric acids	Nesterov et al. (1998)
$\log (1 - f_u)/f_{u(\text{heart})} = \log 0.135 + 0.780 \log P_{\text{o:w}}$	R	Barbituric acids	Nesterov et al. (1998)
$\log (1 - f_u)/f_{u(\text{kidney})} = \log 0.676 + 0.619 \log P_{\text{o:w}}$	R	Barbituric acids	Nesterov et al. (1998)
$\log (1 - f_u)/f_{u(\text{liver})} = \log 1.775 + 0.504 \log P_{\text{o:w}}$	R	Barbituric acids	Nesterov et al. (1998)
$\log (1 - f_u)/f_{u(\text{lung})} = \log 0.164 + 0.841 \log P_{\text{o:w}}$	R	Barbituric acids	Nesterov et al. (1998)
$\log (1 - f_u)/f_{u(\text{muscle})} = \log 0.080 + 0.835 \log P_{\text{o:w}}$	R	Barbituric acids	Nesterov et al. (1998)
$\log (1 - f_u)/f_{u(\text{pancreas})} = \log 0.022 + 1.095 \log P_{\text{o:w}}$	R	Barbituric acids	Nesterov et al. (1998)
$\log (1 - f_u)/f_{u(\text{plasma})} = \log 0.016 + 0.975 \log P_{\text{o:w}}$	R	Barbituric acids	Nesterov et al. (1998)
$\log (1 - f_u)/f_{u(\text{red blood cell})} = \log 0.178 + 0.677 \log P_{\text{o:w}}$	R	Barbituric acids	Nesterov et al. (1998)
$\log (1 - f_u)/f_{u(\text{skin})} = \log 0.271 + 0.736 \log P_{\text{o:w}}$	R	Barbituric acids	Nesterov et al. (1998)
$\log (1 - f_u)/f_{u(\text{spleen})} = \log 0.126 + 0.841 \log P_{\text{o:w}}$	R	Barbituric acids	Nesterov et al. (1998)
$\log (1 - f_u)/f_{u(\text{stomach})} = \log 0.058 + 0.939 \log P_{\text{o:w}}$	R	Barbituric acids	Nesterov et al. (1998)
$\log (1 - f_u)/f_{u(\text{testis})} = \log 0.120 + 0.747 \log P_{\text{o:w}}$	R	Barbituric acids	Nesterov et al. (1998)
$\log K_{\text{plasma protein binding}} = 0.33\Delta R_{\text{mui}} - 0.53l + 4.08$	R	Sulfapyridines	Seydel and Schaper (1982)
$\log (1/f_{u(\text{plasma})} - 1) = 1.016 \log P_{\text{o:w}} - 1.275$	Rb	Organic acids	Laznicek et al. (1987)

[a] K = protein affinity constant (Freundlich isotherm), K_a = protein affinity constant (Scatchard isotherm) and f_u = unbound fraction.
[b] $P_{\text{o:w}}$ = octanol:water partition coefficient, π = molecular hydrophobicity constant, l = family indicator variable, ΔR_{mui} = variable dependant on the resistance constant due to diffusion of the nonionized form in the lipid membrane.
[c] H = humans, Rb = rabbit, and R = rat.

Even if there are no mechanistic algorithms for the prediction of K_a or f_u values, Poulin et al. (1999) proposed a semiquantitative mechanistic algorithm that considers blood protein binding for facilitating the calculation of apparent blood:air PC. The apparent blood:air PC reflects the ratio of steady-state arterial blood concentration ($C_{a(\text{total})}$) to the atmospheric concentration (C_{air}) of the chemical as follows:

$$P_{\text{b:a(app)}} = \frac{C_{a(\text{total})}}{C_{\text{air}}} \tag{40.8}$$

Considering the components of $C_{a(\text{total})}$, the above equation can be rewritten as follows:

$$P_{\text{b:a(app)}} = \frac{C_{a,\text{free}}}{C_{\text{air}}} + \frac{C_{a,\text{bound}}}{C_{\text{air}}} \tag{40.9}$$

Since $C_{a,\text{bound}} = C_{a,\text{free}} K_a C_p / (1 + K_a C_{a,\text{free}})$, where K_a = binding association constant and C_p = concentration of binding proteins.

$$P_{\text{b:a(app)}} = \frac{C_{a,\text{free}}}{C_{\text{air}}} + \left[\frac{C_{a,\text{free}} K_a C_p}{C_{\text{air}} \left(1 + K_a C_{a,\text{free}}\right)} \right] \tag{40.10}$$

The preceding equation can be rewritten as

$$P_{\text{b:a(app)}} = \frac{C_{a,\text{free}}}{C_{\text{air}}} \left(1 + \frac{K_a C_p}{1 + K_a C_{a,\text{free}}} \right) \tag{40.11}$$

The first term of the above equation corresponds to solubility-based $P_{\text{b:a}}$. Therefore, replacing $C_{a,\text{free}}/C_{\text{air}}$ with $P_{\text{b:a}}$, the above equation becomes:

$$P_{\text{b:a(app)}} = P_{\text{b:a(pred)}} \left(1 + \frac{K_a C_p}{1 + K_a C_{a,\text{free}}} \right) \tag{40.12}$$

This equation can be incorporated within PBPK models to calculate the $P_{\text{b,app}}$ as a function of time and exposure concentration. Here, the only additional, chemical-specific parameter that is required relates to K_a. At the present time, there is no validated animal-replacement algorithm for predicting association constants for blood protein binding of organic chemicals. However, based on the analysis presented by Poulin and Krishnan (1996b), it would appear that the average K_a value for rat hemoglobin binding is 1930 M^{-1} for several VOCs (i.e., chemicals with a molecular volume of <300 cubic Angstroms, log $P_{\text{o:w}} > 1$, and lacking oxygen in the molecule). This information may be used, at the present time, to provide a first-cut estimate of K_a and $P_{b:a(app)}$ for purposes of PBPK modeling of VOCs in the absence of experimental data.

In Silico Approaches for Clearance Constants

Hepatic clearance (CL_h) in PBPK models is described as the product of the extraction ratio (E) and liver blood perfusion rate (Q_l). The extraction ratio depends upon the intrinsic clearance (CL_{int}), which is equal to the ratio of V_{max}/K_m for first-order conditions. *In silico* approaches published so far regarding the estimation of CL_h, V_{max}, and K_m are listed in Tables 40.5 to 40.7. Most of the *in silico* models have been developed with data on pharmaceutical products. LFE-type QSARs for benzodiazepines relating CL_h in humans with electrostatic descriptors such as the ionization potential (Lewis, 2000) and such QSARs for V_{max} of *n*-demethylation of ethylamines using molecular length have also been developed (Lewis, 2001). Hydrophobic descriptors have been used to develop QSARs of CL_h of a series of basic drugs in rabbits (Ishizaki et al., 1997; Yokogawa et al., 2002). LFE-type QSARs relating K_m to electrostatic descriptors such as pK_a have been developed for the acetylation of sulfonamides (Table 40.7) (Seydel and Schaper, 1982). Additionally, the Hammet constant has been used to relate demethylation and sulfatation affinity to the structure of halo-nitro and phenol compounds (Hansch and Leo, 1995). K_m has also been related to purely hydrophobic descriptors such as $P_{o:w}$ in the case of demethylation, glucuronidation, hydrolysis, and sulfation of phenols, phenylhippurates, and morphines (Hansch and Leo, 1995). Recent studies have shown, however, that in most cases, a combination of all three types of descriptors—electrostatic, lipophilic, and steric—best describes affinity to metabolizing enzymes in LFE-type models (Lewis and Dickins, 2002).

There have only been a few attempts to develop QSAR models of the hepatic clearance, intrinsic clearance, and metabolism constants (V_{max}, K_m) for environmental pollutants. Waller et al. (1996) developed a three-dimensional QSAR model for estimating intrinsic clearance of a small series of VOCs that are substrates of CYP2E1. Gargas et al. (1988) related the V_{max} of a series of haloalkanes to connectivity indices. Parham and Portier (1998) predicted rates of metabolism of a series of PCB congeners using steric descriptors, although implications of the inclusion of such descriptors were not discussed. Since $k_{cat} = V_{max}/[E_t]$, where $[E_t]$ = total enzyme concentration, some authors explored quantitative relationships between the catalytic rate (k_{cat}) and structural descriptors (Table 40.6). These efforts indicate the varying importance of steric, hydrophobic, and electrostatic processes, depending on the nature of the binding site and enzymes involved (Tables 40.6 and 40.7).

The development of Free–Wilson-type QSARs for V_{max} and K_m of VOCs has been attempted for chloroethanes (Fouchécourt and Krishnan, 2000). No mechanistic algorithms, however, are available for predicting CL_h, CL_{int}, V_{max}, or K_m *a priori* without any experimental work. An interim approach, at least for VOCs, would involve the use of physiological limits of clearance in order to estimate the range of blood (or tissue) concentration possible in an individual (or population). In other words, even without knowing the exact rate of metabolism, it should be possible to

Table 40.5 In Silico Approaches for Estimating Clearances (CL) of Chemicals

Approach[a]	Species[b]	Chemical Class[c]	Reference
QSARs: LFE-type equations			
Electrostatic descriptors			
$\log \mathrm{CL}_{\text{(hepatic)}} = 0.64 \log P_{o:w} - 0.98IP + 9.33$	H	Benzodiazepines	Lewis (2000)
$\log \mathrm{CL}_{\text{(hepatic)}} = 0.055\text{Energy} - 0.95IP - 0.53HBD + 10.63$	H	Benzodiazepines	Lewis (2000)
$\log \mathrm{CL}_{\text{(hepatic)}} = 0.067\text{Energy} - 1.01IP - 0.34HBD - 0.43\Delta E + 14.66$	H	Benzodiazepines	Lewis (2000)
$\log \mathrm{CL}_{\text{(hepatic)}} = 0.094\text{Energy} - 1.18IP - 0.74\Delta E + 18.65$	H	Benzodiazepines	Lewis (2000)
$\log \mathrm{CL}_{\text{(hepatic)}} = 0.65 \log P_{o:w} - 0.40IP - 0.37HBD + 0.0025Hf + 3.63$	H	Benzodiazepines	Lewis (2000)
Metabolic ratio $= 2.72Q_6 + 1.96E_H + 0.014S_N + 6.43$	R	Dichlorobiphenyls	Lewis and Dickins (2002)
Steric descriptors			
$1/\log \mathrm{CL}_{\text{(intrinsic; hepatic)}} = 3.58 - 0.058S\_sCI - 0.57S\_aaO - 0.47\text{Shadow Z length} - 0.75ClC$	H	Commercially available drugs	Ekins and Obach (2000)
$1/\log \mathrm{CL}_{\text{(intrinsic; hepatic)}} = -3.11 - 0.10\text{Dipole} - \text{mag} + 13.25\text{Jurs} - RPCG + 0.57\text{Jurs} - RPCS + 0.00013A_{\text{pol}}$	H	Commercially available drugs	Ekins and Obach (2000)
$\mathrm{CL}_{\text{(intrinsic; hepatic)}} = 25\text{Steric} + 44\text{Electrostatic} + 20\text{LUMO} + 11\text{HINT}$	R	Haloalkanes	Waller et al. (1996)
Hydrophobic descriptors			
$\mathrm{CL}_{\text{(intrinsic; hepatic)}} = 0.0555\,P_{o:w}^{1.05}$	H	Basic drugs	Yokogawa et al. (2002)
$\log \mathrm{CL}_{\text{(renal)}} = -0.24(\log P_{o:w})^2 - 0.04 \log P_{o:w} + 0.58$	H	Probenecid analogs	Seydel and Schaper (1982)
$\log \mathrm{CL}_{\text{(renal)}} = -\log(0.35 + 0.013\,P_{o:w}^{1.12})$	H	Probenecid analogs	Seydel and Schaper (1982)
$\log \mathrm{CL}_{\text{(renal)}} = -0.5 \log P_{o:w} + 3$	H	NSAID	Smith et al. (1996)
$\log \mathrm{CL}_{\text{(renal)}} = -0.5 \log P_{o:w} + 13$	H	β-blockers	Smith et al. (1996)
$\log \mathrm{CL}_{\text{(hepatic)}} = -0.54\Delta R_{\text{mui}} - 0.51$	R	Sulfonamides	Seydel and Schaper (1982)

(continued)

Table 40.5 (continued) *In Silico* Approaches for Estimating Clearances (CL) of Chemicals

Approach[a]	Species[b]	Chemical Class[c]	Reference
$\log CL_{(renal)} = -0.41\Delta R_{mui} - 0.80$	R	Sulfonamides	Seydel and Schaper (1982)
$\log CL_{(renal)} = -0.51 \log P_{o:w} - 0.33$	R	Sulfapyridines	Yamaguchi et al. (1996)
$\log CL_{(renal)} = -\log [0.048 + 6.98 \times 10^{-4}(10^{\Sigma\pi})^{1.394}]$	R	Xylidines	Seydel and Schaper (1982)
$\log CL_{(total)} = -0.74\Delta R_{mui} + 0.22pK_a - 1.73$	R	Sulfonamides	Seydel and Schaper (1982)
$\log E_{(hepatic)} = 0.045 \log P_{o:w} - 0.32$	R	HMWOCs	Yamaguchi et al. (1996)
$CL_{(intrinsic;\ hepatic)} = 3.828\ P_{o:w}^{0.676}$	Rb	Basic drugs	Ishizaki et al. (1997)
$CL_{(intrinsic;\ hepatic)} = 0.0875\ P_{o:w}^{1.338}$	Rb	Basic drugs	Ishizaki et al. (1997)
$CL_{(intrinsic;\ hepatic)} = 0.248\ P_{o:w,\ app}^{1.289}$	Rb	Basic drugs	Ishizaki et al. (1997)

QSARS: Free–Wilson-type equations

$\log CL_{(renal)} = 0.417 R_2(CH_3) - 0.744 R_1(OC_3H_7) + 1.33$	R	Xylidines	Seydel and Schaper (1982)
$\log CL_{(total)} = 0.49 R_2(CH_3) + 0.57\ R_2(C_2H_5) + 0.25 R_1(OC_3H_7) + 1.76$	R	Xylidines	Seydel and Schaper (1982)

[a] ΔE = variable related to molecular orbitals, ΔR_{mui} = variable dependant on the resistance constant due to diffusion of the nonionized form in the lipid membrane, π = molecular hydrophobicity constant, A_{pol} = polar surface area, CIC = complementary information content, Dipole-mag = dipole moment, E_H = HOMO energy, Electrostatic = Coulombic interaction energy, Energy = minimum internal energy, HBD = potential hydrogen bond donor atoms in the molecule, Hf = enthalpy of formation, HINT = hydrophobic field energy, IP = ionization potential, Jurs-RPCG = relative positive charge, Jurs-RPCS = relative positive charge surface area, LUMO = lowest unoccupied molecular orbital energy, $P_{o:w}$ = n-octanol:water partition coefficient (or vegetable oil:water), $P_{o:w,\ app}$ = apparent octanol:water partition coefficient, Q_6 = net atomic charge on carbon atom at biphenyl ring position, $R_2(CH_3)$ = methyl fragment at R_2 position, $R_2(C_2H_5)$ = ethyl fragment at R_2 position, $R_1(OC_3H_7)$ = propyl ether fragment at R_1 position, S_aaO = E-state indices for oxygen atoms with two aromatic bonds, S_sCl = E-state indice for chlorine atoms with a single bond, Shadow Z length = length of the molecule in Z dimension, S_N = total nucleophillic superdelocalizability, and Steric = Van der Waals interaction energy.

[b] F = fish, H = human, and R = rats.

[c] CFCs = chlorofluorocarbons, HMWOCs = high molecular weight organic chemicals, LMWVOCs = low molecular weight volatile organic chemicals, and VOCs = volatile organic chemicals.

Table 40.6 *In Silico* Approaches for Estimating Reaction Rates of Chemicals[a]

Approach[b]	Species[c]	Chemical Class[d]	Reference
QSARs: LFE-type equations			
Electrostatic descriptors			
log $V_{(oxidation)}$ = 0.894 − 0.111diameter − 0.007ΔE	H	Nitriles	Lewis and Dickins (2002)
log $k_{cat\ (oxidation)}$ = 19.97 − 0.024$\Delta H^{\neq}$ − 0.95IP	H	Toluenes	Lewis and Dickins (2002)
log $V_{(oxidation)}$ = 26.90 − 2.58IP	H	Halothanes	Lewis and Dickins (2002)
log $k_{cat\ (oxidation)}$ = 0.024Vol − 0.23μ − 1.14	H	Barbiturates	Lewis and Dickins (2002)
log $k_{cat\ (oxidation)}$ = 1.33 − 0.15μ	H	Anilines	Lewis and Dickins (2002)
log $k_{cat\ (demethylation)}$ = −0.68 σ + 1.06	R	$X\text{-}C_6H_4N(CH_3)_2$	Hansch and Leo (1995)
Steric descriptors			
log $k_{cat}/K_{m(Oxidation)}$ = 0.0347SA − 2.29ΔE + 1.92	H	Toluenes	Lewis and Dickins (2002)
log $V_{max\ (n\text{-}demethylation)}$ = 0.18 Length − 1.94	H	Ethylamines	Lewis (2001)
log $V_{max\ (n\text{-}demethylation)}$ = 3.50 Length − 0.13 Length^2 − 23.9	H	Ethylamines	Lewis (2001)
log $V_{(oxidation)}$ = 2.4861 − 0.1364NPL * NSIDE + 0.5694UNS − 0.2433NOM * NMC + 0.001227MW * NUNSTOT + 0.8242IND − 1.1493MOD	R	PCBs	Parham and Portier (1998)
log $V_{max\ (oxidation)}$ = −1.676^4 x_c^v + 0.424^3 x_c^v − 0.134 x_{pc}^v + 1.622	R	Haloalkanes	Gargas et al. (1988)
$V_{(n\text{-}demethylation)}$ = 0.005SA − 0.52	R	Amines	Lewis and Dickins (2002)
$V_{(n\text{-}demethylation)}$ = 0.038SA − 0.00001SA^2 − 25.64	R	Amines	Lewis and Dickins (2002)
Hydrophobic descriptors			
log $k_{cat}/K_{m(demethylation)}$ = 0.53 log $P_{o:w}$ + 3.47	R	$X\text{-}C_6H_4N(CH_3)_2$	Hansch and Leo (1995)
log V = 0.55 log $P_{o:w}$	R	Barbiturates	Hansch and Leo (1995)

(continued)

Table 40.6 (continued) *In Silico* Approaches for Estimating Reaction Rates of Chemicals[a]

Approach[b]	Species[c]	Chemical Class[d]	Reference
QSARS: Free–Wilson-type equations			
$V_{maxc} = BS_{(C-C)}(51.6) + nH_3(14.6) + nCL(-4.84) + nCL_2(10.2) + nCL_3(-16.9)$	R, H	Chloroethanes	Fouchécourt and Krishnan (2000)

[a] k_{cat} = catalytic rate, K_m = enzyme affinity constant, V = metabolic rate, V_{max} = maximal velocity of metabolism, and V_{maxc} = body weight normalized maximal velocity of metabolism.

[b] ΔE = LUMO energy – HOMO energy, $\Delta H^{\neq}$ = hydrogen abstraction energy, μ = dipolar moment of the molecule, $^4 x_c^v$, $3 x_c^v$, x_{pc}^v = connectivity indices, BS = basic structure, diameter = diameter of the molecule, IND = variable dependant on experimental data used, IP = ionization potential, Length = length of the molecule, MOD = variable dependant on experimental data used, MW = molecular weight, nCL = number of CL fragments, nCL_2 = number of CL_2 fragments, nCL_3 = number of CL_3 fragments, nH_3 = number of H_3 fragments, NMC = number of meta chlorines, NOM = number of adjacent unsubstituted ortho-meta carbon pairs, NPL = variable dependant on the number of chloride atoms in the molecule in ortho position, NSIDE = variable dependant on the number of chloride atoms in the molecule in meta position, NUNSTOT = variable dependant on the number of chloride atoms in the molecule, $P_{o:w}$ = n-octanol:water partition coefficient (or vegetable oil:water), SA = surface area, UNS = variable dependant on the number of atoms in the molecule that are not chloride, Vol = volume of the molecule, and σ^- = Hammet constant.

[c] F = fish, H = human, and R = rats.

[d] PCBs = polychlorobiphenyls.

Table 40.7 *In Silico* Approaches for Estimating the Michaelis–Menten Affinity Constant (K_m) of Chemicals

Approach[a]	Species[b]	Chemical Class[c]	Reference
QSARs: LFE-type equations			
Electrostatic descriptors			
$\log 1/K_{m(\text{demethylation})} = 0.46 \log P_{\text{o:w}} + 0.63\sigma^- + 2.62$	H	$\text{X-C}_6\text{H}_4\text{N(CH}_3)_2$	Hansch and Leo (1995)
$\log 1/K_{m(\text{sulfation})} = 0.92 \log P_{\text{o:w}} - 1.48MR_4 - 0.64MR_3 + 1.04MR_2 + 0.67\sigma^- + 4.01$	H	Phenols	Hansch and Leo (1995)
$\log K_{m(\text{acetylation})} = -0.42 \log P_{\text{ui}} + 0.14pK_a - 2.89$	H	Sulfonamides	Seydel and Schaper (1982)
$K_{m(\text{oxidation})} = [(\mu_a d(\pi_i))/|IP_i - bI|] + c$	R	Alkenes	Csanady et al. (1995)
$\log K_{m(\text{acetylation})} = 0.17pK_a - 0.69$	R	Sulfonamides	Seydel and Schaper (1982)
$\log K_{m(\text{acetylation})} = -0.42\Delta R_{mu,i} + 0.15pK_a - 1.39$	R	Sulfonamides	Seydel and Schaper (1982)
$\log K_{m(\text{acetylation})} = 0.07pK_a + 0.31 \log P_{\text{o:w}} - 0.33$	Rb	Sulfonamides	Seydel and Schaper (1982)
Hydrophobic descriptors			
$\log 1/K_{m(\text{oxidation})} = 1.39 \log P_{\text{o:w}} - 0.22 \log P_{\text{o:w}}^2 - 0.50$	H	Barbiturates	Lewis and Dickins (2002)
$\log 1/K_{m(\text{sulfation})} = 2.93F_2 + 1.16\pi_2 + 0.91\pi_3 + 0.82MR_2 - 0.59I_{\text{pOH}} + 1.29I_{\text{ET}} + 2.59$	H	Phenols	Hansch and Leo (1995)
$-\log K_{m(\text{oxidation})} = 43.27 - 4.03\Delta E - 0.60 \log P_{\text{o:w}}$	H	Toluenes	Lewis and Dickins (2002)
$\log 1/K_{m(\text{glucoronidation})} = 0.83 \log P_{\text{o:w}} + 1.37$	R	Phenols	Hansch and Leo (1995)
$\log 1/K_{m(\text{hydrolysis})} = 0.056Z1_{\text{H2O}} + 0.051Z2_{\text{H2O}} + 0.026Z3_{\text{H2O}} + 0.04Z4_{\text{H2O}} + 4.616$	R	Phenylhippurates	Kim (1993)
$\log 1/K_{m(\text{hydrolysis})} = 0.066Z1_{\text{H2O}} + 4.259$	R	Phenylhippurates	Kim (1993)
$\log 1/K_{m(\text{hydrolysis})} = 0.44\pi + 4.08$	R	Phenylhippurates	Kim (1993)
$\log 1/K_{m(\text{hydrolysis})} = 0.40\pi + 4.40$	R	Phenylhippurates	Kim (1993)
$\log 1/K_{m(\text{NADP-oxidation})} = 0.69 \log P_{\text{o:w}} + 2.90$	R	Drugs	Seydel and Schaper (1982)
$\log K_{m(\text{n-demethylation})} = -0.55 \log P_{\text{o:w}} + 2.67$	R	Morphines	Hansch and Leo (1995)
$\log K_{m(\text{oxidation})} = 0.61 \log P_{\text{o:w}} + 2.23$	R	Carbamates	Hansch and Leo (1995)
$\log K_{m(\text{oxidation})} = 1.02 \log P_{\text{o:w}} + 2.98$	R	Pyrazoles	Hansch and Leo (1995)

(continued)

Table 40.7 (continued) In Silico Approaches for Estimating the Michaelis–Menten Affinity Constant (K_m) of Chemicals

Approach[a]	Species[b]	Chemical Class[c]	Reference
$\log K_{m(oxidation)} = 1.05 \log P_{o:w} + 1.22$	R	4-nitrophenyl alkyl ethers	Hansch and Leo (1995)
$\log K_{m(oxidation)} = 0.79 \log P_{o:w} + 1.46$	R	Alkylbenzenes	Hansch and Leo (1995)
$\log K_{m(oxidation)} = 1.04 \log P_{o:w} + 1.10$	Rb	Toluenes	Hansch and Leo (1995)

QSARs: Free–Wilson-type equations

Approach[a]	Species[b]	Chemical Class[c]	Reference
$K_m = BS_{(C-C)}(3.8) + nH_3(-2.59) + nCL(-0.37) + nCL_2(0.79) + nCL_3(0.19)$	R, H	Chloroethanes	Fouchécourt and Krishnan (2000)

[a] ΔE = LUMO energy – HOMO energy, $\sigma-$ = Hammet constant, μ = dipolar moment of the molecule, π, π_2, π_3 = molecular hydrophobicity constants, ΔR_{mui} = variable dependant on the resistance constant due to diffusion of the nonionized form in the lipid membrane, a = orbital availability, b = LUMO energy, BS = basic structure, c = variable structure, $d(\pi)$ = normalized electron density, F_2 = variable dependant on the electrical field induced by ortho positioned atoms, $|\beta_{OH}$ = variable dependant on the number of β OH groups in the molecule, I_{ET} = variable dependant on the family of the substance, IP = ionization potential, $MR_{2,3,4}$ = molar refractivity indices, nCL = number of CL fragments, nCL_2 = number of CL_2 fragments, nCL_3 = number of CL_3 fragments, nH_3 = number of H_3 fragments, pK_a = log dissociation constant of an acid in water, $P_{o:w}$ = n-octanol:water partition coefficient (or vegetable oil:water), P_{ui} = n-octanol:water partition coefficient for the nonionized form, and Z1, 2, 3, 4_{H2O} = variables corresponding to the potential energy for the interaction between the molecule and water.
[b] F = fish, H = human, and R = rats.
[c] PCBs = polychlorobiphenyls.

establish the theoretical limits of blood concentration curves (Poulin et al., 1999). For example, in the case of chemicals metabolized in the liver, the rate of amount metabolized (RAM) would be equal to

$$\text{RAM} = C_a CL_h \tag{40.13}$$

where C_a = arterial concentration of chemical.

Because $CL_h = Q_l E$ and E cannot be lower than 0 or higher than 1, the envelope of possible concentrations can be obtained by setting CL_h in the above equation to its physiological limits, i.e., Q_l or 0. Although in certain cases this range can be quite large, it can provide a first-cut estimate of the possible effect of metabolism and is especially appropriate for human populations in which the metabolic rate is substantially variable.

There have been limited attempts to develop QSARs for renal and total body clearance of chemicals (e.g., xylidines) using the LFE and Free–Wilson approaches, but the predictive power was limited to the substituents in the dataset (Table 40.5) (Seydel and Schaper, 1982).

In Silico Approaches for Skin Permeability Constants

Table 40.8 provides a list of *in silico* approaches available for predicting the skin permeability constant (K_p). K_p is essential to simulate the pharmacokinetics of chemicals following topical application or dermal contact. The LFE-type QSARs relating K_p to V_x, molecular weight, and connectivity indices have been developed for alcohols, steroids, esters, and several drugs. Recent studies have suggested molecular volume to be the most effective steric descriptor (Patel et al., 2002). However, the most significant overall descriptor is log $P_{o:w}$, as demonstrated by the equations directly relating $P_{o:w}$ and K_p (Table 40.8).

A mechanistic equation for the estimation of K_p in human skin was also developed by Poulin and Krishnan (2001):

$$K_p = \frac{P_{vo:w} 0.028 D_l}{0.0340} + \frac{P_{p:w} 0.88 D_p}{0.0018} \tag{40.14}$$

where $P_{vo:w}$ = vegetable oil:water PC, $P_{p:w}$ = protein:water PC for stratum corneum, D_l = coefficient for diffusion into the lipid fraction of stratum corneum, and D_p = coefficient for diffusion into the protein fraction of stratum corneum.

In the above algorithm, the coefficients 0.028, 0.034, 0.88, and 0.0018 are species-specific and refer to the fractional content of lipid in skin, the path length for a hypothetical tortuous diffusion pathway in stratum corneum, the sum of the fractional content of water and protein in skin, and the path length for a hypothetical transcellular diffusion pathway across the corneocytes of stratum corneum, respectively. The remaining terms are chemical-specific and can be derived from molecular structure. $P_{p:w}$ in stratum corneum has been related to $P_{o:w}$ through an empirical relationship (Poulin and Krishnan, 2001). Validation of this algorithm was

Table 40.8 In Silico Approaches for Estimating the Skin Permeability Coefficient (K_p) of Chemicals

Approach[a]	Species[b]	Chemical Class[c]	Reference
QSARs: LFE-type equations			
Electrostatic descriptors			
$\log K_p = -0.626\Sigma Ca - 23.8\Sigma(Q+)/\alpha\angle\ 0.289SsssCH - 0.0357SsOH - 0.482I_B + 0.405B_R + 0.834$	H	LMWVOCs; HMWOCs	Moss et al. (2002)
$\log K_p = 0.44R_2 - 0.49\ \pi_2^H - 1.48\Sigma\ \alpha_2^H - 3.44\Sigma\ \beta_2^H + 1.94V_x - 5.13$	H	LMWVOCs; HMWOCs	Moss et al. (2002)
$\log K_p = -0.59\ \pi_2^H - 0.63\Sigma\ \alpha_2^H - 3.48\Sigma\ \beta_2^H + 1.79V_x - 5.05$	H	LMWVOCs; HMWOCs	Moss et al. (2002)
$\log K_p = -5.33 - 0.62\ \pi_2^H - 0.38\Sigma\ \alpha_2^H - 3.34\Sigma\ \beta_2^H + 1.85V_x$	H	Alcohols, steroids	Ghafourian and Fooladi (2001)
Steric descriptors			
$K_p = (b_1 + 0.0025/(b_2 + b_3 + P_{o:w}^{b4}))^{-1}MW^{b5}$	H	LMWVOCs; HMWOCs	Moss et al. (2002)
$K_p = (b_1 + b_2 P_{o:w})e^{(b3MW)}$	H	LMWVOCs; HMWOCs	Moss et al. (2002)
$\log K_p = -5.14 - 0.47\Sigma Ca + 0.23\Sigma Cd + 0.038Pol$	H	Alcohols, steroids	Raevsky and Schaper (1998)
$\log K_p = -6.14 - 0.42\Sigma Ca + 0.23\Sigma Cd + 0.21L - 0.11W$	H	Alcohols, steroids	Raevsky and Schaper (1998)
$\log K_p = -7.29 + 0.15Pol$	H	Alcohols	Raevsky and Schaper (1998)
$\log K_p = b_1 + b_2 \log P_{o:w} + b_3 MW^{0.5}$	H	LMWVOCs; HMWOCs	Moss et al. (2002)
$\log K_p = -0.428\delta - 4.80\ ^4X_{PC}^V + 28.06$	H	Hydrocorticone esters	Ghafourian and Fooladi (2001)
$\log K_p = 0.652 \log P_{o:w} - 0.00603MW - 0.623ABSQon - 0.313SsssCH - 2.3$	H	Dermal drugs; LMWVOCs; HMWOCs	Patel et al. (2002)
$\log K_p = 0.77 \log P_{o:w} - 0.0103MW - 2.33$	H	LMWVOCs; HMWOCs	Moss et al. (2002)
$\log K_p = -0.786OT + 0.252^2\kappa - 1.617\ q_s^+ - 5.767$	H	Alcohols, steroids	Ghafourian and Fooladi (2001)
$\log K_p = 0.82 \log P_{o:w} - 0.0093V_m - 0.039MP_t - 2.36$	H	Steroids	Moss et al. (2002)
$\log K_p = 0.84 \log P_{o:w} - 0.07(\log P_{o:w})^2 - 0.27Hb - 1.84 \log MW + 4.39$	H	LMWVOCs; HMWOCs	Moss et al. (2002)

Equation		Group	Reference
$\log K_p = 28.4q^- + 0.018V_m + 2.824$	H	Barbiturates; Isoquinoline; Salicylic acid	Ghafourian and Fooladi (2001)
$\log K_p = 3.99 \log TA + 4.53\, q_s^- - 0.762OT - 11.364$	H	Alcohols, Steroids	Ghafourian and Fooladi (2001)

Hydrophobic descriptors

Equation		Group	Reference
$K_p = 1.17 \times 10^{-7} P_{o:w}^{0.751} + 2.73 \times 10^{-8}$	H	Pharmaceuticals	Moss et al. (2002)
$K_p = b_1(P_{o:w}^{b2}/(b_3 + P_{o:w}^{b2}))$	H	HMWOCs	Moss et al. (2002)
$\log K_p = -0.207 \log P_{o:w}^2 + 1.49 \log P_{o:w} - 5.42$	H	Steroids	Seydel and Schaper (1982)
$\log K_p = -0.37 \log P_{o:w}^2 + 2.39 \log P_{o:w} - 8.71$	H	Phenols	Testa et al. (2000)
$\log K_p = 0.544 \log P_{o:w} - 2.88$	H	Aliphatic alcohols	Seydel and Schaper (1982)
$\log K_p = 0.80 \log P_{o:w} - 8.883$	H	Hydrocorticone esters	Ghafourian and Fooladi (2001)
$\log K_p = -1.46 \Delta\log P_{o:w} + 0.29 \log P_{o:w} - 3.75$	H	Alcohols, steroids	Testa et al. (2000)
$\log K_p = -4.36 - 0.38\Sigma Ca + 0.24\Sigma Cd$	H	Steroids	Raevsky and Schaper (1998)

Mechanistically based equations

Equation		Group	Reference
$K_p = (P_{vo:w}^{*}\, 0.028D_l/0.0340) + (P_{p:w}^{*}\, 0.88D_p/0.0018)$	H	Acids; Alcohols; Hydrocarbons	Poulin and Krishnan (2001)

[a] δ = solubility parameter, π_2^H = dipolarity/polarizability, α_2^H = overall hydrogen-bond acidity, β_2^H = overall hydrogen-bond basicity, ΣCa = hydrogen bond acceptor free energy in the molecule, ΣCd = hydrogen bond donor in the molecule, $^2\kappa$ = molecular shape index, $^4X_{PC}^V$ = connectivity indices, ABSQon = sum of absolute charges on oxygen and nitrogen atoms, b_1, b_2, b_3, b_4, b_5 = regression coefficients without any assigned role, B_R = number of rotatable bonds, D_l = coefficient for diffusion into the lipid fraction of stratum corneum, D_p = coefficient for diffusion into the protein fraction of stratum corneum, Hb = number of hydrogen bonds formed by the substance, I_B = Balaban index, L = molecular length, MP_t = melting point, MW = molecular weight, OT = number of hydrogen bonding heteroatoms, $P_{o:w}$ = n-octanol:water partition coefficient (or vegetable oil:water), Pol = describes bulk or volume related effects, $P_{p:w}$ = protein:water partition coefficient for stratum corneum, $P_{vo:w}$ = vegetable oil:water partition coefficient, q^- = the most negative charge on the hydrogen bond accepting heteroatoms, Q^+/α = positive charge per unit volume, q_s^+ = sum of atomic charges on hydrogen bonding heteroatoms, q_s^+ = sum of atomic charges on hydrogen bonding hydrogens, R_2 = excess molar refraction, SsOH = sum of E-state indices for all hydroxy groups, SsssCH = sum of E-state indices for all methyl groups, TA = total solvent accessible surface, V_m = molar volume, V_x = McGowan characteristic volume, and W = molecular width.
[b] F = fish, H = human, and R = rats.
[c] CFCs = chlorofluorocarbons, HMWOCs = high molecular weight organic chemicals, LMWVOCs = low molecular weight volatile organic chemicals, and VOCs = volatile organic chemicals.

accomplished with human data for a series of structurally unrelated acids, alcohols, and hydrocarbons. While Poulin and Krishnan (2001) suggest that additional processes (metabolism, binding) would probably have to be considered for certain compounds, all predictions using the above equation were within a factor of two of the experimental data. Since hydrogen-bonding effect was not considered in this equation, K_p predicted using the above equation will be limited to organic compounds with weak hydrogen bonding capabilities. Predictions of K_p for chemicals with high hydrogen bonding capabilities (containing at least two important hydrogen bonding groups) can be accomplished by appropriately accounting for this phenomenon.

In Silico Approaches for Oral Absorption Constants

The rate constant for oral absorption of chemicals may be a single number reflecting the sum total of all processes involved, or it may be a set of constants each one of which may describe the rate of absorption along the gastrointestinal tract. The simplest description of oral absorption in PBPK models uses a first-order rate constant ($K_{a\,(oral)}$) to approximate this process. And the value of this parameter is frequently obtained by fitting the model to serial blood concentration data obtained following oral dosing.

In silico efforts in modeling absorption have mainly focused on developing software packages that are capable of predicting the fraction absorbed in humans (Raevsky and Schaper, 1998; Balimane et al., 2000; Agoram et al., 2001; Raevsky et al., 2002). Among these, the ACAT™ and the iDEA™ models are commonly being used for preclinical analysis by the pharmaceutical industry (Agoram et al., 2001; Grass and Sinko, 2002). These models do not provide separate estimates of absorption rate constants, since they also integrate first pass metabolism by the liver in their estimation of fraction absorbed. LFE-type QSARs that have been developed to relate $K_{a\,(oral)}$ to structural descriptors or $P_{o:w}$ are summarized in Table 40.9. Mostly, these equations show the critical importance of lipophilicity in estimating absorption of certain substances, even though this is not necessarily the case for other substances. There is also evidence that partial atomic charge and dipole moment (electrostatic descriptors), as well as surface area and volume (steric descriptors), are related to the percent absorbed in humans (Balimane et al., 2000). However, the role of these parameters, if any, in determining the hepatic first pass effect in addition to the rate of absorption remains unclear (see Tables 40.5 to 40.7). Currently, no mechanistic algorithms are available to provide predictions of $K_{a\,(oral)}$ values of chemicals prior to testing.

The *in silico* approaches described above can be incorporated within PBPK models to obtain simulations of blood and tissue concentrations for new chemicals, prior to testing, as described in the following section.

INTEGRATING *IN SILICO* APPROACHES INTO RISK ASSESSMENT

PBPK models facilitate the incorporation of the estimates of the various chemical-specific parameters with those of physiological parameters to simulate the

Table 40.9 *In Silico* Approaches for Estimating the Oral Absorption Constant (K_a) of Chemicals

Approach[a]	Species[b]	Chemical Class	Reference
QSARs: LFE-type equations			
Electrostatic descriptors			
$\log K_{a(absorption)} = -0.58 \log P_{o:w} + 0.35pK_a - 1.77$	F	Barbiturates	Seydel and Schaper (1982)
Hydrophobic descriptors			
$K_{a(absorption)} = k_m[(1/R_f) - 1]^{r'}/(Q + [(1/R_f) - 1]^{r'})$	R	Sulfonamides	Testa et al. (2000)
$\log K_{a(absorption)} = -0.04 (\log P_{o:w})^2 + 0.22 \log P_{o:w} + 0.04$	R	Sulfonamides	Seydel and Schaper (1982)
$\log K_{a(absorption)} = 0.067 + \log P_{o:w} - \log(1.4 + P_{o:w})$	R	Pharmaceuticals	Yamaguchi et al. (1996)
$\log K_{a(absorption)} = -0.082(\log P_{o:w})^2 + 0.268 \log P_{o:w} + 3.96$	R	Organic acids	Seydel and Schaper (1982)
$\log K_{a(absorption)} = -0.09 (\log P_{o:w})^2 + 0.44 \log P_{o:w} - 0.396$	R	Sulfonamides	Seydel and Schaper (1982)
$\log K_{a(absorption)} = 0.09 \log P_{o:w} + 0.83$	R	Xanthenes	Seydel and Schaper (1982)
$\log K_{a(absorption)} = 0.18 \log P_{o:w} + 0.23$	R	Carbamates	Seydel and Schaper (1982)
$\log K_{a(absorption)} = 0.24 \log P_{o:w} - 1.37$	R	Antihistamines	Seydel and Schaper (1982)
$\log K_{a(absorption)} = 0.30 \log P_{o:w} - 0.07(\log P_{o:w})^2 - 2.38$	R	Sulfonylureas	Seydel and Schaper (1982)
$\log K_{a(absorption)} = 0.3 \log P_{o:w} - 0.57 \log (0.34 P_{o:w} + 1) - 0.15l - 0.74$	R	Carbamates	Seydel and Schaper (1982)
$\log K_{a(absorption)} = 0.46 \log P_{o:w} - 0.36 \log (0.60P_{o:w} + 1) - 0.23$	R	Sulfonylureas	Seydel and Schaper (1982)
$\log K_{a(absorption)} = 0.5 \log P_{o:w} -0.61 \log (0.07P_{o:w} + 1) - 0.39$	R	Sulfonamides	Seydel and Schaper (1982)
$\log K_{a(absorption)} = 0.502 \log P_{o:w} - \log (0.053P_{o:w}^{0.0862} + 1) - 0.384$	R	Sulfonamides	Seydel and Schaper (1982)
$\log K_{a(absorption)} = 0.56 \log P_{o:w} - (0.04P_{o:w}^{0.84} + 1) - 0.63$	R	Phenols; Anilines; Esters	Seydel and Schaper (1982)
$\log K_{a(absorption)} = 1.36 \log P_{o:w} + 0.36$	R	Organic anions	Seydel and Schaper (1982)

(continued)

Table 40.9 (continued) *In Silico* Approaches for Estimating the Oral Absorption Constant (K_a) of Chemicals

Approach[a]	Species[b]	Chemical Class	Reference
QSARs: Free–Wilson type equations			
(see equation below)	R	Sulfonylureas	Seydel and Schaper (1982)

$\log K_{a(\text{absorption})} = BS_{(\text{BEN-SO2-NHCONH})}(-2.272) + nH\,(0) + n2\text{-}CH_3\,(0.088) + n4\text{-}CH_3\,(0.074) + n4\text{-}C_2H_5\,(0.163) + n4\text{-}OCH_3\,(-0.229) + n2\text{-}NO_2\,(-0.324) + n3\text{-}NO_2\,(-0.207) + n4\text{-}NO_2\,(-0.323) + n4\text{-}Cl\,(0.198) + n4\text{-}Br(0.122) + nn\text{-}C_4H_9(0) + nCH_3\,(-0.638) + nC_2H_5\,(-0.361) + nn\text{-}C_3H_7\,(-0.145) + ni\text{-}C_3H_7\,(-0.244) + ni\text{-}C_4H_9(-0.035) + nt\text{-}C_4H_9\,(0.149) + ncy\text{-}C_6H_{11}(0.135) + nallyl\,(-0.419) + nC_6H_5\,(-0.088)$

[a] allyl = allyl group, Br = bromide, BS = basic structure, C_2H_5 = ethyl group, C_6H_5 = aromatic ring group, CH_3 = methyl group, Cl = chloride group, cy-C_6H_{11} = cyclohexyl group, H = hydrogen group, I = family indicator variable, i-C_3H_7 = isopropyl group, i-C_4H_9 = isobutyl group, k_m = rate constant for transfer out of the membrane, n = group occurrence in molecule, n' = constant specific to the equation without any given role, n-C_3H_7 = n-propyl group, n-C_4H_9 = n-butyl group, NO_2 = nitroxide group, OCH_3 = methyl ether group, pK_a = log dissociation constant of an acid in water, $P_{o:w}$ = n-octanol:water partition coefficient (or vegetable oil:water), Q = constant specific to the equation without any given role, R_f = reverse-phase TLC lipophilicity parameter, and t-C_4H_9 = *tert*-butyl group.

[b] F = fish and R = rats.

pharmacokinetics of chemicals in intact animals. The simulations of internal dose measures obtained with these models are increasingly used to replace external dose in risk assessment calculations to enhance the scientific basis of the methodology. For the risk assessment of systemically acting chemicals, PBPK modeling has been used for establishing the internal dose corresponding to the NOAEL in animal and subsequent extrapolation to human safe levels (Reitz et al., 1988), while for the risk assessment of carcinogens, these models have been used to derive unit risk based on internal dose measures and subsequently risk levels in exposed humans (Andersen et al., 1987). The use of *in silico* approaches, presented above, could facilitate risk assessment for *de novo* compounds using only molecular structure as input. However, before applying this to new, untested chemicals, the robustness of such an approach would first have to be studied with known chemicals. The robustness can be studied using a leave-one-out procedure, where one chemical within a dataset is removed from the analysis and new coefficients for the QSAR model parameters are derived. The risk assessment can then be performed for the "left out" chemical, using the derived equations. Such a procedure would be helpful in illustrating the usefulness of the *in silico* approaches for estimating PBPK model parameters in risk assessment. A case study is presented here using the Free–Wilson QSARs for chloroethanes (Fouchécourt and Krishnan, 2000) for the PBPK modeling and health risk assessment of 1,1,1-trichloroethane (methyl chloroform).

Free–Wilson QSARs for Chloroethanes

Quantitative relationships between molecular fragments of eight haloethanes (chloroethane, 1,1 dichloroethane, 1,2 dichloroethane, 1,1,2 trichloroethane, 1,1,1,2 tetrachloroethane, 1,1,2,2 tetrachloroethane, pentachloroethane, and hexachloroethane) and the chemical-specific parameters required for PBPK modeling [tissue:air PC (P_t, subscripts l = liver, f = fat, and s = slowly perfused), blood:air PC (P_b), V_{maxc} (µmol/hr/kg), and K_m (µM)] were established according to an additive model developed by Free and Wilson (1964). Table 40.10 presents the molecular fragments used to describe the chloroethanes. The common basic structure and the substitution positions for the structural fragments are illustrated

Table 40.10 Frequency of Occurrence of Molecular Fragments for Each Chloroethane of the Series

Chemical	BS[a]	H₃	Cl	Cl₂	Cl₃
Chloroethane	1	1	1	0	0
1,1-dichloroethane	1	1	0	1	0
1,2-dichloroethane	1	0	2	0	0
1,1,1-trichloroethane	1	1	0	0	1
1,1,2-trichloroethane	1	0	1	1	0
1,1,1,2-tetrachloroethane	1	0	1	0	1
1,1,2,2-tetrachloroethane	1	0	0	2	0
Pentachloroethane	1	0	0	1	1
Hexachloroethane	1	0	0	0	2

[a] BS = basic structure (C-C).

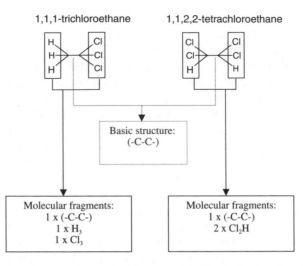

Figure 40.1 Chemical description methodology used in this study. The chemicals are represented as a basic structure (C-C) with substituents on the two carbons. Examples of the description of 1,1,1 trichloroethane and 1,1,2,2 tetrachloroethane are presented.

in Figure 40.1. Fragments consisted of hydrogens (H_3), chloride (ClH_2), dichlorides (Cl_2H), or trichlorides (Cl_3). For simplicity, these will be referred to as H_3, Cl, Cl_2, and Cl_3. Any investigated chloroethane can be reconstituted by assembling the number of appropriate fragments with the basic structure (Figure 40.1). The working hypothesis was that each substituent group in the structure had an additive and constant contribution to the parameter of interest (P_i), as reflected by the following equation (Free and Wilson, 1964):

$$P_i = BS_i + \sum f_s C_{si} \qquad (40.15)$$

where BS_i = contribution of the basic structure to P_i, f_s = frequency of occurrence of the substituent S in the chemical, and C_{si} = contribution of the substituent S to P_i.

By providing experimentally determined rat P_t, P_b, V_{maxc}, and K_m (Gargas et al., 1988, 1989) for the eight chloroethanes, along with the frequency of occurrence of each substituent in each chloroethane (f_s) (Table 40.10) as input to a commercially available software (QSAR®-PC, Biosoft®, Cambridge, U.K.) the parameters of Equation 40.15 were quantified. The output of the multiple linear regression performed by the software provided the contribution of the basic structure and the substituent groups. Any negative value resulting from the application of the QSAR equation was replaced by a default value of 1 (e.g., P_b of chloroethane in rats and humans).

Molecular fragments and their contributions to PBPK model parameters in rats and humans, as developed using the Free–Wilson approach, are presented in Tables 40.11 and 40.12. The correlation between the estimates obtained using the *in silico* approach (i.e., Free–Wilson approach) and experimental data on partition coefficients and metabolic constants is presented in Figures 40.2 and

Table 40.11 Contributions[a] of Chloroethane Structural Features to Rat Partition Coefficients[b] and Metabolic Constants[c]

Fragments	P_b	P_l	P_s	P_f	V_{maxc}	K_m
BS	56.8	2.02	0.746	28.9	52.7	3.75
Cl_2	42.7	−0.319	−0.0181	−1.16	9.40	0.863
Cl_3	7.00	1.60	0.233	14.1	−15.3	−0.0932
Cl	−9.60	−0.506	0.00710	−7.22	−7.22	−0.234
H_3	−50.1	−0.653	−0.0770	−8.56	12.9	−1.65
r^2	0.98	0.91	0.99	0.96	0.82	0.88

[a] Contributions were obtained by multiple linear regression from experimental data on chloroethane, 1,1-dichloroethane, 1,2-dichloroethane, 1,1,2-trichloroethane, 1,1,1,2-tetra-chloroethane, 1,1,2,2-tetrachloroethane, pentachloroethane, and hexachloroethane. BS = basic structure (C-C).

[b] P_b, P_l, P_s, and P_f refer to blood:air, liver:blood, slowly perfused tissue:blood and fat:blood partition coefficients, respectively.

[c] V_{maxc} (μmol/hr/kg) and K_m (μM) refer to maximal velocity of metabolism and affinity constant, respectively.

Table 40.12 Contributions[a] of Chloroethane Structural Features to Human Partition Coefficients[b]

Fragments	P_b	P_l	P_s	P_f
BS	37.4	2.72	1.099	38.9
Cl_2	29.6	−0.365	−0.163	0.105
Cl_3	7.53	2.16	0.166	12.2
Cl	−8.92	−0.446	0.0510	−10.6
H_3	−39.3	−0.699	0.0450	−1.05
r^2	0.83	0.98	0.91	0.94

[a] Contributions were obtained by multiple linear regression from experimental data on chloroethane, 1,1-dichloroethane, 1,2-dichloroethane, 1,1,2-trichloroethane, 1,1,1,2-tetrachloroethane, 1,1,2,2-tetrachloroethane, and hexachloroethane. BS = basic structure (C-C).

[b] P_b, P_l, P_s, and P_f refer to blood:air, liver:blood, slowly perfused tissue:blood and fat:blood partition coefficients, respectively.

40.3. The mean (±SD) of the ratio of experimental values to predicted values in rats was 1.17 ± 1.2 for P_b, 0.96 ± 0.17 for P_l, 0.89 ± 0.21 for P_s, 0.97 ± 0.24 for P_f, 1.03 ± 0.35 for V_{maxc}, and 0.99 ± 0.25 for K_m. The mean (±SD) of the experimental to predicted ratios in humans was 1.08 ± 0.73 for P_b, 0.96 ± 0.19 for P_l, 0.98 ± 0.14 for P_s, and 1.06 ± 0.38 for P_f. These results suggest that both tissue:blood partition coefficients and metabolic constants of structurally related chemicals (e.g., chloroethanes) can be adequately described by a Free–Wilson model. This model was then applied to predict the PBPK model parameters for methyl chloroform (a chemical that was not part of the calibration data set) in rats and humans. Results are presented in Tables 40.13 and 40.14. The ratio of predicted to experimental values in rats ranged from 0.41 (for P_b) to 1.56 (for K_m), whereas the ratio of predicted to experimental values in humans ranged from 0.46 (for P_b) to 2.1 (for P_f). These QSAR predictions were then integrated within a PBPK model to generate simulations of the pharmacokinetics of methyl chloroform in rats and humans.

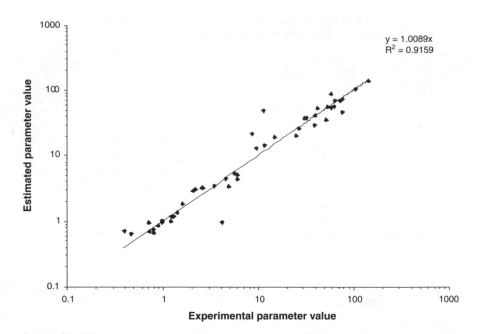

Figure 40.2 Comparison of rat experimental and predicted parameter values. Experimental values from Gargas et al. (1988, 1989).

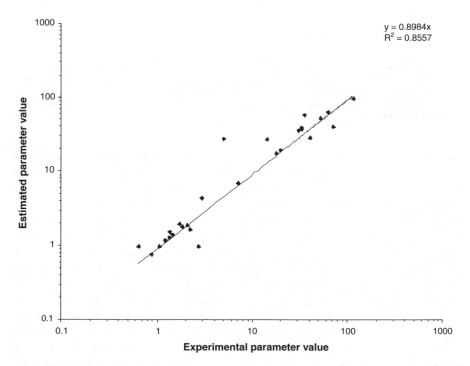

Figure 40.3 Comparison of human experimental and predicted parameter values. Experimental values were derived from Gargas et al. (1988, 1989).

Table 40.13 Comparison of Experimental[a] (Exp) and QSAR-Estimated (Est) Values of Rat Partition Coefficients[b] and Metabolic Constants[c] for 1,1,1-Trichloroethane

Parameter	Exp	Est
P_b	5.67	13.7
P_l	1.52	2.97
P_s	0.56	0.90
P_f	46.4	34.5
V_{maxc}	43.1	50.3
K_m	3.14	2.01

[a] Experimental data from Gargas et al. (1988, 1989).
[b] P_b, P_l, P_s, and P_f refer to blood:air, liver:blood, slowly perfused tissue:blood and fat:blood partition coefficients, respectively.
[c] V_{maxc} (μmol/hr/kg) and K_m (μM) refer to maximal velocity of metabolism and affinity constant, respectively.

Table 40.14 Comparison of Experimental[a] (Exp) and QSAR-Estimated (Est) Values of Human Partition Coefficients[b] for 1,1,1-Trichloroethane

Parameter	Exp	Est
P_b	2.53	5.56
P_l	3.40	4.18
P_s	1.25	1.31
P_f	104	50.1

[a] Data derived from Gargas et al. (1989).
[b] P_b, P_l, P_s, and P_f refer to blood:air, liver:blood, slowly perfused tissue:blood and fat:blood partition coefficients, respectively.

Integrating Free–Wilson QSARs into PBPK Models

The QSARs for parameter estimation were incorporated within a PBPK model that consisted of four compartments (liver, fat, richly perfused and slowly perfused tissues) interrelated by the blood circulation (Ramsey and Andersen, 1984). Tissue uptake was blood flow limited and was determined by the chemical specific tissue:blood PCs:

$$\frac{\partial Ai}{\partial t} = Qi(Ca - Cvi) \tag{40.16}$$

$$Ai = \int_0^t \frac{\partial Ai}{\partial t} \tag{40.17}$$

$$Cvi = \frac{Ai}{ViPi} \tag{40.18}$$

where $\partial Ai/\partial t$ = rate of the amount of chemical entering tissue i (mg/hr), Qi = blood flow to tissue i (L/hr), Ca = arterial blood concentration of chemical (mg/L), Cvi = venous blood concentration of chemical leaving tissue i (mg/L), Ai = quantity of chemical in tissue i (mg), Vi = volume of tissue i (L), and Pi = tissue:blood partition coefficient for tissue i.

In the metabolizing organ (i.e., liver), tissue uptake was determined additionally by the rate of metabolism:

$$\frac{\partial Al}{\partial t} = Ql(Ca - Cvi) - \frac{V_{max}Cvl}{Km + Cvl} \qquad (40.19)$$

The PBPK model was written in advanced continuous simulation language (ACSL®, Aegis Technologies, Huntsville, AL). ACSL® simulation requires two components: a continuous simulation language (CSL) file, which contains the program (i.e., constants, QSAR algorithms for the model parameters, differential equations, and integration algorithms) and a command (CMD) file, which contains simulation conditions (i.e., exposure frequency and duration) and other chemical specific information provided by user input. Since Free–Wilson QSARs along with the values of C_s and BS (Tables 40.11 and 40.12), for the partition coefficients and metabolic constants in rats and humans were included in the CSL file, only the frequencies of the substituents (Table 40.10) needed to be entered as input in the CMD file in order to simulate the kinetics of any given chloroethane (Figure 40.4).

Validation of the integrated Free–Wilson-PBPK model was accomplished by comparing the output of this model to the output of a PBPK model that contained experimentally determined parameter values. Figure 40.5 compares the simulations of steady-state blood and tissue concentrations in rats obtained with the integrated QSAR-PBPK model and the conventional PBPK model for all chloroethanes in the series, following 1 ppm exposure. The steady-state arterial blood and tissue concentrations of 1,1,1-trichloroethanes in rats and humans obtained using the integrated QSAR-PBPK model and the conventional PBPK models are compared in Table 40.15 for a 1 ppm exposure. Ratios were 1.79 ± 0.67 (range: 1.03 in fat to 2.22 in slowly perfused tissues) in rat and 1.42 ± 0.33 (range: 1.06 in fat to 1.85 in richly perfused tissues) in humans.

QSAR-Based Risk Assessment of Methyl Chloroform

The integrated *in silico*-PBPK modeling approach was used to establish the internal dose corresponding to a lifetime exposure to the rat NOAEL of methyl chloroform (875 ppm) (Reitz et al., 1988). For VOCs like methyl chloroform, lifetime exposures are expected to result in steady-state conditions. Therefore, steady-state arterial blood concentrations (Ca_{ss}) were used as internal dose surrogates. The Ca_{ss} in rats during a lifetime of continuous exposure to the NOAEL was obtained using the conventional and QSAR-based PBPK models. The Ca_{ss} given by the QSAR-PBPK model corresponding to the rat NOAEL was 59.3 mg/L, whereas the corresponding value obtained with the experimental data-based PBPK

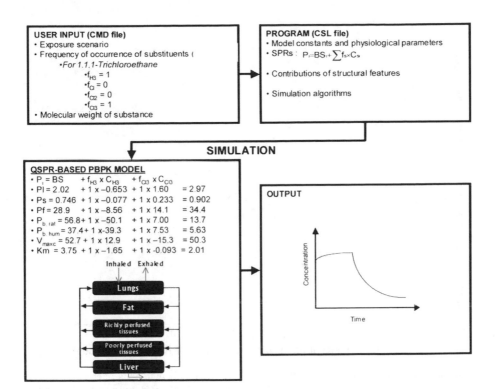

Figure 40.4 Quantitative structure-activity relationship (QSAR) physiologically based pharmacokinetic (PBPK) modeling framework. User input consists of the exposure scenario and chemical structure information such as the number of fragments constituting the molecule. This information is fed to the program that contains the model constants, the Free–Wilson type SPR, the contribution values of each molecular fragment (C_s) and of the basic structure (BS) to the model parameters (P), and the simulation algorithms. The model can then simulate the pharmacokinetics of the chemical in biota and then provide its profile as output. The example of 1,1,1-trichloroethane is shown.

model was 24.9 mg/L. For risk assessment purposes, the human exposure concentration yielding the equivalent internal dose (i.e., Ca_{ss}) was established using the QSAR-PBPK model or alternatively the conventional PBPK model. The human exposure concentrations corresponding to the rat Ca_{ss} of 59.3 mg/L (which is the internal dose during the lifetime exposure to NOAEL) were 6342 ppm and 4252 ppm as obtained with the QSAR-based approach and the experimental data-based PBPK models, respectively.

CONCLUSIONS AND FUTURE DIRECTIONS

Currently, physicochemical and biochemical parameters required for PBPK modeling are obtained by conducting *in vivo* or *in vitro* studies. Alternatively, chemical-specific parameters such as physicochemical and biochemical constants

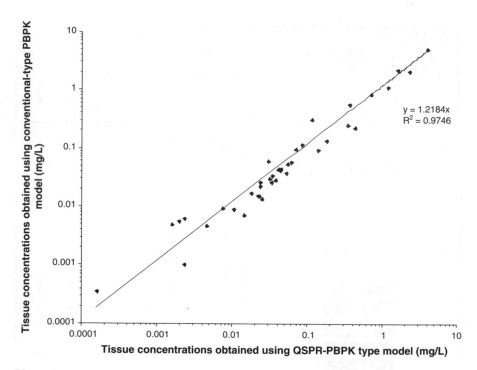

Figure 40.5 Comparison of steady-state blood and tissue concentrations of chloroethanes in rats exposed to 1 ppm, as simulated by conventional and QSAR PBPK models.

Table 40.15 Steady-State Tissue Concentrations (µg/L) of 1,1,1-Trichloroethane in Rat and Humans Estimated Using the Conventional (PBPK) and QSAR-Based (QSAR) Physiologic Model Following a Continuous Exposure to 1 ppm

	Rat		Human	
Tissue	**QSAR**	**PBPK**	**QSAR**	**PBPK**
Blood	22.9	16.6	12.8	8.5
Liver	6.77	4.22	6.23	5.61
Slowly perfused	20.7	9.31	16.7	10.7
Fat	790	770	502	472
Richly perfused	68.1	25.2	53.4	28.9

Table 40.16 Steady-State Arterial Blood Concentration (Ca_{ss}) Obtained Using the Conventional (PBPK) and QSAR-Based (QSAR) Physiological Model in Rats Exposed to the NOAEL of 1,1,1-Trichloroethane (875 ppm) and the Corresponding Environmental Concentration (C_i) in Humans Derived Using the Human Conventional (PBPK) and QSAR-Based (QSAR) Physiological Models

Endpoint	QSAR	PBPK
Rat Ca_{ss} (mg/L)	59.3	24.9
Human C_i (ppm)[a]	6342	4252

[a] Calculated using the QSAR-derived Ca_{ss} (59.3 mg/L).

can be estimated from information on molecular structure. *In silico* approaches for estimating PBPK model parameters have mainly centered on LFE-type QSARs and mechanistically based equations. While LFE QSARs have the advantage of being easily derived, they are limited to the chemical class for which they are developed. Furthermore, resulting parameter estimates cannot be extrapolated across species. There are also growing concerns over the mechanistic relevance of some of the structural descriptors used in these types of equations. The emerging mechanistically based approaches offer the advantage of being relevant regardless of the chemical family and are amenable to interspecies extrapolations. The applicability of these approaches has largely been verified with inhaled VOCs. Even though these approaches are conceptually applicable to nonvolatile organics as well, it becomes more challenging to predict the other PBPK model parameters required for modeling the kinetics of these chemicals (i.e., tissue diffusion coefficients, association constants for binding, oral absorption rates, and dermal permeability coefficients). As our level of understanding of the mechanistic determinants of each of these parameters improves, *in silico* approaches to provide *a priori* predictions of these parameters can be developed.

Direct relationships between number or nature of the molecular fragments and the values of the physicochemical and biochemical parameters used in PBPK modeling can be established using Free–Wilson-type QSARs. This has been done with chloroethanes. The case study presented in this chapter suggests that the development of QSAR-type PBPK models, in which the number or nature of the molecular fragments alone could be varied to provide simulations of the kinetics of chemicals, is feasible. Further, this case study has demonstrated the manner in which QSARs-based PBPK models can be used in human health risk assessment.

If the chemical-specific parameters required for PBPK modeling are related to molecular structure, then the QSARs can be incorporated within a PBPK modeling framework to relate molecular structure to the pharmacokinetics of chemicals. The pharmacokinetic profiles can be generated using only the information on the number of each molecular fragment specific to the chemical as input in the model. With this type of framework, the QSAR-PBPK model can be used to simulate the pharmacokinetic profiles of chemicals for varying exposure scenarios.

Incorporation of species-specific QSARs for parameter estimation allows the prediction of the kinetics and accumulation of chemicals in a variety of species (e.g., fish, rat, mouse, humans) for many different exposure scenarios. Because of this, the internal dose corresponding to a NOAEL or unit risk in one species can be easily extrapolated to another species, using only chemical structure information. The scientific basis of interspecies extrapolation is increased because the resulting extrapolation is based on internal dose and not exposure dose. In this study, this was illustrated by using a QSAR-PBPK model to simulate the internal dose of methyl chloroform in rats and humans. Continued research in this area should facilitate the development and validation of more mechanism based *in silico* approaches for predicting the PBPK model parameters and pharmacokinetic profiles of chemicals, thus reducing the need for animal experiments but still contributing to the cost-efficient conduct of scientifically sound health risk assessments for chemicals of concern.

REFERENCES

Abraham, M., Kamlet, M.J., Taft, R.W., Doherty, R.M., and Weathersby, P.K. (1985) Solubility properties in polymers and biological media. 2. The correlation and prediction of the solubilities of nonelectrolytes in biological tissues and fluids, *J. Med. Chem.*, 28, 865–870.

Abraham, M.H. and Weathersby, P.K. (1994) Hydrogen bonding. 30. Solubility of gases and vapors in biological liquids and tissues, *J. Pharm. Sci.*, 83, 1450–1456.

Agoram, B., Woltosz, W.S., and Bolger, M.B. (2001) Predicting the impact of physiological and biochemical processes on oral drug bioavailability, *Adv. Drug Deliv. Rev.*, 50, s41–s67.

Andersen, M.E., Clewell, H.J., Gargas, M.L., Smith, F.A., and Reitz, R.H. (1987) Physiologically based pharmacokinetics and the risk assessment process for methylene chloride, *Toxicol. Appl. Pharmacol.*, 87, 185–205.

Arms, A.D. and Travis, C.C. (1988) Reference Physiological Parameters in Pharmacokinetic Modeling, Office of Health and Environmental Assessment, EPA, EPA/600/6-88/004, 1-1-7.16, Washington, D.C.

Balimane, P.V., Chong, S., and Morrison, R.A. (2000) Current methodologies used for the evaluation of intestinal permeability and absorption, *J. Pharmacol. Toxicol. Methods*, 44, 301–312.

Batterman, S., Zhang, L., Wang, S., and Franzblau, A. (2002) Partition coefficients for the trihalomethanes among blood, urine, water, milk and air, *Sci. Total Environ.* 284, 237–247.

Bertlesen, S.L., Hoffman, A.D., Gallinat, C.A., Elonen, C.M., and Nichols, J.W. (1998) Evaluation of log Kow and tissue lipid content as predictors of chemical partitioning to fish tissues, *Environ. Toxicol. Chem.*, 17, 1447–1455.

Bird, A.E. and Marshall, A.C. (1967) Correlation of serum binding of penicillins with partition coefficients, *Biochem. Pharmacol.*, 16, 2275–2290.

Cabala, R., Svobodova, J., Feltl, L., and Tichy, M. (1992) Direct determination of partition coefficients of volatile liquids between oil and gas by gas chromatography and its use in QSAR analysis, *Chromatographia*, 34, 601–606.

Clark, D.E. (1999) Rapid calculation of polar molecular surface area and its application to the prediction of transport phenomena. 2. Prediction of blood-brain barrier penetration, *J. Pharm. Sci.*, 88, 815–821.

Connell, D.W., Braddock, R.D., and Mani, S.V. (1993) Prediction of the partition coefficient of lipophilic compounds in the air-mammal tissue system, *Sci. Total Environ. Suppl.*, 2, 1383–1396.

Cowles, A.L., Borgstedt, H.H., and Gillies, A.J. (1971) Solubilities of ethylene, cyclopropane, halothane and diethyl ether in human and dog blood at low concentrations, *Anesthesiol.*, 35, 203–211.

Csanady, G.A. and Laib, R.J. (1990) Use of linear free energy relationships in toxicology: prediction of partition coefficients of volatile lipophilic compounds, *Arch. Toxicol.*, 64, 594–596.

Csanady, G.A., Laib, R.J., and Filser, J.G. (1995) Metabolic transformation of halogenenated and other alkenes — a theoretical approach. Estimation of metabolic reactivities for *in vivo* conditions, *Toxicol. Lett.*, 75, 217–223.

DeJongh, J., Verhaar, H.J., and Hermens, J.L. (1997) A quantitative property-property relationship (QPPR) approach to estimate *in vitro* tissue-blood partition coefficients of organic chemicals in rats and humans, *Arch. Toxicol.*, 72, 17–25.

Eger, E.I. and Larson, C.P., Jr. (1964) Anaesthetic solubility in blood and tissues; values and significance, *Br. J. Anaesth.,* 36, 140–149.

Ekins, S. and Obach, R.S. (2000) Three-dimensional quantitative structure activity relationship computational approaches for prediction of human *in vitro* intrinsic clearance, *J. Pharmacol. Exp. Ther.,* 295, 463–473.

Feher, M., Sourial, E., and Schmidt, J.M. (2000) A simple model for the prediction of blood-brain partitioning, *Int. J. Pharm.* 201, 239–247.

Feingold, A. (1976) Estimation of anesthetic solubility in blood, *Anesth. Analg.,* 55, 593–595.

Fiserova-Bergerova, V., Tichy, M., and Di Carlo, F.J. (1984) Effects of biosolubility on pulmonary uptake and disposition of gases and vapors of lipophilic chemicals, *Drug Metab. Rev.,* 15, 1033–1070.

Fouchécourt, M.-O. and Krishnan, K. (2000) A QSAR-type PBPK model for inhaled chloroethanes, *Toxicol. Sci.,* 54, 88.

Fouchécourt, M.-O., Walker, J., and Krishnan, K. (2000) An integrated QSAR-PBPK model for conducting rat-fish extrapolation of the biokinetics of chloroethanes, in *Handbook on QSARs for Predicting Effects of Chemicals on Environmental-Human Health Interactions,* Walker, J., Ed., SETAC Press, Pensacola, FL.

Free, S.M. and Wilson, J. W. (1964) A mathematical contribution to structure-activity studies, *J. Med. Chem.,* 7, 395–399.

Gargas, M.L., Seybold, P.G., and Andersen, M.E. (1988) Modeling the tissue solubilities and metabolic rate constant (Vmax) of halogenated methanes, ethanes, and ethylenes, *Toxicol. Lett.,* 43, 235–256.

Gargas, M.L., Burgess, R.J., Voisard, D.E., Cason, G.H., and Andersen, M.E. (1989) Partition coefficients of low-molecular-weight volatile chemicals in various liquids and tissues, *Toxicol. Appl. Pharmacol.,* 98, 87–99.

Ghafourian, T. and Fooladi, S. (2001) The effect of structural QSAR parameters on skin penetration, *Int. J. Pharm.,* 217, 1–11.

Grass, G.M. and Sinko, P.J. (2002) Physiologically-based pharmacokinetic simulation modeling, *Adv. Drug Deliv. Rev.,* 54, 433–451.

Hansch, C. and Fujita, T. (1964) ρ-σ-π analysis. A method for the correlation of biological activity and chemical structure, *J. Am. Chem. Soc.,* 86, 1616–1626.

Hansch, C. and Leo, A. (1979) The fragment method of calculating partition coefficients, in *Substituent Constants for Correlation Analysis in Chemistry and Biology,* Hansch, C. and Leo, A., Eds., Wiley, New York, pp. 18–43.

Hansch, C. and Leo, A. (1995) QSAR in metabolism, in *Exploring QSAR: Fundamentals and Applications in Chemistry and Biology,* Hansch, C. and Leo, A., Eds., ACS Professional Reference Book of American Chemical Society, Washington, D.C, pp. 299–343.

Hine, J. and Mookerjee, P.K. (1975) The intrinsic hydrophobic character of organic compounds: correlations in terms of structural contributions, *J. Org. Chem.,* 40, 511–522.

Ishizaki, J., Yokogawa, K., Nakashima, E., and Ichimura, F. (1997) Relationships between the hepatic intrinsic clearance or blood cell-plasma partition coefficient in the rabbit and the lipophilicity of basic drugs, *J. Pharm. Pharmacol.,* 49, 768–772.

Kalizan, R. and Markuszewski, M. (1996) Brain/blood distribution described by a combination of partition coefficients and molecular mass, *Int. J. Pharmacol.,* 145, 9–16.

Kaneko, T., Wang, P.Y., and Sato, A. (1994) Partition coefficients of some acetate esters and alcohols in water, blood, olive oil, and rat tissues, *Occup. Environ. Med.,* 51, 68–72.

Kim, K.H. (1993) 3D-Quantitative structure-activity relationships: describing hydrophobic interactions directly from 3D structures using a comparative molecular field analysis (CoMFA) approach, *Quant. Struct.-Act. Relat.,* 12, 232–238.

Krishnan, K. and Andersen, M.E. (2001) Physiologically based pharmacokinetic modeling in toxicology, in *Principles and Methods of Toxicology,* Hayes, A.W., Ed., Taylor & Francis, Philadelphia, pp. 193–241.

Laass, W. (1987) Estimation of blood/air partition coefficients of organic solvents, in *QSAR in Drug Design and Toxicology* Hadzi, D. and Jerman-Blazic, B., Eds., Elsevier Science Publishers, Amsterdam, pp. 131–134.

Laznicek, M., Kvetina, J., Mazak, J., and Krch, V. (1987) Plasma protein binding-lipophilicity relationships: interspecies comparison of some organic acids, *J. Pharm. Pharmacol.,* 39, 79–83.

Lewis, D.F. (2000) On the recognition of mammalian microsomal cytochrome P450 substrates and their characteristics: towards the prediction of human p450 substrate specificity and metabolism, *Biochem. Pharmacol.,* 60, 293–306.

Lewis, D.F. (2001) COMPACT: a structural approach to the modelling of cytochromes P450 and their interactions with xenobiotics, *J. Chem. Technol. Biotechnol.,* 76, 237–244.

Lewis, D.F. and Dickins, M. (2002) Factors influencing rates and clearance in P450-mediated reactions: QSARs for substrates of the xenobiotic-metabolizing hepatic microsomal P450s, *Toxicology,* 170, 45–53.

Lombardo, F., Blake, J.F., and Curatolo, W.J. (1996) Computation of brain-blood partitioning of organic solutes via free energy calculations, *J. Med. Chem.,* 39, 4750–4755.

Meulenberg, C.J. and Vijverberg, H.P. (2000) Empirical relations predicting human and rat tissue:air partition coefficients of volatile organic compounds, *Toxicol. Appl. Pharmacol.,* 165, 206–216.

Moss, G.P., Dearden, J.C., Patel, H., and Cronin, M.T. (2002) Quantitative structure-permeability relationships (QSPRs) for percutaneous absorption, *Toxicol. In Vitro,* 16, 299–317.

Nestorov, I., Aarons, L., and Rowland, M. (1998) Quantitative structure-pharmacokinetics relationships: II. A mechanistically based model to evaluate the relationship between tissue distribution parameters and compound lipophilicity, *J. Pharmacokinet. Biopharm.,* 26, 521–545.

Norinder, U. and Haeberlein, M. (2002) Computational approaches to the prediction of the blood-brain distribution, *Adv. Drug Deliv. Rev.,* 54, 291–313.

Parham, F.M., Kohn, M.C., Matthews, H.B., DeRosa, C., and Portier, C.J. (1997) Using structural information to create physiologically based pharmacokinetic models for all polychlorinated biphenyls, *Toxicol. Appl. Pharmacol.,* 144, 340–347.

Parham, F.M. and Portier, C. J. (1998) Using structural information to create physiologically based pharmacokinetic models for all polychlorinated biphenyls. II. Rates of metabolism, *Toxicol. Appl. Pharmacol.,* 151, 110–116.

Patel, H., ten Berge, W., and Cronin, M.T. D. (2002) Quantitative structure-activity relationships (QSARs) for the prediction of skin permeation of exogenous chemicals, *Chemosphere,* 48, 603–613.

Paterson, S. and Mackay, D. (1989) Correlation of tissue, blood, and air partition coefficients of volatile organic chemicals, *Br. J. Ind. Med.,* 46, 321–328.

Perbellini, L., Brugnone, F., Caretta, D., and Maranelli, G. (1985) Partition coefficients of some industrial aliphatic hydrocarbons (C5-C7) in blood and human tissues, *Br. J. Ind. Med.,* 42, 162–167.

Poulin, P., Beliveau, M., and Krishnan, K. (1999) Mechanistic animal-replacement approaches for predicting pharmacokinetics of organic chemicals, in *Toxicity Assessment Alternatives: Methods, Issues, Opportunities,* Salem, H. and Katz, S.A., Eds., Humana Press Inc., Totowa, NJ, pp. 115–139.

Poulin, P. and Krishnan, K. (1995a) A biologically-based algorithm for predicting human tissue: blood partition coefficients of organic chemicals, *Hum. Exp. Toxicol.*, 14, 273–280.

Poulin, P. and Krishnan, K. (1995b) An algorithm for predicting tissue: blood partition coefficients of organic chemicals from n-octanol: water partition coefficient data. *J. Toxicol. Environ. Health*, 46, 117–129.

Poulin, P. and Krishnan, K. (1996a) A tissue composition-based algorithm for predicting tissue:air partition coefficients of organic chemicals, *Toxicol. Appl. Pharmacol.*, 136, 126–130.

Poulin, P. and Krishnan, K. (1996b) A mechanistic algorithm for predicting blood:air partition coefficients of organic chemicals with the consideration of reversible binding in hemoglobin, *Toxicol. Appl. Pharmacol.*, 136, 131–137.

Poulin, P. and Krishnan, K. (1996c) Molecular structure-based prediction of the partition coefficients of organic chemicals for physiological pharmacokinetic models, *Toxicol. Methods*, 6, 117–137.

Poulin, P. and Krishnan, K. (2001) Molecular structure-based prediction of human abdominal skin permeability coefficients for several organic compounds, *J. Toxicol. Environ. Health*, 62, 143–159.

Raevsky, O.A. and Schaper, K.-J. (1998) Quantitative estimation of hydrogen bond contribution to permeability and absorption processes of some chemicals and drugs, *Eur. J. Med. Chem.*, 33, 799–807.

Raevsky, O.A., Schaper, K.-J., Artursson, P., and McFarland, J.W. (2002) A novel approach for prediction of intestinal absorption of drugs in humans based on hydrogen bond descriptors and structural similarity, *Quant. Struct.-Act. Relat.*, 20, 402–413.

Ramsey, J. C. and Andersen, M.E. (1984) A physiologically-based description of the inhalation pharmacokinetics of styrene in rats and humans, *Toxicol. Appl. Pharmacol.*, 73, 159–175.

Reitz, R.H., McDougal, J.N., Himmelstein, M.W., Nolan, R.J., and Schumann, A.M. (1988) Physiologically-based pharmacokinetic modeling with methyl chloroform: Implications for interspecies, high-low dose and dose-route extrapolations, *Toxicol. Appl. Pharmacol.*, 95, 185–199.

Saraiva, R.A., Willis, B.A., Steward, A., Lunn, J.N., and Mapleson, W.W. (1977) Halothane solubility in human blood, *Br. J. Anaesth.*, 49, 115–119.

Sato, A. and Nakajima, T. (1979) Partition coefficients of some aromatic hydrocarbons and ketones in water, blood and oil. *Br. J. Ind. Med.*, 36, 231–234.

Seydel, J.K. and Schaper, K.J. (1982) Quantitative structure-pharmacokinetic relationships and drug design, *Pharmacol. Ther.*, 15, 131–182.

Smith, D.S., Jones, B.C., and Walker, D.K. (1996) Design of drugs involving the concepts and theories of drug metabolism and pharmacokinetics, *Medicinal Res. Rev.*, 16, 243–266.

Steward, A., Allott, P.R., Cowles, A.L., and Mapleson, W.W. (1973) Solubility coefficients for inhaled anaesthetics for water, oil and biological media, *Br. J. Anaesth.*, 45, 282–293.

Testa, B., Crivori, P., Reist, M., and Carrupt, P.A. (2000) The influence of lipophilicity on the pharmacokinetic behavior of drugs: concepts and examples, *Perspect. Drug Discov. Des.*, 19, 179–211.

Tichy, M. (1991a) QSAR approach to estimation of the distribution of xenobiotics and the target organ in the body, *Drug Metabol. Drug Interact.*, 9, 191–200.

Tichy, M. (1991b) QSAR approach to target organ estimation, *Sci. Total Environ.*, 109–110, 407–410.

Tichy, M., Fiserova-Bergerova, V., and Di Carlo, F.J. (1984) Estimation of biosolubility of hydrophilic compounds—QSAR study, in *QSAR in Toxicology and Xenobiochemistry*, Tichy, M., Ed., Elsevier Sciences Publishers, Amsterdam, pp. 225–231.

Waller, C.L., Evans, M.V., and McKinney, J.D. (1996) Modeling the cytochrome P450-mediated metabolism of chlorinated volatile organic compounds, *Drug Metab. Dispos.*, 24, 203–210.

Wiester, M.J., Winsett, D.W., Richards, J.H., Doerfler, D.L., and Costa, D.L. (2002) Partitioning of benzene in blood: influence of hemoglobin type in humans and animals, *Environ. Health. Perspect.*, 110, 255–261.

Yamaguchi, T., Yabuki, M., Saito, S., Watanabe, T., Nishimura, H., Isobe, N., Shono, F., and Matsuo, M. (1996) Research to develop a predicting system of mammalian subacute toxicity, (3). Construction of a predictive toxicokinetics model, *Chemosphere*, 33, 2441–2468.

Yokogawa, K., Nakashima, E., Ishizaki, J., Maeda, H., Nagano, T., and Ichimura, F. (1990) Relationships in the structure-tissue distribution of basic drugs in the rabbit, *Pharm. Res.*, 7, 691–696.

Yokogawa, K., Ishizaki, J., Ohkuma, S., and Miyamoto, K. (2002) Influence of lipophilicity and lysosomal accumulation on tissue distribution kinetics of basic drugs: a physiologically based pharmacokinetic model, *Methods Find. Exp. Clin. Pharmacol.*, 24, 81–93.

CHAPTER 41

In Silico Application of Quantum Chemical Methods for Relating Toxicity to Chemical Reactivity

William White

CONTENTS

INTRODUCTION

Serious toxic endpoints such as lethality usually result from a progression of smaller steps. A small number of lesions, adducts, etc. can cascade into a condition with severe physiological distress. Mammalian organisms have so many interrelated systems that inducing stress in one frequently leads to effects on others. To understand the entire process, the individual stages must be separated from each other to the extent possible so that the specific process can be examined with a minimal level of extraneous noise. To become toxic, the molecule must (1) reach its target, (2) interact in a physiologically significant manner with the receptor, and (3) cause damage that is not repaired before the toxic effect is manifested. Phenomena such as exposure, toxicokinetics, and intracellular absorption affect the first step. Electrostatic binding properties and chemical reactivity contribute to the second. Dissociation of the complex, DNA repair, excretion, and synthesis of new proteins are examples of the third.

Enzymes are frequent targets of toxic chemicals. Because of the effectiveness of these proteins in accelerating rates of reaction, only a small number of enzyme molecules is required to maintain requisite concentrations of structural molecules and appropriate levels of metabolic activity. As a result, it only requires inhibition of a few enzyme molecules to alter the normal physiological conditions and the ability of cells and entire systems to respond to external stimuli.

Even though enzymes possess considerable structural and catalytic specificity, their natural substrates are not their only customers. Frequently, similar analogs exist that can serve as substrates. There are two phenomena that contribute to enzyme specificity. First, the substrate must fit within the active site with the correct orientation. If the molecule is too large, it cannot be accommodated in the catalytic center or it will distort the protein sufficiently that the catalytic activity will be lost. Second, the amino acids comprising the catalytic center must be configured around the substrate so that the binding energy of the enzyme-transition structure is greater than for the enzyme-substrate (Pauling, 1946, 1948). If the enzyme stabilizes the ground state more than the transition, then the enzyme would actually inhibit the reaction. In addition, the binding energy for the product must not be so great that the reaction product cannot dissociate from the enzyme (product inhibition). The catalytic center must have requisite components to affect the reaction, i.e., if the mechanism involves base catalysis, an amino acid with a base side chain must be present. It is usually beneficial to the organism if critical enzymes have the minimal catalytic power (i.e., reduction in activation energy is minimally sufficient to maintain an optimal rate of reaction). When this is the case, less reactive analogs will not undergo the specific reaction.

Among the mammalian enzymes, those involved with the nervous system and particularly the transmission of neural signals are critical to the normal functioning of the organism. Acetylcholine is one of the most common neurotransmitters (Taylor and Brown, 1994). At the synapse, acetylcholine is released from the axon, diffuses across the gap, and stimulates the postsynaptic neuron or muscle fiber. Acetylcholine is different from many other neurotransmitters because its activity is terminated quickly by hydrolysis of the ester into two inactive molecules. This hydrolysis is catalyzed by the enzyme acetylcholinesterase, with the formation of acetylcholine into acetate and choline. The enzymatic reaction occurs in two steps. The first is a transesterification reaction in which the acetyl moiety is transferred from choline to a serine residue in the active site of the enzyme with the release of choline. Then water hydrolyzes the new ester bond, generates acetic acid (or acetate), and frees the serine for another cycle. The two-stage mechanism creates a vulnerability for the enzyme if the first reaction is much faster than the second. This situation would not occur with the natural substrate but may occur with artificial substrates. The result is an accumulation of AChE with a blocked active site. Physiologically, this leads to uncontrolled accumulation of acetylcholine at the neuro–neuro and neuro–muscular junctions. Because the neurotransmitter is not removed, the neurons continue to be stimulated until they become depolarized, and if the condition is sufficiently severe, death results from respiratory collapse.

The carbamates and organophosphorus esters are two classes of compounds that have been marketed as insecticides because of their ability to inhibit acetylcholinesterase.

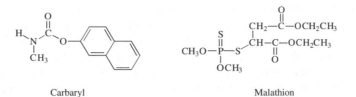

Carbaryl	Malathion

Figure 41.1 Structures of commercial pesticides.

Carbaryl, marketed under the trade name Sevin, is an example of a carbamate insecticide. Malathion is one of the more common organophosphorus pesticides (Figure 41.1).

Because the active site of the enzyme becomes inhibited by formation of a covalent bond rather than by reversible electrostatic, hydrogen bonding, hydrophobic interactions, etc., the reactivity of the inhibitor is crucial. If the molecule is too reactive, either it will be hydrolyzed before it reaches its critical target or the inhibited serine will be hydrolyzed like the normal substrate. If the inhibitor is too stable, it may reach its target but not react sufficiently before it is metabolized or removed by other processes.

The organophosphorus nerve agents are a subclass of the cholinesterase inhibitors. These compounds were discovered in the 1930s as part of a research program at I.G. Farben to develop new pesticides (Borkin, 1978; Croddy, 2002). The chemical warfare (CW) agents used in World War I were principally cytotoxic agents or vessicants (cause blisters). The nerve agents were orders of magnitude more toxic and thereby increased the hazard not only for the military forces who had to combat them, but also for the scientific community, who had to use them routinely in research and development efforts to develop effective defensive equipment and other countermeasures. The mechanism of action for chemical warfare agents and insecticides is the same—the CW agents are quantitatively more potent.

In the past, toxicity of various CW nerve agents was determined by laboratory synthesis of the compounds and measuring lethality in laboratory models like mice, rats, guinea pigs, and rabbits. This is not the most desirable approach because of the hazard posed by the very toxic compounds, the requirement for many laboratory animals, and the costs associated with disposal of chemical and biological wastes. Theoretical approaches relying on computational methods afford the opportunity to reduce the reliance on live animal testing.

Quantitative structure activity relations have been used extensively for many years to condense large quantities of data into manageable formats and to provide mechanistic explanations for physical and chemical properties; they have also been used as a preliminary screen of candidate compounds for novel applications. The first of these activity relations was the Hammet equation that related dissociation constants of a series of benzoic acids to substituents on the phenyl ring. After the substitution constants were determined, Hammet (and subsequently many others) used this equation to interpret and predict useful chemical phenomena. Many but not all of the methods use a series of descriptors whose coefficients are determined mathematically by fitting to a linear equation (Hansch, 1993). As a general rule for prediction, the interpolation of new compounds and properties between existing data is less prone to error than extrapolation beyond the range of measurements. Quantitative structure activity relations (QSAR) studies on inhibitors of acetylcholinesterases and many other enzymes have been reviewed (Gupta, 1987).

Computational chemistry is a valuable tool for studying mechanisms of toxicity. Molecular mechanics and molecular dynamics are useful in identifying the structure and binding energy for ligand–receptor interactions. Quantum chemistry can provide insight into transition structures and other high-energy species that are not accessible by traditional chemical methods (Bruice, 2002). Semiempirical methods as well as more rigorous *ab initio* and density functional methods can generate theoretical descriptors that can be analyzed mathematically to produce QSAR studies.

CHEMICAL REACTIVITY

When a molecule reacts, it moves from one energy minimum (reactant) to another minimum (product) by passing through or over a higher energy region in which the electrons are reorganized. The terms "barrier height" and "energy of activation" are frequently used interchangeably; however, they refer to different phenomena. The activation energy is obtained from the Arrhenius equation and is derived from rates of reaction at different temperatures. The barrier height comes from quantum calculations or other computational methods and refers to the difference between the electronic energies of the reactants and the transition structure (Durant, 1998). Thus, it is not possible to describe reaction rates by examining only the reactants. Both reactants and transition structures must be considered.

PROGRESS OF THE REACTION

Quantum calculations on the hydrolysis of the organophosphorus compounds (White and Wright, 1999) indicated that the reaction passes through a metastable intermediate as indicated in Figure 41.2. As the nucleophile approaches the substrate, the energy rises to a maximum (transition structure 1) before falling to the intermediate. As the leaving group departs, the energy rises to a second transition before falling to the product minimum. Whether the metastable intermediate is a real entity (Uchimaru et al., 1991) or only a computational artifact (Dejaegere et al., 1991, 1994) is a source of conjecture. Regardless of its actuality, this model is a very useful concept because it is representative of the relative energy of the transition (White, 1999).

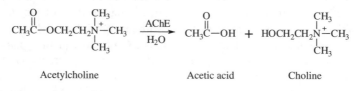

Acetylcholine   Acetic acid   Choline

Figure 41.2 Hydrolysis of acetylcholine.

Semiempirical methods are very useful computational tools because the structure optimization routines are robust and the computation time is short relative to more rigorous methods. The truncated Hamiltonians are too small for accurate absolute energy calculations; however, the errors are usually systematic and tend to cancel. Thus semiempirical methods are ideal for relative comparisons among many different compounds. The activation barriers calculated by semiempirical methods are in the 80 to 90 kcal/mol range in contrast to an experimental value of energy of activation around 30 (Gubaidullin, 1982). *Ab initio* methods generally provide more accurate energies (Wright and White, 1998); however, for phosphorus compounds, it appears that density functional theory is superior to Hartree-Fock and frequently to Møller-Plesset.

STRUCTURE/TOXICITY RELATIONS BASED ON CHEMICAL REACTIVITY

In the procedure described here, the relative reactivity is defined as the energy difference (in kcal/mol) of the heat of formation between the metastable intermediate and the reactants. Technically, the reactants consist of the organophosphorus fluoridate and hydroxide; however, the energy of the hydroxide was eliminated because hydroxide was present in all reactions and the reactivity scale was linear. Heats of formation were calculated with the PM3 (Stewart, 1989a,b) Hamiltonian and associated parameters using the AMPAC (1999) semiempirical computational package. The calculations were run on a small workstation using a UNIX operating system; however, Windows-based systems are available for use on PCs. Other methods such as AM1 (Dewar and Jie, 1989; Dewar et al., 1985), SAM1, MNDO(d), etc. could have been used equally well. Because of differences in parameterization, the various methods usually give different heats of formation. Therefore, it is imperative to use the same method for all calculations. For simple organophosphorus compounds, the default optimization routing was usually sufficient to generate the most stable conformer. For more complex structures, the optimized structure was frequently reconfigured by changing individual dihedral angles and reoptimizing. A pentavalent trigonal bipyramid structure was used for the metastable intermediate. In the input structure, the hydroxide and fluoride groups occupied the two axial positions. Occasionally, upon optimization, the hydroxide moved to an equatorial position. The energy of the optimized intermediate was used in determination of reactivity—regardless of the position of the substituents. It is also prudent to perform force or frequency calculations on the optimized structures to confirm that they are energy minima (no negative vibrational frequencies) and not transition structures (one negative frequency) or higher order structures (more than one negative frequency) on the potential energy surface.

All of the compounds in this study were organophosphorus compounds having a fluoride leaving group. No sulfur analogs were included either as P=S or as a thiol leaving group. The phosphinates containing two P–C bonds were more reactive than the phosphonates (one P–C and one P–O bond), which were more reactive than the phosphates (two P–O bonds). As would be expected, introduction of electron withdrawing halogen atoms on the alkyl substituents reduced the reactivity of the molecule. The effect of a nitrogen molecule was more complex. Sometimes, the amidates (P–N bonds) appeared to be more reactive than the carbon analogs. In other compounds, they appeared to be less reactive. The electronic nature of the P–N bond is not completely understood and has been the subject of considerable controversy (Gilheany, 1990, 1992)—especially the role of d orbitals on the phosphorus and the potential backbonding with the nitrogen lone pair (Gilheany, 1994).

Figure 41.3 is a semilog plot of the toxicity of the various compounds as a function of relative reactivity. The lethality data were determined in mice via intravenous injection. This route minimizes effects on toxicity resulting from differences in absorption, metabolism, etc. and thereby provides more comparable data with which to compare chemical reactivity. The most reactive compounds on the left have low toxicity. These compounds react too rapidly with water and therefore have been hydrolyzed into inactive species before they reach the synaptic region. As the reactivity increases, the toxicity increases to a maximum before decreasing. The phosphonates are among the most effective inhibitors because they are sufficiently stable to reach the synapse in an active state. The enzyme is capable of catalyzing the nucleophilic phosphonalation rapidly, so the active site becomes blocked. In contrast, the phosphates are too stable for maximal inhibition. They reach the site intact; however, the catalytic site of the enzyme is not able to reduce the energy of activation sufficiently to effect a rapid reaction, and, thus, few covalent adducts are formed. The phosphates are among the least reactive of the compounds studied and have lower toxicity. The phosphonates are among the optimal inhibitors and have been studied extensively as chemical warfare agents because of their high toxicity.

The parabolic shape of the curve suggests that there is a maximal toxicity for compounds whose mechanism of action is the covalent attachment to AChE. Increasing the reactivity causes greater hydrolysis and decreased toxicity. Decreasing the reactivity of the agent leads to less inhibition. Thus, it seems unlikely that new agents whose toxicity is orders of magnitude greater will be discovered. It is possible that

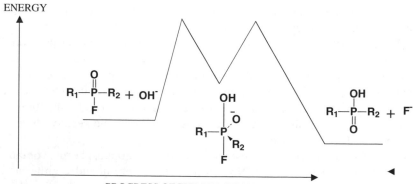

Figure 41.3 Progress of the reaction (x-axis) mapped against energy (y-axis).

modifications could increase binding specificity and thereby increase toxicity slightly. This study has no relevance to poisons whose target is other receptors or whose chemical mechanism is different. There is a continuing effort to identify analogs of huperzine (Camps et al., 1999; Kozikowski and TuckMantel, 1999), tetrahydroacridines, benzylamines, and other reversible inhibitors of AChE for treatment of Alzheimer's disease. The goal of this effort is identification of effective inhibitors of the enzyme that have a wide safety margin. It is not surprising that QSAR methods identified hydrophobic, electronic, and steric effects as important contributors to binding (Recanatini et al., 1997).

The curve in Figure 41.3 can also be used to explain outliers. The toxicity of n-decyl methylphosphonofluoridate (6.1 μg/kg IV rabbit) is considerably less than would be suggested by its reactivity. This compound is a long chain analog of GB (or sarin) and has almost the same relative reactivity (i.e., 78.2 vs. 78.3 kcal/mol for GB). Inhibitors of cholinesterase must be of appropriate size to fit into the catalytic site with the correct orientation. On the ester side, AChE can accommodate about eight heavy atoms—depending on their arrangement. The phosphonate with the C_{10} chain is too large for optimal inhibition. Failure to follow the curve is an indication of adverse steric interactions.

Quantum chemistry using computationally inexpensive semiempirical methods was able to generate chemical reactivities with sufficient accuracy to construct a smooth structure–toxicity graph. This parabolic curve is a quantitative representation of a concept that had been discussed anecdotally for many years, but had not been formalized because of difficulty quantitating the reactivity of the toxic compounds. The needed data could have been obtained empirically; however, laborious synthesis of numerous compounds and experimental measurement of their rates of hydrolysis would have been prohibitively expensive. Furthermore, laboratory workers would have been subjected to substantial risk to generate data that were obtained quickly with essentially no hazard using theoretical methods.

For poisons whose mechanism of toxicity involves the formation of covalent bonds, chemical reactivity of the inhibitor is an important criterion. Quantum chemistry is a useful tool for estimating chemical reactivity because it is capable of determining the relative energies of the substrate and the transition structure and, therefore, can provide a good estimate of the activation barrier.

REFERENCES

AMPAC 6.55 (1999) Semichem Inc., Box 1649, Shawnee, KS 66216.

Borkin, J. (1978) *The Crime and Punishment of I.G. Farben,* Barnes and Noble, New York.

Bruice, T.C. (2002 A view at the millennium: the efficiency of enzymatic catalysis, *Accounts Chem. Res.,* 35, 139–148.

Camps, P., Achab, R.E., Gorbig, D.M., Morral, J., Munoz-Torrero, D., Badia, A., Banos, J.E., Vivas, N.M., Barril, X., Orozco, M., and Luque, F.J. (1999) Synthesis, *in vitro* pharmacology, and molecular modeling of the very potent tacrine-huperzine A hybrids as acetylcholinesterase inhibitors of potential interest for the treatment of Alzheimer's disease. *J. Med. Chem.,* 42.

Croddy, E. (2002) *Chemical and Biological Warfare,* Copernicus Books, New York.

Dejaegere, A., Liang, X. and Karplus, M. (1994) Phosphate ester hydrolysis: calculation of gas-phase reaction paths and solvation effects, *J. Chem. Soc. Faraday Trans.*, 90, 1763–1770.

Dejaegere, A., Lim, C., and Karplus, M. (1991) Dianionic pentacoordinate species in the base-catalyzed hydrolysis of ethylene and dimethyl phosphate, *J. Am. Chem. Soc.*, 113, 4353–4355.

Dewar, M.J.S. and Jie, C. (1989) AM1 parameters for phosphorus, *J. Mol. Structure (Theochem)*, 187, 1–13.

Dewar, M.J.S., Zoebisch, E.G., Healy, E.F., and Stewart, J.J.P. (1985) AM1: a new general purpose quantum mechanical molecular model, *J. Am. Chem. Soc.*, 107, 3902–3909.

Durant, J.L. (1998) Computational Thermochemistry and Transition States, in *Computational Thermochemistry: Prediction and Estimation of Molecular Thermodynamics*, Irkura, K.K. and Frurip, D.J., Eds., American Chemical Society, Washington, D.C., pp. 267–284.

Gilheany, D.G. (1990) Structure and Bonding in Organophosphorus (III) Compounds, in *Primary, Secondary, and Tertiary Phosphines, Polyphosphines and Heterocyclic Organophosphorus (III) Compounds*, Hartley, F.R., Ed., John Wiley & Sons, New York, pp. 9–49.

Gilheany, D.G. (1992) Structure and Bonding in Tertiary Chalcogenides, in *Phosphine Oxices, Sulfides, Selenides, and Tellurides*, Hartley, F.R., Ed., John Wiley & Sons, New York, pp. 1–44.

Gilheany, D.G. (1994) No d orbitals but Walsh diagrams and maybe banana bonds: chemical bonding in phosphines, phosphine oxides, and phosphonium ylides, *Chem. Rev.*, 94, 1339–1374.

Gubaidullin, M.G. (1982) Some relations holding with respect to the effects of substituents on the reactivity of phosphorus compounds, *J. Gen. Chem. U.S.S.R.*, 52, 2182–2184.

Gupta, S.P. (1987) QSAR studies on enzyme inhibitors, *Chem. Rev.*, 87, 1183–1253.

Hansch, C. (1993) Quantitative structure-activity relationships and the unnamed science, *Acc. Chem. Res.*, 26, 147–153.

Kozikowski, A.P. and TuckMantel, W. (1999) Chemistry pharmacology, and clinical efficacy of the Chinese noontropic agent huperzine A, *Acc. Chem. Res.*, 32, 641–650.

Pauling, L. (1946) Molecular architecture and biological reactions, *Chem. Eng. News*, 24, 1375–1377.

Pauling, L. (1948) Nature of forces between large molecules of biological interest, *Nature* 161, 707–709.

Recanatini, M., Cavalli, A., and Hansch, C. (1997) A comparative QSAR analysis of acetyl-cholinesterase inhibitors currently studied for the treatment of Alzheimer's disease, *Chem. Biol. Int.*, 105, 199–228.

Stewart, J.J.P. (1989a) Optimization of parameters for semiempirical methods: I methods, *J. Comput. Chem.*, 10, 209–220.

Stewart, J.J.P. (1989b) Optimization of parameters for semiempirical methods: II applications, *J. Comput. Chem.*, 10, 221–264.

Taylor, P. and Brown, J. H. (1994) Acetylcholine, in *Basic Neurochemistry. Molecular, Cellular, and Medical Aspects*, Siegel, G.J. et al., Eds., Raven Press, New York, pp. 231–260.

Uchimaru, T., Tanabe, K., Nishikawa, S., and Taira, K. (1991) Ab initio studies of a marginally stable intermediate in the base-catalyzed methanolysis of dimethyl phosphate and nonexistence of the stereoelectronically unfavorable transition state, *J. Am. Chem. Soc.*, 113, 4351–4353.

White, W.E. (1999) Effects of chemical reactivity on the toxicity of phosphorus fluoridates, *SAR QSAR Environ. Res.,* 10, 207–213.

White, W.E. and Wright, J.B. (1999) A comparison of semi-empirical, and ab initio methods on the hydrolysis of phosphinates, phosphonates, and phosphates, *Phosphorus, Sulfur, Silicon and Related Elements,* 144–146, 785–788.

Wright, J.B. and White, W.E. (1998) A neutral gas phase mechanism for the reaction of methanol with dimethylphosphinic fluoride, *J. Mol. Struct. (Theochem),* 454, 259–265.

CHAPTER 42

In Silico Cardiac Toxicity: Increasing the Discovery of Therapeutics through High-Performance Computing

Csaba K. Zoltani and Steven I. Baskin

CONTENTS

INTRODUCTION

The explosive improvements in the processing speed and storage capability of computers have opened an ancillary path for gathering and analyzing information on biological processes. This technology in conjunction with developments in software technology has revolutionized and measurably shortened the development time for new drugs and therapeutic agents. Computer studies are now viable and cost-effective alternatives to many *in vivo* animal studies. Indeed, bioinformatics has become an indispensable tool for efficient drug discovery.

In principle, most drugs act by binding to specific receptors of cells or soluble sites and thereby alter the pharmacology/toxicology of cellular or extracellular processes. Computer models can shed considerable insight on ligand-receptor interactions, i.e., how and under what conditions molecules, both agonists and antagonists, bind to receptors, and which receptors are the most likely to be bound. Cell functions depend heavily on the coordinated action of processes controlled by genes. The signaling and metabolic pathways, an expression of the "genetic circuit," thus play a crucial role and should be understood in detail before the pathophysiology of the cell can be modified. Computer simulations can be well suited to study these issues.

Drug discovery commences with the identification of biomolecules with potential suitability for drug targets, i.e., receptors, enzymes, or ion channels. Modulation of the target site, by the selective binding of the introduced chemical, the drug, then constitutes the therapy. *In silico* models, the study of living organisms on the computer, would be very beneficial in searching for these sites. Typically, through combinatorial synthesis, tens of thousands of compounds are exposed to the target by high-throughput screening. Compounds that show target modulation are termed lead compounds and are given closer scrutiny.

Terstappen et al. (2001) quote a study published in 1996 that showed that the number of molecular targets known is still very limited, of the order of 500. Cell membrane receptors, G protein-coupled receptors, make up 45% of all targets, with enzymes accounting for 28%. Yet of the 30,000 human genes, an estimated 6,500 constitute target classes of receptors, enzymes, or ion channels. The number of genes that are thought to contribute to a multifactorial disease is thought to be around 10. The total number of relevant genes may be around 1,000.

Only about 3% of the three billion bases of the human genome actually encode proteins. Currently 1.6 million human sequences are stored in expressed sequence tag databases, i.e., contain short sequence information from expressed genes. Structural genomics plays an important role here. It has been estimated that the number of globular protein folds, i.e., distinct spatial arrangements, may be less than 5,000. *In silico* techniques are excellent for comparing the levels of gene expression in affected and normal genes. *In silico* database searches can identify up- or down-regulation of the genes.

For example, deCode genetics (Soares, 2001), a research firm in Iceland, is in the process of creating the first "phenotype database." It is a collection of the health records of the population of Iceland, a country not known for its ethnic diversity. This database is used to try to find disease-causing genes. Though laborious, it is straightforward in a disease such as Huntington's disease, where a single gene is responsible, but much more difficult where several genes, as is usually the case, are thought to be involved.*

---

* Effort is underway to put together a database of toxicophores. These are to be used with catalysts. The idea, in part, is that the molecular space might mathematically predict the molecular space for toxic moieties.

Ancillary use of *in silico* techniques is the determination of gene function leading to target discovery. It is based on comparative genomics. Here, chromosomal localization using *in silico* polymerase chain reaction (PCR) has been used to see whether a potential target is close to a position that has been previously associated with a pathological or toxicological condition.

Data are accumulating at an unprecedented rate from the Human Genome Project on sequence and structural information. Listed below are four of the hundreds of depository sites:

GenBank (http://www.ncbi.nlm.nih.gov/Genbank)
Protein Data Bank (http://www.rcsb.org/pdb)
The National Center for Biotechnology Information (http://www.ncbi.nlm.nih.gov/)
Metabolic Pathways Database (http://wit.mcs.anl.gov/MPW/)

Tools to extract information from these databases for modeling disease processes are still rudimentary. There is a great need to organize biological data to support drug design and gene targeting. A database describing 2,034 genes, 306 enzymes encoded by these genes, and the associated metabolic reactions organized into 100 metabolic pathways that occur in *E. coli* is now available in EcoCyc (Karp et al. 1996) from SRI, Inc. It allows wide-ranging *in silico* experiments.

According to PricewaterhouseCoopers (Pharma 2005, 2002), it takes 15 years and an investment of $500 million to develop and test a new drug. By FDA estimates, 75% of the new formulations never make it past the testing phase. Thus, there is a constant search by drug developers for cost reduction and for approaches that shorten the development cycle (Drews, 2000).

In silico models and data mining are two of the new resources at the disposal of the drug developer. The PricewaterhouseCoopers study (Pharma 2005, 2002) estimates that typically these techniques can save several years and approximately $200 million in development costs of a new drug over traditional approaches. In this study we will provide an overview of the *in silico* approach. First, we outline a thumbnail sketch of several promising computational cellular models with brief comments on their use. Then, we give guidelines to available software in data mining. Then, by means of an example, we describe how an *in silico* model is used in unraveling cellular processes in organophosphonate (soman)-caused cardiac toxicity. The analysis points to possible antidote strategies.

Clearly, the future of therapy discovery depends on bioinformatics, proteomics, and structural genomics. *In silico* techniques will be an indispensable part of this effort.

IN SILICO MODELS

This section illustrates some of the successful approaches to the study of biological processes at the cellular level on the computer. Experimental validation gives confidence in the prediction of these models.

E-Cell

Proteome analysis, the understanding of how proteins work collectively as a system, is now possible with the emerging understanding of genomics. Models of cells that incorporate gene regulation, metabolism, and signaling have been developed by Masaru Tomita (Tomita et al., 1999; Tomita, 2001) of Keio University in Fujisawa, Japan. E-Cell is a modeling environment for genetic and biochemical processes. The computer model of this hypothetical cell has 127 genes and allows the most fundamental genetic functions, including transcription, translation, and energy production. Since humans have an estimated 30,000 genes, E-Cell, available at http://www.e-cell.org, is a caricature of the real world, but a promising first step that allows computer experiments that can help to decipher many cellular processes. It allows the user to define functions of proteins, protein–protein interactions, regulation of gene expression, and cellular metabolism in terms of a set of reaction rules. The user of the simulation package can observe the dynamic changes within the virtual cell.

The code allows "dry" (i.e., *in silico*) experiments, such as depriving the cell of glucose by turning off the appropriate gene. Analogously, cell processes in the presence of toxic chemicals can be simulated.

Virtual Cell Environment

This computational spatial modeling framework (Schaff et al., 2001) for simulating cellular biochemical processes is under development at the National Resource for Cell Analysis and Modeling at the University of Connecticut Health Center (http://www.nrcam.uchc.edu). It incorporates the idea to study subcellular domains and map the physical observation in terms of a system of equations describing the membrane fluxes, kinetics, and diffusion. The reaction–diffusion equations are then solved, and the predictions are correlated with and analyzed by image processing tools. The front-end graphical user interface runs in a web browser and is combined with a database, visualization capability, and numerical algorithms for data processing. An interesting feature is that the user performs his experiments on the Internet, i.e., the "Virtual Cell" (Schaff and Loew, 1999) software is used remotely, run on Compaq DS20 computers.

This model is based upon subcellular compartments and the interaction of the molecular and chemical species within and as they cross the cellular compartments. In this model, a compartment represents a cellular structure. The web-based interface allows the specified compartment topology to be associated with molecular species and chemical reactions. This information, coupled with the topology, results in a system of differential equations that can be viewed on the graphical interface. The solutions of the equations can then be compared with experimental data and analyzed with statistical and image analysis tools. The attractive feature of Virtual Cell is its ability to specify cellular geometry using experimental images and to change the geometry without modifying this physiological model.

Virtual Cell has been successfully used to model calcium oscillations, a prerequisite for triggering processes such as hormone secretion and muscle contraction.

An important step is the calcium release from the endoplasmic reticulum (ER), the internal calcium store, through calcium channels that can be activated by cytoplasmic calcium.

CellML Language and Other Resources

CellML (Hedley, 2001) is an XML-based language developed by Physiome Sciences and the University of Auckland in New Zealand. It is designed to enable researchers at different sites to exchange models over the World Wide Web. Models based on this approach consist of discrete connected components that constitute a network. A component represents a functional unit that may be represented by mathematical relationships and metadata. MathML content markup is used to describe the interactions between the variables of a compartment.

Complementary efforts to create virtual cells have also been launched by the Alliance for Cellular Signaling (AFCS), and a Microbial Cell Project to create a virtual microbe *in silico* (http://www.microbialcellproject.org) has also been launched by the U.S. Department of Energy. Undoubtedly, *in silico* techniques are expected to shed considerable insight into the functioning of living organisms.

DATA MINING

The Human Genome Project has yielded undreamed of quantities of data yielding information that may point to techniques that have the potential to reverse most pathological conditions. But tools to extract the necessary information from these databases, even to answer the most basic questions, are still in a very rudimentary state. Data mining, first used in classical statistical analysis, has gained prominence in this effort.

Data mining is computer-assisted sieving of data for information (McCulloch, 2000; Miled et al., 2000). This information then forms the first step in the development of new drugs. Drug discovery relies on the collection of the structural, chemical, and physical attributes of compounds and cataloging the information in huge databases, sometimes referred to as data warehouses. Data mining is used to detect patterns in the data sets of seemingly unrelated fields. Drug researchers usually establish combinatorial libraries of products reflecting all possible combinations of ingredients. Data mining and sequence analysis are used to look for characteristic protein binding sites and similar features in other protein structures of known structure. Software is now available to comb through large volumes of data looking for drug candidates. An example of such software is MSI's Insight II, which performs binding site analysis (http://www.msi.com).* It automatically locates potential binding sites on the basis of the protein's shape alone. To solve this problem, the software tries to detect structure-to-activity relationships. Such analysis is but the first step in developing pharmacokinetic and toxicity profiles of compounds.

---

* Now a subsidiary of Accelrys Inc. of Princeton, NJ.

Techniques used in data mining include cluster analysis, learning classification rules, and finding dependency relations and statistics to measure associations and relationships between attributes. Often, the available data is imprecise and heterogeneous. Conventional statistical analysis is not yet possible; discoveries may be counterintuitive.

Algorithms have also been developed to search and identify peptides that bind to HLA (human leukocyte antigen) and activate T cells. Pockets in human leukocyte antigen group DR(HLA-DR) have distinct chemical size in alleles of HLA-DR, also called a pocket. The interaction of amino acid residues with a pocket are used to generate HLA-DR matrices, the HLA-DR peptide binding specificity. This data has been incorporated in TEPITOPE, software capable of predicting HLA Class II ligands. The software scans for genes for HLA-DR binding sites. The protein sequences are parsed into overlapping peptides and subsequently screened for predetermined patterns representative of peptides that bind to HLA molecules. Promising leads are then used in vaccine development. Tepitope-2000, virtual matrix-based T cell epitope prediction software (www.vaccinoma.com), is now commercially available. Details can be found in Sturniolo et al. (1999) and Schultz et al. (2000).

A PRACTICAL EXAMPLE

The power of *in silico* methods is well illustrated by a simulation of the changes in the electrophysiology of cardiac tissue due to soman (organophosphorus compound)-produced toxicity. The approach is to describe the electrophysiology of atrial tissue and study the pathology as a result of the presence of toxins in the environment. In this example we show how such a model is used to identify the conditions that precipitate atrial fibrillation (AF). By manipulating the membrane currents, the action potential cycle length and other observables can be modulated, enabling the processes leading to AF to be antagonized. Results are verified by experimental observations. Such studies suggest the properties required of therapeutic agents.

Soman toxicity, reviewed by Baskin et al. (1991), produces an overload of acetylcholine (ACh) in the body. In the atria it decreases the action potential duration and shortens the effective refractory period. As reported by Schuessler et al. (1991), application of ACh (acetylcholine) to atrial tissue induces arrhythmia (Allessie et al., 1984) that often degenerates into AF and irregular ventricular function (Scheinman, 2000). Above a certain critical rate, regular organized wave motion cannot be sustained. Once initiated by rapid pacing, AF remains self-sustained even after the pacing is removed. The wave accelerates and slows down as it enters the tissue at various stages of excitability and recovery. AF can culminate in ventricular fibrillation (VF) and sudden cardiac death (SCD).

Our understanding of atrial fibrillation is based on the hypothesis of Moe (Moe and Abildskov, 1959; Moe et al., 1964), which states that fibrillation is generated by multiple atrial random reentrant waves that persist and culminate in arrhythmia instead of dying out. Reentry is the presence of self-perpetuating, circulating wave fronts of electrical activity. Typically, reentry is a circus movement, where the wave travels in a ring-shaped structure, one that is long enough so that by the time the head of the ring returns to the starting point, the tissue has had time to recover, allowing the wave to reenter. Reentry waves are spirals in a plane or scrolls in three dimensions. Spirality develops because wave speed depends on the curvature of the wave front. Presence of an inhomogeneity is presumed necessary for the initiation of the spiral-wave activity.

Four to six circulating reentrant waves are necessary for maintenance of AF. An accurate description of the wave motion is complicated by the fact that the walls of the atria are complex, with a thin sheet attached to relatively thick bundles of tissue called the pectinate muscle network. Age and state of toxic involvement and disease influence the action potential dynamics.

Reentrant waves may also circulate around anatomical regions, such as an infarct scar, a region that has electrical properties different from its surroundings. There are several manifestations of reentry where the spiral may be drifting or have a stationary core. Hypoxia or other disease states have a strong influence on the evolution of reentry dynamics. Reentry persists as long as the wavelength of the tachycardia is less than the tachycardia path length. Maintenance of AF depends on adequate atrial mass to encompass sufficient wavelets to perpetuate the arrhythmia. The fact that AF produces electrophysiological changes in the heart that, in turn, promote AF maintenance complicates its management (Gray et al., 2000). The changes produced include a reduced transient outward K^+ current that results in a substrate that supports maintenance of AF. The activation of $i_{K(ACh, Ado)}$ is a common ionic mechanism underlying the proarrhythmic effect of ACh in supraventricular (atrial) tissue. Since organophosphates (OPs) increase ACh concentration by inhibiting ACh hydrolysis, it is thought that $i_{K,ACh}$ is also increased. This mechanism exacerbates the atrial cardiotoxicity from OPs.

Therapeutics rely on the ability to modulate membrane currents and thus reverse or antagonize anomalous electrophysiological behavior. Potent Na^+ channel blockers that prolong atrial refractoriness and calcium channel blockers that attenuate the abnormal shortening of the atrial action potential have been tried with some success in regular, but not in soman-induced, AF therapeutics.

In Silico Simulation of Atrial Action Potential Propagation in the Presence of Soman

The simulation reported here uses the Nygren et al. (1998, 2001) electrophysiological model of the atrial cell. Built on earlier work of Lindblad et al. (1996), the model consists of equations expressing the movement of charged ions across a cell's membrane, including the gating mechanisms of the ionic channels and changes in the ion concentrations. The model is used to track the action potential as it spreads over atrial tissue* that includes a region of inhomogeneity due to toxicity or disease. The encounter between the wave and the regional inhomogeneity generates reentry, which can lead to AF (Pertsov et al., 1993).

---

* *In vivo*, the activation spreads from the terminal crest at the superior vena cava to the atrio ventricular groove and septum into the left atrium. Envelopment of the right atrium usually precedes that of the left atrium.

Toxins change the myocyte's environment and the electrophysiology of the cell. Modulating these changes by enhancing, diminishing, or blocking membrane currents and thereby changing the dynamics of the action potential within the tissue is the basic approach to therapeutics. The computer model allows identifying those cellular parameters that can be most effective in controlling these changes. Toward these ends, the movement and concentration changes of Na$^+$, K$^+$, and Ca^{++} ions are the most important targets of therapeutics.

The model starts from the observation that within the tissue, Kirchhoff's law of the conservation of electrical charge holds. This is described by equations expressing the movement of the participating ions and the gating mechanism. Opening and closing of the ion channels are controlled by molecules whose conformation changes in response to voltage changes. In the Hodgkin–Huxley formalism, the gating equation typically is written as

$$\frac{dn}{dt} = \alpha(1-n) - \beta n$$

where α and β are constants whose values depend on the membrane potential and n designates the fraction of occupied sites.

The equations for the currents generated by the ion movement are obtained by fitting data from patch clamp experiments. Since there are considerable differences between species and even between single and multi-cell experiments within the same species, the experimental data need to be interpreted with caution.

Typically, the individual currents, due to the movement of the ions, are of the form

$$I_t = g_t rs(V - E_K)$$

where r and s are the activation and deactivation variables, g_t the conductance, V the membrane voltage, and E_K the Nernst potential for the ion whose identity is signified by the subscript.

For example, the temporal change of the potassium ion concentration in the intracellular space is given as

$$\frac{d[K^+]_c}{dt} = -\sum \text{currents} / (V_c F)$$

while in the extracellular space it is

$$\frac{d[K^+]_c}{dt} = \frac{[K^+]_b - [K^+]_c}{\tau_K} + \sum \text{currents} / \left(V_c F\right)$$

where $[K^+]$ is the concentration of potassium ions, V_c is the volume of the cell, F is the Faraday constant, and τ_K activation time constant for potassium ions.

Analogous equations are written for the Na$^+$ and the Ca^{2+} ion transport. A total of eleven ion current equations need to be solved. For additional details, including the complete set of equations, initial and parameter values, the reader is referred to Nygren et al. (1998, 2001), Lindblad et al. (1996), and Courtemanche, 1998).

To describe the propagation of the electrical impulse, the cardiac tissue is assumed to be a syncytium, a multinucleated mass of protoplasm from the fusion of cells. Its electrical properties can be described in terms of the bidomain theory where the intracellular space and the interstitium are assumed to be two interpenetrating domains separated by the cell membrane. The bidomain equations are derived by applying conservation of the charge movement between the extra- and intracellular domains. Computationally, a major simplification accrues when it is possible to assume that the longitudinal and transverse diffusion constants are equal. The monodomain model has been widely used for electrophysiological simulations.

For the calculations reported here, the monodomain model of cardiac tissue was assumed to be valid. The properties of the cells are averaged over the whole domain without taking the anisotropy of the cardiac tissue into account. The action potential propagation is determined from the solution of the following equation:

$$\frac{\partial v}{\partial t}(\bar{x},t) = \frac{1}{C_m}\left[-i_{\text{ion}}(\bar{x},t) - i_{\text{stim}}(\bar{x},t) + \frac{1}{\beta}\left(\frac{\kappa}{\kappa+1}\right)\nabla\circ\left(D_i(\bar{x})\nabla v(\bar{x},t)\right)\right].$$

In the equation, v is the membrane voltage, i_{stim} is the applied stimulus current per unit area, i_{ion} is the ionic current, and β is the ratio of the membrane area to volume. C_m is the membrane capacitance per unit area and D_i the intracellular conductivity tensor, while t represents time and x the position vector. Neumann boundary conditions were applied in solving the equation.

The equations were solved using the code CardioWave (2002). Calculations were performed on atrial tissue sizes of 3 cm × 3 cm. The time step was 0.001 sec and the spatial discretization was 0.01 cm.

A stimulus of 40 µA/cm^2 was applied at $t = 0$ to the leftmost column of computational nodes of the sheet of tissue for 2 ms. A region of inhomogeneity of the tissue, resulting from the presence of a toxic agent, was simulated by higher than normal potassium concentration in a block of cells in the center of the region. Inhibition of AChE by soman is an example of such an inhomogeneity.

This formalism allows parametric studies that can take pathological conditions into account. For example, it is known that in soman poisoning, ACh overload manifests itself, leading to hyperkalemia (that is also a sign of ischemia) and to changes in the T-wave in an ECG. Hyperkalemia can be simulated by changes in the ionic potassium concentration in the model. T-wave changes that result are modeled by changes in the dynamics of the repolarization, i.e., the dynamics of the phase 3 in the cell cycle. See Zoltani and Baskin (2000) for some of the details.

Solution of the Monodomain Equations on the MSRC Assets

The calculations were carried out using CardioWave (2002) on the ARL Major Shared Resource Center's Origin 3000 and IBM SP3 assets. To obtain a typical solution (i.e., the time-resolved electrophysiological state of the atria) for 300 μs real time in a tissue of 3 cm × 3 cm required 7 hr of nondedicated time using 16 processors. The machine used was an SGI, with a total of 256 shared processors, rated at 300 MHz using the R12K chip. It is capable of a peak performance of 600 MFlops. The machine has the cc-NUMA architecture* where all memory is logically shared with local memory shared by two processors. The local cache is 8 MB. In separate calculations, up to 96 processors were used. Speedup was observed, but it was less than linear.

Both the Origin 3000 and the SP3 were used in the calculations. For the calculations reported here, up to 96 nodes were used. Data from the simulation was stored at 5 ms intervals, and TIFF files were constructed of the voltage as a function of position in the two-dimensional plane of the tissue. The panels displayed were constructed using Tecplot, version 8.01.

RESULTS

The power of the *in silico* approach is shown in the results presented in the figures. Figure 42.1 shows the action potential wave propagation through atrial tissue, 3cm × 3cm in size, represented by $300 \times 300 \times 1$ computational nodes. Two subregions, each 1 cm^2 in size, were included and had $[K^+]_0 = 10.8$ mM. The first, along the central axis of the tissue, started at the left-hand boundary. The second, 1 cm from the left-hand boundary, was located along the bottom edge of the tissue. As the region of higher concentration is encountered, the wave speeds up and its front distorts, a precursor to breakup and eventual atrial fibrillation.

In Figure 42.2, the case where the action potential encounters a square patch of tissue, centrally located at the potassium concentration level of 25.0 mM is shown. At 25 ms, the wave in the affected region shows an almost threefold velocity increase over the adjacent tissue.

DISCUSSION

We issue a clarion call to the research community to consider shifting the emphasis from animal experimentation to using computers in searching for and developing new therapeutics. Outlined was one of the possible scenarios in taking advantage of the tremendous benefits of *in silico* techniques to gain understanding of aspects of cardiac toxicity without *in vivo* animal studies. *In silico* techniques are powerful, predictive, dry experiments. They allow parametric studies to fathom the effect of environmental changes on the electrophysiology of cells.

* SGI Numaflex modular technology is a snap-together server system concept that allows reconfiguration of the computer to meet requirements of the application.

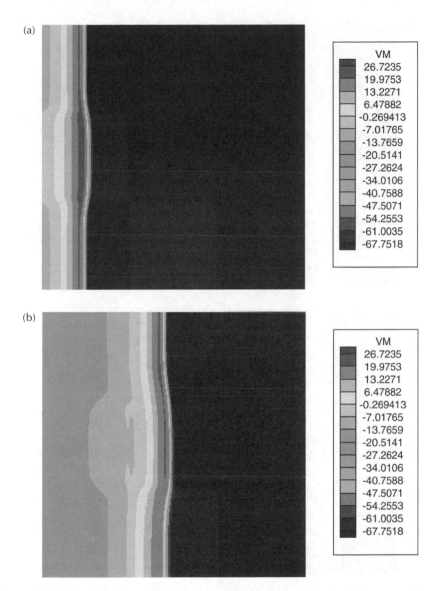

Figure 42.1 Frame sequence showing the evolution of the action potential in an atrial tissue using the Nygren model for the electrophysiology of the tissue. The times of the frames going clockwise are (a) 50 ms, (b) 100 ms, (c) 150 ms, and (d) 200 ms. The stimulus consisted of a current pulse of 40 μA/cm² delivered to the leftmost column of atrial cells. The stimulus lasted for 2 ms and VM in the legend is the voltage in mV. (continued)

Our computer simulations showed how changes in membrane currents in tissue with an overload in ACh can culminate in reentry and subsequently establish conditions that are favorable to atrial fibrillation. The computer model predicts the time-resolved electrophysiological state of the tissue and allows the simulation experiments to study the means by which membrane currents may be modulated, suggest-

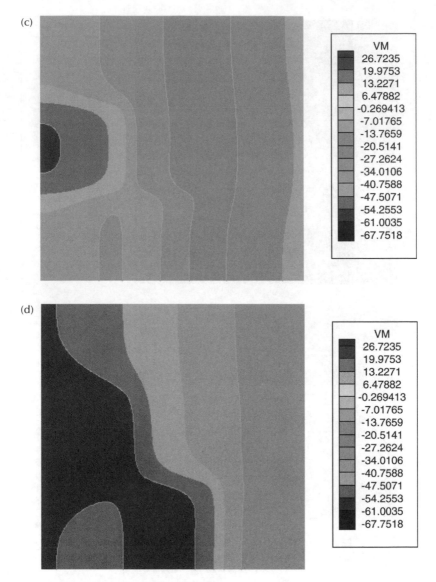

Figure 42.1 (continued) Frame sequence showing the evolution of the action potential in an atrial tissue using the Nygren model for the electrophysiology of the tissue. The times of the frames going clockwise are (a) 50 ms, (b) 100 ms, (c) 150 ms, and (d) 200 ms. The stimulus consisted of a current pulse of 40 $\mu A/cm^2$ delivered to the leftmost column of atrial cells. The stimulus lasted for 2 ms and VM in the legend is the voltage in mV.

ing avenues to therapeutics. This approach eliminates the need for certain *in vivo* studies and confers considerable savings in research expenditures.

The coming of age of the use of computer simulations in the health sciences was underlined by Thomas B. Kepler, Vice President for Academic Affairs at the Santa Fe Institute. He was quoted in the *New York Times* (Johnson, 2001) as saying

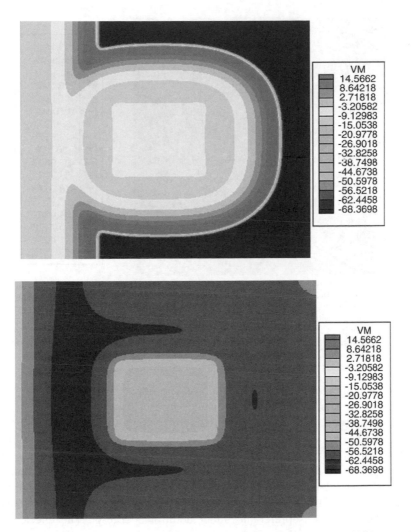

Figure 42.2 Action potential, entering from the left and encountering a region of high potassium concentration region at *t* = 40 and 250 ms, respectively. The hyperkalemic region is along the tissue central axis, in the center taking up 1 cm² of the 3 cm × 3 cm tissue.

that "Physics is almost entirely computational now, nobody would dream of doing these big accelerator experiments without a tremendous amount of computer power to analyze the data." But the biggest change, he said, was in biology. "Ten years ago biologists were very dismissive of the need for computation, now they are aware that you can't really do biology without it."

A case in point is the human genome project. The Celera Genomics map of the human gene required 80 trillion bytes of data to be analyzed. This was accomplished using the largest commercial supercomputer. Indeed, biologists in trying to figure out how genes are expressed are now requiring more computing power than other scientific disciplines.

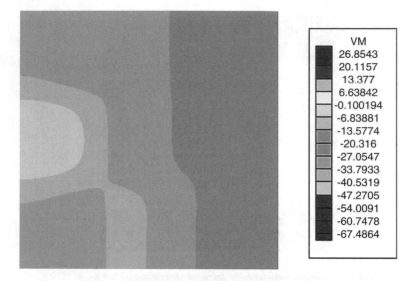

Figure 42.3 This figure contrasts the effect of potassium current blockers on the action potential. The left-hand panel shows the voltage, that is, the action potential in the tissue without modulation of the currents. The effect of reducing the i_{Kr} and i_{Ks}, such as is effected by newer antiarrhythmic drugs such as azimilide, is shown in the right-hand panel. Modulation of the wave distortion and erratic behavior should be noted.

The development that will have the greatest impact on furthering the understanding of cellular processes and developing antidotes to pathologies is the emerging ability to tailor artificial enzymes for producing novel protein structures (Street and Mayo, 1999; Dahiayat and Mayo, 1997; Desmet et al., 1992). The strategy is to predict protein sequences that are likely to possess the desired fold. Then by means of the dead end elimination theorem, a method in combinatorial optimization (Holtzman, 2000), the globally optimal sequence and geometry are determined. A Monte Carlo search is executed, starting with the optimal sequence to find the one that is preferable under additional criteria. The check on the computed sequence consists of inserting a section of synthetic DNA into bacteria and testing the catalytic power of the created enzyme. Initial results using this approach have been favorable. For example, the technique could also be used to design an enzyme that could theoretically rapidly hydrolyze the excess ACh in soman-induced ACh overload.

Herein lies a future path of cardiac toxicology research, already exemplified by the research of Holtzman (2000), which suggests that *in silico* toxicology can improve the process of drug discovery. Extensive investment in supercomputer use and algorithmic development will accelerate the discovery process and obviate the need for costly wet experiments. *In silico* approaches to toxicity assessment and physiological modeling have become indispensable tools for therapeutic and drug development. In the near future, computerized toxicology could move to center stage and replace a sizeable portion of *in vivo* studies.

ACKNOWLEDGMENTS

It is a pleasure to thank Dr. John Pormann of Duke University for making Cardiowave available and giving expert advice in its use. This work has benefited from computer time made available by the Department of Defense High Performance Computing Modernization Program. The computer calculations were made at the Major Shared Resource Center at ARL, Aberdeen Proving Ground, MD, on the SGI Origin 3000 and the IBM SP3.

REFERENCES

Allessie, M., Lammers, W., Smeets, J., Bonke, F., and Hollen, J. (1982) Total mapping of atrial excitation during acetylcholine-induced atrial flutter and fibrillation in the isolated canine heart, in *Atrial Fibrillation,* Kulbertus, H.E. et al. Eds., AB Hassle, Sweden.

Allessie, M.A., Lammers, W.J., Borke, I.M., and Hollen, J. (1984) Intra-atrial reentry as a mechanism for atrial flutter induced by acetylcholine and rapid pacing in the dog, *Circulation,* 70, 123–135.

Baskin, S.I. and Whitmer, M.P. (1991) The cardiac toxicology of organophosphorus agents, in *Cardiac Toxicology,* Baskin, S.I. Ed., CRC Press, Boca Raton, FL.

CardioWave (2002) (www.ee.duke.edu/~jpormann/simsys/CardioWave.html).

Courtemanche, M., Ramirez, R.J., and Nattel, S. (1998) Ionic mechanisms underlying human atrial action potential properties: insights from a mathematical model, *Am. J. Physiol.,* 275, H301–H321.

Dahiyat, B.I. and Mayo, S.L. (1997) *De novo* protein design: fully automated sequence selection, *Science* 278, 82–87.

Desmet, J., DeMaeyer, M., Hazes, M., and Lasters, I. (1992) The dead end elimination theorem and its use in protein side-chain positioning, *Nature,* 356, 539–542.

Drews, J. (2000) Drug discovery: a historical perspective, *Science,* 287, 1960–1964.

Gray, R.A., Takkellapati, K., and Jalife, J. (2000) Dynamics and anatomical correlates of atrial flutter and fibrillation, in *Cardiac Electrophysiology from Cell to Bedside,* 3rd ed., W.B. Saunders Co., Philadelphia, pp. 356–363.

Hedley, W.J., Nelson, M.R., Bullivant, D.P., and Nielsen, P.F. (2001) A short introduction to CellML, *Phil. Trans. R. Soc. Lond. A,* 359, 1073–1089.

Holtzman, S. (2000) *In silico* toxicology, *Ann. NY Acad. Sci.,* 919, 68–74.

Johnson, G. (2001) All science is computer science, *New York Times,* March 25, 2001.

Karp, P.D., Riley, M., Paley, S.M., Pellegrini-Toole, A. (1996) EcoCyc: an encyclopedia of Escherichia coli genes and metabolism, *Nucleic Acids Res.,* 24, 32–39.

Lindblad, D.S., Murphey, C.R., Clark, J.W., and Giles, W.R. (1996) A model of the action potential and underlying membrane currents in a rabbit atrial cell, *Am. J. Physiol.,* 271, H1666–H1691.

McCulloch, A.D. (2000) Modeling the human cardiome in silico, *J. Nucl. Cardiol.,* 7, 496–499.

Miled, Z.B., Liu, Y., Powers, D., Bukhres, O., Bem, M., Jones, R., Oppelt, R., and Milosevich, S. (2000) Data access performance in a large and dynamical pharmaceutical drug candidate database, paper presented in the Proceedings of Supercomputing 2000, IEEE Computer Society.

Moe, G.K. and Abildskov, J.A. (1959) Atrial fibrillation as a self-sustaining arrhythmia independent of focal discharge, *Am. Heart J.,* 58, 59–70.

Moe, G.K., Rheinboldt, W.C., and Abildskov, J.A. (1964) A computer model of atrial fibrillation, *Am. Heart J.,* 67, 200–220.

Nygren, A., Leon, L.J., and Giles, W.R. (2001) Simulations of the human atrial action potential, *Phil. Trans. R. Soc. Lond. A,* 359, 1073–1089.

Nygren, A., Fiset, C., Firek, L., Clark, J.W., Lindblad, D.S., Clark, R.B., and Giles, W.R. (1998) Mathematical model of an adult human atrial cell. The role of K^+ currents in repolarization, *Circ. Res.,* 82, 63–81.

Pertsov, A.M., Davidenko, J.M., Salomonsz, R., Baxter, W.T., and Jalife, J. (1993) Spiral waves of excitation underlie reentrant activity in isolated cardiac muscle, *Circ. Res.,* 72, 631–650.

Pharma 2005 (2002) Silicon Rally: The race to e-R&D, PricewaterhouseCoopers (www.pwc-global.com).

Schaff, J. and Loew, L.M. (1999) The virtual cell, *Pac. Symp. Biocomput.,* 4, 228–239.

Schaff, J.C., Slepchenko, B.M., Choi, Y., Wagner, J., Resasco, D., and Loew, L.M. (2001) Analysis of nonlinear dynamics on arbitrary geometries with the virtual cell, *Chaos,* 11, 115–131.

Scheinman, M.M. (2000) Mechanism of atrial fibrillation: is a cure at hand? *J. Am. Coll. Cardiol.,* 35, 1687–1692.

Schuessler, R.B., Rosenshtraukh, L.V., Boineau, J.P., Bromberg, B.I., and Cox, J.L. (1991) Spontaneous tachyarrhythmias after cholinergic suppression in the isolated perfused canine right atrium, *Circ. Res.,* 69, 1075–1087.

Schultz, J., Doerks, T., Ponting, C.P., Copley, R.R., and Bork, P. (2000) More than 1,000 putative new human signaling proteins revealed by EST data mining, *Nat Genet.* 25, 201–204.

Soares, J. (2001) Population, *Inc. Technol. Rev.,* 104, 50–55.

Street, A.G. and Mayo, S.L. (1999) Computational protein design, *Structure,* 7, R105–R109.

Sturniolo, T., Bono, E., Ding, J., Raddrizzani, L., Tuereci, O., Sahin, U., Braxenthaler, M., Gallazzi, F., Protti, M.P.. Sinigaglia, F., and Hammer, J. (1999) Generation of tissue-specific and promiscuous HLA ligand databases using DNA microarrays and virtual HLA class II matrices, *Nat. Biotechnol.,* 17, 555–561.

Terstappen, G.C. and Reggiani, A. (2001) *In silico* research in drug discovery, *Trends Pharmacol. Sci.,* 22, 23–26.

Tomita M. (2001) Whole-cell simulation: a grand challenge of the 21st century, *Trends Biotechnol.,* 19, 205–210.

Tomita, M., Hashimoto, K., Takahashi, K., Shimizu, T.S., Matsuzaki, Y., Miyoshi, F., Saito, K., Tanida, S., Yugi, K., Venter, J.C., and Hutchison, C.A. (1999) E-Cell: software environment for whole-cell simulation, *Bioinformatics,* 15, 72–84.

Zoltani, C.K. and Baskin, S.I. (2000) Simulation of acetylcholine cardiac overload caused by soman, a cholinesterase inhibitor, paper presented at the Proceedings of Computers in Cardiology 2000, IEEE, pp. 243–246.

CHAPTER **43**

Submillimeter-Wave Frequency Studies of the Vibrational Modes of Deoxyribonucleic Acid: A Metric for Mutagenicity?

T.R. Globus, B.L. Gelmont, M. Bykhovskaia, J. Hesler, D.L. Woolard,
A.C. Samuels, J.O. Jensen, H. Salem, and W.R. Loerop

CONTENTS

INTRODUCTION

Deoxyribonucleic acid (DNA) is a ubiquitous and vitally important biopolymer in all living organisms (Sinden, 1994). In addition to transmitting the genetic code in the chromosomes, the molecule ultimately dictates protein synthesis via ribonucleic acid (RNA) transcription. As such, any materials that specifically damage DNA may be mutagenic or carcinogenic. Recent experimental evidence of the interaction of low-frequency radiation with chromosomal DNA (Belyaev et al., 1995, 1996) has prompted the interest in studying the spectroscopic interaction of submillimeter and microwave frequency electromagnetic radiation with the biopolymer. The nature of the interaction has been suggested by theoretical studies to be due at least in part to the occurrence of phonon modes in the biomolecule. The phenomenology and measurement of phonon modes in large biomolecules has been the subject of a large body of theoretical studies and a reasonable number of preliminary experimental investigations. The predicted eigenvectors of a phonon with respect to a long polymeric chain such as DNA are expected to occur in the millimeter and submillimeter region of the electromagnetic spectrum. The phenomena responsible for these eigenvectors include, but are not limited to, longitudinal motion along the axis of the nucleic acid, transverse motions normal to the axis, rotations ("twisting") about the axis, and combinations of these motions (notably those involved in the winding and unwinding of the double helix during replication) (Mei et al., 1981). Defects in biopolymers are also expected to produce unique associated eigenvectors (Saxena and van Zandt, 1994a,b). Systematic investigations on the nature of these interactions are scarce; most involve few molecular species in a limited wavelength regime. Notable investigations include early far infrared studies (Wittlin et al., 1986), Brillouin scattering studies (Maret et al., 1979; Tao et al., 1988), neutron scattering, (Grimm et al., 1987), and neutron spectroscopy (Middendorf et al., 1995). Swicord et al. undertook extensive study of the interaction of microwave radiation in the 8 to 12 GHz regime (Swicord and Davis, 1982; Edwards et al., 1984, 1985) but found an intimate dependence of the observed phenomena on sample preparation processes (Swicord et al., 1983).

METHODS AND MATERIALS

Computational Studies

Well-known computational methods for studying the dynamics of biopolymers are molecular dynamics (reviewed in McCammon and Harvey, 1986) and normal mode analysis (Noguti and Go, 1982; Brooks and Karplus, 1983; Levitt et al., 1985; Lin et al., 1997; Duong and Zakrzewska, 1997). Normal mode analysis allows calculations of molecular vibrations around an energy minimum by making a harmonic approximation to the local energy hypersurface. The advantages of the normal mode analysis for studying macromolecular dynamics are that (1) it is a relatively rapid computational technique and (2) the calculated vibrational frequencies can be compared with resonance frequencies found by spectroscopy methods, whether Raman (Melchers et al., 1996) or direct absorption. DNA absorption measurements (Wittlin et al., 1986; Powell et al., 1987) coupled with lattice dynamics analysis (Young et al., 1989) has demonstrated that DNA low-frequency vibrations produce characteristic absorption bands in the far infrared (IR) region (between 40 and 300 cm^{-1}), which are sensitive both to DNA composition and to environment (Powell et al., 1987).

Experimental Measurements

Free-standing DNA films were prepared from the gelatinous mixtures of herring and salmon DNA sodium salts in glass-distilled water with a mass ratio between

1:5 and 1:10. This gel was brought to the desired thickness by placing it inside an arbor shim between two 50-µm thick Teflon sheets. The assembly was dried at room temperature for several days. The samples were then completely separated from the mold. These free-standing films are extremely fragile and are not oriented by intention. Herring DNA sodium salt (type XIV from herring testes, lot 14H7121 with 6.5% Na content) and salmon DNA sodium salt (type XIV from salmon testes, lot 44H7020 with 6% Na content) were obtained from Sigma Chemical Company and used without further purification.

The spectral studies reported were performed on a commercial Fourier Transform Spectrometer (Bruker IFS-66) system equipped with mercury-lamp and liquid-helium-cooled Si-bolometer (1.7 K) for signal detection. All the measurements are made in vacuum to eliminate any influence of water-absorption lines. The resolution was set between 0.2 and 2 cm^{-1}, and up to 512 interferograms were accumulated, coadded, and Fourier transformed. Each sample was measured several times in the same position, and the procedure was repeated for several different sample positions.

RESULTS AND DISCUSSION

Computational Studies

Typical computational results for a representative oligomer that was studied as a helical double-stranded DNA polymer analog are shown in Figure 43.1 for two values of the linewidth parameter. A notable feature of the predicted spectra is the fine structure, which is predicted on the basis of low-frequency vibrational modes

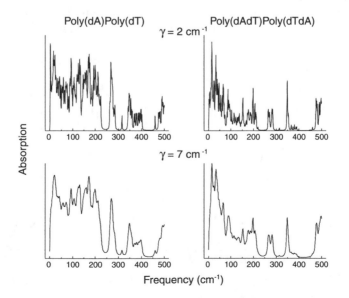

Figure 43.1 Calculated spectra of Poly(dA)Poly(dT) and of Poly(dAdT)Poly(dTdA) at two line-widths: 2-wavenumber and 7-wavenumber.

Table 43.1 Comparison of Predicted Vibrational Band Positions (in Wavenumbers) of Poly(dA)Poly(dT) with Values Observed by Experiments in the Literature

Calculations	Experiment (Powell, 1987)	Calculations	Experiment (Powell, 1987)
20	Unknown	172	170
43	Unknown	199	200
57	62	211	214
71	80	—	238
94	95	270	—
106	106	348	—
131	136	400	—
160	—	459	—

in the polymer. A comparison of predicted line positions with those observed in early experimental measurements by Powell et al. (1987) serves as an initial validation of the model used for the computational studies (see Table 43.1).

Experimental Studies

Typical results of infrared measurement of DNA materials are shown in Figures 43.2 and 43.3. The mid-infrared region (regions I and II in Figure 43.2) is home to the bond vibrations (bending, stretching, puckering, etc.) of the constituent chemical bases, nucleotides, and the sugar-phosphate polymer backbone of the oligomer. Below around 400 wavenumbers (the far infrared region, region III in Figure 43.2), the spectrum of the biopolymers is relatively featureless, with interference effects of the film with the radiation dominating the spectrum. However, close examination of the fine structure in the very far infrared region, from 25 wavenumbers down, reveals the low-energy, low-frequency modes of interest (Figure 43.3).

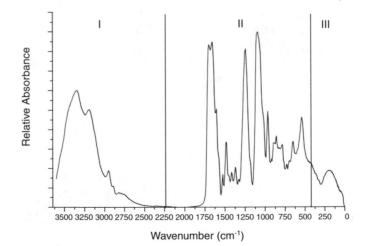

Figure 43.2 Experimental absorbance spectra of herring DNA in the mid-infrared through the very far infrared region.

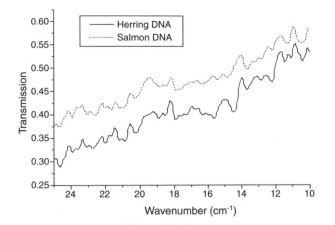

Figure 43.3 Fine structure in the absorbance spectra of herring and salmon DNA in the very far infrared region.

The phenomenology associated with the fine structure observed below 25 wave-numbers is not nearly as well understood as the molecular vibrations that are responsible for the absorption bands in regions I and II of Figure 43.2. The low frequency vibrational modes may be associated with lattice modes in the biopolymer or phonon modes that run the length of the oligomer or accompany motions associated with base pair hydrogen bonds, for example.

We have demonstrated that the very far infrared spectra of nucleic acids are characterized by a significant amount of fine structure. The origin of this spectroscopic structure is believed to lie in the long-range molecular deformations and dynamics of the secondary nucleic acid structure as opposed to the internal vibrational modes of the constituent chemical bonds.

While the experimental procedure for acquiring and analyzing the far infrared spectra of these materials is indeed very involved, advances in high frequency electronics circuits, driven in part by the need for higher bandwidth in the communications industry, are producing circuits that can synthesize and analyze signals upward of the terahertz range, which begins to overlap the region of highest interest revealed in this study.

Initial proof-of-principle experiments were performed by Woolard et al. (1997) using a Vector Network Analyzer (Hewlett-Packard/Agilent Technologies) operating at 75 to 110 GHz frequencies, which corresponds to 2.5 to 3.7 wavenumbers. The results, shown in Figure 43.4, are promising. Frequency synthesizers can be used to detect very low levels of signal using compact electronics, and the potential for *in situ* study of the interaction of genomic DNA exists. Studies have already appeared in the literature that detail the results of millimeter-wave transmission studies on microbial cells (Belyaev et al., 1995, 1996), with emphasis on the extinction in this region resulting from the extinction of the polynucleotides.

As an alternative to studies with live animals, a direct metric for genomic DNA damage through mutagen activity may be realized using an extension of the spectroscopic characterization technique. Experiments are currently in progress

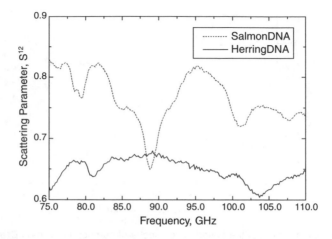

Figure 43.4 Transmission scattering parameter (S_{12}) measurement of herring and salmon DNA in the microwave (W-band) region.

that will help to elucidate the phenomena and validate the interpretation, including a systematic study of controlled DNA damage using the spectroscopic measurement approach.

REFERENCES

Belyaev, I.Y., Alipov, Y.D., Matronchik, A.Y., and Radko, S.P. (1995) Cooperativity in *E. coli* cell response to resonance effect of weak extremely low frequency electromagnetic field, *Bioelectrochem. Bioenerg.*, 37, 85–90.

Belyaev, I.Y., Shcheglov, V.S., Alipov, Y.D., and Polunin, V.A. (1996) Resonance effect of millimeter waves in the power range from 10^{-19} to 3×10^{-3} W/cm² on *Escherichia coli* cells at different concentrations, *Bioelectromagn.*, 17, 312–321.

Brooks, B. and Karplus, M. (1983) *Proc. Natl. Acad. Sci.*, 80, 6571–6575.

Duong, T.H. and Zakrzewska, K. (1997) *J. Comp. Chem.*, 18, 796–811.

Edwards, G.S., Davis, C.C., Saffer, J.D., and Swicord, M.L. (1984) Resonant microwave absorption of selected DNA molecules, *Phys Rev. Lett.*, 53(13), 1284–1287.

Edwards, G.S., Davis, C.C., Saffer, J.D., and Swicord, M.L. (1985) Microwave-field-driven acoustic modes in DNA, *Biophys. J.*, 47, 799–807.

Grimm, H., Stiller, H., Majkrzak, C.F., Rupprecht, A., and Dahlborg, U. (1987) Observation of acoustic Umklapp phonons in water-stabilized DNA by neutron scattering, *Phys. Rev. Lett.*, 59, 1780–1783.

Levitt, M., Sander, C., and Stern, P.S. (1985) *J. Mol. Biol.*, 181, 423–447.

Lin, D., Matsumoto, A., and Go, N. (1997) *J. Chem. Phys.*, 107, 3684–3690.

Maret, G., Oldenbourg, R., Winterling, G., Dransfeld, K., and Rupprecht, A. (1979) Velocity of high frequency sound waves in oriented DNA fibres and films determined by Brillouin scattering, *Colloid Polymer Sci.*, 257, 1017–1020.

McCammon, J.A. and Harvey, S.C. (1986) *Dynamics of Proteins and Nucleic Acids,* Cambridge University Press, Cambridge.

Mei, W.N., Kohli, M., Prohovsky, E.W., and van Zandt, L.L. (1981) Acoustic modes and nonbonded interactions of the double helix, *Biopolymers*, 20, 833.

Melchers, P., Knapp, E.W., Parak, F., Cordone, L., Cupane, A., and Leone, M. (1996) *Biophys. J.,* 70, 2092–2099.

Middendorf, H.D., Hayward, R.L., Parker, S.F., Bradshaw, J., and Miller, A. (1995) Vibrational neutron spectroscopy of collagen and model polypeptides, *Biophys. J.,* 69, 660–673.

Noguti, T. and Go, N. (1982) *Nature,* 226, 776–778.

Powell, J.W., Edwards, G.S., Genzel, L., Kremer, F., Wittlin, A., Kubasek, W., and Peticolas, W. (1987) *Phys. Rev. A,* 35, 3929–3939.

Saxena, V.K. and van Zandt, L.L. (1994a) Vibrational local modes in DNA polymer, *J. Biomolec. Struct. Dyn.,* 11, 1149–1159.

Saxena, V.K. and van Zandt, L.L. (1994b) Local modes in a DNA polymer with hydrogen bond defect, *Biophys. J.,* 67, 2448–2453.

Sinden, R.R. (1994) *DNA Structure and Function,* Academic Press, San Diego.

Swicord, M.L. and Davis, C.C. (1982). Microwave absorption of DNA between 8 and 12 GHz, *Biopolymers,* 21, 2453–2460.

Swicord, M.L., Edwards, G.S., Sagripanti, J.L., and Davis, C.C. (1983) *Biopolymers,* 22, 2513–2516.

Tao, N.J., Lindsay, S.M., and Rupprecht, A. (1988) Dynamic coupling between DNA and its primary hydration shell studied by brillouin scattering, *Biopolymers,* 27, 1655–1671.

Wittlin, A., Genzel, L, Kremer, F., Häseler, S., and Poglitsch, A. (1986) Far-infrared spectroscopy on oriented films of dry and hydrated DNA, *Phys. Rev. A,* 34, 493–500.

Woolard, D.L., Koscica, T., Rhodes, D.L., Cui, H.L., Pastore, R.A., Jensen, J.O., Jensen, J.L., Loerop, W.R., Jacobsen, R.H., Mittleman, D., and Nuss, N.C. (1997) Millimeter wave-induced vibrational modes in DNA as a possible alternative to animal tests to probe for carcinogenic mutations, *J. Appl. Toxicol.,* 17, 243–246.

Young, L., Prabhu, V.V., and Prohofsky, E.W. (1989) *Phys. Rev.,* 39, 3173–3179.

CHAPTER 44

Trophoblast Toxicity Assay (TTA): A Gestational Toxicity Test Using Human Placental Trophoblasts

Harvey J. Kliman

CONTENTS

HUMAN TROPHOBLASTS *IN VIVO*: THREE DIFFERENTIATION PATHWAYS

Trophoblasts are unique cells derived from the outer cell layer of the blastocyst that mediate implantation and placentation. Depending on their external environment, undifferentiated cytotrophoblasts can develop into (1) hormonally active villous syncytiotrophoblasts, (2) extravillous anchoring trophoblastic cell columns, or (3) invasive intermediate trophoblasts (Kliman and Feinberg, 1992) (Figure 44.1).

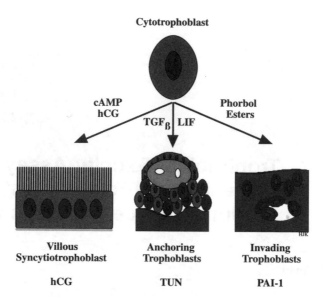

Cytotrophoblast

cAMP
hCG
TGF$_\beta$ | LIF
Phorbol
Esters

Villous
Syncytiotrophoblast

Anchoring
Trophoblasts

Invading
Trophoblasts

hCG   TUN   PAI-1

Figure 44.1 Pathways of trophoblast differentiation. Just as the basal layer of the skin gives rise to keratinocytes, the cytotrophoblast — the stem cell of the placenta — gives rise to the differentiated forms of trophoblasts. (Left) Within the chorionic villi, cytotrophoblasts fuse to form the overlying syncytiotrophoblast. The villous syn-cytiotrophoblast makes the majority of the placental hormones, the most studied being hCG. cAMP, EGF, and even hCG itself have been implicated as stimulators of this differentiation pathway. In addition to upregulating hCG secretion, cAMP has also been shown to down-regulate trophouteronectin (TUN) synthesis. (Center) At the point where chorionic villi make contact with external extracellular matrix (decidual stromal ECM in the case of intrauterine pregnancies), a popu-lation of trophoblasts proliferates from the cytotrophoblast layer to form the second type of trophoblast — the junctional trophoblast. These cells form the anchoring cell columns that can be seen at the junction of the placenta and endometrium throughout gestation. Similar trophoblasts can be seen at the junction of the chorion layer of the external membranes and the decidua. The junctional tropho-blasts make a unique fibronectin — trophouteronectin — that appears to mediate the attachment of the placenta to the uterus. TGF$_\beta$ and LIF have been shown to induce cultured trophoblasts to secrete increased levels of trophouteronectin, while down-regulating hCG secretion. (Right) Finally, a third type of trophoblast differentiates toward an invasive phenotype and leaves the placenta entirely — the invasive intermediate trophoblast. In addition to making human placental lactogen, these cells also make urokinase and plasminogen activator inhibitor-1 (PAI-1). Phorbol esters have been shown to increase trophoblast invasiveness in *in vitro* model systems and to upregulate PAI-1 in cultured trophoblasts. The general theme that comes from these observations is that specific factors are capable of shifting the differentiation pathway of the cytotrophoblast toward one of the above directions while turning off differentiation toward the other pathways. See text for details.

Studies using cultured cytotrophoblasts are beginning to elucidate the specific factors that mediate these pathways of trophoblast differentiation. This chapter will review the differentiation pathways of the cytotrophoblast, what is known about the factors that regulate trophoblast differentiation, the model systems used to study trophoblast biology, and the various hormones that have been shown to be made by these trophoblasts, both *in vitro* and *in vivo*.

Villous Syncytiotrophoblast

The hormones secreted by the villous syncytiotrophoblast are critical for maintaining pregnancy (Conley and Mason, 1990; Petraglia et al., 1990). Early in gestation, human chorionic gonadotropin (hCG) is essential to maintain corpus luteum progesterone production. Near the end of the first trimester, the mass of villous syncytiotrophoblast is large enough to make sufficient progesterone and estrogen to maintain the pregnancy. During the third trimester, large quantities of placental lactogen are produced, a hormone purported to have a role as a regulator of lipid and carbohydrate metabolism in the mother. Other syncytiotrophoblast products, to name a few, include pregnancy specific β_1-glycoprotein (Kliman et al., 1986), plasminogen activator inhibitor type 2 (Feinberg et al., 1989), growth hormone (Jara et al., 1989), collagenases (Moll and Lane, 1990), thrombomodulin (Maruyama et al., 1985; Ohtani et al., 1989), and growth factor receptors (Posner, 1974; Uzumaki et al., 1989; Kawagoe et al., 1990). The factors responsible for the regulated synthesis of these compounds have been the subject of a great deal of investigation, some of which will be reviewed below.

In vitro experiments have identified several compounds that are capable of differentiating cultured cytotrophoblasts toward an endocrine phenotype. These include cAMP (Feinman et al., 1986; Ringler et al., 1989b; Ulloa-Aguirre et al., 1987), epidermal growth factor (EGF) (Maruo et al., 1987), and hCG itself (Shi et al., 1993). Cyclic AMP has been shown to up-regulate hCG and progesterone secretion. In the case of hCG, the mechanism appears to be a direct up-regulation of hCG gene transcription via a cAMP regulatory region of the genome. For progesterone, increased synthesis appears to be due to a concerted up-regulation of a number of enzymes responsible for progesterone biosynthesis, including the side chain cleavage enzyme and adrenodoxin complex — the first steps in the conversion of cholesterol to progesterone. Not only do these compounds up-regulate hormone secretion, they also appear to down-regulate the synthesis of markers of the other pathways of trophoblast differentiation. For example, in the presence of 8-bromo-cAMP, cultured trophoblasts are induced to secrete large quantities of hCG (Feinman et al., 1986). At the same time, their synthesis and secretion of the trophoblast form of fibronectin, trophouteronectin (Feinberg et al., 1991) — a marker of junctional trophoblasts (see Figure 44.1) — is turned off (Ulloa-Aguirre et al., 1987). This result suggests that mutually exclusive differentiation pathways result from stimulation by appropriate factors.

Trophoblasts seem to make more than one hormone at the same time — a difficult task for a cell. Once stimulated to become hormonally active, the trophoblast seems capable of producing at least two glycoproteins simultaneously (Kliman et al., 1987), although electron microscopic immunochemistry has demonstrated that these products are located in different secretory vacuoles within the same cell (Hamasaki et al., 1988). This synchronous hormone production may help to explain why the syncytiotrophoblast is multinucleated: multiple copies of the genome may be necessary to allow this complex cell to make numerous products simultaneously while it continues to perform its other functions of absorption and waste excretion.

Anchoring Trophoblasts

It has been generally accepted that some form of cell-extracellular matrix interaction takes place at the attachment interface between the anchoring trophoblasts and the uterus. Recently, a specific type of fibronectin — *trophouteronectin (TUN)* — has been implicated as the protein responsible for the attachment of anchoring, extravillous trophoblasts to the uterus throughout gestation (Feinberg et al., 1991; Feinberg and Kliman, 1993). This specialized form of fibronectin appears to be made wherever trophoblasts contact extracellular matrix proteins. The factors that may be responsible for activating trophoblast TUN production include transforming growth factor-β (TGF_β) (Feinberg et al., 1994) and leukemia inhibitory factor (LIF) (Nachtigall et al., 1993). TGF_β has been identified in the region of the uteroplacental junction, possibly made by both decidual cells in that area and by the trophoblasts themselves (Lysiak et al., 1992). LIF has been identified in human endometrium (Stewart, 1994) but has not been shown to be made by trophoblasts. Interestingly, both TGF_β and LIF have been shown to upregulate TUN secretion from cultured trophoblasts while down-regulating hCG secretion (Figure 44.1) (Feinberg et al., 1994; Nachtigall et al., 1993).

Invading Trophoblasts

As human gestation progresses, invasive populations of extravillous trophoblasts attach to and interdigitate through the extracellular spaces of the endometrium and myometrium. The endpoint for this invasive behavior is penetration of maternal spiral arteries within the uterus (Pijnenborg, 1990). Histologically, trophoblast invasion of maternal blood vessels results in disruption of extracellular matrix components and development of dilated capacitance vessels within the uteroplacental vasculature. Biologically, trophoblast-mediated vascular remodeling within the placental bed allows for marked distensibility of the uteroplacental vessels, thus accommodating the increased blood flow needed during gestation. Abnormalities in this invasive process have been correlated with early- and mid-trimester pregnancy loss, preeclampsia and eclampsia, and intrauterine growth retardation (Robertson et al., 1986).

As would be anticipated when considering invasive cells, these trophoblasts produce a variety of proteases (Queenan et al., 1987; Fisher et al., 1989; Milwidsky et al., 1993) and protease inhibitors (Feinberg et al., 1989) that are used to regulate the invasive process. In addition to the protease systems, invasive trophoblasts also make protein hormones, most notably human placental lactogen (Kurman et al., 1984).

IN VITRO MODEL SYSTEMS TO STUDY
TROPHOBLAST DIFFERENTIATION

The most commonly used approaches for examining the regulation of hormone production by trophoblasts have come from *in vitro* studies. Model systems developed to study placental and trophoblast function have included placental organ and explant culture, trophoblast culture, chorion laeve culture, choriocarcinoma cell line culture, and placental perfusion studies (Kliman and Feinberg, 1992). Recently, most investigators

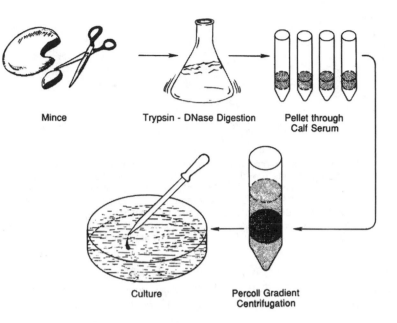

Figure 44.2 Purification of cytotrophoblasts from term placenta. A term placenta is minced and digested with trypsin and DNAse. The supernatant is passed through calf serum to inactivate the digestive enzymes; then these pellets are pooled and placed on a Percoll gradient to separate out the cytotrophoblasts. (From Kliman et al. (1986) *Endocrinology*, 118(4), 1567–1582. With permission.)

have turned to trophoblast cell culture since it eliminates the complications of more heterogeneous cell systems (Figure 44.2). Since the cytotrophoblast is the precursor of all other trophoblasts, a variety of methods have been proposed to purify this cell type from the human placenta (Belisle et al., 1986; Kliman et al., 1986; Bax et al., 1989; Loke et al., 1989; Truman et al., 1989; Yagel et al., 1989a; Branchaud et al., 1990; Dodeur et al., 1990; Fisher et al., 1990; Loke, 1990; Shorter et al., 1990).

We have demonstrated by time-lapse cinematography that when these mononuclear cytotrophoblasts are placed in Dulbecco's Modified Eagles' Medium (DMEM) containing 20% (v/v) heat-inactivated fetal calf serum (FCS), they flatten onto the culture surface within 3 to 12 hr, migrate toward each other to form aggregates within the first 24 hr, and form syncytiotrophoblasts over the next 24 hr of culture (Figure 44.3) (Kliman et al., 1986). Concomitant with these morphologic changes, these trophoblasts synthesize and secrete a number of cell products, including protein hormones, peptide hormones, steroid hormones, growth factors, and cytokines. We and others have used these cells to elucidate the products of trophoblast differentiation and to explore the mechanisms by which their synthesis and secretion is regulated.

TROPHOBLASTS AS ENDOCRINE CELLS

Trophoblasts synthesize and secrete a vast array of endocrine products (for reviews see Blay and Hollenberg, 1989; Jones, 1989; Sirinathsinghji and Heavens,

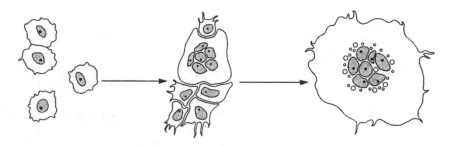

Figure 44.3 *In vitro* morphologic differentiation of cytotrophoblasts. After purification, the cytotrophoblasts are dispersed as individual cells (left). When plated in culture media containing serum, these cells flatten out and begin to move toward each other. After 24 hr in culture, aggregates begin to appear, with some evidence of cell fusion (center). After 72 hr in culture, most of the trophoblasts have fused and formed large, multinucleated syncytiotrophoblasts. (From Kliman et al. (1986) *Endocrinology*, 118(4), 1567–1582. With permission.)

1989; Conley and Mason, 1990; Petraglia et al., 1990; Ringler and Strauss, 1990; Cunningham et al., 1997). Collectively, these hormones function to regulate tropho-blast growth and differentiation; affect fetal growth and homeostasis; modulate maternal immunologic, cardiovascular, and nutritional status; protect the fetus from infection; and prepare the uterus and mother for parturition.

PROTEIN HORMONES

Chorionic Gonadotropin

The most widely studied trophoblast hormone product is chorionic gonadotropin. This glycoprotein is critical to pregnancy since it rescues the corpus luteum from involution, thus maintaining progesterone secretion by the ovarian granulosa cells. Its usefulness as a diagnostic marker of pregnancy stems from the fact that it may be one of the earliest secreted products of the conceptus. Ohlsson et al. (1989) have demonstrated by *in situ* hybridization that β-hCG transcripts are present in human blastocyst trophoblasts prior to implantation. Placental production of hCG peaks during the eighth to the tenth week of gestation and tends to plateau at a lower level for the remainder of pregnancy. This difference in the rate of hCG secretion may be mimicked to some extent by trophoblasts cultured from first vs. third trimester placentae. Kato and Braunstein (1990) have demonstrated that trophoblasts from first trimester placentae secrete greater amounts of hCG than trophoblasts purified from term placentae, suggesting that cultured trophoblasts may retain the regulatory effects of their *in situ* milieu even after several days of culture (Figure 44.4).

What regulates hCG synthesis and secretion in the trophoblast? Workers have attempted to discover what regulates hCG synthesis and secretion by examining likely factors *in vitro*. Table 44.1 summarizes our current knowledge of the regulatory factors that appear to modulate hCG secretion in trophoblasts. The sensitivity of human trophoblasts to exogenous regulation is clearly demonstrated by examination

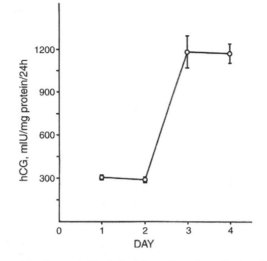

Figure 44.4 hCG secretion by trophoblasts in culture. Percoll-gradient purified cytotrophoblasts were cultured in DMEM media for four days. Media was changed daily and assayed for hCG by radioimmunoassay. hCG was not detectable at the time of initial plating. (From Kliman et al. (1986) *Endocrinology*, 118(4), 1567–1582. With permission.)

Table 44.1 Regulation of Trophoblast hCG Secretion

Factor	Trophoblasts (Trimester)	Effect on hCG Secretion	References
CAMP	Term	Stimulates	(Feinman et al., 1986)
HCG	Term	Stimulates	(Shi et al., 1993)
GnRH	Term	Stimulates	(Belisle et al., 1989; Szilagyi et al., 1992)
GnRH	First, Term	Not clear	(Kelly et al., 1991)
β-Adrenergic agonists	First	Stimulates	(Oike et al., 1990)
Dexamethasone	Term	Stimulates	(Ringler et al., 1989a)
Inhibin	Term	Inhibits	(Petraglia et al., 1987, 1989, 1991)
Activin	Term	Potentiates GnRH stimulation of hCG secretion	(Petraglia et al., 1991)
Activin	First	Stimulates	(Steele et al., 1993)
EGF	First, Term	Stimulates	(Maruo et al., 1987)
Thyroid hormone	First, Term	Stimulates	(Maruo et al., 1991)
Thyroid stimulating hormone	Term	Inhibits	(Beckmann et al., 1992)
Interleukin-1	First	Stimulates	(Yagel et al., 1989b)
Interleukin-6	First	Stimulates	(Nishino et al., 1990)
Basement membrane	First	Stimulates	(Truman and Ford, 1986)
Decidual protein	Term	Inhibits	(Ren and Braunstein, 1991)
Prolactin	Term	Inhibits	(Yuen et al., 1986)

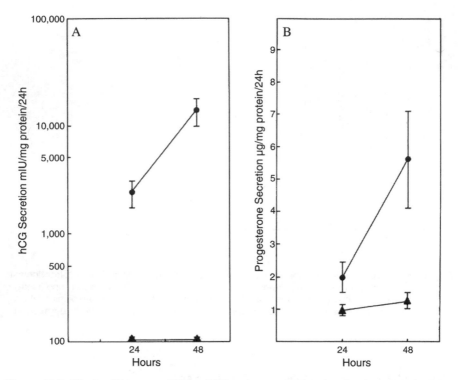

Figure 44.5 Effects of 8-bromo-cAMP on hCG and progesterone secretion by cultured cytotrophoblasts. Percoll-gradient purified cytotrophoblasts were cultured for 48 hr in the
absence (▲) or presence (●) of 8-bromo-cAMP. hCG (A) and progesterone (B)
were quantitated in the medium at 24-hr intervals. Values presented are the mean
± SE from six separate experiments. At each time point, 8-bromo-cAMP-treated
cultures secreted significantly more (*p* < 0.014, by the Wilcoxon signed rank test)
progesterone and hCG than did control cultures. (From Feinman et al. (1986) *J.
Clin. Endocrinol. Metab.*, 63(5), 1211. With permission.)

of the marked stimulatory effect of cAMP on hCG and progesterone secretion by
cultured trophoblasts (Figure 44.5).

Human Placental Lactogen (hPL)

This potent glycoprotein is made throughout gestation, increasing progressively
until the 36th week, where it can be found in the maternal serum at a concentration
of 5 to 15 μg/ml, the highest concentration of any known protein hormone. The
major source of hPL appears to be the villous syncytiotrophoblasts, where it is made
at a constant level throughout gestation (Sakbun et al., 1987). In addition to the
villous syncytiotrophoblast, hPL has been identified in invasive intermediate trophoblasts during the first trimester (Heyderman et al., 1981; Kurman et al., 1984), as
well as the third trimester (Gosseye and van, 1992). In addition to identifying hPL
within trophoblasts *in situ*, experiments have shown that cultured first trimester
trophoblasts secrete hPL *in vitro* (Dodeur et al., 1990). Petraglia et al. (1989) have
also identified hPL mRNAs in cultured trophoblasts. Hoshina et al. (1984), working

with choriocarcinoma cell lines, have proposed that hPL gene expression occurs after α-hCG and β-hCG gene expression, which suggests that hPL is a product of a more differentiated trophoblast. Kliman et al. have also shown that intracytoplasmic α-hCG appears prior to intracytoplasmic hPL in cultured term trophoblasts (Kliman et al., 1987).

The factors that regulate hPL synthesis and secretion are not as well studied as for hCG. Kato and Braunstein (1989) have demonstrated that the secretion of hCG and hPL are discordant during the first 5 d of term trophoblast culture, which suggests different regulatory pathways for these hormones. Dodeur et al. (1990) demonstrated that dibutyryl cAMP stimulated hPL secretion from cultured first trimester trophoblasts. Maruo et al. (1987) have shown that EGF, in addition to increasing hCG secretion by cultured human trophoblasts, also augments hPL secretion by these cells. Handwerger et al. (1987) showed that high-density lipoproteins (HDL) stimulate the release of hPL from human placental explants, while Wu and Handwerger showed that HDL stimulates hPL release from cultured trophoblasts via a protein kinase-C-dependent pathway (Wu and Handwerger, 1992). Finally, Petit et al. (1989) have demonstrated that angiotensin II stimulates hPL release by cultured trophoblasts, while opioids stimulate hPL release via a calcium influx mechanism (Petit et al., 1993).

TROPHOBLAST TOXICITY ASSAY

Using the *in vitro* assay systems and the secreted products described above, an assay to assess the toxicologic potential of chemicals, both natural and synthesized, can be developed. The trophoblast toxicity assay focuses on the three major differentiated forms of trophoblasts described above. To perform this assay, we have chosen characteristic markers for each of these trophoblasts: amino acid uptake and secretion of β-hCG and progesterone for villous syncytiotrophoblasts; trophouteronectin secretion for anchoring trophoblasts; and PAI-1 secretion for invasive intermediate trophoblasts. We have studied all of these products and have used standard assay methods to measure these trophoblast markers. The goal of the trophoblast toxicity assay will be to evaluate the effects of chemicals on the ability of cultured human trophoblasts to take up amino acids and secrete these markers. Dose-response curves will be generated for agents as a function of trophoblast differentiation in culture over a 72 to 96 hr period. Statistical methods will be employed to accurately evaluate the differences seen in the treated cultures compared to controls. In concert with the biochemical aspects of the trophoblast toxicity assay, the cultures will be evaluated cytologically to assess for gross effects of these chemicals and immunocytochemically to assess for cell to cell variability for each of the markers examined.

CONCLUSIONS

As well as becoming a practical and useful assay to assess drugs and environmental toxins, the further development of the trophoblast toxicity assay may have significant impact on the evaluation of compounds that have exposure potential during pregnancy and could possibly become a standard safety assay for gestational therapeutics.

REFERENCES

Bax, C.M., Ryder, T.A., Mobberley, M.A., Tyms, A.S., Taylor, D.L., and Bloxam, D.L. (1989) Ultrastructural changes and immunocytochemical analysis of human placental trophoblast during short-term culture, *Placenta*, 10, 179–194.

Beckmann, M.W., Wurfel, W., Austin, R.J., Link, U., and Albert, P.J. (1992) Suppression of human chorionic-gonadotropin in the human placenta at term by human thyroid-stimulating hormone in vitro, *Gynecol. Obstet. Invest.*, 34, 164–170.

Belisle, S., Bellabarba, D., Gallo Payet, N., Lehoux, J.G., and Guevin, J.F. (1986) On the role of luteinizing hormone-releasing hormone in the *in vitro* synthesis of bioactive human chorionic gonadotropin in human pregnancies, *Can. J. Physiol. Pharmacol.*, 64, 1229–1235.

Belisle, S., Petit, A., Bellabarba, D., Escher, E., Lehoux, J.G., and Gallo Payet, N. (1989) Gallo Payet N, Ca2+, but not membrane lipid hydrolysis, mediates human chorionic gonadotropin production by luteinizing hormone-releasing hormone in human term placenta, *J. Clin. Endocrinol. Metab.*, 69, 117–121.

Blay, J. and Hollenberg, M.D. (1989) The nature and function of polypeptide growth factor receptors in the human placenta, *J. Dev. Physiol.*, 12, 237–248.

Branchaud, C., Goodyer, C.G., Guyda, H.J., and Lefebvre, Y. (1990) A serum-free system for culturing human placental trophoblasts, *In Vitro Cell. Dev. Biol.*, 26, 865–870.

Conley, A.J. and Mason, J.I. (1990) Placental steroid-hormones. *Baillieres Clin. Endocrinol. Metab.*, 4, 249–272.

Cunningham, F.G., MacDonald, P.C., Gant, N.F., Leveno, K.J., Gilstrap, L.C.I., Hankins, G.D.V., et al. (1997) *Williams Obstetrics,* Appleton & Lange, Stamford.

Dodeur, M., Malassine, A., Bellet, D., Mensier, A., and Evain Brion, D. (1990) Characterization and differentiation of human first trimester placenta trophoblastic cells in culture, *Reprod. Nutr. Dev.*, 30, 183–192.

Feinberg, R. and Kliman, H.J. (1993) Human trophoblasts and tropho-uteronectin (TUN): a model for studying early implantation events, *Assisted Reprod. Rev.*, 3, 19–25.

Feinberg, R., Kliman, H.J., and Lockwood, C. (1991) Oncofetal fibronectin: a trophoblast "glue" for human implantation? *Am. J. Pathol.*, 138, 537–543.

Feinberg, R.F., Kliman, H.J., and Wang, C.L. (1994) Transforming growth factor-beta stimulates trophoblast oncofetal fibronectin synthesis *in vitro*: implications for trophoblast implantation in vivo, *J. Clin. Endocrinol. Metab.*, 78, 1241–1248.

Feinberg, R.F., Wun, T.C., Strauss, J.F., Queenan, J.T., Kliman, H.J., Kao, L.C., et al. (1989) Plasminogen-activator inhibitor type-1 and type-2 in human trophoblasts — PAI-1 is an immunocytochemical marker of invading trophoblasts, *Lab. Invest.*, 61, 20–26.

Feinman, M.A., Kliman, H.J., Caltabiano, S., and Strauss, J.F.D. (1986) 8-Bromo-3,5-adenosine monophosphate stimulates the endocrine activity of human cytotrophoblasts in culture, *J. Clin. Endocrinol. Metab.*, 63, 1211–1217.

Fisher, S.J., Cui, T.Y., Zhang, L., Hartman, L., Grahl, K., Zhang, G.Y., et al. (1989) Adhesive and degradative properties of human placental cytotrophoblast cells *in vitro, J. Cell Biol.*, 109, 891–902.

Fisher, S.J., Sutherland, A., Moss, L., Hartman, L., Crowley, E., Bemfield, M., et al. (1990) Adhesive interactions of murine and human trophoblast cells, *Trophoblast Res.,* 4, 115–138.

Gosseye, S. and van, d.F. (1992) HPL-positive infiltrating trophoblastic cells in normal and abnormal pregnancy, *Eur. J. Obstet. Gynecol. Reprod. Biol.,* 44, 85–90.

Hamasaki, K., Ueda, H., Okamura, Y., and Fajimoto, S. (1988) Double immunoelectron microscopic labeling of human chorionic gonadotropin and human placental lactogen in human chorionic villi, *Sangyo Ika Daigaku Zasshi,* 10, 171–177.

Handwerger, S., Quarfordt, S., Barrett, J., and Harman, I. (1987) Apolipoproteins AI, AII, and CI stimulate placental lactogen release from human placental tissue. A novel action of high density lipoprotein apolipoproteins, *J. Clin. Invest.,* 79, 625–628.

Heyderman, E., Gibbons, A.R., and Rosen, S.W. (1981) Immunoperoxidase localisation of human placental lactogen: a marker for the placental origin of the giant cells in 'syncytial endometritis' of pregnancy, *J. Clin. Pathol.,* 34, 303–307.

Hoshima, M., Hussa, R., Pattillo, R., Camel, H.M., and Boime, I. (1984) The role of trophoblast differentiation in the control of the hCG and hPL genes, *Adv. Exp. Med. Biol.,* 176, 299–312.

Jara, C.S., Salud, A.T., Bryantgreenwood, G.D., Pirens, G., Hennes, G., and Frankenne, F. (1989) Immunocytochemical localization of the human growth hormone variant in the human placenta, *J. Clin. Endocrinol. Metab.,* 69, 1069–1072.

Jones, C.T. (1989) Endocrine function of the placenta, *Baillieres Clin. Endocrinol. Metab.,* 3, 755–780.

Kato, Y. and Braunstein, G.D. (1989) Discordant secretion of placental protein hormones in differentiating trophoblasts *in vitro, J. Clin. Endocrinol. Metab.,* 68, 814–820.

Kato, Y. and Braunstein, G.D. (1990) Purified first and third trimester placental trophoblasts differ in *in vitro* hormone secretion, *J. Clin. Endocrinol. Metab.,* 70, 1187–1192.

Kawagoe, K., Akiyama, J., Kawamoto, T., Morishita, Y., and Mori, S. (1990) Immunohistochemical demonstration of epidermal growth factor (EGF) receptors in normal human placental villi, *Placenta,* 11, 7–15.

Kelly, A.C., Rodgers, A., Dong, K.W., Barrezueta, N.X., Blum, M., and Roberts, J.L. (1991) Gonadotropin-releasing hormone and chorionic gonadotropin gene expression in human placental development, *DNA Cell Biol.,* 10, 411–421.

Kliman, H.J. and Feinberg, R.F. (1992) Trophoblast differentiation, in *The First Twelve Weeks of Gestation,* Barnea, E., Hustin, J., and Jauniaux, E., Eds., Springer-Verlag, New York.

Kliman, H.J., Feinman, M.A., and Strauss, J.F. (1987) Differentiation of human cytotrophoblasts into syncytiotrophoblasts in culture, *Trophoblast Res.,* 2, 407–421.

Kliman, H.J., Nestler, J.E., Sermasi, E., Sanger, J.M., and Strauss, J.F.D. (1986) Purification, characterization, and *in vitro* differentiation of cytotrophoblasts from human term placentae, *Endocrinology,* 118, 1567–1582.

Kurman, R.J., Main, C.S., and Chen, H.C. (1984) Intermediate trophoblast: a distinctive form of trophoblast with specific morphological, biochemical and functional features, *Placenta,* 5, 349–369.

Loke, Y.W. (1990) New developments in human trophoblast cell culture, *Colloque INSERM* 199, 110–116.

Loke, Y.W., Gardner, L., and Grabowska, A. (1989) Isolation of human extravillous trophoblast cells by attachment to laminin-coated magnetic beads, *Placenta,* 10, 407–415.

Lysiak, J., McCrae, K., and Lala, P.K. (1992) Localization of transforming growth factor-beta at the human fetal-maternal interface: role in trophoblast growth and differentiation, *Biol. Reprod.,* 46, 561–572.

Maruo, T., Matsuo, H., and Mochizuki, M. (1991) Thyroid hormone as a biological amplifier of differentiated trophoblast function in early pregnancy, *Acta Endocrinologica,* 125, 58–66.

Maruo, T., Matsuo, H., Oishi, T., Hayashi, M., Nishino, R., and Mochizuki, M. (1987) Induction of differentiated trophoblast function by epidermal growth factor: relation of immunohistochemically detected cellular epidermal growth factor receptor levels, *J. Clin. Endocrinol. Metab.,* 64, 744–750.

Maruyama, I., Bell, C.E., and Majerus, P.W. (1985) Thrombomodulin is found on endothelium of arteries, veins, capillaries, and lymphatics, and on syncytiotrophoblast of human placenta, *J. Cell Biol.,* 101, 363–371.

Milwidsky, A., Finciyeheskel, Z., Yagel, S., and Mayer, M. (1993) Gonadotropin-mediated inhibition of proteolytic-enzymes produced by human trophoblast in culture, *J. Clin. Endocrinol. Metab.,* 76, 1101–1105.

Moll, U.M. and Lane, B.L. (1990) Proteolytic Activity of 1st trimester placenta-localization of interstitial collagenase in villous and extravillous trophoblast, *Histochemistry,* 94, 555–560.

Nachtigall, M.J., Kliman, H.J., Feinberg, R.F., Meaddough, E.I., and Arici, A. (1993) Potential role of leukemia inhibitory factor (LIF) in human implantation, paper presented at the 41st Annual Meeting of the Society for Gynecologic Investigation, p. 96.

Nishino, E., Matsuzaki, N., Mashuhiro, K., Kameda, T., Taniguchi, T., Takagi, T., et al. (1990) Trophoblast-derived interleukin-6 (IL-6) regulates human chorionic gonadotropin release through IL-6 receptor on human trophoblast, *J. Clin. Endocrinol. Metab.,* 71, 436–441.

Ohlsson, R., Larsson, E., Nilsson, O., Wahlstrom, T., and Sundstrom, P. (1989) Blastocyst implantation precedes induction of insulin-like growth factor II gene expression in human trophoblasts, *Development,* 106, 555–559.

Ohtani, H., Maruyama, I., and Yonezawa, S. (1989) Ultrastructural immunolocolization of thrombomodulin in human placenta with microwave fixation, *Acta Histochem.,* 22, 393–395.

Oike, N., Iwashita, M., Muraki, T., Nomoto, T., Takeda, Y., and Sakamoto, S. (1990) Effect of adrenergic agonists on human chorionic-gonadotropin release by human trophoblast cells obtained from 1st-trimester placenta, *Horm. Metab. Res.,* 22, 188–191.

Petit, A., Guillon, G., Tence, M., Jard, S., Gallo Payet, N., Bellabarba, D., et al. (1989) Angiotensin II stimulates both inositol phosphate production and human placental lactogen release from human trophoblastic cells, *J. Clin. Endocrinol. Metab.,* 69, 280–286.

Petit, A., Gallo, P.N., Bellabarba, D., Lehoux, J.G., and Belisle, S. (1993) The modulation of placental lactogen release by opoids: a role for extracellular calcium, *Mol. Cell. Endocrinol.,* 90, 165–170.

Petraglia, F., Sawchenko, P., Lim, A.T., Rivier, J., and Vale, W. (1987) Localization, secretion, and action of inhibin in human placenta, *Science,* 237, 187–189.

Petraglia, F., Calza, L., Garuti, G.C., Giardino, L., De, R.B., and Angioni, S. (1990) New Aspects of placental endocrinology, *J. Endocrinol. Invest.,* 13, 353–371.

Petraglia, F., Angioni, S., Coukos, G., Uccelli, E., DiDomenica, P., De, R.B.M., et al. (1991) Neuroendocrine mechanisms regulating placental hormone production, *Contrib. Gynecol. Obstet.,* 18, 147–156.

Petraglia, F., Vaughan, J., and Vale, W. (1989) Inhibin and activin modulate the release of gonadotropin-releasing hormone, human chorionic gonadotropin, and progesterone from cultured human placental cells, *Proc. Natl. Acad. Sci. U.S.A.,* 86, 5114–5117.

Pijnenborg, R. (1990) Trophoblast invasion and placentation in the human-morphological aspects, *Trophoblast Res.,* 4, 33–47.

Posner, B.I. (1974) Insulin receptors in human and animal placental tissue, *Diabetes,* 23, 209–217.

Queenan, J.T., Jr., Kao, L.C., Arboleda, C.E., Ulloa Aguirre, A., Golos, T.G., Cines, D.B., et al. (1987) Regulation of urokinase-type plasminogen activator production by cultured human cytotrophoblasts, *J. Biol. Chem.,* 262, 10903–10906.

Ren, S.G. and Braunstein, G.D. (1991) Decidua produces a protein that inhibits choriogonadotropin release from human trophoblasts, *J. Clin. Invest.,* 87, 326–330.

Ringler, G.E., Kallen, C.B., and Strauss, J.F.D. (1989a) Regulation of human trophoblast function by glucocorticoids: dexamethasone promotes increased secretion of chorionic gonadotropin, *Endocrinology,* 124, 1625–1631.

Ringler, G.E. and Strauss, J.F.D. (1990) In vitro systems for the study of human placental endocrine function, *Endocrine Rev.,* 11, 105–123.

Ringler, G.E., Kao, L.C., Miller, W.L., and Strauss, J.F.D. (1989b) Effects of 8-bromo-cAMP on expression of endocrine functions by cultured human trophoblast cells. Regulation of specific mRNAs, *Mol. Cell. Endocrinol.,* 61, 13–21.

Robertson, W.B., Khong, T.Y., Brosens, I., De Wolf, F., Sheppard, B., and Bonnar, J. (1986) The placental bed biopsy: review from three European centers, *Am. J. Obstet. Gynecol.,* 155, 401–412.

Sakbun, V., Koay, E.S., and Bryant Greenwood, G.D. (1987) Immunocytochemical localization of prolactin and relaxin C-peptide in human decidua and placenta, *J. Clin. Endocrinol. Metab.,* 65, 339–343.

Shi, Q.J., Lei, Z.M., Rao, C.V., and Lin, J. (1993) Novel role of human chorionic gonadotropin in differentiation of human cytotrophoblasts, *Endocrinology,* 132, 1387–1395.

Shorter, S.C., Jackson, M.C., Sargent, I.L., Redman, C.W., and Starkey, P.M. (1990) Purification of human cytotrophoblast from term amniochorion by flow cytometry. *Placenta,* 11, 505–513.

Sirinathsinghji, D.J. and Heavens, R.P. (1989) Stress-related peptide hormones in the placenta: their possible physiological significance, *J. Endocrinol.,* 122, 435–437.

Steele, G., Currie, W., Yuen, B., Jia, X., Perlas, E., and Leung, P. (1993) Acute stimulation of human chorionic gonadotropin secretion by recombinant human activin-A in first trimester human trophoblast, *Endocrinology,* 133, 297–303.

Stewart, C.L. (1994) A cytokine regulating embryo implantation, *N.Y. Acad. Sci.*

Szilagyi, A., Benz, R., and Rossmanith, W.G. (1992) The human first-term placenta *in vitro*: regulation of hCG secretion by GnRH and its antagonist, *Gynecol. Endocrinol.,* 6, 293–300.

Truman, P. and Ford, H.C. (1986) The effect of substrate and epidermal growth factor on human placental trophoblast cells in culture, *In Vitro Cell. Dev. Biol.,* 22, 525–528.

Truman, P., Ford, H.C., and Pomare, L. (1989) Human placental cytotrophoblast cells-identification and culture, *Arch. Gynecol. Obstet.,* 246, 39–49.

Ulloa-Aguirre, A., August, A.M., Golos, T.G., Kao, L.C., Sakuragi, N., Kliman, H.J., et al. (1987) 8-Bromo-adenosine 3,5-monophosphate regulates expression of chorionic gonadotropin and fibronectin in human cytotrophoblasts, *J. Clin. Endocrinol. Metab.,* 64, 1002–1009.

Uzumaki, H., Okabe, T., Sasaki, N., Hagiwara, K., Takaku, F., Tobita, M., et al. (1989) Identification and characterization of receptors for granulocyte colony-stimulating factor in human placenta and trophoblastic cells, *Proc. Natl. Acad. Sci. U.S.A.,* 86, 9323–9326.

Wu, Y.Q. and Handwerger, S. (1992) High density lipoproteins stimulate molecular weight 80K protein phosphorylation in human trophoblast cells: evidence for a protein kinase-C-dependent pathway in human placental lactogen release, *Endocrinology,* 131, 2935–2940.

Yagel, S., Casper, R.F., Powell, W., Parhar, R.S., and Lala, P.K. (1989a) Characterization of pure human first-trimester cytotrophoblast cells in long-term culture: growth pattern, markers, and hormone production, *Am. J. Obstet. Gynecol.,* 160, 938–945.

Yagel, S., Lala, P.K., Powell, W.A., and Casper, R.F. (1989b) Interleukin-1 stimulates human chorionic gonadotropin secretion by first trimester human trophoblast, *J. Clin. Endocrinol. Metab.,* 68, 992–995.

Yuen, B.H., Moon, Y.S., and Shin, D.H. (1986) Inhibition of human chorionic gonadotropin production by prolactin from term human trophoblast, *Am. J. Obstet. Gynecol.,* 154, 336–340.

Index